CURRENT CLINICAL UROLOGY

ERIC A. KLEIN, MD, SERIES EDITOR

For further volumes:
http://www.springer.com/series/7635

J. Stephen Jones

Editor

Prostate Cancer Diagnosis

PSA, Biopsy and Beyond

Humana Press

Editor
J. Stephen Jones, MD, FACS, MBA
Cleveland Clinic
Cleveland Clinic Lerner College of Medicine
  at Case Western Reserve
Cleveland, OH, USA

ISBN 978-1-62703-187-5   ISBN 978-1-62703-188-2 (eBook)
DOI 10.1007/978-1-62703-188-2
Springer New York Heidelberg Dordrecht London

Library of Congress Control Number: 2012950793

Printed on acid-free paper

Humana Press is a brand of Springer
Springer is part of Springer Science+Business Media (www.springer.com)

For the patients that have entrusted me with their care and the colleagues – physician and otherwise – with whom I have shared the journey. We have learned much together and are better for it.
— J. Stephen Jones, MD, FACS, MBA

Preface

The final chapter of this book arrived the day that the US Preventive Services Task Force issued its recommendation that men should forego PSA screening for early diagnosis of prostate cancer. What a mess! Not the chapter – it was brilliant – but rather the firestorm created by this stance taken by individuals that have never had primary responsibility caring for patients with the second most common cause of cancer death in men.

This controversy may play out for a long time, but the information contained herein makes clear that we are actually preventing tens of thousands of men from dying of prostate cancer through early diagnosis and improved treatments. That fact won't go away with a dismissive remark by a group that interprets the data very differently from most experts in the field, including those who came together for this book on the topic. Despite the opinions of some critics outside the field, most urologists do prioritize avoidance of morbidity and cost of treatment for men with low-risk prostate cancer. Those men are now often managed conservatively with active surveillance – 25 % of the patients that I personally diagnose – and our treatments continue to improve for those patients who either chose or essentially have to undergo therapy. This concept of individualized care with no, appropriately delayed, or minimally invasive treatment for patients who appear to have low risk from disease morbidity or death is not new, as summarized several years ago. Nevertheless, we do acknowledge that some clinicians pursue strategies outside those described in this book, just like there is deviation in all fields of medicine and otherwise, but the fact that this behavior is outside the standards of care described by the authors in this book should not be ignored by the Task Force.

The prostate diagnostics field has witnessed a remarkable transformation in the 5 years since *Prostate Biopsy: Indications, Techniques, and Complications* was published. At that time, the standard "sextant" biopsy was still used in some quarters despite missing up to half of cancers, and the role and best technique for periprostatic local anesthesia were still occasionally debated. Now we define the biopsy standard of care as a minimum of 12 cores with at least half being from the apical and lateral aspects of the gland. Using a periprostatic anesthetic block, 20 or more core transrectal saturation biopsies can be performed routinely in an office setting, if desired, for repeat or cancer staging biopsy. Transperineal template mapping biopsy is now used in a number of centers for both diagnostics as well as quantification and qualification of disease status for patients being considered for active surveillance or focal therapy. Prostate MRI has advanced from novelty status in a few centers to routine use in many of the world's top institutions, and a number of investigators are developing biopsy techniques that may be performed under a variety of imaging guidance modalities in the near future. Finally, we are departing an era where PSA drove most biopsy decisions to one where it becomes only one of a number of factors that determine diagnostic strategy. Hence, we have titled this edition *Prostate Cancer Diagnostics: PSA, Biopsy, and Beyond* to reflect the breadth of this growing field.

As you read the chapters that follow, it may be difficult to recall that only a few short years ago, prostate cancer diagnostics seemed relatively straightforward. All men over 50 years old were believed to need PSA screening, and if its level was over 4.0, a biopsy inevitably ensued (a change the Task Force seems to have missed completely). A negative biopsy was previously regarded as definitive and further investigation was felt unnecessary unless the PSA value rose substantially. However, we now know that there is no truly meaningful threshold PSA value. Furthermore, PSA velocity appears to be less significant from a purely diagnostic standpoint than is intuitive, and a single negative biopsy still leaves a significant chance that a small-volume cancer remains unrecognized. Pathological findings on the initial biopsy, such as high-grade prostatic intraepithelial neoplasia or atypical small acinar proliferation, carry potentially significant implications to the likelihood that the patient will be found to have cancer during further investigation. Despite all these observations, prediction of prostate cancer risk remains elusive based on variations in the target populations, especially in the repeat biopsy setting. These complexities call for further efforts to optimize cancer diagnosis.

The authors in this book represent the highest levels of expertise in this discipline. They have been key drivers that have defined the science of prostate cancer diagnostics. Their body of work continues to transform the field, improving the decision process, patient experience, accuracy, and safety. The book includes intentional overlap of several chapters to acknowledge the controversial nature and existence of differing viewpoints by authorities considered the masters of their fields. I trust you will learn as much from their contributions as I have. I am deeply indebted to them all.

Cleveland, OH, USA   J. Stephen Jones, MD, FACS, MBA

Contents

Contributors

Hashim Uddin Ahmed Department of Urology, University College London Hospitals, NHS Foundation Trust, London, UK

Division of Surgery and Interventional Science, University College London, London, UK

Christopher L. Amling Department Urology, Oregon Health & Science University, Portland, OR, USA

Gerald L. Andriole Division of Urologic Surgery, Washington University School of Medicine, St. Louis, MO, USA

William J. Aronson Department of Urology, School of Medicine, University of California-Los Angeles, Los Angeles, CA, USA

Al B. Barqawi Division of Surgery/Urology, University of Colorado Hospital, University of Colorado Denver School of Medicine, Denver, CO, USA

Ronald S. Boris Department of Urology, Indiana University, Indianapolis, IN, USA

David G. Bostwick Bostwick Laboratories, Glen Allen, VA, USA

Jason Burnette Department of Urology, Georgia Health Sciences University, Augusta, GA, USA

H. Ballentine Carter Department of Urology, Marburg 403, Johns Hopkins School of Medicine, Baltimore, MD, USA

Benjamin Challacombe Urology Department, Guy's and St Thomas' Hospitals NHS Foundation Trust, London Bridge Hospital, London Bridge, London, UK

Sam S. Chang Department of Urologic Surgery, Vanderbilt University Medical Center, Nashville, TN, USA

Jonathan A. Coleman Department of Surgery/Urology, Memorial Sloan Kettering Cancer Center, New York, NY, USA

Michael S. Cookson Department of Urologic Surgery, Vanderbilt University Medical Center, Nashville, TN, USA

E. David Crawford Division of Urology, School of Medicine, University of Colorado Denver, Denver, CO, USA

Ahmed El-Shafei Glickman Urological and Kidney Institute, Cleveland Clinic, Cleveland, OH, USA

Mark Emberton Department of Urology, University College London Hospitals, NHS Foundation Trust, London, UK

Division of Surgery and Interventional Science, University College London, London, UK

John Fitzpatrick Department of Surgery, The Mater Misericordiae Hospital, University College, Dublin, Ireland

Allison Glass Department of Urology, Helen Diller Family Comprehensive Cancer Center, University of California, San Francisco, CA, USA

Kiran Gollapudi Department of Urology, School of Medicine, University of California-Los Angeles, Los Angeles, CA, USA

Leonard G. Gomella Department of Urology, Kimmel Cancer Center, Thomas Jefferson University, Philadelphia, PA, USA

William M. Hilton Department of Urology, University of Texas Health Science Center at San Antonio, San Antonio, TX, USA

J. Stephen Jones Cleveland Clinic, Cleveland Clinic Lerner College of Medicine at Case Western Reserve, Cleveland, OH, USA

Adam J. Jung Department of Radiology and Biomedical Imaging, University of California, San Francisco, CA, USA

Christopher J. Kane Division of Urology, C. Lowell and JoEllen Parsons Endowed Chair in Urology, University of California San Diego Medical Center, San Diego, CA, USA

Michael W. Kattan Department of Quantitative Health Sciences, Cleveland Clinic, Cleveland, OH, USA

Arjun Khosla Department of Urology, Kimmel Cancer Center, Thomas Jefferson University, Philadelphia, PA, USA

Adam S. Kibel Division of Urology, Brigham and Woman's Hospital, Dana Farber Cancer Institute, Boston, MA, USA

Roger Kirby The Prostate Centre, London, UK

Eric Klein Glickman Urological and Kidney Institute, Cleveland Clinic Lerner College of Medicine, Cleveland, OH, USA

Joseph C. Klink Glickman Urological and Kidney Institute, Cleveland Clinic Lerner College of Medicine, Cleveland, OH, USA

Michael O. Koch Department of Medicine, Indiana University, Indianapolis, IN, USA

Ryan P. Kopp Division of Urology, University of California San Diego Medical Center, San Diego, CA, USA

John Kurhanewicz Department of Radiology and Biomedical Imaging, University of California, San Francisco, CA, USA

Jeffrey C. La Rochelle Department of Urology, Oregon Health & Science University, Portland, OR, USA

Herbert Lepor Division of Urologic Oncology, Department of Urology, New York University Langone Medical Center (NYULMC), New York, NY, USA

Stacy Loeb Department of Urology, New York University, New York, NY, USA

Carmen Maccagnano Department of Urology, San Raffaele Hospital, Milan, Italy

Francesco Montorsi Department of Urology, San Raffaele Hospital, Milan, Italy

Ayman S. Moussa Glickman Urological and Kidney Institute, Cleveland Clinic, Cleveland, OH, USA

Kenneth G. Nepple Division of Urologic Surgery, Washington University School of Medicine, St. Louis, MO, USA

Carvell T. Nguyen Urologic Oncology, Glickman Urological & Kidney Institute, Cleveland Clinic, Cleveland, OH, USA

Adriana Olar Department of Pathology and Genomic Medicine, The Methodist Hospital, Houston, TX, USA

Dipen J. Parekh Department of Urology, University of Texas Health Science Center at San Antonio, San Antonio, TX, USA

Kellogg Parsons Division of Urology, University of California San Diego Medical Center, San Diego, CA, USA

Joseph C. Presti Jr Department of Urology, Stanford University School of Medicine, Stanford, CA, USA

Philippe Puech Department of Radiology, CHRU, Hospital Huriez, University Lille Nord de France, Lille, France

Sanoj Punnen Department of Urology, Helen Diller Family Comprehensive Cancer Center, University of California, San Francisco, CA, USA

Krishna Ramaswamy Division of Urologic Oncology, Department of Urology, New York University Langone Medical Center (NYULMC), New York, NY, USA

Gurdarshan S. Sandhu Division of Urologic Surgery, Washington University School of Medicine, St. Louis, MO, USA

Vincenzo Scattoni Department of Urology, San Raffaele Hospital, Milan, Italy

Douglas S. Scherr Department of Urology and Division of Medical Oncology, Weill Cornell Medical College, New York Presbyterian Hospital, New York, NY, USA

Shahrokh F. Shariat Department of Urology and Division of Medical Oncology, Weill Cornell Medical College, New York Presbyterian Hospital, New York, NY, USA

Katsuto Shinohara Department of Urology, Helen Diller Family Comprehensive Cancer Center, University of California, San Francisco, CA, USA

Vassilis J. Siomos Division of Urology, University of Colorado Hospital, Denver, CO, USA

Samir S. Taneja Division of Urologic Oncology, Department of Urology, New York University Langone Medical Center (NYULMC), New York, NY, USA

Martha K. Terris Department of Urology, Georgia Health Sciences University, Charlie Norwood VA Medical Center, Augusta, GA, USA

Ian M. Thompson III Department of Urologic Surgery, Vanderbilt University Medical Center, Nashville, TN, USA

Ian M. Thompson Jr., Department of Urology, University of Texas Health Science Center at San Antonio, San Antonio, TX, USA

Edouard J. Trabulsi Department of Urology, Kimmel Cancer Center, Thomas Jefferson University, Philadelphia, PA, USA

Arnauld Villers Department of Urology, Hospital Huriez, University Lille Nord de France, Lille, France

Daniel B. Vigneron Department of Radiology and Biomedical Imaging, University of California, San Francisco, CA, USA

Lily C. Wang Department of Urology and Division of Medical Oncology, Weill Cornell Medical College, New York Presbyterian Hospital, New York, NY, USA

Thomas M. Wheeler Department of Pathology & Immunology, Baylor College of Medicine, Houston, TX, USA

Osama Zaytoun Department of Urology, Cleveland Clinic, Cleveland, OH, USA

Defining the Problem

Kenneth G. Nepple and Gerald L. Andriole

Introduction

Prostate cancer detection and management continues to be an area of immense study, debate, and controversy. Despite the best efforts of urologists, radiation oncologists, and medical oncologists, some men will die of prostate cancer despite the currently available options for prostate cancer treatment. On the opposite end of the spectrum from that aggressive form of prostate cancer is the indolent prostate cancer that never affects the man who bears the diagnosis. Thus, this creates a primary problem in the use of prostate cancer screening: some men with aggressive prostate cancer may not be readily identified and treated despite efforts at prostate cancer screening and biopsy; however, other men who have an indolent small volume prostate cancer are unlikely to be harmed from the prostate cancer itself but are subjected to the side effects associated with treatment.

In this chapter, we will define the contemporary burden of prostate cancer and then focus on what is known about the general prevalence of prostate cancer in the aging male from autopsy series which identified that the pathologic presence of prostate cancer far exceeded the clinical prevalence of prostate cancer at any age.

K.G. Nepple, M.D. (✉) • G.L. Andriole
Division of Urologic Surgery, Washington University
School of Medicine, 4960 Children's Place,
Campus Box 8242, St. Louis, MO 63110, USA
e-mail: nepplek@wustl.edu

These findings in men who had the presence of unidentified prostate cancer but died of causes unrelated to prostate cancer will then allow for discussion of the potential for overdiagnosis and overtreatment of prostate cancer. We will then conclude with a discussion of how prostate cancer risk assessment influences the interpretation of large screening and prevention trials and the decision about whether to proceed with prostate screening or a prostate biopsy.

The Burden of Prostate Cancer

Prostate cancer is the most common cancer in males in the United States (excluding skin cancer) and accounted for 28% of all new cancer in men in 2010 [1]. Prostate cancer has an incidence of 155.5 per 100,000 in the year 2010 with an estimated 217,730 new cases with 1 in 6 men diagnosed with prostate cancer during the course of a lifetime [1]. With the introduction of PSA as a screening test in the 1980s, the incidence of prostate cancer dramatically increased and peaked in 1992 (Fig. 1.1), which corresponds to the addition of clinically asymptomatic men with prostate cancer to the population of men who were diagnosed based on the presence of clinical findings [1]. Such a rise in prostate cancer incidence did not occur in regions where PSA-based screening was less common [2]. Subsequent to that time, the diagnosis of prostate cancer has decreased (by 2.4% per year from 2000 to 2006) but remains at levels higher than before the use of PSA screening [1].

J.S. Jones (ed.), *Prostate Cancer Diagnosis: PSA, Biopsy and Beyond*, Current Clinical Urology,
DOI 10.1007/978-1-62703-188-2_1, © Springer Science+Business Media New York 2013

Fig. 1.1 Cancer incidence rates from 1975 to 2006 in the SEER cancer registry (Used with permission from Jemal et al. 2010)

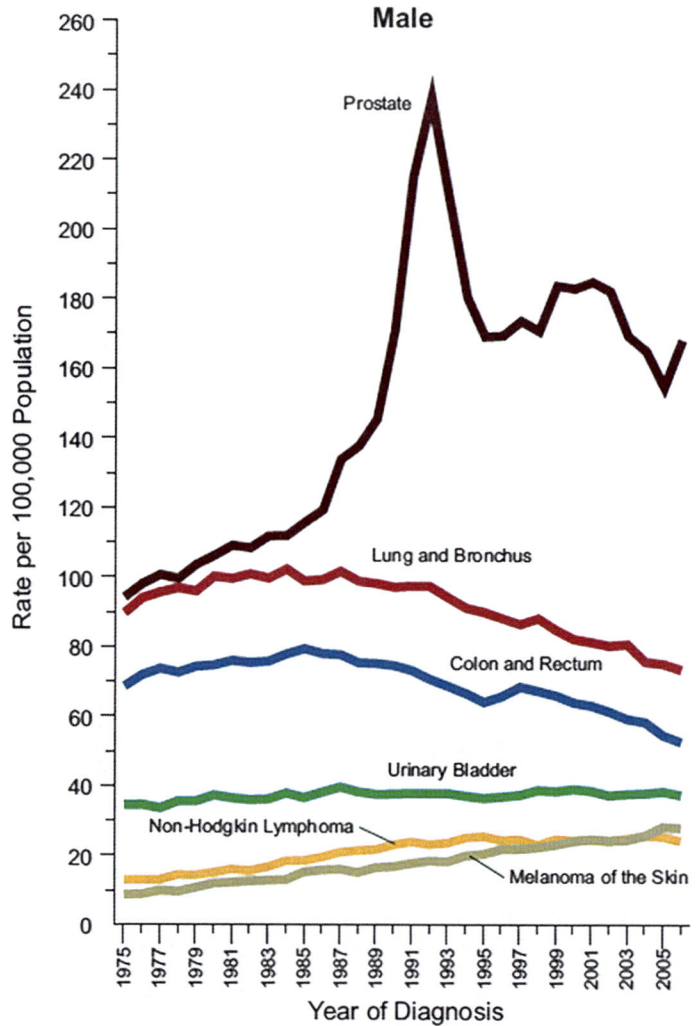

Male

Prostate

Lung and Bronchus

Colon and Rectum

Urinary Bladder

Non-Hodgkin Lymphoma

Melanoma of the Skin

Rate per 100,000 Population

Year of Diagnosis

Mortality from prostate cancer is the second most common cause of cancer death in men (Fig. 1.2) at a rate of 23.6 per 100,000 in 2006, which accounts for 11% of cancer-related deaths [1]. However, it is often said that many men die with, but not of, prostate cancer. In contrast to the relatively frequent diagnosis of prostate cancer during a man's lifetime (1 in 6 men), death from prostate cancer is substantially less common as only 2.8% of all men (1 in 36) will have prostate cancer as their cause of death which is much less common than cardiovascular causes or death from lung cancer. Albertsen et al. [3] evaluated coexisting medical comorbidity and competing causes of death from non-prostate cancer causes and confirmed that death from prostate cancer was a relatively infrequent occurrence. They evaluated mortality in men over age 65 years with T1c prostate cancer who did not receive initial treatment. In men with low grade prostate cancer, overall mortality dwarfed the risk of prostate cancer mortality especially in men with increased medical comorbidity (Table 1.1). Prostate cancer mortality was more sizable in men with high grade prostate cancer, particularly in men with minimal medical comorbidity, but remained less common than other cause mortality.

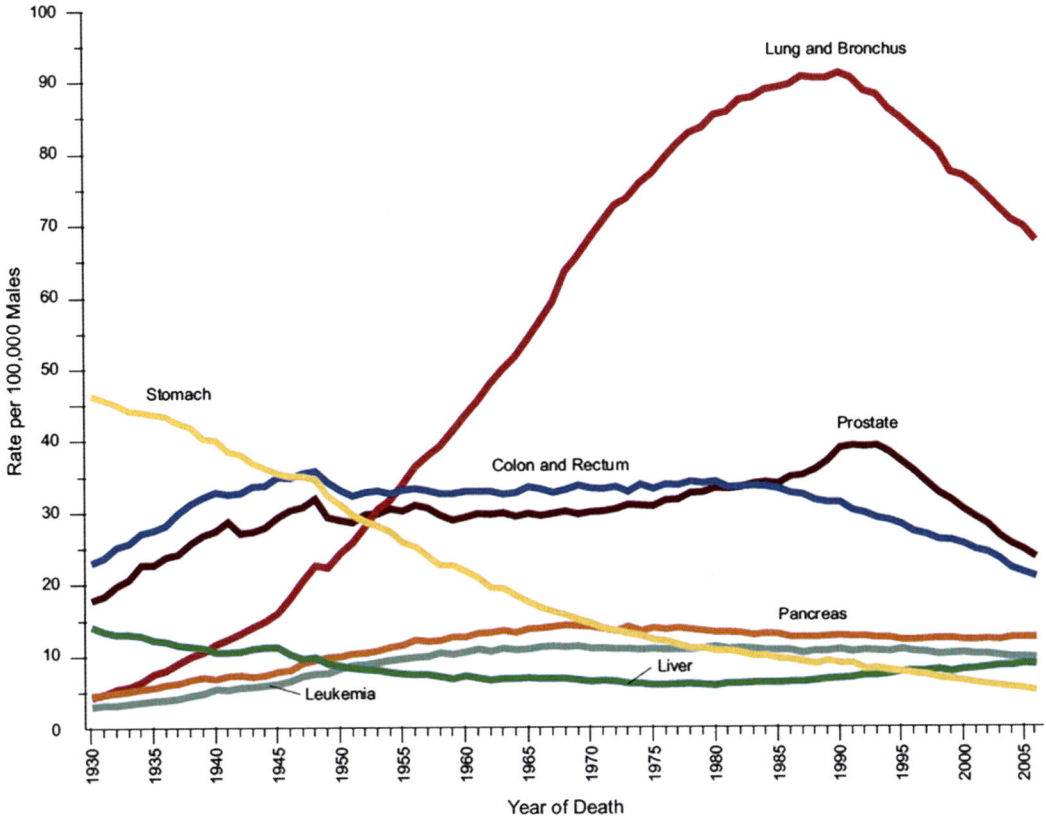

Fig. 1.2 Cancer death rates from 1975 to 2006 in the SEER cancer registry (Used with permission from Jemal et al. 2010)

Table 1.1 Risk of prostate cancer and overall mortality in men without initial treatment for prostate cancer (Adapted from Albertsen et al.)

Gleason grade	Medical comorbidity	10-year prostate cancer mortality (%)	10-year overall mortality (%)
5–7	0	4.8	28.8
	1	2.0	50.5
	>1	5.3	83.1
8–10	0	25.7	55.0
	1	20.2	52.0
	>1	13.7	64.3

The combination of a common diagnosis, effective treatment options, and an often indolent disease course has created a large pool of men who are alive with prostate cancer. Prostate cancer survivors compromise approximately one-fifth of the 11.7 million cancer survivors in the United States [4]. The number of prostate cancer survivors in the future is also likely to increase in the future as life expectancy increases. In those men who ultimately die from prostate cancer, the risk of death is more common in men with a Gleason grade 8–10 tumor, advanced clinical stage, or PSA greater than 20 ng/mL [5, 6].

The introduction of PSA as a screening test in the United States also leads to a population-based trend toward diagnosis of a less aggressive prostate cancer over time, which has been called the stage migration. Most contemporary tumors are now smaller and clinically localized at diagnosis, which contrasts to the often clinically advanced or overtly metastatic tumors before the introduction of screening. In the CAPSURE tumor registry, the proportion of tumor classified as low risk (PSA≤10 ng/ml, Gleason score≤6, clinical stage≤T2a) increased from 27.5% in 1990–994 to 46.4% in 2000–2001 then remained stable to 2006 [7]. In men who are newly diagnosed with prostate cancer, 94% of men are diagnosed with T1 or T2 prostate cancer [8]. The subsequent earlier diagnosis of prostate cancer because of screening (lead time) and treatment has improved the 5-year relative survival rate from 69% in 1975–1977, 76% in 1984–1986, to nearly 100% in 1999–2005 [1]. Additionally, contemporary men diagnosed with prostate cancer are also younger than historic cohorts, as the average age at diagnosis decreased from 72 to 67 years [8].

The burden of prostate cancer exists not only from mortality or symptoms associated with the disease. The diagnosis of prostate cancer increases patient anxiety and stress. A population-based analysis revealed an increased risk of cardiovascular events (including mortality) and suicide within the first year, and especially the first week, after the diagnosis of prostate cancer regardless of whether or not men received treatment [9]. Men also experience the burden of toxicity and side effects from treatments. Prostate cancer treatments are associated with varying degrees of effects on quality of life domains related to urinary, sexual, and bowel function [10, 11] which may never return to baseline after treatment [12]. In addition, the use of androgen deprivation therapy may have a detrimental effect on quality of life and medical conditions including bone health [13].

The economic costs of prostate cancer are also sizable. While the costs of prostate cancer management are less than most other cancers [14], the high prevalence of prostate cancer contributes to a significant economic burden. In the United States, the annual costs of prostate cancer have increased from $2.7 billion in 1996 to $4.5 billion in 2000 and then $6.8 billion in 2005 [15]. Future expenditures are likely to increase as costlier treatment alternatives are adopted [16]. The growth in medical expenditures for prostate cancer evaluation and treatment is in addition to the expense of prostate cancer screening, which is far less costly than the costs of prostate cancer treatment [17]. With respect to mortality, the value of lives lost to prostate cancer deaths is estimated to amount to nearly $35 billion dollars per year.

Incidental Diagnosis of Prostate Cancer

Sakr et al. [18] shed light onto the true prevalence of prostate cancer. While it was previously known that the majority of elderly men harbor clinically unapparent prostate cancer [19], it had not been established how early the prostate cancer was present. Using an autopsy series of men under 50 years of age who died from other causes, they reported in 1993 that histological prostate cancer was not seen frequently in men under 30 years but surprisingly was found in 27% of men in their 30s, and 34% of men in their 40s had small foci of histological cancer [18]. With their finding of cancer at a remarkably young age, it was realized that a long latency period (years or even decades) exists from the presence of prostate cancer to the development of clinically apparent prostate cancer. In a recent updated autopsy report from the Sakr et al. which now comprises 1,056 men [20], tumors were identified in even some younger men in their 20s (Table 1.2).

A separate estimate of the prevalence of latent undiagnosed preclinical prostate cancer comes from the evaluation of prostate specimens in radical cystoprostatectomy specimens. One report of 121 men (median age 68 years) undergoing cystoprostatectomy from Revello et al. found that 41% had unsuspected prostate cancer [21]. Of these prostate tumors, 48% met the criteria defining pathological significance based on size, Gleason score, or stage. A report from Pettus et al. similarly found that 48% of cystectomy

Table 1.2 Percentage of men with prostate cancer at autopsy (Adapted from Powell et al. Journal of Urology, 2010)

Age group	Percentage with prostate cancer at autopsy	
	Black	White
20–29	8	11
30–39	31	31
40–49	43	38
50–59	46	44
60–69	72	68
70–79	77	68

specimens harbored prostate cancer. Of those tumors, 29% had Gleason score ≥7; prostate cancer tumor volume was >0.5 cc in 22% of patients, and 13% had extracapsular extension [22]. Other series have reported rates of incidental prostate cancer in 27–60% of cystoprostatectomy specimens with clinically significant prostate cancer in 18–53% [22–26].

Overdiagnosis

The finding of a discrepancy between the large reservoir of asymptomatic prostate cancer in men as they age and the relatively infrequent occurrence of death by prostate cancer helps to explain the concept of overdiagnosis. Overdiagnosis refers to the concept that a proportion of men with screening-detected prostate cancers would have never progressed to cause symptoms or death without the use of the screening test. An aspect of prostate cancer which makes it susceptible to overdiagnosis includes the use of a screening test (PSA) which has a low specificity, and an inability to distinguish indolent from aggressive

prostate cancer results in a substantial number of men who are overdiagnosed with prostate cancer. The overdiagnosis of subclinical prostate cancer often leads to overtreatment due to the inability to distinguish between aggressive prostate cancer with a high risk of progression to symptoms and death from those prostate cancers that are destined to have no clinical sequela. It has been estimated that the introduction of prostate cancer screening has lead to over 1.3 million cancer diagnoses from 1986 to 2005 and over 1 million additional men treated during that time period [27]. The inherent nature of early detection with a screening test creates the possibility of overdiagnosis, as not every diagnosed patient would have progressed to diagnosis, and even in those who are diagnosed, death from other causes may occur before death from prostate cancer. The success of PSA as a screening test depends on the ability to find disease that requires cure.

One way to think of overdiagnosis of prostate cancer is to place it in the context of the risk the prostate cancer poses to the individual patient on the basis of the possible effect of prostate cancer (Fig. 1.3). In those men destined to have prostate

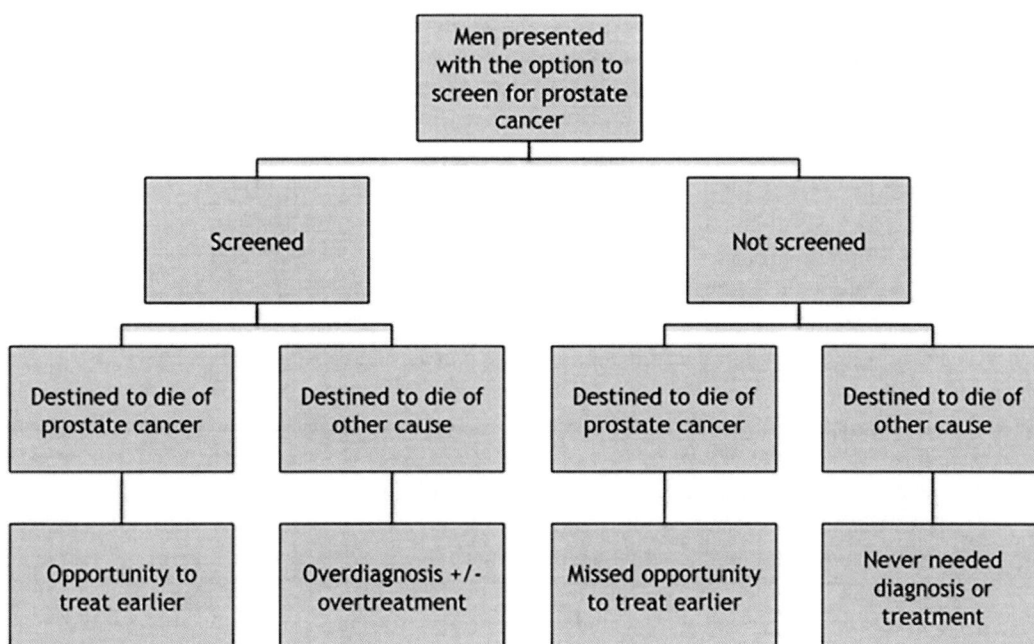

Fig. 1.3 Possible effects of prostate cancer in screened and unscreened men

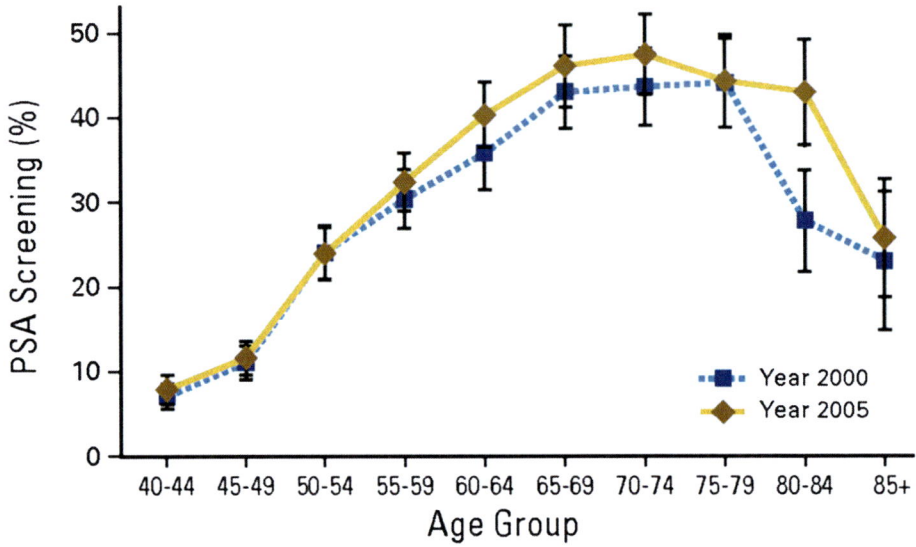

Fig. 1.4 Population-based prevalence of PSA screening in the United States (Used with permission from Drazer et al.)

	40-44	45-49	50-54	55-59	60-64	65-69	70-74	75-79	80-84	85+
2000	7.1%	11.0%	24.1%	30.4%	35.8%	43.0%	43.6%	44.1%	27.8%	23.1%
2005	7.9%	11.6%	23.9%	32.4%	40.3%	46.1%	47.4%	44.3%	43.0%	25.8%
Total	7.5%	11.3%	24.0%	31.5%	38.2%	44.6%	45.5%	44.2%	35.7%	24.6%
No. interviewed	2,688	2,517	2,204	1,887	1,497	1,191	1,070	756	507	290

cancer shorten their life, screening provides an opportunity to possibly treat the prostate cancer more effectively if caught at an earlier stage, while lack of screening may miss this opportunity. In contrast, those men with an indolent tumor who would not die of prostate cancer are at risk of overdiagnosis if they were to undergo screening, and the man with indolent cancer would not be harmed if he never underwent screening. Thus, the concept of overdiagnosis hinges on the ability to detect who will and who will not die of prostate cancer. However, currently available methods for prognostication at diagnosis are moderately accurate but do not allow definitive categorization of indolent versus aggressive prostate cancer.

Overdiagnosis of prostate cancer is particularly a concern when PSA screening is utilized in patient populations who are unlikely to benefit. The patient populations who are most likely to benefit from PSA screening and thus would be less prone to overdiagnosis would be men without medical comorbidity [28] as seen in PLCO or

perhaps more broadly in men ages 55–69 years as seen in ERSPC [29]. Similarly, in the Swedish randomized trial of prostatectomy versus watchful waiting, the survival benefit of prostatectomy was limited to men less than 65 years of age [30]. However, PSA screening in the United States is actually most commonly utilized in men ages 70–74 years (Fig. 1.4).[31]

Several authors have estimated the rate of overdiagnosis. The difficulty with quantifying overdiagnosis is that it is not apparent at the time of diagnosis. To truly establish overdiagnosis, an individual diagnosed with cancer must not receive treatment and subsequently die of an unrelated cause. Because the majority of cancers that are diagnosed are treated, the reported estimates of overdiagnosis rely on epidemiologic data, computational models, or a combination of both. Using data from the ERSPC trial, Welch and Black estimated that 60% of screening-detected prostate cancers met the definition of overdiagnosis [32]. This calculation was based on the finding that of the 58 prostate cancers per

1,000 men screened, there were an extra 34 prostate cancers per 1,000 men compared to no screening.

Others' estimates of overdiagnosis have varied widely from 27% to 84%. Draisma et al. [33] used a simulation analysis and reported that age at diagnosis heavily influenced the estimate of overdiagnosis, which was estimated at 27% at age 55 years compared to 56% at age 75 years. Etzioni et al. [34] evaluated racial differences and estimated overdiagnosis was more common in black men than white men (44% vs. 29%). They also estimated that of the asymptomatic reservoir of prostate cancer that would only be identified at autopsy, the use of PSA would identify up to 15% of that reservoir in white men and 37% in black men. McGregor et al. [35] used a more stringent definition of overdiagnosis (prostate cancer mortality, not just prostate cancer symptoms) and reported an overdiagnosis rate of 84%. More recently, three independent mathematical models were recalibrated and reported in one publication, which estimated the rate of overdiagnosis ranged from 23% to 42% of prostate cancers detected by screening [36].

In the context of a discussion of prostate cancer overdiagnosis and overtreatment, it may be perhaps too easy to lump all prostate cancers into the indolent group. However, it has been shown that even in the contemporary PSA era, prostate cancer has the potential to impact longevity. However, estimating the current risk natural history of prostate cancer without screening or treatment is difficult as many men pursue prostate cancer treatment. Gulati and colleagues [37] addressed this issue by developing models to project the outcomes using the best available data and assumptions to evaluate the risks of PSA-detected prostate cancer. They estimated that only 10–13% of PSA-detected cancers would develop a clinical diagnosis during a lifetime, which implies an overdiagnosis rate of 87–90%. They estimated that 20–33% of men in the absence of PSA would have a biopsy-detectable prostate cancer (a lower rate that would be detectable at autopsy) and of these men that tumor would be clinically diagnosed in 67–93% without screening and cause death in 23–34%

without treatment. The risks in younger men or higher Gleason grade were more pronounced and reported that these groups are less prone to overdiagnosis.

Some authors have taken a different approach and attempted to estimate overdiagnosis and underdiagnosis based on the assessment of pathology specimens from prostatectomy. Graif et al. [38] evaluated prostatectomy specimens in men with T1c prostate cancer over time from 1989 to 2005 and defined pathologic criteria for underdiagnosis (non-organ confined, pathologic pT3 or greater, positive surgical margin) and overdiagnosis (tumor volume <0.5 cm [3], negative margins, and no Gleason 4 or 5). They reported pathologic overdiagnosis in only 1.3–7.1% compared to underdiagnosis in 25–30%.

Pelzer et al. [39] evaluated whether a PSA cut point of 4.0 ng/mL could be used to discriminate whether patients would experience overdiagnosis based on the pathology outcomes at prostatectomy. They used a pathologic definition of overdiagnosis as Gleason score <7, pathologic stage pT2a, and negative surgical margins and compared men with PSA below and above 4 ng/mL. They reported that pathologic overdiagnosis was present in 19.7% of patients with PSA <4 ng/mL and 16.5% of men with PSA >4 ng/mL. However, pathologic underdiagnosis is also a concern as 18.9% of men with PSA< 4 ng/mL and 36.7% of men with PSA >4 ng/mL had pathologic stage pT3 or higher or positive surgical margins.

Prostate Cancer Risk Assessment

When balancing the risks of overdetection versus the potential benefits of the early detection of prostate cancer, it becomes important to recognize the background of a large asymptomatic disease reservoir, as evidenced by the autopsy studies previously noted. Several factors have contributed to a contemporary man's risk of detected prostate cancer beginning to more closely resemble the small indolent prostate cancers that are identified at autopsy rather than large aggressive prostate cancers. The widespread use of screening PSA and prostate biopsy and the

Table 1.3 Prostate cancer diagnosis in the PLCO and ERSPC prostate cancer screening trials

	PLCO		ERSPC[a]	
	Screened arm	Usual care arm	Screened arm	Usual care arm
Cancers	3,452	2,974	5,990	4,307
Rate[b] (per 10,000 person-years)	103	88	93	55
Rate ratio (95% CI)	1.17 (1.11–1.22)		1.71 (1.32–2.33)	

[a]Core age group
[b]Rates estimated from ERSPC

practice of obtaining prostate biopsy with a lower threshold for abnormal PSA, obtaining more prostate biopsies per session, and pursuing further biopsies after an initial prostate biopsy over time have likely all contributed to the identification of many aggressive tumors which have been removed from the reservoir and have left a predominantly low risk disease appearance in the population of newly diagnosed patients.

Subsequent chapters will discuss making a decision about whether to proceed with prostate cancer screening, deciding whether to pursue a prostate biopsy, or utilizing a medication for prostate cancer risk reduction. To place these studies in context, it is useful to consider a man's risk of prostate cancer in the control arms of screening studies relative to the likelihood of prostate cancer seen at autopsy.

With respect to risk assessment, two large prostate cancer screening trials have been conducted (Table 1.3). In the United States, no mortality benefit was seen with screening in the PLCO study where the rate of prostate cancer was 116 per 10,000 person-years in the screening group (vs. 95 per 10,000 person-years in the control group) after 7 years of follow-up [40]. In contrast, the ERSPC (European Randomized Study of Screening for Prostate Cancer) trial reported a 20% decrease in prostate cancer mortality at 9-year follow-up, where 9.2% of the screened group was diagnosed with prostate cancer (vs. 4.8% of the control group) with an absolute prostate cancer death risk of 0.71 death per 1,000 men. It was estimated that 1,410 men

would need to be screened 48 prostate cancers treated to save one death from prostate cancer during that time frame. While the two studies differ somewhat in their methodology, the results of both further shed light on the potential for overdiagnosis. From a population-bases perspective, the use of prostate cancer screening clearly leads to an increase in the number of prostate cancers diagnosed while the incremental gain in prostate cancer mortality is less well established. Additionally, the rates of clinically detected prostate cancer are markedly lower than the rates identified at autopsy in men who died of causes not related to prostate cancer. Thus, the important question in future studies of screening and prostate biopsy is not whether more prostate cancers can be detected (because based on the autopsy series, we know that a large detectable asymptomatic reservoir is present) but rather whether methods can be developed to preferentially detect high risk prostate cancer while not detecting indolent prostate cancers that have a much higher chance of overdiagnosis.

The high prevalence of prostate cancer detected at autopsy has an even more apparent influence on studies which include a protocol-mandated prostate biopsy, such as the trial designs used to evaluate the use of 5-alpha-reductase inhibitors for prostate cancer risk reduction. The PCPT (Prostate Cancer Prevention Trial) and REDUCE (Reduction by Dutasteride of Prostate Cancer Events) trials were performed in the context of two populations with substantial differences in the risk of prostate cancer. PCPT was performed in a lower risk population of men with entry PSA < 3 ng/mL, while REDUCE was in a higher risk population of men with a prior negative biopsy. The absolute prostate cancer risk reduction with 5-alpha-reductase inhibition was 24.4% (placebo arm risk) to 18.4% (intervention arm risk) in PCPT and from 25.1% to 19.9% in REDUCE. It is notable that in both studies, the rate of prostate cancer diagnosis was greater than the 17% (1 in 6 men) chance of prostate cancer diagnosis during a man's lifetime, even in the intervention arms and in light of the fact that the REDUCE trial patients had already undergone one prior negative prostate biopsy. These two studies are influential as they show that the decision to proceed with a prostate biopsy (even in a normal male with low PSA as was seen in the PCPT trial) increases a man's chance of prostate cancer diagnosis to approximately 25%. One can imagine that as the accuracy of prostate biopsy improves, perhaps with the assistance of imaging technology, rates of prostate cancer detection will continue to rise and start to more closely approximate the high prevalence of prostate cancer seen at autopsy, which again highlights the close linkage between the increased diagnosis of prostate cancer and the potential for overdiagnosis.

In conclusion, when considering the contemporary risks of prostate cancer, it is important to place the discussion in the context of the histological presence of prostate cancer as the adult male ages. From studies on the incidental diagnosis of prostate cancer, we know now that the histological presence of prostate cancer is relatively common even in younger men and with time is present in the majority of men over age 60 years. This finding is important to consider when interpreting studies of prostate cancer screening and risk reduction studies.

Editorial Commentary:
As Dr. Ian Thompson has observed, the greatest risk factor for being diagnosed with prostate cancer is undergoing a prostate biopsy. This is because prostate cancer prevalence is immense, as demonstrated by both multiple autopsy series and the prevention trials that involved empiric biopsy regardless of clinical suspicion.

Thus, the goal must not be identification of disease that we know is probably present based simply on our knowledge of prevalence. It must not be to increase detection. It must be to improve detection.

This should start with focusing on the cancers that have potential to cause harm to the patient. Then, recognizing that no current methods allow us to reliably avoid detecting the other cancers that pose little if any risk to the patient, it is also critical that we follow the advice of Dr. Peter Carroll, who advocates the position that diagnosis and management should be regarded as separate issues. Subsequent chapters will explore how to achieve this safely and in a manner that allows

patients to be managed effectively based on the spectrum of risk posed by this amazingly heterogeneous disease.

–J. Stephen Jones

References

1. Jemal A, Siegel R, Xu J, Ward E. Cancer statistics, 2010. CA Cancer J Clin. 2010;60(5):277–300. Sep–Oct.
2. Kvale R, Auvinen A, Adami HO, et al. Interpreting trends in prostate cancer incidence and mortality in the five Nordic countries. J Natl Cancer Inst. 2007;99(24):1881–1887. Dec 19.
3. Albertsen PC, Moore DF, Shih W, Lin Y, Li H, Lu-Yao GL. Impact of comorbidity on survival among men with localized prostate cancer. J Clin Oncol. 2011;29(10):1335–1341. Apr 1.
4. Centers For Disease Control and Prevention. Cancer survivors – United States, 2007. *Morbidity and Mortality* weekly report. 2011.
5. D'Amico AV, Whittington R, Malkowicz SB, et al. Biochemical outcome after radical prostatectomy, external beam radiation therapy, or interstitial radiation therapy for clinically localized prostate cancer. JAMA. 1998;280(11):969–974. Sep 16.
6. Boorjian SA, Karnes RJ, Rangel LJ, Bergstralh EJ, Blute ML. Mayo clinic validation of the D'amico risk group classification for predicting survival following radical prostatectomy. J Urol. 2008;179(4):1354–1360. discussion 1360–1351.
7. Cooperberg MR, Broering JM, Kantoff PW, Carroll PR. Contemporary trends in low risk prostate cancer: risk assessment and treatment. J Urol. 2007;178(3 Pt 2):S14–19. Sep.
8. Shao YH, Demissie K, Shih W, et al. Contemporary risk profile of prostate cancer in the United States. J Natl Cancer Inst. 2009;101(18):1280–1283. Sep 16.
9. Fall K, Fang F, Mucci LA, et al. Immediate risk for cardiovascular events and suicide following a prostate cancer diagnosis: prospective cohort study. PLoS Med. 2009;6(12):e1000197.
10. Sanda MG, Dunn RL, Michalski J, et al. Quality of life and satisfaction with outcome among prostate-cancer survivors. N Engl J Med. 2008;358(12):1250–1261. Mar 20.
11. Gomella LG, Johannes J, Trabulsi EJ. Current prostate cancer treatments: effect on quality of life. Urology. 2009;73(5 Suppl):S28–35.
12. Gore JL, Kwan L, Lee SP, Reiter RE, Litwin MS. Survivorship beyond convalescence: 48-month quality-of-life outcomes after treatment for localized prostate cancer. J Natl Cancer Inst. 2009;101(12):888–892. Jun 16.
13. Sharifi N, Gulley JL, Dahut WL. Androgen deprivation therapy for prostate cancer. JAMA. 2005;294(2):238–244. Jul 13.

14. Yabroff KR, Lamont EB, Mariotto A, et al. Cost of care for elderly cancer patients in the United States. J Natl Cancer Inst. 2008;100(9):630–641. May 7.

15. Roehrig C, Miller G, Lake C, Bryant J. National health spending by medical condition, 1996–2005. Health Aff (Millwood). 2009;28(2):w358–367. Mar–Apr.

16. Nguyen PL, Gu X, Lipsitz SR, et al. Cost implications of the rapid adoption of newer technologies for treating prostate cancer. J Clin Oncol. 2011;29(12):1517–1524. Apr 20.

17. Shteynshlyuger A, Andriole GL. Cost-effectiveness of prostate specific antigen screening in the United States: extrapolating from the European study of screening for prostate cancer. J Urol. 2011;185(3): 828–32.

18. Sakr WA, Haas GP, Cassin BF, Pontes JE, Crissman JD. The frequency of carcinoma and intraepithelial neoplasia of the prostate in young male patients. J Urol. 1993;150(2 Pt 1):379–385.

19. Sheldon CA, Williams RD, Fraley EE. Incidental carcinoma of the prostate: a review of the literature and critical reappraisal of classification. J Urol. 1980;124(5):626–31.

20. Powell IJ, Bock CH, Ruterbusch JJ, Sakr W. Evidence supports a faster growth rate and/or earlier transformation to clinically significant prostate cancer in black than in white American men, and influences racial progression and mortality disparity. J Urol. 2010;183(5):1792–1796.

21. Revelo MP, Cookson MS, Chang SS, Shook MF, Smith Jr JA, Shappell SB. Incidence and location of prostate and urothelial carcinoma in prostates from cystoprostatectomies: implications for possible apical sparing surgery. J Urol. 2004;171(2 Pt 1): 646–651.

22. Pettus JA, Al-Ahmadie H, Barocas DA, et al. Risk assessment of prostatic pathology in patients undergoing radical cystoprostatectomy. Eur Urol. 2008;53(2): 370–375.

23. Winkler MH, Livni N, Mannion EM, Hrouda D, Christmas T. Characteristics of incidental prostatic adenocarcinomaincontemporaryradicalcystoprostatectomy specimens. BJU Int. 2007;99(3): 554–558.

24. Gakis G, Schilling D, Bedke J, Sievert KD, Stenzl A. Incidental prostate cancer at radical cystoprostatectomy: implications for apex-sparing surgery. BJU Int. 2010;105(4):468–71.

25. Abdelhady M, Abusamra A, Pautler SE, Chin JL, Izawa JI. Clinically significant prostate cancer found incidentally in radical cystoprostatectomy specimens. BJU Int. 2007;99(2):326–329.

26. Kouriefs C, Fazili T, Masood S, Naseem MS, Mufti GR. Incidentally detected prostate cancer in cystoprostatectomy specimens. Urol Int. 2005;75(3):213–216.

27. Welch HG, Albertsen PC. Prostate cancer diagnosis and treatment after the introduction of prostate-specific antigen screening: 1986–2005. J Natl Cancer Inst. 2009;101(19):1325–1329. Oct 7.

28. Crawford ED, Grubb 3rd R, Black A, et al. Comorbidity and mortality results from a randomized prostate cancer screening trial. J Clin Oncol. 2011;29(4):355–361. Feb 1.

29. Schroder FH, Hugosson J, Roobol MJ, et al. Screening and prostate-cancer mortality in a randomized European study. N Engl J Med. 2009;360(13):1320–1328. Mar 26.

30. Bill-Axelson A, Holmberg L, Ruutu M, et al. Radical prostatectomy versus watchful waiting in early prostate cancer. N Engl J Med. 2011;364(18):1708–1717. May 5.

31. Drazer MW, Huo D, Schonberg MA, Razmaria A, Eggener SE. Population-based patterns and predictors of prostate-specific antigen screening among older men in the United States. J Clin Oncol. 2011;29(13): 1736–1743. May 1.

32. Welch HG, Black WC. Overdiagnosis in cancer. J Natl Cancer Inst. 2010;102(9):605–613. May 5.

33. Draisma G, Boer R, Otto SJ, et al. Lead times and overdetection due to prostate-specific antigen screening: estimates from the European randomized study of screening for prostate cancer. J Natl Cancer Inst. 2003;95(12):868–878. Jun 18.

34. Etzioni R, Penson DF, Legler JM, et al. Overdiagnosis due to prostate-specific antigen screening: lessons from U.S. prostate cancer incidence trends. J Natl Cancer Inst. 2002;94(13):981–990. Jul 3.

35. McGregor M, Hanley JA, Boivin JF, McLean RG. Screening for prostate cancer: estimating the magnitude of overdetection. CMAJ. 1998;159(11):1368–1372. Dec 1.

36. Draisma G, Etzioni R, Tsodikov A, et al. Lead time and overdiagnosis in prostate-specific antigen screening: importance of methods and context. J Natl Cancer Inst. 2009;101(6):374–383. Mar 18.

37. Gulati R, Wever EM, Tsodikov A, et al. What if I don't treat my PSA-detected prostate cancer? Answers from three natural history models. Cancer Epidemiol Biomarkers Prev. 2011;20(5):740–750.

38. Graif T, Loeb S, Roehl KA, et al. Under diagnosis and over diagnosis of prostate cancer. J Urol. 2007; 178(1):88–92.

39. Pelzer AE, Bektic J, Akkad T, et al. Under diagnosis and over diagnosis of prostate cancer in a screening population with serum PSA 2 to 10 ng/ml. J Urol. 2007;178(1):93–97. discussion 97.

40. Andriole GL, Bostwick DG, Brawley OW, et al. Effect of dutasteride on the risk of prostate cancer. N Engl J Med. 2010;362(13):1192–1202. Apr 1.

Prostate Cancer Screening: Navigating the Controversy

William M. Hilton, Ian M. Thompson Jr., and Dipen J. Parekh

Despite advances in diagnosis, treatment, and patient outcomes, prostate cancer remains an important public health problem. In the United States in 2010, an estimated 217,730 new cases of prostate cancer were diagnosed and 32,050 men died as a result of this disease [1]. Prostate cancer is the second leading cause of cancer death in US men. The natural history of prostate cancer is remarkably heterogeneous, ranging from clinically silent tumors never destined to impact a patient to aggressive, metastatic cancers which cause considerable morbidity and patient death. A recent autopsy study revealed a prostate cancer prevalence of 1 in 3 for men aged 60–69 [2]. However, the risk of death from prostate cancer is only 3.4%, highlighting the variable natural history of prostate cancer.

Estimates of US national health-care expenditures for prostate cancer care are expected to increase dramatically between now and 2020 from $11.85 billion to $16.35 billion [3]. Zhang et al. analyzed the growth of prostate cancer spending by analyzing Surveillance, Epidemiology, and End Results (SEER)-Medicare data from 1992 to 2003 and concluded that Medicare spending for prostate cancer care increased by 20% [4]. Effective strategies of prevention, screening, and treatment are paramount to reduce the burden and cost of this disease. The goal of early detection by screening is to reduce morbidity and mortality of prostate cancer.

PSA-based screening has been controversial since it was first introduced in the late 1980s. Although PSA testing was originally intended to assess tumor recurrence or progression after treatment, it began to be used as a screening test despite the absence of level I evidence after publication of guidelines from the American Cancer Society and the American Urological Association beginning in the early 1992 [5, 6]. The adoption of PSA as a screening test has been associated with stage migration with a reduction in mortality and incidence of metastatic prostate cancer [7, 8]. However, many prostate cancers diagnosed based on PSA-based screening may have remained clinically indolent, never causing any symptoms. This phenomenon has resulted in overdiagnosis and overtreatment of clinically insignificant prostate cancer. Screening-related complications resulting in hospital admission from transrectal ultrasound-guided prostate biopsy have also risen sharply in the past 10 years, primarily due to infection but also due to bleeding and urinary obstruction [9]. The challenge in prostate cancer screening is to develop a sensitive and specific test that differentiates between cancers that would remain clinically indolent and those that would cause morbidity or death to the patient.

W.M. Hilton, M.D. • I.M. Thompson Jr., M.D.
• D.J. Parekh (✉)
Department of Urology, University of Texas Health Science Center at San Antonio, 7703 Floyd Curl Dr, Mail Code 7845, San Antonio, TX 78229, USA
e-mail: hiltonw@uthscsa.edu; thompsoni@uthscsa.edu; parekhd@uthscsa.edu

J.S. Jones (ed.), *Prostate Cancer Diagnosis: PSA, Biopsy and Beyond*, Current Clinical Urology, DOI 10.1007/978-1-62703-188-2_2, © Springer Science+Business Media New York 2013

Principles of Screening for Cancer

In 1907, Charles Childe developed the paradigm for cancer screening in a book titled *The Control of a Scourge, Or How Cancer is Curable*. Childe argued for the aggressive pursuit of the subtlest deviations from normal to identify asymptomatic latent cancers for curative treatment, stating that delay in cancer diagnosis is what makes cancer lethal [10]. Although it may seem intuitive that early diagnosis and treatment of an asymptomatic cancer would logically result in a benefit to patients, not all cancers are destined to become symptomatic or result in death, especially low-grade and low-stage cancers. In the 1960s, medicine began to question the linear model of carcinogenesis and the overall utility in widespread cancer screening. The United States Preventive Services Task Force was created in 1984 and has shifted the paradigm by examining the medical evidence for cancer screening. The USPTF has shifted away from the intuitive approach and developed a rigorous analytical framework for developing screening recommendations.

Cancer screening is defined as testing for cancer in a patient when no signs or symptoms exist. The principles of an effective prostate cancer screening test are important to review. An effective screening test must have the following attributes:

- It must capture a larger number of earlier stage prostate cancers
- It must improve prostate-cancer-specific survival
- It must improve overall patient survival
- It must decrease cancer-related morbidity

The introduction of PSA-based screening has certainly led to an increase in the diagnosis of a larger proportion of clinically localized prostate cancer. Mettlin and colleagues demonstrated the effectiveness of PSA-based screening in a study of 2,999 men and concluded that PSA testing resulted in the diagnosis of a more favorable stage distribution [11]. Additionally, Catalona et al. demonstrated that PSA-based serial screening resulted in the diagnosis of less advanced, clinically localized prostate cancer in a study of more

than 10,251 men [12]. This study compared 266 patients who underwent biopsy for an abnormal DRE versus an initial and serially PSA-screened population and concluded that PSA-based serial screening results in the diagnosis of a larger proportion of clinically localized, less advanced prostate cancer compared to those patients with an abnormal DRE alone.

Since the introduction of PSA-based prostate cancer screening in the United States, prostate cancer mortality has steadily declined. An analysis of the Surveillance, Epidemiology, and End Results (SEER) Program database revealed a 37% decrease in prostate-cancer-specific mortality since 1992. However, it is not clear that PSA-based screening is the only reason for the observed marked decline in mortality. Overdiagnosis of insignificant prostate cancers, lead-time bias, and healthy screened bias, as well as advances in the treatment of prostate cancer, may contribute to an improved prostate-cancer-specific mortality. In a provocative study that examined two regional cohorts from Seattle and Connecticut which experienced markedly different PSA-based screening, Lu-Yao et al. concluded that although the rate of PSA testing in Seattle was 5 times higher than Connecticut, the rate of prostate cancer mortality at 11 years of follow-up was virtually the same. Etzoni and colleagues used a surveillance modeling approach to quantify the association between PSA-based screening and the decline in distant stage incidence, as has been observed since the introduction of PSA testing [13]. This study concluded that PSA-based screening is likely accounted for 14% of the observed decline since 1990, accounting for 2/3 of the overall decline. The results from large randomized trials, the European Randomized Study of Screening for Prostate Cancer (ERSPC), and the Prostate, Lung, Colorectal, and Ovarian Cancer Screening Trial have recently been reported and show efficacy to screening. However, screening-related overdiagnosis and attendant overtreatment were common to both trials. The Holy Grail for prostate cancer continues to be measures to differentiate indolent from aggressive cancers.

History of Prostate Cancer Screening

Hugh Hampton Young was the first urologist to advocate screening for prostate cancer in 1905 with the digital rectal examination (DRE). DRE was advocated as a method to identify early changes in the prostate consistent with prostate cancer, suitable for curative radical prostatectomy. Unfortunately, most cancers were found to be advanced at the time of diagnosis.

Prostate cancer screening did not change significantly for the next 80 years. A digital rectal examination is known to be insensitive as a screening tool for the detection of low-grade, low-stage prostate cancer. In 1994, Catalona et al. conducted a large prospective trial involving 6,630 patients to compare the efficacy of DRE and serum PSA [12]. Quadrant biopsies were performed if the PSA was >4 ng/l or if the DRE was suspicious. This study demonstrated that DRE was less sensitive than PSA for the detection of prostate cancer. Combining DRE and PSA as a screening test for prostate cancer improved the detection of organ-confined disease by 78% over DRE alone.

The introduction of PSA-based prostate cancer screening in 1987 by Stamey et al. resulted in a "harvest effect," and the observed incidence of prostate cancer rose dramatically, peaking in 1992 (Fig. 2.1)[14]. The abrupt increase in prostate cancer incidence between 1987 and 1992 is attributable largely to the introduction and rapid dissemination of PSA-based prostate cancer screening [15].

SEER Observed Incidence, SEER Delay Adjusted Incidence and US Death Rates[a]
Cancer of the Prostate, by Race

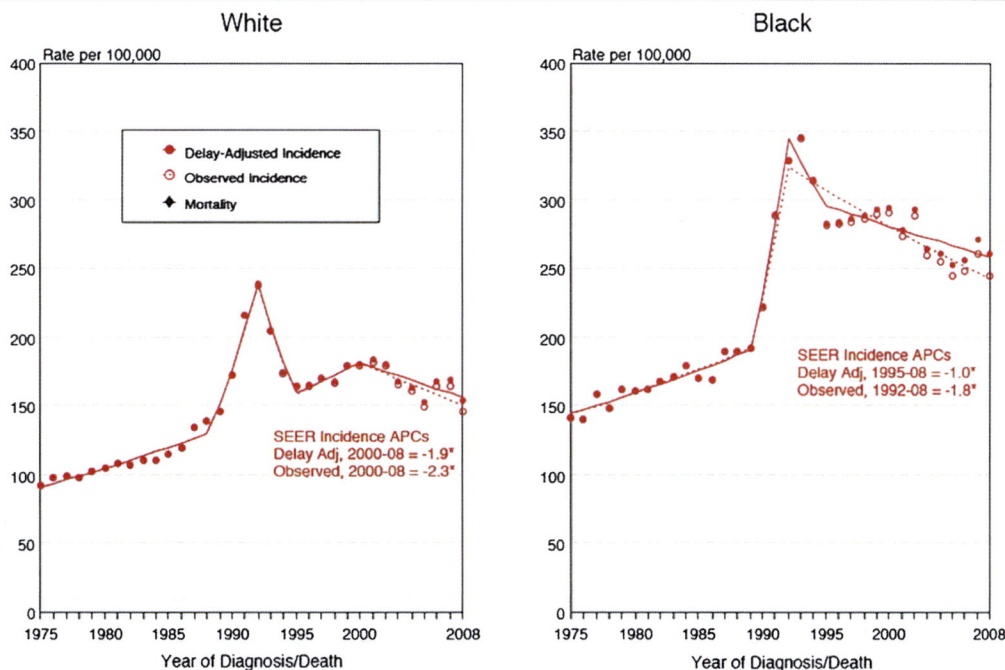

a   Source: SEER 9 areas and US Mortality Files (National Center for Health Statistics, CDC).
    Rates are age-adjusted to the 2000 US Std Population (19 age groups - Census P25-1103).
    Regression lines and APCs are calculated using the Joinpoint Regression Program Version 3.5, April 2011, National Cancer Institute.
    The APC is the Annual Percent Change for the regression line segments. The APC shown on the graph is for the most recent trend.
*   The APC is significantly different from zero (p < 0.05).

Fig. 2.1 SEER observed incidence, SEER delay-adjusted incidence, and US death rates (Adapted from: http://seer.cancer.gov/csr/1975_2008/sections.html)

PSA-Based Screening for Prostate Cancer

In 1970, Ablin et al. characterized what is now known as PSA. The first application of PSA analysis was to utilize the test in sex crimes due to its high concentration in human semen [16]. PSA is a member of the human kallikrein gene family and is a serine protease produced by prostatic epithelium. Nadji and colleagues demonstrated that PSA is specific to the prostate, and researchers then began to investigate if PSA could be used as a biomarker for prostate cancer [17]. Prior to using PSA for prostate cancer screening, serum prostatic acid phosphatase (PAP) was utilized as a marker for prostate cancer. However, in comparison to PSA, PAP was not found to be a sensitive marker for clinically localized disease and was not used for prostate cancer screening. Seamonds and colleagues compared PSA and PAP and concluded that for clinically localized disease, PSA was more sensitive than PAP [18]. In 1987, Stamey et al. confirmed the improved sensitivity of PSA by evaluating 699 patients, 378 of whom had prostate cancer and concluded that PSA is more sensitive for prostate cancer, but both PSA and PAP are not specific [14]. Beginning in the early 1990s, the first of many large PSA screening studies began to appear in the medical literature [19–22]. In 1991, Catalona et al. ushered in PSA-based prostate cancer screening. In this landmark paper, Catalona and colleagues demonstrated the utility of PSA-based prostate cancer screening by concluding that the combination of serum PSA and digital rectal examination provides an improved method of detecting prostate cancer. This finding led to widespread adoption of PSA-based screening in the United States and an explosion in the number of prostate cancer diagnoses. A 1995 analysis of SEER and Medicare claims data concluded that the exponential increase in prostate cancer detection was due to widespread rapid adoption of PSA-based screening. Importantly, this study raised serious concerns regarding overdetection of a large pool of latent disease, never destined to cause harm to the patient. Furthermore, Potosky and colleagues stated that the implementation of a highly sensitive test such as PSA was a "double-edged sword" because it uncovered a broader spectrum of disease that may have never been detected and whose natural course and response to radical treatment we know little about [23].

Operating Characteristics of PSA

Central to understanding screening tests is a thorough knowledge of the performance characteristics of the test. A receiver operating curve (ROC) is a plot of the true-positive rate (sensitivity) versus the false-positive rate (1 – specificity). A perfect screening test would, as seen in the upper left of the graph in Fig. 2.2, have 100% sensitivity and 100% specificity. Graphically, an ROC plot demonstrates the trade-off between true-positive and false-positive results. In 2005, Thompson et al. analyzed Prostate Cancer Prevention Trial (PCPT) data and illustrated important operating characteristics of PSA-based prostate cancer screening, as seen in Fig. 2.3 [24]. This study showed that PSA is more sensitive for higher Gleason grade cancers and concluded that lowering the threshold for prostate biopsy would increase the detection of insignificant prostate cancers.

Applying ROC analysis to PSA has been challenging because of verification bias and spectrum bias. Verification bias is introduced in cancer screening when verification of disease status (prostate biopsy) is determined by a positive test (abnormal PSA or DRE). Punglia et al. determined the impact of verification bias by modeling and demonstrated that adjustment for verification bias improved the area under the curve (AUC) from 0.69 to 0.86 for men <60 years old and implied that lowering the PSA threshold for prostate biopsy from 4.1 to 2.6 ng/mL in men <60 years old would double the cancer detection rate from 18% to 36% [25].

Spectrum bias refers to a change in performance of a screening test based on a change in patient population. Ransohoff and colleagues first described spectrum bias in 1978 and stated that "unless an appropriately broad spectrum is chosen for the diseased and non-diseased patients who comprise the study population,"

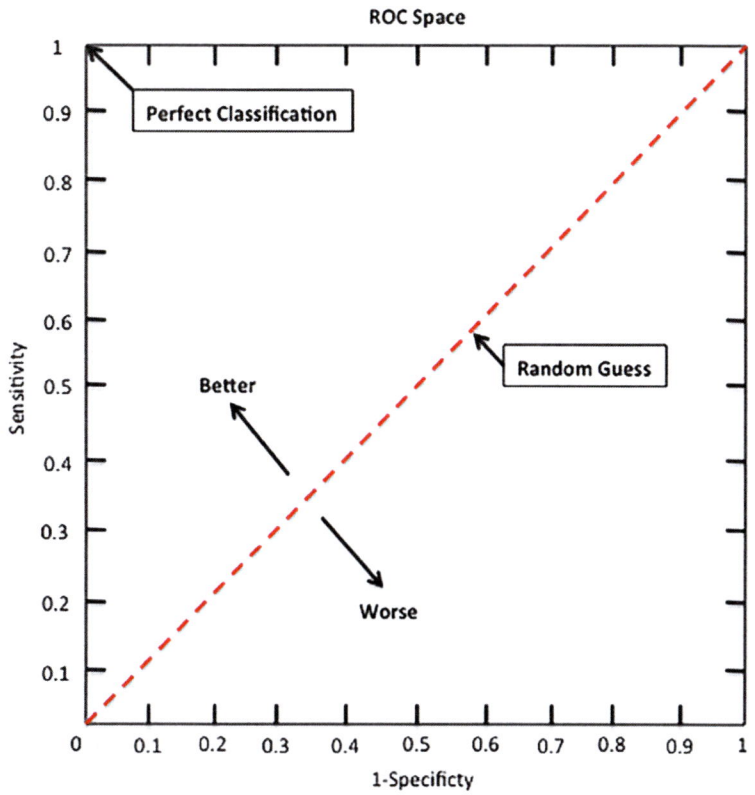

Fig. 2.2 Receiver operating characteristic curve

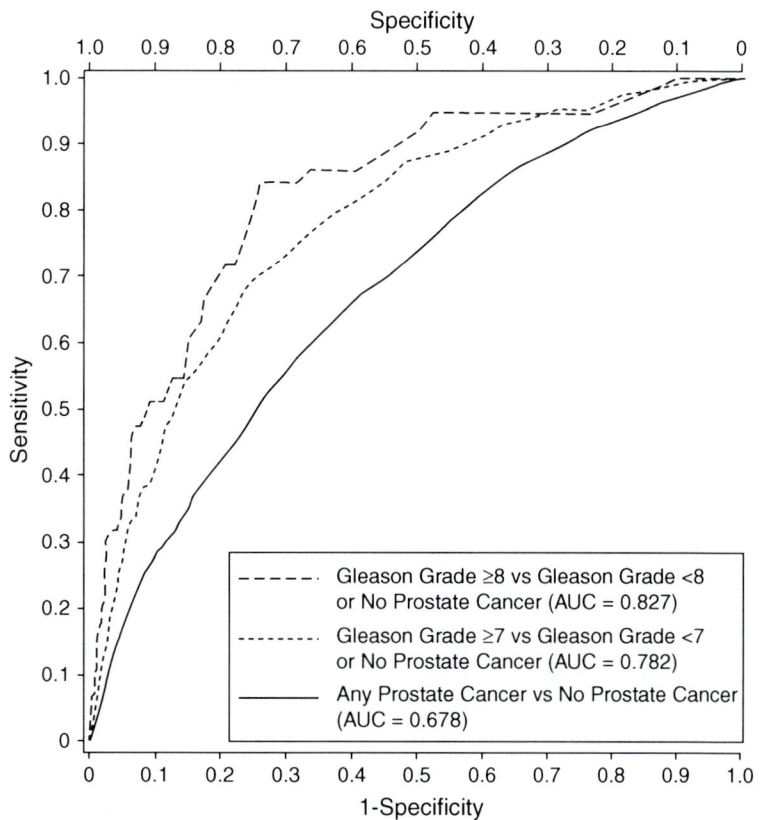

Fig. 2.3 Receiver operating characteristic curve for PSA. As Gleason grade increases, PSA becomes more sensitive and specific for the detection of prostate cancer

diagnostic accuracy of the test may be biased and overestimated if a test is evaluated in a population known to have the disease but applied to a group of normal subjects, as in annual PSA-based prostate cancer screening [26]. A method to reduce spectrum bias in the development of screening tests is to include a broad range of disease severity in the population undergoing the test.

PSA Derivatives

In order to enhance the sensitivity and specificity of PSA-based screening, researchers have investigated multiple PSA derivatives, including age-specific PSA, PSA velocity (PSAV), PSA density (PSAD), %free PSA (fPSA), and PSA isoforms. PSA derivatives attempt to differentiate elevated PSA from benign prostatic hyperplasia.

Age-specific PSA has been used in an attempt to detect potentially fewer clinically insignificant cancers. Serum PSA increases an average of age-specific PSA as men age due to a higher volume of tissue associated with benign prostatic hyperplasia. Annually, serum PSA has been observed to increase in men with and without benign prostatic hyperplasia (BPH). The rate of change in serum PSA for men without BPH has been observed to be 0.04 ng/mL/year, while for those with BPH, the rate of change of PSA was higher at 0.07–0.27 ng/mL/year [27]. Age-specific ranges for normal PSA were proposed by Oesterling in 1996 [28]. Regarding the clinical utility of using age-adjusted PSA, studies have reported conflicting results. Catalona et al. prospectively evaluated 6,630 men to determine the effect of using age-specific PSA ranges on biopsy and cancer detection rates and noted that if biopsy criteria were lowered to 3.5 ng/mL in men aged 50–59, a 45% increase in biopsies would be performed with a calculated 15% increase in prostate cancer detection [29]. On the other hand, if the PSA threshold were increased to 4.5 ng/mL in the 60–69 age group, 15% fewer biopsies would be performed, resulting in a decrease in the cancer detection rate by 8%. Most interestingly, increasing the PSA threshold in men more than 70 years old would result in 44% fewer biopsies and would not detect 47% of organ-confined cancers. This study

concluded that the general guideline for performing a biopsy should remain at 4.0 ng/mL.

In a pathological review of 4,597 men with clinically localized prostate cancer, Partin and colleagues analyzed the effect of using age-adjusted PSA and concluded that age-specific PSA increased the detection of clinically localized, potentially curable prostate cancer in younger men by 18% and decreased the detection rate in older men by 22% but that 95% of these tumors had favorable pathology. These studies point to common problems associated with age-specific PSA, that using different PSA thresholds results in overdetection of prostate cancer in younger men and underdetection of potentially significant tumors in older men.

PSA velocity has been studied to improve screening for prostate cancer. In 1992, one of the first research groups to investigate PSA velocity reported results after studying 16 men with no evidence of prostate cancer, 20 men with BPH, and 18 men with prostate cancer [30]. Their analysis revealed important characteristics of PSA metrics in the years prior to a diagnosis of prostate cancer; noting an association with an increased PSA velocity >0.75 ng/mL/year is a specific marker for prostate cancer. In this study, 72% of men with prostate cancer were noted to have a PSAV>0.75 ng/mL/year for men with a PSA between 4 and 10 ng/mL/year. Additionally, serial PSA measurements over a minimum of 18 months are required to estimate PSAV [31–33].

PSA may be elevated due to benign prostatic hyperplasia, and adjustment for this phenomenon has been used to increase the specificity. PSA density is defined as PSA/prostate gland volume, and use of this PSA metric may predict which patients are at risk for extracapsular extension in the setting of a PSA< 10 ng/mL[34]. Furthermore, Kang et al. demonstrated that for patients with a PSA between 4 and 10 ng/mL, adjustment of PSA for the volume of transition zone tissue may reduce unnecessary prostate biopsies [35].

Additional methods to increase specificity of PSA rely on the fact that PSA exists in two fractions in serum: complexed PSA, which is bound to plasma proteins, and unbound or free PSA. Jung et al. demonstrated that %free PSA could be used to distinguish between BPH-associated elevated PSA and prostate cancer but could not be used reliably to differentiate between chronic prostatitis and prostate cancer [36]. In men with a PSA <2.5 ng/mL, %free PSA and DRE were shown to be the only reliable independent predictors of prostate cancer [37].

PSA alone has a limited ability to aid in the diagnosis of prostate cancer because of its low specificity. The discovery of free and complexed forms of PSA led to an increase in specificity for prostate cancer by demonstrating that the ratio of free to complexed PSA was inversely proportional to the risk of harboring prostate cancer. It was also observed that serum PSA is composed of a diverse array of PSA isoforms. Over the last decade, investigators have discovered several free PSA isoforms. Four free PSA isoforms have been well characterized: BPSA, [−5/−7] proPSA, [−4] proPSA, and [−2] proPSA. In 2003, Mikolajczyk et al. discovered that proPSA is associated with prostate cancer by showing that in the 4–10 ng/mL PSA range, an analysis of the receiver operating characteristic area under the curve 0.689 versus 0.637 for %free PSA and 0.538 for complexed PSA [38]. In the largest retrospective study to date, Catalona et al. studied 1,091 patients by concluding that [−2] proPSA or "pan" proPSA (total of −2, −4, −5, and −7 proPSA) expressed as a ratio of with free-PSA-improved specificity for prostate cancer in patients with a PSA range between 2 and 10 ng/mL. The ratio of panproPSA

to free PSA reduced the need for prostate biopsy by 21%, while %free PSA reduced the biopsy rate by 13%[39]. Although analysis of PSA isoforms has been shown in the literature to improve the specificity for prostate cancer, more evaluation is necessary before clinical application.

Individual Risk Assessment for Prostate Cancer

Prostate cancer risk calculators have been shown to be superior to PSA and DRE in deciding whom to biopsy. Thompson et al. evaluated 5,519 men from the placebo group of the PCPT who underwent prostate biopsy and had a PSA test and DRE within a year preceding the biopsy and at least two prior annual PSA tests [40]. Using logistic regression, four variables were found to be significantly associated with risk for prostate cancer: PSA, family history of prostate cancer, abnormal DRE, and a previous negative biopsy result. The strength of this risk calculator is that it is based on a large sample of patients across a wide spectrum of PSA levels. As such, the Prostate Cancer Risk Calculator allows a man to assess his individual prostate cancer risk threshold and decide whether or not to undergo a prostate biopsy. Depending on the patient's personal risk tolerance, he can decide whether or not to pursue a prostate biopsy. Figure 2.4 shows the

Individualized Risk Assessment of Prostate Cancer

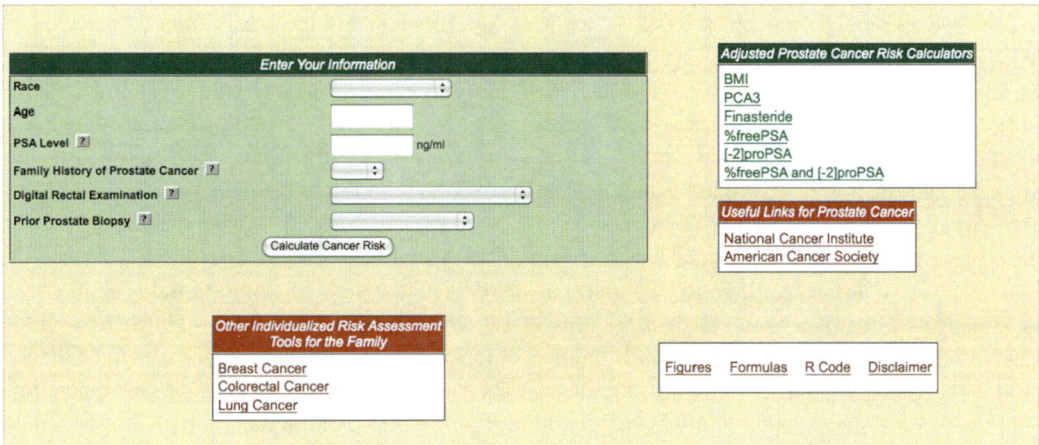

Fig. 2.4 Prostate cancer risk calculator (http://deb.uthscsa.edu/URORiskCalc/Pages/calcs.jsp)

PCPT-based Prostate Cancer Risk Calculator, which can be accessed at http://deb.uthscsa.edu/URORiskCalc/Pages/uroriskcalc.jsp. However, when counseling patients regarding the decision to undergo a prostate biopsy, it is important to understand the limitations of risk calculators. Vickers et al. analyzed data from five European and three United States cohorts of men undergoing prostate biopsy and concluded that reliance on a single cohort to determine risk of prostate cancer based on PSA can have significant variation when applied to other clinical cohorts [41].

Risk of Overdiagnosis and Overtreatment of Prostate Cancer

The frequency of overdiagnosis is related to the time that screening advances diagnosis of prostate cancer, which is defined as lead time. Given the natural history of prostate cancer, there is the potential to overdiagnose and overtreat a significant number of what would have been clinically indolent prostate cancers that were never destined to cause symptoms or contribute to a patient's death. Draisma et al. mathematically modeled prostate cancer detection and progression calibrated to Surveillance, Epidemiology, and End Results program data and also performed microsimulation screening analysis (MISCAN) of the United States and ERSPC Rotterdam data and concluded that among screen-detected cancers that would have been diagnosed, the estimated mean lead time was 5.4–6.9 years and overdiagnosis ranged from 23% to 42%, while MISCAN modeling predicted a mean lead time of 7.9 years and an overdiagnosis rate of 66% [42]. Welch and colleague analyzed SEER data for the period from 1986 to 2005 and noted that after the introduction of PSA-based screening in 1987, more than one million additional men were diagnosed and treated for prostate cancer [43]. The rate of prostate cancer diagnosis was particularly increased for men younger than 50 years. Lead time in the ERSPC was analyzed by Finne et al. [44]. Using a cutoff of 4 ng/mL, the mean lead time in the study population was 6.8 years, and overdiagnosis or detection of nonprogressive tumors may significantly contribute to lead time.

Overdiagnosis and overtreatment are arguably the most pressing problems associated with PSA-based prostate cancer screening. In the future, improved biomarkers may have a significant impact in reducing this problem.

Prostate Cancer Prevention Trial

In 2003, the Prostate Cancer Prevention Trial (PCPT) significantly expanded our understanding of prostate cancer across a broad range of PSA values and changed our perception about PSA [45]. The PCPT was a phase 3, randomized, double-blind, placebo-controlled trial to determine if daily finasteride could reduce the risk of prostate cancer over a 7-year period. A total of 18,882 men were randomized to either placebo or 5 mg of finasteride. Men underwent annual PSA and DRE. During the study, men with a PSA of >4.0 ng/mL or an abnormal DRE underwent prostate biopsy. All patients underwent an end-of-study sextant prostate biopsy if they had never been diagnosed with prostate cancer during the trial.

The PCPT markedly shifted our perception of PSA. Prior to the trial, the PSA test was considered a dichotomous test, either normal or abnormal. The PCPT demonstrated that there is no "normal" PSA and that prostate cancer exists at all PSA levels. It is now widely recognized that a high prevalence of prostate cancer exists at a PSA < 4.0 ng/mL [46]. While it had been known that prostate cancer incidence rates in the aging male population were quite high, it was assumed that these generally small tumors detected at autopsy were generally not found with prostate biopsies employing 6–12 cores [47]. In the PCPT, for the first time, a group of men all underwent prostate biopsy regardless of PSA level. In this study, 2,950 men in the placebo group that had a normal DRE and PSA, who had never had an abnormal DRE or PSA over the 7 years of the study, underwent an end-of-study biopsy, and 24.4% of men were found to have cancer on biopsy [46]. Further analysis demonstrated a 24.5% sensitivity for PSA using an upper limit of 4 ng/mL. Additionally, to achieve a 90% sensitivity for cancer detection, a PSA of approximately 1 ng/mL would be necessary [48].

The performance of PSA was found to be better for higher grade tumors, but a cut point of 4.0 ng/mL would still miss 60% of Gleason 7 or higher tumors [48].

ERSPC and PLCO

Two large randomized controlled trials designed to investigate the benefit of prostate cancer screening were published in March 2009. The European Randomized Study of Screening for Prostate Cancer (ERSPC) was a multi-institutional study of 162,000 men randomized to PSA-based prostate cancer screening every 4 years versus no screening [7]. Different screening intervals and follow-up routines were used in different countries. The ERSPC may be viewed not necessarily as a single study with a common protocol but as an amalgam of different studies. This study concluded that PSA-based screening without DRE resulted in an absolute reduction of 0.71 prostate cancer deaths per 1,000 men after a follow-up period of 8.8 years. This study also concluded that PSA-based screening results in a 20% relative risk reduction in prostate cancer death. With an average follow-up of 8.8 years, there were 214 prostate cancer deaths in the screening cohort versus 326 in the control group. Therefore, in order to prevent one prostate cancer death within an initial 10-year period, 1,410 men would need to be screened with the number needed to treat would be 48. Additionally, the age group found to benefit the most from prostate cancer screening was restricted to the 55–69 age group, which benefited the most in mortality reduction. Additionally, after adjustment for nonattendance and contamination effects, Roobol and colleagues determined that PSA-based prostate cancer screening actually reduces the risk of dying from prostate cancer by 31% [49]. Hugosson and colleagues reported results of the Goteborg cohort of the ERSPC, which had a longer follow-up period and shorter screening interval of 2 years [50]. It would be expected that the benefits of screening should increase beyond the 10-year trial period, and indeed the authors concluded that with increased follow-up, PSA-based screening demonstrated a larger decrease in prostate cancer

mortality than was seen in the ERSPC trial. In order to prevent one death from prostate cancer, 293 men would have to be screened, significantly lower than reported by the ERSPC trial. Loeb et al. performed a thoughtful analysis of ERSPC data and concluded that number needed to screen (NNS) and number needed to treat (NNT) are highly sensitive to the time-dependent effect of screening on prostate cancer mortality, implying that with longer follow-up, it is likely that the NNS and NNT to prevent a death from prostate cancer will decrease [51].

The screening interval in the ERSPC was predominantly every 4 years, but the Belgium cohort, which consisted of 8,562 patients, had a much broader screening interval, from 4 to 7 years. Nelen et al. reported the effect of screening interval on the screening outcome in 1,660 men from the screening arm of the Antwerp ERSPC cohort with an average screening interval of 6.1 years with a mean follow-up time of 8.4 years [52]. Interval cancers were defined as clinically diagnosed prostate cancers between two screening visits, while aggressive interval cancers were defined as stage M1 or N1 or a Gleason score of 7 or higher or a WHO grade of 3. Compared to the Rotterdam and Goteborg cohorts, the Antwerp cohort had a higher incidence of interval cancers (50, 3.0%) versus 0.43% in Rotterdam and 0.7% in Goteberg. The aggressiveness of these interval cancers was low with 36% detected at clinical stage T1 and 34% with clinical stage T2. The authors concluded that a 6-year screening interval may miss some aggressive prostate cancers, while a 4-year screening interval may be more effective at diagnosing aggressive interval cancers.

The Prostate, Lung, Colorectal, and Ovarian (PLCO) Screening Trial randomly assigned 76,000 men to annual PSA testing for 6 years and annual DRE for 4 years [53]. This study concluded that screening is associated with no reduction in prostate cancer mortality at 7 years. However, the control arm of this trial was significantly contaminated by PSA screening. Men in the control group were made aware of screening but were not actively screened. Forty-four percent of the study participant's arm had already undergone a PSA test within 3 years of study entry, which effectively prescreened the control group and likely diluted the effect on mortality of PSA-based screening. Despite a common protocol at each site, the PLCO trial essentially compares a rigorously screened group versus a cohort screened less rigorously. Considering the power required to show a significant difference between the two groups, it is easy to see why the PLCO trial failed to show a screening benefit, as prostate cancer deaths in the screening cohort were 50 versus 44 in the control group. Additionally, the prostate biopsy rate in men with a serum PSA of >4.0 ng/mL or an abnormal DRE was only 40%. It is likely that a substantial number of significant prostate cancers remained undetected in the screening arm. The control group was further contaminated because a significant number of men underwent PSA testing during the trial. Additionally, the median follow-up of 7 years is likely not long enough to demonstrate a significant difference between the two groups. It is interesting to note that all causes of mortality increased in the screened cohort of the PLCO. It is possible that the risk of mortality related to treatment may increase as may be seen with hormonal ablation with increased risk of heart disease, stroke, and diabetes [54].

Both the ERSPC and the PLCO trial address the significant problem of overdiagnosis and attendant overtreatment. The rate of overdiagnosis is far higher than was previously estimated. The ERSPC provides justification for screening, although at a cost of overdetection, and highlights the need for a well-informed decision after careful counseling by the patient's physician. The ERSPC and PLCO also stress the need for a sensitive and specific biomarker to differentiate between indolent and virulent prostate cancer, which is urgently needed.

Side Effects from Treatment of Screen-Detected Prostate Cancer

The ERSPC reported a 20% reduction in prostate-cancer-specific cancer mortality at the 10-year time frame, but it is unclear if this reduction in mortality outweighs the morbidity of treatment.

Carlsson et al. reported treatment side effects in the Goteborg cohort of the ERSPC and concluded that the excess burden of treatment-related side effects after population-based screening may be regarded as relatively low when compared to the number of men saved from prostate cancer death [55]. In the Goteborg trial, the number needed to treat to prevent 1 prostate cancer death was 12, significantly lower than the overall 48 reported by the combined ERSPC results. Erectile dysfunction and urinary incontinence were both evaluated in patients undergoing radical prostatectomy, and the authors concluded that despite the high risk of erectile dysfunction and incontinence, the burden of these complications was relatively low in comparison to the lives saved from prostate cancer screening.

Future Biomarkers for Prostate Cancer Screening

Prostate cancer gene 3 (PCA3) was originally described in 1999. Bussemakers and colleagues analyzed mRNA expression patterns in normal versus prostate tumor tissue and concluded that PCA3 is a noncoding RNA and is highly overexpressed in 53 of 56 tumors [56]. After DRE, a voided urine is collected and measurement of PCA3 mRNA is measured and normalized to PSA mRNA which results in a PCA3 score. Marks et al. calculated PCA3 scores in 233 men prior to repeat biopsy after initial negative biopsy in men with a PSA>2.5 ng/mL and determined that a PCA3 score cutoff of 35 resulted in a receiver operating characteristic curve area under the curve of 0.68, while the serum PSA AUC was 0.52 [57]. Additionally, at PCA3 scores<5, 12% of men were noted to have prostate cancer, and if the PCA3 score was>100 ng/mL, 50% of men were diagnosed with prostate cancer. In a prospective study of 533 men, Deras and colleagues calculated PCA3 score after a standardized DRE before prostate biopsy and observed that the probability of positive prostate biopsy increased directly with the PCA3 score [58]. Men with a PCA3 score of<5 had a positive biopsy rate of 14%. If the PCA3 score was more than 100, 69%

of patients were noted to have a positive biopsy. ROC analysis revealed that a history of prior negative biopsy did not influence the diagnostic accuracy of this test. Prostate volume was also not seen to influence the performance characteristics of PCA3. In the REDUCE trial, a subset of the placebo arm comprising 1,140 patients was evaluated with PCA3 at year 2 and year 4 prior to scheduled prostate biopsy [59]. PCA3 score performance characteristics were validated in the largest repeat biopsy study to date. The most interesting finding in this study was that PCA3 scores were predictive of repeat biopsy at year 4 and suggested that prostate biopsy at year 2 had missed tumors, while PCA3 had, in fact, detected their presence. Nakanishi and colleagues were able to demonstrate that tumor volume and Gleason score significantly correlated with PCA3 score and may be useful in predicting low volume tumors (<0.5 cc)[60]. De la Taille et al. evaluated PCA3 by studying more than 500 men scheduled for prostate biopsy with a serum PSA between 2.5 and 10.0 ng/mL [61]. Mean PCA3 scores were found to be significantly higher for men with a positive biopsy than those with a negative biopsy, 69.6 versus 31.0. A PCA3 cutoff score of 35 was found to have optimal sensitivity (64%) and specificity (76%), and men with a PCA3 score of 35 or higher had a 2.7-fold higher probability of a positive biopsy (64%) than those with a PCA3 score of less than 35 (24%).

Using a panel of kallikrein markers may reduce unnecessary prostate biopsies. In 2008, Vickers and colleagues demonstrated that using free PSA, intact PSA, and human kallikrein 2 (hK2) by studying the Goteborg cohort from the ERSPC and concluded that biopsies could be reduced by 57% using a 20% threshold of risk for prostate cancer [62]. Benchikh et al. independently validated this method to reduce unneeded prostate biopsies by analyzing the French cohort of the ERSPC in 2010 [63]. Again, using a 20% threshold of risk for prostate cancer, this study found that prostate biopsies could be reduced by 49.2% at a cost of 61 missed prostate cancers, the majority of which would be low stage and low grade. Vickers and colleagues again replicated this method to reduce the need for biopsy by

studying the Rotterdam cohort of the ERSPC and were able to reduce prostate biopsies by 51.3% at a relatively low cost of missing 12 high-grade cancers [64].

Early prostate cancer antigen (EPCA) and early prostate cancer antigen-2 (EPCA-2) were first reported by Getzenberg et al. [65]. EPCA, a nuclear structural protein, is found in prostate cancer tissue but not observed in benign prostatic tissue or benign prostatic hyperplasia tissue. Leman and colleagues studied 385 patients with PSA<2.5 ng/mL, PSA equal to or>2.5 ng/mL with a negative biopsy, BPH, organ-confined prostate cancer, non-organ-confined disease, and prostate cancer with PSA<2.5 ng/mL [66]. An epitope of EPCA-2 and EPCA-2.22 was set at a cutoff of 30 ng/mL and found to have a 94% sensitivity and a 92% specificity for men with and without BPH for prostate cancer. Additionally, EPCA-2.22 was highly accurate for differentiating between localized and extracapsular disease with an AUC of 0.89, while PSA demonstrated an AUC of 0.62. EPCA holds promise as a biomarker for prostate cancer screening but requires more study before a final conclusion can be made.

Hypermethylation of CpG islands has been associated with a variety of different tumors [67]. Several genes have been identified in prostate cancer that have undergone abnormal hypermethylation: GSTP1, APC, MGMT, RASSF1A, PTGS2, and RAR-beta [68–71]. Aberrantly hypermethylated GSTP1 is the most well-characterized biomarker for prostate cancer. Changes to GSTP1 are seen in 70% of high-grade prostatic intraepithelial neoplasia and 90% of prostate cancers, implying that GSTP1 hypermethylation is an early event in the carcinogenesis of prostate cancer [72]. Roupret and colleagues investigated aberrant promoter hypermethylation in prostatic fluid in 95 patients, of which 63 patients had pT1 prostate cancer, 31 patients with pT2, and 1 with pT3, as well as 38 controls [73]. A combination of four genes, GSTP1, RASSF1a, RAR-beta2, and APC, were found to be the best markers to differentiate between benign and malignant cases. Prostate cancer patients demonstrated a markedly higher degree of hypermethylation of these four genes, see Fig. 2.5. The sensitivity and specificity of the

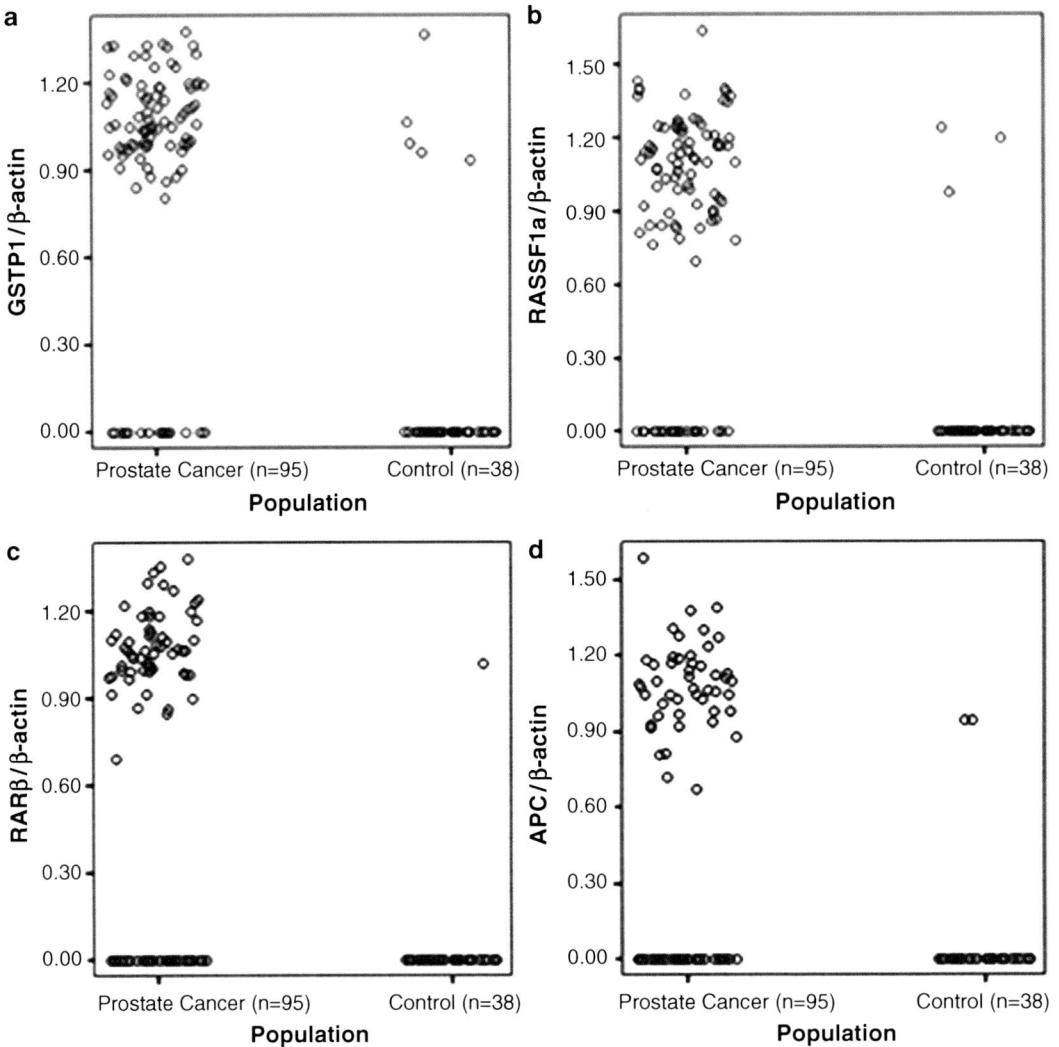

Fig. 2.5 Methylation levels of GSTP1, RASSF1a, RARbeta2, and APC in prostate cancer patients

four-gene set were 86% and 89%, respectively. Additional research into this area is underway, and future biomarkers for prostate cancer screening may include these potential biomarkers.

The most common type of fusion gene in prostate cancer is the fusion of TMPRSS2 and ERG. Perner et al. identified a significant association between higher stage tumors and TMPRSS2:ERG rearranged tumors [74]. This fusion gene has been found in approximately 50% of prostate cancers. Recently, Tomlins and colleagues investigated a urine-based assay for TMPRSS2:ERG rearrangement. In 187 prostatectomy patients,

TMPRSS2:ERG score positively correlated with markers of tumor volume, such as number of positive cores and maximum percentage of tumor involvement of a single core in the biopsy. Additionally, TMPRSS2:ERG score was also positively associated with maximum tumor dimension but was not associated with prostate weight, serum PSA, or PSA density. TMPRSS2:ERG score was additionally significantly higher in patients with high prostatectomy Gleason score and tumor upgrading at prostatectomy. Finally, TMPRSS2:ERG score was higher in men with significant versus insignificant cancer at prostatectomy as well as biopsy. Tomlins et al. also combined PSA3 score with the TMPRSS2:ERG score to individualize prostate cancer risk and found that this combined score predicted risk of prostate cancer diagnosis and higher Gleason score. Urine assays for TMPRSS2:ERG score and PCA3 score may have utility in determining the urgency for biopsy and may individually risk stratify men. Further study is needed to determine the clinical utility of this new biomarker.

One method to reduce unnecessary prostate biopsies is to target patients at higher risk for prostate cancer. Lilja et al. analyzed blood samples from 21,277 Swedish men from the Malmo Preventive Project which was a cardiovascular study from 1974 to 1986[75]. In Sweden, national guidelines advise against routine PSA-based prostate cancer screening and most prostate cancers are diagnosed clinically. This study concluded that a single PSA drawn at age 44–50 is a very strong predictor of prostate cancer clinically diagnosed decades later. These findings were not restricted to insignificant prostate cancers and pertain to clinically palpable and advanced or metastatic at diagnosis. The risk of clinically diagnosed prostate cancer was low (1–5%) for men with a PSA<0.5 ng/mL and was 8–15% for men with a PSA of 0.75–1.25 ng/mL. For a PSA above 1.5 ng/mL, the risk of prostate cancer was significantly higher. The clinical implication of this study is that a single early PSA could be used to individualize later screening for prostate cancer. In men with a low initial PSA of less than the median (0.6 ng/mL), annual screening could be expected to be of little clinical benefit and, likewise, men with high initial PSA could be advised that they are at a significant increased risk for developing clinically significant prostate cancer. Risk stratifying prostate cancer screening could retain many of the benefits of screening such as reducing mortality while avoiding harm of unnecessary screening and overdiagnosis. Unfortunately, without appropriate screening biomarkers validated to separate indolent from aggressive prostate cancers, the phenomena of overdiagnosis and subsequent overtreatment will continue to be a problem.

Individualizing PSA values may lead to a decrease in overdiagnosis and overtreatment. Gudmondsson and colleagues analyzed six genetic loci and their association with PSA levels and risk of prostate cancer [76].

Prostate Cancer Screening Today

In 2009, the American Urological Association released a PSA Best Practice Statement [77]. Updated from 2000, this statement had two important changes:
- A recommendation that initial PSA-based prostate cancer screening begins at age 40
- A recommendation that no single threshold PSA value be used to trigger a prostate biopsy

The authors of this best practice statement concluded that all men at risk for prostate cancer should be counseled regarding the relative risks and benefits of prostate cancer screening. Additionally, improved biomarkers are urgently needed to improve the detection of clinically significant prostate cancers and reduce overdiagnosis and overtreatment of insignificant cancers.

The United States Preventive Services Task Force (USPSTF) has concluded that there is convincing evidence of harms of detection and early treatment [78]. The task force concluded that treatment for screen-detected prostate cancer causes moderate to substantial harms such as erectile dysfunction, urinary incontinence, bowel dysfunction, and death, especially since many screen-detected prostate cancers are never destined to cause symptoms or death of the patient and adequate evidence that screening causes pain and discomfort from a prostate biopsy as well as psychological effects from a false-positive test. Controversially, the USPSTF changed its previous position and recommended against prostate cancer screening in 2011.

The American Cancer Society (ACS) recommends that men make an informed decision with their health-care provider about prostate cancer screening after a careful consideration of the risks, uncertainties, and benefits beginning at age 50 in men with average risk for prostate cancer and expected to live at least 10 years [79]. For men at high risk for prostate cancer, such as African-American men and men with a first-degree relative diagnosed with prostate cancer earlier than age 65, a discussion about screening should occur at age 45. For those men at an even higher risk, such as a man with several first-degree relatives with prostate cancer at an early age, a discussion about screening should occur at age 40. The recommended screening interval for a PSA <2.5 ng/mL should be every 2 years, and for those with a PSA >2.5 ng/mL, the interval should be annual.

Editorial Commentary:

No other topic in prostate cancer diagnostics generates as much controversy as screening. This exploded as this book was going to print based on the highly controversial position taken by the United States Preventive Services Task Force (USPSTF). Their interpretation of the published data led to a recommendation not to screen.

This position does have some justification based on a literal and narrow view of the published data, but in my (also controversial) opinion, it ignores the complexity of this issue. Most importantly, the large trials discussed in this chapter do demonstrate an undeniable and significant decrease in prostate cancer mortality when screening is performed. Furthermore, the impact is even more obvious when taking into account the decrease in mortality among men that actually were screened, regardless of group that they were randomized to. This is most likely related to the degree of cross-contamination in the groups, for example, that many men randomized to screening did not undergo screening, and of those, many with abnormal PSA did not undergo biopsy and/or treatment. Furthermore, larger numbers of men randomized to the non-screening arm actually did undergo screening outside the protocol either during or before the study periods, so their results cannot be considered controls representative of non-screening status.

Finally, the benefits of screening are clearly most influential over time based on the natural history of prostate cancer. Thus, follow-up studies from two of the ERSPC centers have now predictably shown that the benefit continues to become more exaggerated as the patients go beyond 10 years, and the numbers needed to screen and treat become far more justifiable.

Thus, it becomes clear that screening is mostly beneficial for men with a life expectancy of over 10 years. Furthermore, a single PSA at some point in mid-life – 40 years is the AUA recommendation – serves as a significant predictor of future prostate cancer risk. If it is very low (<1.0 ng/dl), the patient is unlikely to develop prostate cancer in the foreseeable future. If it is even slightly elevated (>1.0 ng/dl) at that age, the patient should undergo serial evaluation and may require biopsy if it continues to rise.

References

1. Jemal A, et al. Cancer statistics, 2010. CA Cancer J Clin. 2010;60(5):277–300.
2. Yin M, et al. Prevalence of incidental prostate cancer in the general population: a study of healthy organ donors. J Urol. 2008;179(3):892–5. discussion 895.
3. Mariotto AB, et al. Projections of the cost of cancer care in the United States: 2010–2020. J Natl Cancer Inst. 2011;103(2):117–28.
4. Zhang Y, et al. Understanding prostate cancer spending growth among Medicare beneficiaries. Urology. 2011;77(2):326–31.
5. A.U. Association. Early detection of prostate cancer and use of transrectal ultrasound. In: American Urological Association 1992 policy statement book. Baltimore: LWW; 1992.
6. Mettlin C, et al. Defining and updating the American Cancer Society guidelines for the cancer-related checkup: prostate and endometrial cancers. CA Cancer J Clin. 1993;43(1):42–6.
7. Schroder FH, et al. Screening and prostate-cancer mortality in a randomized European study. N Engl J Med. 2009;360(13):1320–8.
8. Jhaveri FM, et al. Declining rates of extracapsular extension after radical prostatectomy: evidence for continued stage migration. J Clin Oncol. 1999;17(10):3167–72.
9. Nam RK, et al. Increasing hospital admission rates for urological complications after transrectal ultrasound guided prostate biopsy. J Urol. 2010;183(3):963–8.
10. Childe C. The control of a scourge, or how cancer is curable. New York: E.P. Dutton; 1907.
11. Mettlin C, et al. Characteristics of prostate cancer detected in the American Cancer Society-National Prostate Cancer Detection Project. J Urol. 1994;152 (5 Pt 2):1737–40.
12. Catalona WJ, et al. Comparison of digital rectal examination and serum prostate specific antigen in the early detection of prostate cancer: results of a multicenter clinical trial of 6,630 men. J Urol. 1994; 151(5):1283–90.

13. Etzioni R, et al. Impact of PSA screening on the incidence of advanced stage prostate cancer in the United States: a surveillance modeling approach. Med Decis Making. 2008;28(3):323–31.

14. Stamey TA, et al. Prostate-specific antigen as a serum marker for adenocarcinoma of the prostate. N Engl J Med. 1987;317(15):909–16.

15. Jacobsen SJ, et al. Incidence of prostate cancer diagnosis in the eras before and after serum prostate-specific antigen testing. JAMA. 1995;274(18):1445–9.

16. Ablin RJ, et al. Precipitating antigens of the normal human prostate. J Reprod Fertil. 1970;22(3):573–4.

17. Nadji M, et al. Prostatic-specific antigen: an immuno-histologic marker for prostatic neoplasms. Cancer. 1981;48(5):1229–32.

18. Seamonds B, et al. Evaluation of prostate-specific antigen and prostatic acid phosphatase as prostate cancer markers. Urology. 1986;28(6):472–9.

19. Cooner WH, et al. Prostate cancer detection in a clinical urological practice by ultrasonography, digital rectal examination and prostate specific antigen. J Urol. 1990;143(6):1146–52. discussion 1152–4.

20. Catalona WJ, et al. Measurement of prostate-specific antigen in serum as a screening test for prostate cancer. N Engl J Med. 1991;324(17):1156–61.

21. Brawer MK, et al. Screening for prostatic carcinoma with prostate specific antigen. J Urol. 1992;147(3 Pt 2):841–5.

22. Brawer MK, et al. Screening for prostatic carcinoma with prostate specific antigen: results of the second year. J Urol. 1993;150(1):106–9.

23. Potosky AL, et al. The role of increasing detection in the rising incidence of prostate cancer. JAMA. 1995;273(7):548–52.

24. Thompson IM, et al. Operating characteristics of prostate-specific antigen in men with an initial PSA level of 3.0 ng/ml or lower. JAMA. 2005;294(1):66–70.

25. Punglia RS, et al. Effect of verification bias on screening for prostate cancer by measurement of prostate-specific antigen. N Engl J Med. 2003;349(4):335–42.

26. Ransohoff DF, Feinstein AR. Problems of spectrum and bias in evaluating the efficacy of diagnostic tests. N Engl J Med. 1978;299(17):926–30.

27. Carter HB, et al. Longitudinal evaluation of prostate-specific antigen levels in men with and without prostate disease. JAMA. 1992;267(16):2215–20.

28. Oesterling JE. Age-specific reference ranges for serum PSA. N Engl J Med. 1996;335(5):345–6.

29. Catalona WJ, et al. Selection of optimal prostate specific antigen cutoffs for early detection of prostate cancer: receiver operating characteristic curves. J Urol. 1994;152(6 Pt 1):2037–42.

30. Carter HB, et al. Estimation of prostatic growth using serial prostate-specific antigen measurements in men with and without prostate disease. Cancer Res. 1992;52(12):3323–8.

31. Smith DS, Catalona WJ. Rate of change in serum prostate specific antigen levels as a method for prostate cancer detection. J Urol. 1994;152(4):1163–7.

32. Carter HB, et al. Prostate-specific antigen variability in men without prostate cancer: effect of sampling interval on prostate-specific antigen velocity. Urology. 1995;45(4):591–6.

33. Carter HB, et al. Detection of life-threatening prostate cancer with prostate-specific antigen velocity during a window of curability. J Natl Cancer Inst. 2006;98(21):1521–7.

34. Zlotta AR, et al. Prostate specific antigen density of the transition zone for predicting pathological stage of localized prostate cancer in patients with serum prostate specific antigen less than 10 ng/ml. J Urol. 1998;160(6 Pt 1):2089–95.

35. Kang SH, et al. Prostate-specific antigen adjusted for the transition zone volume as a second screening test: a prospective study of 248 cases. Int J Urol. 2006;13(7):910–4.

36. Jung K, et al. Ratio of free-to-total prostate specific antigen in serum cannot distinguish patients with prostate cancer from those with chronic inflammation of the prostate. J Urol. 1998;159(5):1595–8.

37. Walz J, et al. Percent free prostate-specific antigen (PSA) is an accurate predictor of prostate cancer risk in men with serum PSA 2.5 ng/mL and lower. Cancer. 2008;113(10):2695–703.

38. Mikolajczyk SD, Rittenhouse HG. Pro PSA: a more cancer specific form of prostate specific antigen for the early detection of prostate cancer. Keio J Med. 2003;52(2):86–91.

39. Catalona WJ, et al. Serum pro prostate specific antigen improves cancer detection compared to free and complexed prostate specific antigen in men with prostate specific antigen 2 to 4 ng/ml. J Urol. 2003;170(6 Pt 1):2181–5.

40. Thompson IM, et al. Assessing prostate cancer risk: results from the Prostate Cancer Prevention Trial. J Natl Cancer Inst. 2006;98(8):529–34.

41. Vickers AJ, et al. The relationship between prostate-specific antigen and prostate cancer risk: the Prostate Biopsy Collaborative Group. Clin Cancer Res. 2010;16(17):4374–81.

42. Draisma G, et al. Lead time and overdiagnosis in prostate-specific antigen screening: importance of methods and context. J Natl Cancer Inst. 2009;101(6):374–83.

43. Welch HG, Albertsen PC. Prostate cancer diagnosis and treatment after the introduction of prostate-specific antigen screening: 1986–2005. J Natl Cancer Inst. 2009;101(19):1325–9.

44. Finne P, et al. Lead-time in the European randomised study of screening for prostate cancer. Eur J Cancer. 2010;46(17):3102–8.

45. Thompson IM, et al. The influence of finasteride on the development of prostate cancer. N Engl J Med. 2003;349(3):215–24.

46. Thompson IM, et al. Prevalence of prostate cancer among men with a prostate-specific antigen level < or =4.0 ng per milliliter [see comment][erratum appears in N Engl J Med. 2004 Sep 30;351(14):1470]. N Engl J Med. 2004;350(22):2239–46.

47. Sirovich BE, Schwartz LM, Woloshin S. Screening men for prostate and colorectal cancer in the United States: does practice reflect the evidence? JAMA. 2003;289(11):1414–20.

48. Thompson IM, et al. Operating characteristics of prostate-specific antigen in men with an initial PSA level of 3.0 ng/ml or lower. JAMA. 2005;294(1):66–70.

49. Roobol MJ, et al. Prostate cancer mortality reduction by prostate-specific antigen-based screening adjusted for nonattendance and contamination in the European Randomised Study of Screening for Prostate Cancer (ERSPC). Eur Urol. 2009;56(4):584–91.

50. Hugosson J, et al. Mortality results from the Goteborg randomised population-based prostate-cancer screening trial. Lancet Oncol. 2010;11(8):725–32.

51. Loeb S, et al. What is the true number needed to screen and treat to save a life with prostate-specific antigen testing? J Clin Oncol. 2011;29(4):464–7.

52. Nelen V, et al. Interval cancers in the Antwerp European randomised study of screening for prostate cancer study, using a 6 year screening interval. Eur J Cancer. 2010;46(17):3090–4.

53. Andriole GL, et al. Mortality results from a randomized prostate-cancer screening trial. N Engl J Med. 2009;360(13):1310–9.

54. Efstathiou JA, et al. Cardiovascular mortality after androgen deprivation therapy for locally advanced prostate cancer: RTOG 85-31. J Clin Oncol. 2009;27(1):92–9.

55. Carlsson S, et al. The excess burden of side-effects from treatment in men allocated to screening for prostate cancer. The Goteborg randomised population-based prostate cancer screening trial. Eur J Cancer. 2011;47(4):545–53.

56. Bussemakers MJ, et al. DD3: a new prostate-specific gene, highly overexpressed in prostate cancer. Cancer Res. 1999;59(23):5975–9.

57. Marks LS, et al. PCA3 molecular urine assay for prostate cancer in men undergoing repeat biopsy. Urology. 2007;69(3):532–5.

58. Deras IL, et al. PCA3: a molecular urine assay for predicting prostate biopsy outcome. J Urol. 2008;179(4):1587–92.

59. Aubin SM, et al. PCA3 molecular urine test for predicting repeat prostate biopsy outcome in populations at risk: validation in the placebo arm of the dutasteride REDUCE trial. J Urol. 2010;184(5):1947–52.

60. Nakanishi H, et al. PCA3 molecular urine assay correlates with prostate cancer tumor volume: implication in selecting candidates for active surveillance. J Urol. 2008;179(5):1804–9. discussion 1809–10.

61. de la Taille A, et al. Clinical evaluation of the PCA3 assay in guiding initial biopsy decisions. J Urol. 2011;185(6):2119–25.

62. Vickers AJ, et al. A panel of kallikrein markers can reduce unnecessary biopsy for prostate cancer: data from the European randomized study of prostate cancer screening in Goteborg, Sweden. BMC Med. 2008;6:19.

63. Benchikh A, et al. A panel of kallikrein markers can predict outcome of prostate biopsy following clinical work-up: an independent validation study from the European randomized study of prostate cancer screening, France. BMC Cancer. 2010;10:635.

64. Vickers A, et al. Reducing unnecessary biopsy during prostate cancer screening using a four-kallikrein panel: an independent replication. J Clin Oncol. 2010;28(15):2493–8.

65. Getzenberg RH, et al. Identification of nuclear matrix proteins in the cancer and normal rat prostate. Cancer Res. 1991;51(24):6514–20.

66. Leman ES, et al. EPCA-2: a highly specific serum marker for prostate cancer. Urology. 2007;69(4):714–20.

67. Herman JG, Baylin SB. Gene silencing in cancer in association with promoter hypermethylation. N Engl J Med. 2003;349(21):2042–54.

68. Nakayama M, et al. GSTP1 CpG island hypermethylation as a molecular biomarker for prostate cancer. J Cell Biochem. 2004;91(3):540–52.

69. Enokida H, et al. Multigene methylation analysis for detection and staging of prostate cancer. Clin Cancer Res. 2005;11(18):6582–8.

70. Kuzmin I, et al. The RASSF1A tumor suppressor gene is inactivated in prostate tumors and suppresses growth of prostate carcinoma cells. Cancer Res. 2002;62(12):3498–502.

71. Woodson K, et al. CD44 and PTGS2 methylation are independent prognostic markers for biochemical recurrence among prostate cancer patients with clinically localized disease. Epigenetics. 2006;1(4):183–6.

72. Nelson WG, De Marzo AM, Isaacs WB. Prostate cancer. N Engl J Med. 2003;349(4):366–81.

73. Roupret M, et al. Molecular detection of localized prostate cancer using quantitative methylation-specific PCR on urinary cells obtained following prostate massage. Clin Cancer Res. 2007;13(6):1720–5.

74. Perner S, et al. TMPRSS2:ERG fusion-associated deletions provide insight into the heterogeneity of prostate cancer. Cancer Res. 2006;66(17):8337–41.

75. Lilja H, et al. Prediction of significant prostate cancer diagnosed 20 to 30 years later with a single measure of prostate-specific antigen at or before age 50. Cancer. 2011;117(6):1210–9.

76. Gudmundsson J, et al. Genetic correction of PSA values using sequence variants associated with PSA levels. Sci Transl Med. 2010;2(62):62ra92.

77. American Urological Association Web site. 2011. http://www.auanet.org/content/guidelines-and-quality-care/clinical-guidelines.cfm. Accessed 15 Aug 2011.

78. U.S. Preventive Services Task Force Web site. 2011. http://www.uspreventiveservicestaskforce.org/uspstf08/prostate/prostaters.htm. Accessed 15 Aug 2011.

79. American Cancer Society Web site. 2011. http://www.cancer.org/Cancer/ProstateCancer/MoreInformation/ProstateCancerEarlyDetection/prostate-cancer-early-detection-acs-recommendations. Accessed 15 Aug 2011.

Is the PSA Era Over?

3

Ronald S. Boris and Michael O. Koch

Introduction

Tom Stamey has recently challenged the utilization of PSA in the management of prostate cancer. According to Stamey, PSA remains a surrogate for BPH and prostate size and with little impact on prostate cancer volume [1]. Stamey's explanation for increasing positive biopsy rates in men with increasing PSA levels is secondary to the many years required for BPH to produce increase in PSA, years that allow the presence of microscopically small cancers to grow enough to be detected by the ever-increasing number of performed prostate biopsies [2]. These concepts are supported, according to Stamey, by autopsy studies documenting prostate cancer incidence in men dying of accidental causes, correlating the critical relationship of prostate cancer with age [3]. Stamey has stressed the urgency for the identification of superior molecular markers to better select the presence of clinically significant

disease in this large cohort of men forced to bear the burden of their diagnosis.

Despite shortcomings, serum prostate-specific antigen remains the most sensitive serum marker in men with prostatic diseases. It is generally accepted that for practical purposes PSA is produced exclusively by the prostatic epithelial cells. As Stamey suggests, there is a strong correlation between PSA, the presence of BPH, and prostate size which confounds interpretation when evaluating the relationship between serum PSA and the presence and extent of prostate cancer. Although there is little question that PSA falls short as a perfect screening tool for prostate cancer, it appears that PSA population screening increases detection rates and decreases prostate cancer death rates. In a large number of studies, PSA is still related to overall tumor volume and has usefulness as a prostatic cancer marker. Analyzing PSA cutoff points and PSA kinetics has allowed us to detect more clinically significant cancers and make more accurate predictions of the efficacy of different treatment approaches. As we will demonstrate, the utility of PSA at the very least remains an enduring marker after primary therapy, guiding the initiation of salvage therapy and the management of metastatic prostate cancer. By reviewing the literature, we hope to show that the serum PSA era is not over as Stamey has suggested. In fact, PSA has a growing and expanding role in the total management of prostate cancer through detection, prognosis, and management.

R.S. Boris
Department of Urology, Indiana University, Indianapolis, IN, USA
e-mail: rboris@iuhealth.org

M.O. Koch, M.D. (✉)
Department of Medicine, Indiana University, 525 N Barnhill Drive, Suite 420, Indianapolis, IN 46202, USA
e-mail: miokoch@iupui.edu

J.S. Jones (ed.), *Prostate Cancer Diagnosis: PSA, Biopsy and Beyond*, Current Clinical Urology, DOI 10.1007/978-1-62703-188-2_3, © Springer Science+Business Media New York 2013

Background

The introduction of serum prostate-specific antigen (PSA) as a marker for prostate cancer and its use beginning in the late 1980s has led to a dramatic increase in prostate cancer detection. Prostate cancer is the most commonly diagnosed visceral cancer in men in the United States with an estimated incidence of 240,000 with 33,000 deaths in 2011, the second leading cause of cancer death in men [4]. Since the advent of the PSA era, however, a stage migration has led to diagnoses in younger men with lower PSA with less aggressive disease more likely to be organ confined [5]. Although the intent of screening is to identify disease which poses a biologic threat to the patient and decrease the morbidity and mortality associated with prostate cancer, annual screening has increased the likelihood that detected tumors will be low grade and localized. This has led to an increase in aggressive local therapy, including radical prostatectomy (RP) and radiotherapy, with intention to eradicate a population, which in some cases would never have suffered significant prostate cancer mortality.

Dr. Stamey emphasized that prostate cancer is a ubiquitous disease with a very low death rate both nationally and internationally. In a 5-year analysis of RP specimens at Stanford ending in 2003, serum PSA related to prostate cancer volume in only 15% of the specimens and correlated only significantly with prostate weight on multiple regression analyses. Stamey's explanation for increasing positive biopsy rates in men with increasing PSA levels is secondary to the many years required for BPH to produce increased in PSA, years that allow the presence of microscopically small cancers to grow enough to be detected by the ever-increasing number of performed prostate biopsies [2]. These concepts are supported, according to Stamey, by autopsy studies documenting prostate cancer incidence in men dying of accidental causes, correlating the critical relationship of prostate cancer with age [3]. Stamey has stressed the urgency for the identification of superior molecular markers to better select the presence of clinically significant disease in this large cohort of men forced to bear the burden of their diagnosis.

PSA and Benign Prostatic Hyperplasia

It has been suggested that serum PSA may be used as a reliable tool for estimating prostate volume (PV) in men with lower urinary tract symptoms (LUTS) [6, 7]. Other research has suggested that the effect of pharmacotherapy (5-alpha-reductase inhibitors and alpha blockers) in men with LUTS can be related to baseline prostate volume [8–10]. Stamey has suggested that BPH is the major contributor to serum PSA between 2 and 10 μg/L [11]. This relationship between PSA and transition zone prostatic volume does remain consistent across several studies. Mochtar et al. demonstrated that PV and PSA have an age-dependent log-linear relationship, where 42% of the variance of PV can be explained by PSA and age. Area under the curves (AUC) revealed that PSA had good predictive value with AUC around 82% in the overall age group irrespective of PV cutoff values [12]. Results of holmium laser enucleation of the prostate or HoLEP, a technique designed to remove the entire transitional zone adenoma for the treatment of BPH, have demonstrated reduction of PSA by an average of 86%, again reemphasizing the correlation of PV and PSA [13]. Several other therapies for BPH (KTP laser, transurethral microwave therapy (TUMT), and even traditional transurethral resection of the prostate (TURP)) have shown a less dramatic reduction in PSA compared with HoLEP and simple prostatectomy suggesting that post-procedure PSA for BPH may be an accurate surrogate for amount of tissue treated [14, 15]. Elmansy et al. analyzed 335 men undergoing HoLEP concluding that both absolute PSA reduction and PSA velocity (PSAV) after treatment could significantly predict men who would subsequently develop prostate cancer in follow-up. Large discrepancies were observed in the PSAV between the malignant and benign groups at 1 and 3 years (1.28 vs. 0.13 ng/mL/year and 2.4 vs. 0.09 $P<0.022$, $P<0.001$) [16]. Based on studies such as these, it seems clear that there is a strong correlation between prostate volume and PSA and furthermore that the accuracy of PSA as a predictor of prostate cancer may be improved in men with prior transurethral procedures, especially those undergoing complete extirpation of the transition zone adenoma.

PSA and Prostate Cancer Volume

Historically, prostate cancer volume was reported to be the primary contributor to serum PSA with PSA production at least 10× higher per cc cancer compared to that of BPH [17, 18]. As we described above, prostate gland volume has been shown to be independently linked to PSA. Since PSA was originally described as a screening test for prostate cancer over three decades ago, concomitant tumor volume in prostatectomy specimens has decreased linearly, that is to say that there has been a "stage migration" to lower volume prostate cancers [19] Stamey has suggested that while the relationship between PSA and prostate size remains consistent, the correlation between PSA and prostate cancer volume has diminished. This, however, may not be completely accurate.

Ochiai et al. selected 200 men undergoing RP early (1991–1994) and 200 men undergoing RP recently (2000–2003) to examine this relationship [20]. They found that while noncancerous tissue remained consistent in both groups, PSA, tumor volume, higher Gleason scores, and higher level of extraprostatic extension were observed in the earlier group. Multiple regression analyses revealed that tumor volume, BPH volume, and Gleason score were significant independent variables for predicting log PSA in the two groups. The correlation of PSA and tumor volume was somewhat stronger, however, in the earlier group. A similar study was published by Figler et al. in a series of 2067 patients undergoing RP at Cleveland Clinic [21]. Their results demonstrated that the preoperative PSA level correlated positively with the percentage of Gleason pattern 4/5, surgical Gleason score, and prostate volume with nearly identical findings in both the early and late groups. They concluded that even in the late PSA era, PSA continues to have prognostic value for men with clinically localized prostate cancer and that the relationship between serum PSA and prostate volume very much exists today.

PSA Calculations and Kinetics in Prostate Cancer Detection

Recent research has been devoted to improving performance characteristics of serum PSA. Adjusting PSA cutoff points, PSA density, and PSA velocity and the analysis of PSA in complexed and free molecular forms have all been investigated for their use in prostate cancer detection and prognostication. In addition, there is now recognition that prostate cancers are prevalent at PSA levels below 4.0 ng/mL [22]. Catalona et al. suggested that utilizing cutoffs below 4.0 will improve sensitivity of detection and avoid missing potentially clinically significant cancers [23]. Other authors have confirmed that a substantial portion of cancers will be missed by withholding prostate biopsies until the PSA reaches 4.0 and that more men will be diagnosed with treatable disease by lowering the PSA cutoff point to a threshold of 2.5 ng/mL [24].

The relative contributions of total PSA as it relates to benign and malignant tissue are the major confounding variable in interpreting PSA results. As prostate cancer stage migration has occurred, this problem has become magnified. The concept of PSA density was developed to account for this issue. A direct relationship between PSA density and the chance of cancer has been documented [25, 26]. A PSA density of 0.15 or greater was proposed as a threshold for recommending prostate biopsy in men with PSA levels between 4 and 10 and a negative digital rectal exam (DRE). The major predictor of serum PSA in men without prostate cancer is the transition zone epithelium, not the epithelium of the peripheral zone of the prostate, where prostate cancer is usually found [27]. Unfortunately, most studies have now shown that PSA density has predictive accuracy only equal to or slightly better than total PSA in predicting positive prostate biopsies.

Carter and colleagues showed that a rate of change in PSA more than 0.75 ng/mL per year was a positive marker for the presence of prostate cancer and that men with cancer had significantly more rapid rates of PSA rise than men without prostate cancer when the PSA levels were in the normal range [28]. Thus, PSA velocity was introduced. Initially this was thought to be a useful predictive model in men with elevated PSA ranges. Recently, however, it has been demonstrated that PSA velocity may be useful for prostate cancer detection among men with PSA levels below 4 [29, 30]. Fang et al. demonstrated in a longitudinal aging study that freedom from prostate cancer at 10 years in men with PSA values between 2 and 4 was 97% and 35% when the PSA velocity was less than and greater than 0.1 ng/mL per year, respectively [31]. Thompson et al. also found that in men with PSA <4 and a negative DRE, the annual change in PSA was positively associated with prostate cancer over a 7-year period [22]. According to several authors, the minimal length of time to determine PSAV should be 18 months, and more measurements appear to improve the accuracy of cancer detection [32, 33].

It has been well accepted that men with prostate cancer have a greater fraction of serum PSA that is bound to protease inhibitors, that is a lower percent of PSA that is free, than men without prostate cancer [34, 35]. Free PSA levels can vary with age and volume and total PSA levels. Percent cutoffs of free PSA and its correlation with prostate cancer can vary with respect to these variables. Free and total PSA both decrease in men taking 5-alpha-reductase inhibitors allowing the percent free PSA to remain mostly unchanged in men taking these medications [36]. Christensson et al. reported that a cutoff of 18% free/total PSA value would significantly improve the ability to distinguish between cancer and noncancer PSA values [34]. In 1995, Catalona found that a free PSA cutoff of 23% would have eliminated almost one third of unnecessary biopsies in men with PVs >40 g, whereas a free PSA cutoff of 14% would have eliminated 76% of unnecessary biopsies in men with glands smaller than 40 g [37]. In men with PSA values between 3 and 10, Gann and associates found that using a free PSA cutoff

of 20% to detected an additional 10% more cancers with 13% fewer false-positive tests [38].

PSA and Prostate Cancer Screening

While it is generally accepted that serum PSA is a useful biomarker for prostate cancer detection, the impact of PSA population-based screening on prostate cancer-specific mortality (PCSM) remains unclear. A retrospective nonrandomized study by Efstathiou et al. looked at outcomes in a dedicated screened and community population of 1,492 patients with clinically localized prostate cancer who underwent RP and experienced PSA failure [39]. Men in the unscreened group were followed regularly starting from the time of their surgery. When compared with the community population of patients who also underwent radical prostatectomy, the screened men with PSA failure had a lower PSA at diagnosis, were less likely to have Gleason score 7–10, and were more likely to have low-risk disease. After a median follow-up of 4.5 and 4.1 years after PSA failure in the screened and community cohorts, the PCSM was significantly lower in the screened group (10-year estimate 3.6% vs. 11.3% $P < 0.001$) [39]. Despite acknowledging obvious limitations of the study including its retrospective nature, selection bias, and proportion of men treated with radiotherapy, this was one of the first publications linking PSA screening and PCSM laying the foundation for larger, randomized trials that were soon to follow.

The first report from the Prostate, Lung, Colorectal, and Ovarian (PLCO) Cancer Screening Trial on prostate cancer mortality randomly assigned 76,693 mean between 1993 and 2001 to either annual screening or usual care [40]. Screened men were offered annual PSA testing for 6 years and DRE for 4 years. After 7 years of follow-up, the incidence of prostate cancer per 10,000 was 116 in the screening group and 95 in the control group with a rate ratio of 1.22. The incidence of death per 10,000 was 2 (50 deaths) in the screening group and 1.7 (44 deaths) in the control group with the study concluding that the rate of death from prostate cancer was very low and did not differ significantly between the two study groups.

The European Randomized Study of Screening for Prostate Cancer was initiated in the early 1990s with similar intentions of the PLCO trial. It included 162,243 men between 55 and 69 with the primary outcome being death from prostate cancer [41]. Eighty-two percent of men in the screening group accepted at least one offer of screening. After a median of 9 years of follow-up, the incidence of prostate cancer was 8.2% in the screening group and 4.8% in the control group, and ratio of death from prostate cancer in the screened group compared to the control group was 0.8. The absolute risk difference was 0.71 deaths per 1,000 men suggesting that 48 prostate cancers would need to be treated to prevent one death. The overall rate reduction of death from prostate cancer was 20% in the screened group with a high risk of overdiagnosis.

Despite the evidence that PSA population-based screening will diagnose more cancers but have minimal impact on PCSM, numerous limitations of these large-scale studies require mentioning that may significantly temper their conclusions. The PLCO trial had major problems in both the control and screened arms. Firstly, the apparent negative result of the PLCO trial may be in part because many of the control group patients were "prescreened" with 44% and 55% having had prior recent PSAs or DREs before entry into the trial. Approximately 2/3 of the cancers in the non-screened group had clinical stage T1c prostate cancer indicating that these patients pursued screening outside of the study protocol. The cumulative biopsy rate of men with a PSA over 4 was only 40%, potentially leaving a number of clinically significant prostate cancers undiagnosed and greatly impacting detection rates between screened and non-screened groups. Finally, the median follow-up of 7 years in the PLCO trial and 9 years in the ERSPC is relatively short to be able to show differences between groups in a cancer that has been established to have its greatest impact at 10- and 15-year outcomes. Individuals with localized disease are more likely to benefit from early detection; however their survival, even if untreated, might

exceed 10 years. Hopefully, these results will be revisited at later time points to assess if the author's earlier conclusions remain accurate. Preliminary reports from the European trial suggest that much greater benefit will be apparent with more prolonged follow-up.

What reasonable conclusions can be made from these trials? Firstly, PSA cutoff points remain unreliable. Data from the Prostate Cancer Prevention Trial show that probability of detecting cancer with a sextant biopsy is 24.7% in men with PSA values between 2.1 and 4 and 17% at 1.1–2.0, with many significant cancers (high Gleason score) being found in patients with these lower PSA values. Secondly, there is a need for an adjunctive biomarker in addition to PSA to help differentiate clinically significant from clinically insignificant cancer, thereby reducing overtreatment of clinically insignificant prostate cancer. Unfortunately, as of this time it remains unclear whether prostate cancer population PSA screening has an impact on disease-specific death. Hopefully, as data matures and future studies emerge, the exact role of PSA, prostate cancer screening, and disease-specific mortality will be better delineated.

PSA and Active Surveillance (AS)

In addition to its role in prostate cancer detection, serum PSA and PSA kinetics are extensively integrated in the management of patients weighing options of primary therapy for localized disease. Many urologists, radiation oncologists, and medical oncologists use PSA to impact treatment decision making, predict outcomes, and drive follow-up whether it be for active surveillance (AS), radical prostatectomy, or radiotherapy in both the primary and salvage settings.

Good risk prostate cancer, by most criteria being Gleason score 6 or less, T1c-T2a, and PSA < 10, has been demonstrated by many large-scale series to have a slow and indolent course and is highly subject to overtreatment. Patients with favorable risk prostate cancer are candidates for active surveillance with selective delayed intervention offered to those with disease progression as they are followed over time.

Proponents of active surveillance defend this management strategy as a compromise between radical therapy (subjected to overtreatment) and watchful waiting with palliation (subjected to under-treatment for aggressive disease).

As described by Klotz, patients placed on AS protocol are evaluated with estimation of PSA doubling time (PSADT) and repeat biopsy to stratify risk of progression. Patients who have a PSADT of ≤3 years (based on three values over at least 6 months) are offered radical intervention. The remaining patients are closely monitored with serial PSA and biopsies at 1, 4, 7, and 10 years. At 8 years of follow-up, 65% remained free of treatment with a prostate cancer-specific survival of entire cohort of 99.3% [42]. The median PSADT was 7 years. Twenty-one percent of the patients had a PSADT < 3 years. Forty-two percent had a PSADT of >10 years. Short PSADT in this series was associated with a more aggressive phenotype. Patients with a DT of <2 years with otherwise favorable clinical features had a higher likelihood of locally advanced disease than patients with longer doubling times. Clearly, in this series of almost 300 patients placed on AS, PSA and PSA DT play a critical role in not only selecting patients better served with radical intervention but also predicting which patients requiring definitive treatment would have high-risk features which might necessitate adjuvant therapy [43].

PSA and Radical Prostatectomy

The predictive impact of serum PSA in patients undergoing radical prostatectomy has been extensively studied and published in the literature. As previously described in this chapter, PSAV has been demonstrated in several studies to be a predictive tool for the diagnosis of prostate cancer. Several other studies have suggested that PSAV can predict tumor stage, grade, and even the time to recurrence [32, 44]. D'Amico et al. studied 1,095 men with localized prostate cancer and determined that an annual PSA velocity of > 2.0 ng/mL in the year prior to diagnosis was associated with a significantly shorter time to death from both prostate cancer and death from any cause [45]. Sengupta et al. identified 2,290 men treated with RP between 1990 and 1999 with multiple preoperative PSA measurements available and calculated PSADT and PSAV using linear regression models. At a median follow-up of 7.1 years, the hazard ratio for death from prostate cancer was 6.22 in men with PSADT less than 18 months compared with men having a doubling time >18 months and 6.54 in men with PSAV ≥3.4 ng/mL yearly compared with men having an annual PSA velocity of less than 3.4 ng/mL [46]. They concluded that PSAV was a significant predictor of biochemical failure while PSADT predicted both risk of clinical progression and cancer death.

Southwick et al. investigated the predictive role of percent free PSA in 268 men undergoing RP for localized prostate cancer [47]. They determined that higher percent free PSA levels were associated with more favorable pathologic findings at the time of RP and that a value of 15% or more free PSA provided the greatest discrimination in predicting favorable outcome. Multivariate analysis revealed percent free PSA to be the strongest predictor of postoperative pathologic outcome following by biopsy Gleason sum and patient age. In this cohort, total PSA was not predictive of outcome. A follow-up study by Shariat et al. confirmed these findings when evaluating over 400 patients undergoing RP and bilateral pelvic lymph node dissection [48]. They determined that lower percent free PSA was significantly associated with higher amounts of extracapsular extension, seminal vesicle invasion, positive surgical margins, and higher pathologic Gleason sum. In 22 patients with biochemical recurrence, lower percent free PSA was correlated with shorter PSADT and was predictive of patients who failed salvage radiotherapy. Again, preoperative total PSA was not associated with prostate cancer outcomes in this patient cohort.

Despite the aforementioned studies, preoperative total PSA has been shown to play a predictive role in RP outcomes in several series. Freedland et al. evaluating 900 men found that higher preoperative PSA values were associated with increased odds of extracapsular extension, positive surgical margins, seminal vesicle invasion, and an increased risk of biochemical progression [49]. Even when the analyses were limited to men with PSA< 10 (690 patients) or men with PSA< 10 and T1c disease (448 patients), preoperative PSA was associated with a significantly increased risk of biochemical recurrence. The association between PSA and risk of biochemical recurrence has been demonstrated in other large single series, patients with Gleason 8–10 disease, and patients undergoing robotic-assisted radical prostatectomy [50–53]. Mitchell et al. at Columbia University identified 1,782 patients who underwent RP and pelvic LND between 1988 and 2003 [54]. Patients were classified by year of surgery to determine if the predictive ability of PSA has changed over time. Using a Cox model including PSA and year of surgery and correcting the model for the effects of stage and grade, there was no significant change in the impact of PSA over time. The authors concluded that the predictive ability of PSA has remained relatively constant during the PSA era. Without question, serum total PSA and the calculation of various PSA kinetics and PSA compounds can play a predictive role in the management of patients undergoing RP for prostate cancer. Counseling patients regarding the risk of recurrence based on these values remains warranted.

PSA, Radiotherapy, and the PSA Bounce Effect

As described above for radical prostatectomy, the prognostic significance of PSA levels can play a role in both pretreatment and posttreatment settings for men receiving radiotherapy for prostate cancer. As mentioned previously, a pre-therapy PSAV of greater than 2.0 ng/mL/year has been shown to impact PCSM for men after radical prostatectomy. Nguyen et al. evaluated 358 men undergoing external beam radiotherapy and concluded that PSAV, especially the PSAV within 18 months prior to treatment, was strongly associated with the interval to PSA recurrence, PSCSM, and all-cause mortality (Nguyen J Urol 2007) [33]. The relationship between PSA, PSAV, and PSADT and prostate cancer-specific death after radiation treatment for prostate cancer has been well supported in the literature [55].

The prostate-specific antigen definition of treatment success for radiation therapy for prostate cancer has been heavily debated over recent years. Unlike radical prostatectomy, where PSA levels are expected to reach negligible values within weeks of surgery, both traditional external beam and brachytherapy work through a slower process of tumor-cell death, resulting in a gradual decrease of PSA reaching nadir levels in 2–5 years. PSA nadir and time to PSA nadir have been surrogates for successful treatment after radiation. Vicini et al. evaluated 685 patients who experience biochemical failure after RT over an 18-year period that included over 2,100 treated patients [56]. They reported a 37% failure rate after five years and that increasing time to nadir was associated with increased time to BCR. On multivariate analysis, factors significantly associated with 10-year BCR included both PSA nadir levels and time to nadir. The authors concluded that PSA nadir and nadir time represent potential factors in the future definition of biochemical cure after radiation.

In 1997, the American Society for Therapeutic Radiology and Oncology (ASTRO) conference recommended the definition of biochemical failure to be three consecutive PSA rises after nadir, spaced 3–6 months apart. Disagreements with interpretation of ASTRO led to the "Phoenix" definition which specifies a PSA increase of >2 ng/mL after achieving a nadir as failure of radiotherapy. The Phoenix criteria is often misunderstood and utilized incorrectly. The Phoenix criteria were developed from a consensus conference that included urologists and medical oncologists with the expressed purpose of predicting those patients who were most likely to progress with failures that were most likely to result in prostate cancer mortality. These criteria were never intended to measure disease eradication, and it was assumed that there would be many people with disease persistence but not failure by the Phoenix definition and therefore not likely to suffer from prostate cancer mortality. The Phoenix criteria were specifically developed to compare various forms of radiotherapy to one another and also account for whether or not adjuvant radiotherapy was administered.

Others have tried to simplify this by relying on PSA nadir rather than utilizing rises in PSA by either criteria. Stock et al. determined that achieving a PSA nadir of ≤0.2 ng/mL significantly predicted 10-year freedom from failure rates after radiotherapy [57]. Patients who reached a nadir of ≤0.2 corresponded to a 99% freedom from failure rate using ASTRO criteria and a 98% with the Phoenix definition compared to 86% and 81%, respectively, when a PSA level of 0.2 was not achieved. Despite these definition dynamics, post-radiation PSA levels remain the driving force in interpreting success or failure of treatment and whether salvage measures should be considered in each instance.

An interesting phenomenon worth mentioning is the concept of "PSA bounce," seen mostly in men undergoing brachytherapy who document a transient elevation or "bounce" in PSA levels occurring between 1 and 2 years after treatment and occurring in roughly a third of patients [58, 59]. The bounce phenomenon, hypothesized to be a result of membrane instability, prostate infarct, or radiation prostatitis, has been associated with both younger men and men with larger prostate volumes [60, 61]. Despite the potential anxiety for both physician and patient, multiple centers have reported that patients who experience PSA bounce after brachytherapy for prostate cancer were less likely to experience biochemical failure [58, 59, 61]. Recognizing these PSA fluctuations and trends, post-therapy can reassure the patients and avoid premature initiation of salvage therapy.

PSA and Salvage Therapy

Recent data suggests that roughly 35% of men treated with local therapy for prostate cancer will experience a PSA recurrence within 10 years leaving approximately 70,000 men per year with this circumstance. As described with the ASTRO and now Phoenix criteria, defining PSA failure after radiation therapy continues to evolve.

Historically, definition of PSA failure after radical prostatectomy has ranged between 0.1 and 0.4 ng/mL before a recent consensus decision of 0.2 ng/mL as the AUA guideline definition of biochemical recurrence. In any event, despite the accepted recognition that patients with a PSA recurrence after primary therapy remain a higher risk group than patients with "sub-failure" levels, PSA failure is not necessarily a surrogate for prostate cancer-specific death and remains a highly variable group of patients. Pound et al. described 304 men with PSA recurrence after RP who did not receive hormonal treatment until the time of metastasis [62]. Median time from PSA recurrence was 8 years and from metastasis to death was 5 years. A more recent follow-up study by Freedland et al. noted median time from PSA BCR to prostate cancer death was not reached after 16 years [63]. As radical treatment for prostate cancer in younger and healthier men continues to increase, it is possible that identifying early biochemical failure and potential candidates for salvage therapy may ultimately demonstrate a larger overall effect on cancer death.

Multiple studies in the literature have demonstrated that absolute PSA levels and PSA kinetics play a strong role in both the timing of salvage radiation after radical prostatectomy as well predicting outcomes. Trock et al. evaluated 635 patients with BCR after RP and determined that salvage therapy within 2 years of PSA recurrence and initiated in men with PSADT of less than 6 months experienced improvement in prostate cancer-specific survival [64]. Only PSA levels, independent of pathologic stage or Gleason score, were statistically significant predictors of outcome in this patient population. Stephenson et al. in a separate study concluded that men receiving salvage radiation with a PSA 2 ng/mL or less had significantly better outcomes than men with PSA >2, and this was further subdivided to men with low risk (less than 0.6 ng/mL) and men with intermediate risk (0.6–2 ng/mL) [65].

Prostate-specific antigen levels and kinetics have also played a predictive role in men with biochemical recurrence after primary radiotherapy. Bianco et al. published on long-term results of salvage prostatectomy observing the 5-year progression-free survival at 86%, 55%, and 28% for patients with preoperative PSA levels less than 4, 4–10, and greater than 10, respectively [66]. Stephenson et al. found that a rapid doubling time prior to salvage RP is a significant risk factor for metastatic disease [67]. Spiess et al. identified that pre-salvage PSA and PSADT predicted biochemical failure of salvage cryotherapy, reflecting the aggressive tumor biology in this patient subset [68].

Souhami et al. investigated the timing of hormonal therapy (HT) in prostate cancer patients after radiation failure and determined that the early hormone group (PSA less than 10 ng/mL) compared with the late hormone group (PSA greater than 10) demonstrated significantly improved overall survival but not cancer-specific mortality [69]. Moul et al. evaluated the role of early hormonal therapy after biochemical failure following radical prostatectomy in a cohort of 1,352 men. They found that early HT was associated with delayed clinical metastasis in men with a PSA doubling time of less than 12 months; however, PSA levels at diagnosis had no effect on metastasis-free survival [70].

PSA, Hormonal Therapy, and Locally Advanced or Metastatic Prostate Cancer

Androgen suppression therapy remains an important treatment and the primary therapy for patients with metastatic prostate cancer. Prostate-specific antigen as described earlier remains an excellent serum marker for the detection of recurrent prostate cancer after potentially curative treatments for localized disease and for the detection of tumor progression after palliative treatment for prostate cancer metastasis. In most circumstances, PSA declines after androgen suppression and then stabilizes for varying intervals [71]. Subsequent elevation can predict tumor progression and generally precedes objective evidence of disease by about 6–12 months [72]. The magnitude and rate of decline in PSA has been utilized to predict the duration of response to androgen deprivation therapy. In metastatic prostate cancer

patients, a PSA nadir after initiating androgen deprivation therapy of less than 10 ng/mL and less than 4 ng/mL has been demonstrated to correlate with improved progression-free and overall survival [73–75].

A rising PSA after androgen deprivation may be used as a surrogate of androgen-independent progression or hormone refractory prostate cancer (HRPC). Morote et al. evaluated 283 patients who were treated with HT as their only treatment until HRPC [76]. They analyzed predictive variables of those who survived less than or greater than 24 months before biochemical progression. On multivariate analysis, nadir PSA and the time to reach nadir were the most significant predictors of time until failure. The odds ratio of responding for greater than 24 months was 20 times higher in patients who achieved PSA values of 0.2 ng/mL (or less with androgen deprivation). In accordance with these findings, Huang et al. in a group of patients with advanced or metastatic prostate cancer also identified PSA nadir and time to PSA nadir as independent and significant predictors of disease progression [77]. Loberg et al. observed that PSADT significantly decreases once a patient converts from hormone-sensitive to hormone-refractory metastatic prostate cancer [78].

In the pre-PSA era, up to one third of men diagnosed with prostate cancer presented with metastatic disease. Traditional screening to evaluate for prostate cancer metastasis at the time of diagnosis includes a bone scan and CT scan of the abdomen and pelvis. The discovery of serum PSA and its role in prostate cancer screening has resulted in earlier prostate cancer detection and higher volumes of men being diagnosed with clinically localized disease. This diagnostic migration suggests that the routine staging workup for prostate cancer may require reevaluation. Gleave et al. reviewed 683 patients with prostate cancer and found that only 6% had positive bone scans on initial evaluation. No patient with PSA levels below 10 ng/mL had a positive bone scan. This increased to 40% for men with PSA greater than 50 ng/mL [79]. Chybowski et al. found PSA to be the best overall predictor of bone scan findings and calculated a negative predictive value of 99.7% in patients with PSA <20 ng/mL [80]. A larger report from Oesterling et al. determined false-negative rates of PSA cutoffs for positive bone scans to be 0 for PSA <8, 0.5 for PSA <10, and 0.8 for PSA less than 20 ng/mL [81]. Many of these authors conclude that significant cost savings could be achieved by PSA-driven staging studies for newly diagnosed prostate cancer.

Conclusions

Is the PSA era over? Since the discovery of prostate-specific antigen in 1970 by Ablin et al., routine PSA has become the mainstay of prostate cancer detection [82]. Concurrent with the well-established increase in PSA screening, prostate cancer incidence has increased, while mortality rates have decreased. Yet despite these trends, the utility and role of PSA continues to be debated. Much of the concern surrounds the risks of over-diagnosis of a potentially indolent disease. Despite these questions, PSA remains an invaluable tool for both physician and patient when faced with decisions regarding detection, management, and follow-up for prostate cancer. This review has demonstrated the extensive role that PSA still plays today in the total scope of this disease – from diagnosis through therapy. The search for new prostate cancer biomarkers should be embraced as an opportunity not to replace PSA, but to improve upon it, potentially identifying a battery of urine, serum, or tissue-based studies that can be utilized to better differentiate indolent versus clinically significant disease. Our review has demonstrated that the accuracy of PSA to predict cancer outcome has not decreased over time. In fact, in the analysis of each vital aspect of prostate cancer, the contribution of PSA remains highly valuable and should clearly not be abandoned.

Editorial Commentary:

Is PSA the best or worst thing to ever happen in urology? Its limitations have been widely reported, including the potential cascade that begins with identifying a high PSA level, leading to biopsy and possibly to treatment. Both steps carry the risk of complications in some set of patients, and there is significant potential to identify a very low-risk cancer that ultimately would pose little if any danger to the patient if unrecognized, so the cascade can lead to no good for some patients.

Nevertheless, the authors describe a wide number of areas in which PSA serves a critical role in patient management, including for screening and diagnosis. Thus, discarding PSA would be a huge mistake unless some other marker or markers are identified to improve upon its performance both diagnostically and for assessment of therapeutic effects. For the foreseeable future, the PSA era is alive and well, and we must strive to better understand the information this molecule provides us.

–J. Stephen Jones

References

1. Stamey TA. The central role of prostate specific antigen in diagnosis and progression of prostate cancer. J Urol. 1995;154:1418.
2. Stamey TA. Preoperative serum prostate-specific antigen (PSA) below 10 microg/l predicts neither the presence of prostate cancer nor the rate of postoperative PSA failure. Clin Chem. 2001;47:631.
3. Sakr WA, Grignon DJ, Crissman JD, et al. High grade prostatic intraepithelial neoplasia (HGPIN) and prostatic adenocarcinoma between the ages of 20–69: an autopsy study of 249 cases. In Vivo. 1994;8:439.
4. Jemal A, Siegel R, Xu J, et al. Cancer statistics, 2010. CA Cancer J Clin. 2010;60:277.
5. Catalona WJ, Smith DS, Ratliff TL, et al. Detection of organ-confined prostate cancer is increased through prostate-specific antigen-based screening. JAMA. 1993;270:948.
6. Roehrborn CG, Boyle P, Bergner D, et al. Serum prostate-specific antigen and prostate volume predict long-term changes in symptoms and flow rate: results of a four-year, randomized trial comparing finasteride versus placebo. PLESS Study Group. Urology. 1999;54:662.
7. Morote J, Encabo G, Lopez M, et al. Prediction of prostate volume based on total and free serum prostate-specific antigen: is it reliable? Eur Urol. 2000;38:91.
8. Boyle P, Gould AL, Roehrborn CG. Prostate volume predicts outcome of treatment of benign prostatic hyperplasia with finasteride: meta-analysis of randomized clinical trials. Urology. 1996;48:398.
9. Roehrborn CG, Boyle P, Gould AL, et al. Serum prostate-specific antigen as a predictor of prostate

volume in men with benign prostatic hyperplasia. Urology. 1999;53:581.

10. de la Rosette JJ, Kortmann BB, Rossi C, et al. Long-term risk of re-treatment of patients using alpha-blockers for lower urinary tract symptoms. J Urol. 2002;167:1734.

11. Stamey TA, Yang N, Hay AR, et al. Prostate-specific antigen as a serum marker for adenocarcinoma of the prostate. N Engl J Med. 1987;317:909.

12. Mochtar CA, Kiemeney LA, van Riemsdijk MM, et al. Prostate-specific antigen as an estimator of prostate volume in the management of patients with symptomatic benign prostatic hyperplasia. Eur Urol. 2003;44:695.

13. Tinmouth WW, Habib E, Kim SC, et al. Change in serum prostate specific antigen concentration after holmium laser enucleation of the prostate: a marker for completeness of adenoma resection? J Endourol. 2005;19:550.

14. Te AE, Malloy TR, Stein BS, et al. Impact of prostate-specific antigen level and prostate volume as predictors of efficacy in photoselective vaporization prostatectomy: analysis and results of an ongoing prospective multicentre study at 3 years. BJU Int. 2006;97:1229.

15. Walden M, Dahlstrand C, Petersson S, et al. Effect of transurethral microwave thermotherapy on serum concentrations of total and free prostate-specific antigen. Scand J Urol Nephrol. 1997;31:173.

16. Elmansy HM, Elzayat EA, Sampalis JS, et al. Prostatic-specific antigen velocity after holmium laser enucleation of the prostate: possible predictor for the assessment of treatment effect durability for benign prostatic hyperplasia and detection of malignancy. Urology. 2009;74:1105.

17. Blackwell KL, Bostwick DG, Myers RP, et al. Combining prostate specific antigen with cancer and gland volume to predict more reliably pathological stage: the influence of prostate specific antigen cancer density. J Urol. 1994;151:1565.

18. Babaian RJ, Troncoso P, Steelhammer LC, et al. Tumor volume and prostate specific antigen: implications for early detection and defining a window of curability. J Urol. 1995;154:1808.

19. Stamey TA, Caldwell M, McNeal JE, et al. The prostate specific antigen era in the United States is over for prostate cancer: what happened in the last 20 years? J Urol. 2004;172:1297.

20. Ochiai A, Troncoso P, Babaian RJ. The relationship between serum prostate specific antigen level and tumor volume persists in the current era. J Urol. 2007;177:903.

21. Figler BD, Reuther AM, Dhar N, et al. Preoperative PSA is still predictive of cancer volume and grade in late PSA era. Urology. 2007;70:711.

22. Thompson IM, Pauler DK, Goodman PJ, et al. Prevalence of prostate cancer among men with a prostate-specific antigen level < or =4.0 ng per milliliter. N Engl J Med. 2004;350:2239.

23. Catalona WJ, Loeb S. Prostate cancer screening and determining the appropriate prostate-specific antigen cutoff values. J Natl Compr Canc Netw. 2010;8:265.

24. Punglia RS, D'Amico AV, Catalona WJ, et al. Effect of verification bias on screening for prostate cancer by measurement of prostate-specific antigen. N Engl J Med. 2003;349:335.

25. Seaman E, Whang M, Olsson CA, et al. PSA density (PSAD). Role in patient evaluation and management. Urol Clin North Am. 1993;20:653.

26. Bazinet M, Meshref AW, Trudel C, et al. Prospective evaluation of prostate-specific antigen density and systematic biopsies for early detection of prostatic carcinoma. Urology. 1994;43:44.

27. Lepor H, Wang B, Shapiro E. Relationship between prostatic epithelial volume and serum prostate-specific antigen levels. Urology. 1994;44:199.

28. Carter HB, Morrell CH, Pearson JD, et al. Estimation of prostatic growth using serial prostate-specific antigen measurements in men with and without prostate disease. Cancer Res. 1992;52:3323.

29. Ham WS, Kang DR, Kim YS, et al. Prostate-specific antigen velocity in healthy Korean men with initial PSA levels of 4.0 ng/mL or less. Urology. 2008;72:99.

30. Makarov DV, Loeb S, Magheli A, et al. Significance of preoperative PSA velocity in men with low serum PSA and normal DRE. World J Urol. 2011;29:11.

31. Fang J, Metter EJ, Landis P, et al. Low levels of prostate-specific antigen predict long-term risk of prostate cancer: results from the Baltimore longitudinal study of aging. Urology. 2001;58:411.

32. Carter HB, Pearson JD, Metter EJ, et al. Longitudinal evaluation of prostate-specific antigen levels in men with and without prostate disease. JAMA. 1992;267:2215.

33. Nguyen PL, Chen MH, Renshaw AA, et al. Effect of definition of preradiotherapy prostate-specific antigen velocity on its association with prostate cancer-specific mortality and all-cause mortality. Urology. 2007;70:288.

34. Christensson A, Bjork T, Nilsson O, et al. Serum prostate specific antigen complexed to alpha 1-antichymotrypsin as an indicator of prostate cancer. J Urol. 1993;150:100.

35. Stenman UH, Hakama M, Knekt P, et al. Serum concentrations of prostate specific antigen and its complex with alpha 1-antichymotrypsin before diagnosis of prostate cancer. Lancet. 1994;344:1594.

36. Keetch DW, Andriole GL, Ratliff TL, et al. Comparison of percent free prostate-specific antigen levels in men with benign prostatic hyperplasia treated with finasteride, terazosin, or watchful waiting. Urology. 1997;50:901.

37. Catalona WJ. Screening for prostate cancer. JAMA. 1995; 273:1174; author reply 1175.

38. Gann PH, Ma J, Catalona WJ, et al. Strategies combining total and percent free prostate specific antigen for detecting prostate cancer: a prospective evaluation. J Urol. 2002;167:2427.

39. Efstathiou JA, Chen MH, Catalona WJ, et al. Prostate-specific antigen-based serial screening may decrease

prostate cancer-specific mortality. Urology. 2006; 68:342.

40. Andriole GL, Crawford ED, Grubb 3rd RL, et al. Mortality results from a randomized prostate-cancer screening trial. N Engl J Med. 2009;360:1310.

41. Schroder FH, Hugosson J, Roobol MJ, et al. Screening and prostate-cancer mortality in a randomized European study. N Engl J Med. 2009;360:1320.

42. Klotz L. Active surveillance with selective delayed intervention for favorable risk prostate cancer. Urol Oncol. 2006;24:46.

43. Klotz L. Active surveillance with selective delayed intervention using PSA doubling time for good risk prostate cancer. Eur Urol. 2005;47:16.

44. Goluboff ET, Heitjan DF, DeVries GM, et al. Pretreatment prostate specific antigen doubling times: use in patients before radical prostatectomy. J Urol. 1997;158:1876.

45. D'Amico AV, Chen MH, Roehl KA, et al. Preoperative PSA velocity and the risk of death from prostate cancer after radical prostatectomy. N Engl J Med. 2004;351:125.

46. Sengupta S, Myers RP, Slezak JM, et al. Preoperative prostate specific antigen doubling time and velocity are strong and independent predictors of outcomes following radical prostatectomy. J Urol. 2005;174:2191.

47. Southwick PC, Catalona WJ, Partin AW, et al. Prediction of post-radical prostatectomy pathological outcome for stage T1c prostate cancer with percent free prostate specific antigen: a prospective multi-center clinical trial. J Urol. 1999;162:1346.

48. Shariat SF, Abdel-Aziz KF, Roehrborn CG, et al. Pre-operative percent free PSA predicts clinical outcomes in patients treated with radical prostatectomy with total PSA levels below 10 ng/ml. Eur Urol. 2006;49:293.

49. Freedland SJ, Hotaling JM, Fitzsimons NJ, et al. PSA in the new millennium: a powerful predictor of prostate cancer prognosis and radical prostatectomy outcomes—results from the SEARCH database. Eur Urol. 2008;53:758.

50. Gonzalez CM, Roehl KA, Antenor JV, et al. Preoperative PSA level significantly associated with interval to biochemical progression after radical retropubic prostatectomy. Urology. 2004;64:723.

51. Pierorazio P, Desai M, McCann T, et al. The relationship between preoperative prostate-specific antigen and biopsy Gleason sum in men undergoing radical retropubic prostatectomy: a novel assessment of traditional predictors of outcome. BJU Int. 2009;103:38.

52. Boorjian SA, Karnes RJ, Rangel LJ, et al. Impact of prostate-specific antigen testing on the clinical and pathological outcomes after radical prostatectomy for Gleason 8–10 cancers. BJU Int. 2008;101:299.

53. Liss M, Osann K, Ornstein D. Positive surgical margins during robotic radical prostatectomy: a contemporary analysis of risk factors. BJU Int. 2008;102:603.

54. Mitchell RE, Desai M, Shah JB, et al. Preoperative serum prostate specific antigen remains a significant prognostic variable in predicting biochemical failure after radical prostatectomy. J Urol. 2006;175:1663.

55. D'Amico AV, Renshaw AA, Sussman B, et al. Pretreatment PSA velocity and risk of death from prostate cancer following external beam radiation therapy. JAMA. 2005;294:440.

56. Vicini FA, Shah C, Kestin L, et al. Identifying differences between biochemical failure and cure: incidence rates and predictors. Int J Radiat Oncol Biol Phys. 2011;81(4):e369–75.

57. Stock RG, Klein TJ, Cesaretti JA, et al. Prognostic significance of 5-year PSA value for predicting prostate cancer recurrence after brachytherapy alone and combined with hormonal therapy and/or external beam radiotherapy. Int J Radiat Oncol Biol Phys. 2009;74:753.

58. Mitchell DM, Swindell R, Elliott T, et al. Analysis of prostate-specific antigen bounce after I(125) permanent seed implant for localised prostate cancer. Radiother Oncol. 2008;88:102.

59. Patel C, Elshaikh MA, Angermeier K, et al. PSA bounce predicts early success in patients with permanent iodine-125 prostate implant. Urology. 2004; 63:110.

60. Crook J, Gillan C, Yeung I, et al. PSA kinetics and PSA bounce following permanent seed prostate brachytherapy. Int J Radiat Oncol Biol Phys. 2007; 69:426.

61. Thompson A, Keyes M, Pickles T, et al. Evaluating the Phoenix definition of biochemical failure after (125)I prostate brachytherapy: can PSA kinetics distinguish PSA failures from PSA bounces? Int J Radiat Oncol Biol Phys. 2010;78:415.

62. Pound CR, Partin AW, Eisenberger MA, et al. Natural history of progression after PSA elevation following radical prostatectomy. JAMA. 1999;281:1591.

63. Freedland SJ, Humphreys EB, Mangold LA, et al. Risk of prostate cancer-specific mortality following biochemical recurrence after radical prostatectomy. JAMA. 2005;294:433.

64. Trock BJ, Han M, Freedland SJ, et al. Prostate cancer-specific survival following salvage radiotherapy vs observation in men with biochemical recurrence after radical prostatectomy. JAMA. 2008;299:2760.

65. Stephenson AJ, Shariat SF, Zelefsky MJ, et al. Salvage radiotherapy for recurrent prostate cancer after radical prostatectomy. JAMA. 2004;291:1325.

66. Bianco Jr FJ, Scardino PT, Stephenson AJ, et al. Long-term oncologic results of salvage radical prostatectomy for locally recurrent prostate cancer after radiotherapy. Int J Radiat Oncol Biol Phys. 2005;62:448.

67. Stephenson AJ, Eastham JA. Role of salvage radical prostatectomy for recurrent prostate cancer after radiation therapy. J Clin Oncol. 2005;23:8198.

68. Spiess PE, Lee AK, Leibovici D, et al. Presalvage prostate-specific antigen (PSA) and PSA doubling time as predictors of biochemical failure of salvage cryotherapy in patients with locally recurrent prostate cancer after radiotherapy. Cancer. 2006; 107:275.

69. Souhami L, Bae K, Pilepich M, et al. Timing of salvage hormonal therapy in prostate cancer patients

with unfavorable prognosis treated with radiotherapy: a secondary analysis of Radiation Therapy Oncology Group 85–31. Int J Radiat Oncol Biol Phys. 2010; 78:1301.

70. Moul JW, Wu H, Sun L, et al. Early versus delayed hormonal therapy for prostate specific antigen only recurrence of prostate cancer after radical prostatectomy. J Urol. 2004;171:1141.

71. Stamey TA, Kabalin JN, Ferrari M. Prostate specific antigen in the diagnosis and treatment of adenocarcinoma of the prostate. III. Radiation treated patients. J Urol. 1989;141:1084.

72. Miller JI, Ahmann FR, Drach GW, et al. The clinical usefulness of serum prostate specific antigen after hormonal therapy of metastatic prostate cancer. J Urol. 1992;147:956.

73. Ercole CJ, Lange PH, Mathisen M, et al. Prostatic specific antigen and prostatic acid phosphatase in the monitoring and staging of patients with prostatic cancer. J Urol. 1987;138:1181.

74. Daver A, Soret JY, Coblentz Y, et al. The usefulness of prostate-specific antigen and prostatic acid phosphatase in clinical practice. Am J Clin Oncol. 1988;11(Suppl 2):S53.

75. Morote J, Vila J, Lopez-Pacios MA, et al. Clinical course of hormone refractory cancer of the prostate. Actas Urol Esp. 1992;16:722.

76. Morote J, Trilla E, Esquena S, et al. Nadir prostate-specific antigen best predicts the progression to androgen-independent prostate cancer. Int J Cancer. 2004;108:877.

77. Huang SP, Bao BY, Wu MT, et al. Impact of prostate-specific antigen (PSA) nadir and time to PSA nadir on disease progression in prostate cancer treated with androgen-deprivation therapy. Prostate. 2011;71:1189.

78. Loberg RD, Fielhauer JR, Pienta BA, et al. Prostate-specific antigen doubling time and survival in patients with advanced metastatic prostate cancer. Urology. 2003;62(Suppl 1):128.

79. Gleave ME, Coupland D, Drachenberg D, et al. Ability of serum prostate-specific antigen levels to predict normal bone scans in patients with newly diagnosed prostate cancer. Urology. 1996;47:708.

80. Chybowski FM, Keller JJ, Bergstralh EJ, et al. Predicting radionuclide bone scan findings in patients with newly diagnosed, untreated prostate cancer: prostate specific antigen is superior to all other clinical parameters. J Urol. 1991;145:313.

81. Oesterling JE, Martin SK, Bergstralh EJ, et al. The use of prostate-specific antigen in staging patients with newly diagnosed prostate cancer. JAMA. 1993;269:57.

82. Ablin RJ, Soanes WA, Bronson P, et al. Precipitating antigens of the normal human prostate. J Reprod Fertil. 1970;22:573.

PSA Dynamics

4

Stacy Loeb and H. Ballentine Carter

Prostate-specific antigen (PSA) is widely used today for the diagnosis and management of men with prostate cancer. It is well known that PSA screening has led to a major stage migration, with most prostate cancers now diagnosed at a localized, curable stage [1]. Epidemiologic studies have also shown that prostate cancer mortality rates are lowest in areas where the rates of distant-stage disease are lowest, and distant-stage disease is lowest in areas with the highest PSA utilization [2]. Finally, randomized trials of PSA screening have recently been reported. The European Randomized Study of Screening for Prostate Cancer (ERSPC) and the Goteborg population-based screening trial (including a subset of Swedish ERSPC participants) reported a 21% and 44% relative reduction in prostate cancer mortality with screening at 11 and 14 years, respectively [3, 4]. The US Prostate, Lung, Colorectal and Ovarian (PLCO) Cancer Screening Trial reported no difference in mortality with screening in the overall results [5].

In addition to its use in screening, PSA is also widely used for assessing disease extent after diagnosis of prostate cancer and for monitoring

patients who have undergone treatment for the disease [6]. Even though widely used for two decades, interpretation of PSA values can be confusing both when used for diagnosis and management. There is increasing recognition of a wide variety of influences on PSA, including genetic variations, certain classes of medications (e.g., statins), obesity, and differences in assay standardization [7–11].

Correspondingly, there has been increasing interest in PSA changes (dynamics), which may provide important information beyond an absolute PSA value for assessing the risk of cancer, cancer significance, and death from prostate cancer after curative intervention. This chapter will review the role of PSA dynamics in the diagnosis and management of men with prostate cancer with an emphasis on diagnosis and assessment of disease significance.

Introduction to PSA Dynamics

The most commonly used metrics to describe changes in PSA are PSA velocity and PSA doubling time. PSA velocity (PSAV) is the rate of change in PSA or the change corrected for the elapsed time usually expressed in ng/ml per year (i.e., annualized), whereas PSA doubling time (PSADT) reflects "growth" of PSA and is the time to double the marker, usually expressed in months or years. PSADT is calculated from the slope of the regression of the log-transformed PSA on time and thus assumes an exponential

S. Loeb, M.D.
Department of Urology, New York University,
New York, NY, USA

H.B. Carter, M.D. (✉)
Department of Urology, Marburg 403,
Johns Hopkins School of Medicine, 600 N Wolfe Street,
Baltimore, MD 21287, USA
e-mail: hcarter@jhmi.edu

J.S. Jones (ed.), *Prostate Cancer Diagnosis: PSA, Biopsy and Beyond*, Current Clinical Urology,
DOI 10.1007/978-1-62703-188-2_4, © Springer Science+Business Media New York 2013

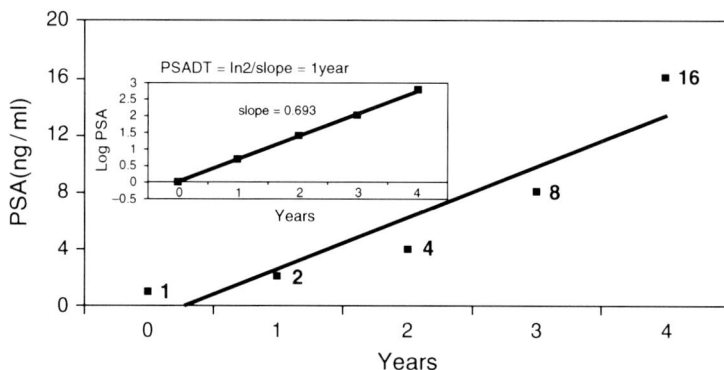

Fig. 4.1 Prostate-specific antigen (PSA) as a function of time (years). *Line* represents regression of PSA on time. *Inset* is log transformation of PSA as a function of time. *PSADT* PSA doubling time, *ln* natural logarithm

relationship between PSA and time. PSADT could be constant while PSA is increasing exponentially (see Fig. 4.1).

The slope of the line of the regression of PSA on time is the rate of change in PSA or PSA velocity (PSAV). The equation that describes a straight line is $y = mx + b$, where m is the slope and b is the intercept. This approach assumes a linear relationship between PSA and time as shown in Fig. 4.1. The slope (PSAV) in this example is 3.6 ng/ml per year over 4 years. Another method for calculating PSAV is the running average or the simple PSAV (change divided by time) between 2 points, plus the PSAV between the next 2 points, all divided by 2. For example, the average rate of change in Fig. 4.1 for year 2–4 is ([8 ng/ml-4 ng/ml]/1 year)+([16 ng/ml-8 ng/ml]/1 year)/2 = 6 ng/ml/year. For PSADT, one can plot the log-transformed PSA on time for the above example (see figure inset), then apply the following formula: ln (2)/slope = PSADT. The ln2 = 0.693 and the slope = 0.693 giving a PSADT of 1 year.

Some studies have suggested that PSAV should be calculated using three repeated PSA measurements over an interval of at least 18 months to optimize its accuracy for prostate cancer detection [12–14] whereas more recent studies have shown predictive value using PSAV calculated over a 12-month time interval [15]. Prior studies have compared the different methods of PSAV calculation and demonstrated how the measurement will differ depending upon the time interval over which it is calculated (e.g., 12 vs. 18 months or longer) [16].

PSA Dynamics: Predicting the Presence of Prostate Cancer

There can be substantial changes or variability in serum PSA between measurements in the presence or absence of prostate cancer [17–20]. The short-term changes in PSA are primarily a result of physiologic variation [18]. Numerous studies have shown that men who harbor prostate cancer have more rapid rises in PSA when compared to those without the disease [12, 13, 21–26], which is useful for assessing the risk that prostate cancer is present.

Using frozen sera to measure PSA from many years earlier, Carter and colleagues found that at 5–10 years before clinical diagnosis, the median PSAV for men with localized prostate cancer (0.27 ng/ml/year) and metastatic disease (1.33 ng/ml/year) were significantly greater when compared to those men with BPH (0.09 ng/ml/year) and controls (0.01 ng/ml/year) (see Fig. 4.2) [12]. Even at 10–15 years prior to clinical diagnosis, the median PSAV for men with localized prostate cancer (0.14 ng/ml/year) and metastatic disease (0.30 ng/ml/year) were significantly greater when compared to controls (0.02 ng/ml/year) but not those with BPH (0.09 ng/ml/year). In that study,

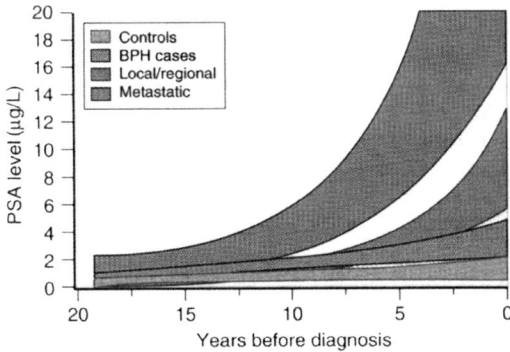

Fig. 4.2 The *curves* represent the average PSA levels and the 95% confidence limits of PSA among men without prostate disease (*bottom curve*), men with BPH who underwent simple prostatectomy (*next to bottom*), localized prostate cancer (*third from bottom*), and metastatic prostate cancer (*top curve*) as a function of years before diagnosis (prostate cancer), simple prostatectomy (BPH), or last visit to the BLSA indicated by time 0. Men in this study were diagnosed prior to the PSA era and were more likely to have life-threatening disease when compared to men diagnosed today (Adapted from Carter et al. [12])

72% of men with cancer and 5% of men without cancer had a PSAV >0.75 ng/ml/year. The specificity of PSA velocity using a cut point of 0.75 ng/ml/year remained high (over 90%) when PSA levels were between 4 and 10 ng/ml or below 4 ng/ml, but sensitivity for cancer detection was 11% at levels below 4 ng/ml compared with 79% for levels between 4 and 10 ng/ml.

More recent studies have demonstrated that PSA velocity might be useful for prostate cancer detection among men with PSA levels below 4.0 ng/ml. In a longitudinal aging study, the cumulative probability of freedom from prostate cancer at 10 years after a baseline PSA between 2 and 4 ng/ml was 97.1% (range 91.4–100%) and 35.2% (range 14.0–56.4%) when the PSAV was less than and greater than 0.1 ng/ml/year, respectively [27]. However, Roobol et al. did not find that PSAV was an independent predictor of a prostate cancer diagnosis at the second screening round of the Rotterdam ERSPC when PSA was less than 4.0 ng/ml, although the calculations were based upon two PSA measurements separated by a 4-year screening interval [28]. By contrast, in 22,019 men with PSA <4 ng/ml from a

large PSA screening study in the US, a PSAV >0.4 ng/ml/year was a stronger predictor of prostate cancer on multivariate analysis than age, race, or family history [29].

The 2012 National Comprehensive Cancer Network Guidelines recommend considering a biopsy for men with a PSA ≤2.5 ng/ml and PSAV ≥0.35 ng/ml/year [30]. This was recently challenged by one study using data from the Prostate Cancer Prevention Trial (PCPT), in which PSAV was a significant independent predictor of biopsy outcome but was associated with only a small improvement in predictive accuracy [31]. Thus, the authors concluded that biopsy should be based on total PSA rather than a PSAV indication. However, emerging data suggest that men with a PSAV >0.4 ng/ml/year prior to a prostate cancer diagnosis are 50% less likely to meet published criteria for insignificant disease [32]. Another recent study from the Baltimore Longitudinal Study of Aging (BLSA) showed that the probability of life-threatening prostate cancer was 3% for men with a PSA <3 ng/ml; however, this increased to 13.6% if the PSAV was greater than 0.4 ng/ml/year [33]. Thus, PSAV may be more useful in enhancing the specificity of screening for clinically significant prostate cancer, as will be discussed in the next section.

Overall, Table 4.1 compares the PSAV findings in men with and without prostate cancer from several studies with different designs (i.e., prospective and retrospective). Differences in PSAV between studies may reflect differences in cohort age, absolute PSA levels, and cancer grade and extent—all of which can influence PSAV. Indeed, PSAV increases directly with PSA [34], which should be taken into consideration for proper clinical interpretation. For example, among men without prostate cancer from the BLSA, the mean PSAV was 0.02±0.29 ng/ml/year for observations at PSA levels <3 ng/ml compared to 0.3±0.59 ng/ml/year at a PSA of 3–10 ng/ml [33]. PSAV may also be influenced by age [13], with some data suggesting improved performance characteristics in young men [35]. However, age-related differences in the prevalence of confounding conditions (such as BPH and prostatitis [36]) may be more important determinants than age

Table 4.1 Average PSA velocity (PSAV) in men with and without prostate cancer

		PSAV (ng/ml per year)	
Study	Study design	No cancer	Cancer
Carter et al. [12, 13]	Longitudinal aging study	0.04	0.75
Oesterling et al. [26]	Longitudinal BPH study	0.04	–
Berger et al. [25]	Invitational screening over 10 years	0.03	0.4
Raaijmakers et al. [24]	Randomized screening at 4-year interval	0.09	0.62
Loeb et al. [35]	Invitational screening over 10 years	0–0.1	0.6–0.7[a]

[a]Depending upon age decade

itself. Finally, changes in PSA are greater for men with high-grade cancers when compared to low-grade cancers [37, 38].

Of note, there is also evidence that PSA kinetics are useful for prostate cancer risk assessment in men taking medications known to affect PSA levels, such as 5-alpha-reductase inhibitors (5-ARIs). For example, Etzioni et al. demonstrated that in contrast to the expected decreasing PSA levels for men taking finasteride, those diagnosed with prostate cancer had a rising annual PSA by approximately 15% for interval cases and 7% for cases diagnosed on empiric biopsy at the end of the trial [37]. Thus, a rise in the PSA level during treatment with 5ARIs can indicate the need for prompt biopsy.

PSA Dynamics: Prediction of Life-Threatening Disease

Before Curative Intervention

D'Amico et al. demonstrated that PSAV in the year prior to treatment of presumed localized prostate cancer was associated with the probability of prostate cancer death after curative intervention [15, 39]. In a landmark study, the authors evaluated PSAV in the year prior to surgery for men with clinically localized disease [15]. They found that when compared to a PSA velocity below 2 ng/ml/year in the year prior to diagnosis, a PSA velocity greater than 2 ng/ml/year was associated with a tenfold greater risk of prostate cancer death in the 7 years after surgery. Thus, failure of local therapy among men with presumed localized disease was associated with a

higher PSAV. This seminal observation suggested that PSA velocity could be useful in assessing the biological behavior of prostate cancer prior to treatment. The authors have made the same observations after radiation therapy for prostate cancer [39]. In addition, Sengupta et al. showed that both PSAV and PSADT were significant predictors of radical prostatectomy outcomes at a median follow-up of 7 years [40].

It seems intuitive that PSA would rise faster in those men with high-grade cancer when compared to those with lower-grade cancers if PSA gains access to the systemic circulation by alterations in prostatic architecture caused by cancer. In addition, PSA may have greater access to the circulation in men with micrometastatic deposits compared to those with organ confined disease. Data from the PCPT have shown that men with high-grade cancers have faster PSA rises (annual percent change in PSA) in PSA compared to those with lower-grade cancers [37]. In the end of study biopsies (biopsies done not for elevated PSA or abnormal digital rectal examination) in the PCPT, men with high-grade cancers (Gleason score 7 and above) had an annual PSA change of 11–12% compared to those with low-grade cancers (Gleason score ≤6) where annual changes were 5–6% (i.e., twofold higher for high-grade cancers vs. low-grade cancers). For a man with a PSA of 2.5 ng/ml, this would translate into a PSAV of 0.3 ng/ml/year for high-grade cancer and 0.15 ng/ml/year for low-grade cancer.

Overall, the data from D'Amico et al. demonstrated that a higher PSAV in the year before diagnosis was associated with a greater likelihood that presumed localized disease would not be cured with local therapy (radiation and surgery) [15, 39]. This leads to the question whether PSAV could help identify those men with life-threatening cancers at a time when cure might still be possible. Among men enrolled in a longitudinal aging study, PSAV evaluated 10–15 years prior to diagnosis (when absolute PSA levels were below 4.0 ng/ml in most men) predicted cancer-specific survival 25 years later [41]. Using a PSAV cutoff of 0.35 ng/ml/year, cancer-specific survival was 92% (84–96) for those with a PSAV of 0.35 ng/ml/year or less compared to 54% (15–82) for men with a PSAV more than 0.35 ng/ml per year ($p = 0.0001$). The relative risk of prostate cancer death was 4.7 (1.3–16.5) for participants with a PSAV more than 0.35 ng/ml/year compared to those whose PSAV $\leq$0.35 ng/ml/year ($p = .02$). These data suggest that even among men with PSA levels that are traditionally considered to be low (below 4.0 ng/ml), the rate of rise in PSA may provide an early warning sign to identify those men at risk for life-threatening disease. This suggests that overdiagnosis and overtreatment might be reduced through an evaluation of the rate at which PSA rises (PSAV) rather than relying on a single dichotomous PSA cut point.

PSADT has also been studied in relation to treatment outcomes. Among men undergoing active surveillance, some groups have used PSADT after diagnosis to assess for progressive disease [42], whereas others have found a poor correlation between PSADT with adverse pathology on repeat surveillance biopsy or subsequent radical prostatectomy [43].

For men undergoing definitive treatment, the data are similarly controversial. In the study by Sengupta et al., PSADT was a robust predictor of clinical progression and prostate cancer death after radical prostatectomy [40]. By contrast, other studies have found that PSAV during the 5 years prior to prostate cancer diagnosis improved the prediction of life-threatening disease, while PSADT did not [44].

A systematic review of studies published prior to 2007 concluded that there was little evidence that pretreatment PSA kinetics provide incremental value above PSA alone [45]. However, the negative findings in this study may reflect the outcome of combining together studies using PSAV or PSADT in heterogeneous patient populations to predict a divergent set of endpoints. In this regard, an updated systematic review of studies focusing on a single PSA dynamic to predict clinically significant or life-threatening prostate cancer would be useful, particularly given the rapidly expanding literature on this topic.

After Failed Curative Intervention

It has been estimated that 20–40% of men who undergo curative intervention for presumed localized prostate cancer with radiotherapy or surgery will have evidence of biochemical failure over the 10 years after treatment [46]. Because a detectable or rising PSA after treatment is not a valid surrogate for clinical relapse (radiographic or physical evidence of disease) or more importantly overall survival, it is difficult to identify which patients will benefit from further treatment [46–51]. In a series of men with a detectable PSA after surgical treatment of prostate cancer followed without additional treatments, 34% developed metastatic disease at a median of 8 years after PSA failure, and of these 43% (or 15% of those with metastatic disease) died of prostate cancer at a median of 5 years later [47]. Ward et al. found that 29% of men who experienced biochemical failure progressed to clinical failure, and 8% died of prostate cancer at a median of 10 years after clinical failure was documented [48]. Thus, biochemical failure after curative intervention is not synonymous with death from prostate cancer but instead represents a heterogeneous state that is a continuum from insignificant disease to the development of metastatic disease and death.

The management of biochemical failure after curative intervention is complicated by this uncertainty regarding future progression to clinically apparent disease and the inability to accurately determine by imaging if microscopic disease is localized or distant. Since salvage therapy is associated with potential morbidity and most men with biochemical failure after definitive therapy will not develop metastatic disease or die

Table 4.2 Distributions of PSA doubling time (PSADT) after failure of local therapy

Study (# of subjects)	PSADT (months)	Distribution (%) of subjects
D'Amico et al. [49] (n = 8,669)	<3	12
	3–5.9	16
	6–11.9	28
	≥12	44
Freedland et al. [50] (n = 379)	<3	6
	3–5.9	15
	6–11.9	29
	≥12	50
Stephenson et al. [51] (n = 501)	<7.4	50
	>7.4	50
Ward et al. [48] (n = 211)	<7.3	50
	>7.3	50

from prostate cancer within 10 years [47, 48], it is important to identify those with a significant recurrence for whom further treatment may be most beneficial.

In this regard, D'Amico et al. showed that PSADT is a surrogate endpoint for prostate cancer mortality and overall mortality among men with biochemical failure, independent of curative treatment received (radiation or surgery) [49]. In their study, the posttreatment PSADT was statistically significantly associated with time to prostate cancer-specific and all-cause mortality. A PSADT of less than 3 months was associated with a median time to prostate cancer-specific mortality of 6 years and a hazard ratio of 19.6 for prostate cancer-specific mortality. These results were confirmed by Freedland et al. who followed untreated men with biochemical failure after radical prostatectomy [50]. Overall, the proportion of patients with postoperative biochemical failure with a PSADT less than 3 months is around 10% (Table 4.2). However, due to the imminent risk of metastatic disease in these men, a PSADT <3 months may be a useful marker for a subset who would benefit from early salvage therapy.

In fact, the continuum of PSADT provides a useful surrogate endpoint for prostate cancer-specific mortality for those with biochemical failure after curative intervention [49]. In the study by Freedland et al., PSADT, pathological Gleason score, and time from surgery to biochemical recurrence were all significant risk factors for time to prostate cancer-specific mortality [50]. However, a PSADT below 9 months was associated with a higher risk of prostate cancer death when compared to time from surgery to recurrence (≤3 vs. >3 years) and pathological Gleason score (≥8 vs. <8). Thus, PSADT should be used in the decision-making process when determining the need for salvage treatments in those with biochemical failure after curative intervention. Accordingly, the authors calculated estimates of the risk of biochemical recurrence at 15 years after biochemical failure as a function of PSADT, grade, and time from surgery to recurrence to help physicians and patients choose management options (Table 4.3) [50].

Conversely, D'Amico et al. identified a subset of patients who appear to have clinically insignificant PSA failure and might be spared from salvage therapy [52]. A PSADT ≥12 months and a pretreatment PSAV <0.5 ng/ml/year (12% of population) were associated with maintenance of a minimally detectable PSA and associated with pathological features at surgery that were not different from those who did not sustain PSA failure. Further follow-up may identify a larger proportion of patients with biochemical failure after curative intervention who should consider surveillance instead of salvage therapy.

Conclusions

Evaluation of PSA changes over time (PSA dynamics) is a method that can be used to help assess the risk of prostate cancer detection. Accumulating data suggest that there is no PSA level below which we can reassure a man that prostate cancer is not present. Therefore, instead of performing a biopsy on all men who reach a given PSA threshold, another approach would be to evaluate the rate at which the PSA rises and use this information as part of the decision-making process regarding the need for biopsy. Although the data on PSAV as a predictor of overall prostate cancer risk are more controversial, a large body of evidence demonstrates that PSAV correlates with the likelihood that life-threatening

Table 4.3 Estimated risk of prostate cancer-specific survival 15 years after biochemical failure following surgery

| PSADT (mo) | Risk estimate, % (95% confidence interval) | | | |
| | Recurrence >3 year after surgery | | Recurrence ≤3 year after surgery | |
	Gleason score <8	Gleason score ≥8	Gleason score	Gleason <8 score ≥8
≥15	94(87–100)	87(79–92)	81(57–93)	62(32–85)
9–14.9	86(57–97)	72(35–92)	59(24–87)	31(7–72)
3–8.9	59(32–81)	30(10–63)	16(4–49)	1(<1–51)
<3	19(5–51)	2(<1–38)	<1(<1–26)	<1(<1–2)

Adapted from Freedland et al. [50]

disease is present. Thus, a PSAV-based screening approach might help reduce the overdiagnosis and overtreatment of prostate cancer that has occurred with PSA screening. PSA dynamics are also useful predictors of treatment outcomes. Finally, among men with biochemical recurrence after curative intervention, PSA doubling time is a surrogate for survival and can be used to help identify those men with life-threatening recurrence who are most likely to benefit from salvage treatments.

Editorial Commentary:

If fraternal twins present to different urologists with PSA values of 4.1 and 3.9, respectively, the traditional threshold (4.0) would lead to a recommendation for biopsy in the first one but reassurance and a recommendation to repeat the laboratory test in 1 year in the second. Obviously this would be flawed thinking, as their actual likelihood of having cancer is essentially—if not exactly—the same.

Thus, it has become clear that thresholds or cutoffs are artificial and misleading. Delving deeper using tools such as PSAV allows us to more fully explore and understand prostate cancer risk assessment. Although a recent study has challenged empiric use of this concept, the authors demonstrate that taking PSA dynamics into account improves our ability to identify real risk, even if incrementally. Even more importantly, PSAV appears to improve identification of the higher-grade cancers whose detection has the potential to improve outcomes.

–J. Stephen Jones

References

1. National Cancer Institute Surveillance Research Program SEER*Stat software, 6.2.4 edn. Available at: http://www.seer.cancer.gov/seerstat.
2. Jemal A, Ward E, Wu X, et al. Geographic patterns of prostate cancer mortality and variations in access to medical care in the United States. Cancer Epidemiol Biomarkers Prev. 2005;14(3):590–5.
3. Schröder FH, Hugosson J, Roobol MJ, et al. ERSPC Investigators. Prostate-cancer mortality at 11 years of follow-up. N Engl J Med. 2012; 366(11):981–90. Erratum in: N Engl J Med. 2012;366(22):2137. PMID: 22417251.
4. Hugosson J, Carlsson S, Aus G, et al. Mortality results from the Goteborg randomised population-based prostate-cancer screening trial. Lancet Oncol. 2010; 11(8):725–32.
5. Andriole GL, Crawford ED, Grubb RL 3rd, et al. Prostate cancer screening in the randomized Prostate, Lung, Colorectal, and Ovarian Cancer Screening Trial: mortality results after 13 years of follow-up. PLCO Project Team. J Natl Cancer Inst. 2012;104(2):125–32. Epub 2012 Jan 6. PMID: 22228146.
6. Ercole CJ, Lange PH, Mathisen M, et al. Prostatic specific antigen and prostatic acid phosphatase in the monitoring and staging of patients with prostatic cancer. J Urol. 1987;138(5):1181–4.
7. Jansen FH, Roobol M, Bangma CH, van Schaik RH. Clinical impact of new prostate-specific antigen WHO standardization on biopsy rates and cancer detection. Clin Chem. 2008;54(12):1999–2006.
8. Loeb S, Carter HB, Walsh PC, et al. Single nucleotide polymorphisms and the likelihood of prostate cancer at a given prostate specific antigen level. J Urol. 2009;182(1):101–4. Discussion 105.
9. D'Amico AV, Roehrborn CG. Effect of 1 mg/day finasteride on concentrations of serum prostate-specific antigen in men with androgenic alopecia: a randomised controlled trial. Lancet Oncol. 2007;8(1):21–5.
10. Hamilton RJ, Goldberg KC, Platz EA, Freedland SJ. The influence of statin medications on prostate-

specific antigen levels. J Natl Cancer Inst. 2008; 100(21):1511–8.

11. Banez LL, Hamilton RJ, Partin AW, et al. Obesity-related plasma hemodilution and PSA concentration among men with prostate cancer. JAMA. 2007; 298(19):2275–80.

12. Carter HB, Pearson JD, Metter EJ, et al. Longitudinal evaluation of prostate-specific antigen levels in men with and without prostate disease. JAMA. 1992; 267(16):2215–20.

13. Carter HB, Morrell CH, Pearson JD, et al. Estimation of prostatic growth using serial prostate-specific antigen measurements in men with and without prostate disease. Cancer Res. 1992;52(12):3323–8.

14. Carter HB, Pearson JD, Waclawiw Z, et al. Prostate-specific antigen variability in men without prostate cancer: effect of sampling interval on prostate-specific antigen velocity. Urology. 1995;45(4):591–6.

15. D'Amico AV, Chen MH, Roehl KA, Catalona WJ. Preoperative PSA velocity and the risk of death from prostate cancer after radical prostatectomy. N Engl J Med. 2004;351(2):125–35.

16. Yu X, Han M, Loeb S, et al. Comparison of methods for calculating prostate specific antigen velocity. J Urol. 2006;176(6 Pt 1):2427–31. Discussion 2431.

17. Riehmann M, Rhodes PR, Cook TD, Grose GS, Bruskewitz RC. Analysis of variation in prostate-specific antigen values. Urology. 1993;42(4):390–7.

18. Prestigiacomo AF, Stamey TA. Physiological variation of serum prostate specific antigen in the 4.0 to 10.0 ng./ml. range in male volunteers. J Urol. 1996;155(6):1977–80.

19. Roehrborn CG, Pickens GJ, Carmody 3rd T. Variability of repeated serum prostate-specific antigen (PSA) measurements within less than 90 days in a well-defined patient population. Urology. 1996;47(1): 59–66.

20. Eastham JA, Riedel E, Scardino PT, et al. Variation of serum prostate-specific antigen levels: an evaluation of year-to-year fluctuations. JAMA. 2003;289(20):2695–700.

21. Smith DS, Catalona WJ. Rate of change in serum prostate specific antigen levels as a method for prostate cancer detection. J Urol. 1994;152(4):1163–7.

22. Kadmon D, Weinberg AD, Williams RH, et al. Pitfalls in interpreting prostate specific antigen velocity. J Urol. 1996;155(5):1655–7.

23. Lujan M, Paez A, Sanchez E, et al. Prostate specific antigen variation in patients without clinically evident prostate cancer. J Urol. 1999;162(4):1311–3.

24. Raaijmakers R, Wildhagen MF, Ito K, et al. Prostate-specific antigen change in the European randomized study of screening for prostate cancer, section Rotterdam. Urology. 2004;63(2):316–20.

25. Berger AP, Deibl M, Steiner H, et al. Longitudinal PSA changes in men with and without prostate cancer: assessment of prostate cancer risk. Prostate. 2005;64(3):240–5.

26. Oesterling JE, Jacobsen SJ, Chute CG, et al. Serum prostate-specific antigen in a community-based population of healthy men. Establishment of age-specific reference ranges. JAMA. 1993;270(7):860–4.

27. Fang J, Metter EJ, Landis P, Carter HB. PSA velocity for assessing prostate cancer risk in men with PSA levels between 2.0 and 4.0 ng/ml. Urology. 2002;59(6):889–93. Discussion 893–4.

28. Roobol MJ, Kranse R, de Koning HJ, Schroder FH. Prostate-specific antigen velocity at low prostate-specific antigen levels as screening tool for prostate cancer: results of second screening round of ERSPC (ROTTERDAM). Urology. 2004;63(2):309–13. Discussion 313–5.

29. Loeb S, Roehl KA, Nadler RB, Yu X, Catalona WJ. Prostate specific antigen velocity in men with total prostate specific antigen less than 4 ng/ml. J Urol. 2007;178(6):2348–52. Discussion 2352–3.

30. National Comprehensive Cancer Network Clinical Practice Guidelines in Oncology. http://www.nccn. org/professionals/physician_gls/pdf/prostate_detection.pdf (2012). Accessed 4 Sep 2012.

31. Vickers AJ, Till C, Tangen CM, Lilja H, Thompson IM. An empirical evaluation of guidelines on prostate-specific antigen velocity in prostate cancer detection. J Natl Cancer Inst. 2011;103(6):462–9.

32. Loeb S, Roehl KA, Helfand BT, Kan D, Catalona WJ. Can prostate specific antigen velocity thresholds decrease insignificant prostate cancer detection? J Urol. 2010;183(1):112–6. PMID: 19913814.

33. Loeb S, Carter HB, Schaeffer EM, et al. Distribution of PSA velocity by total PSA levels: data from the Baltimore Longitudinal Study of Aging. Urology. 2011;77(1):143–7.

34. Yu X, Loeb S, Roehl KA, Han M, Catalona WJ. The association between total prostate specific antigen concentration and prostate specific antigen velocity. J Urol. 2007;177(4):1298–302. Discussion 1301–2.

35. Loeb S, Roehl KA, Catalona WJ, Nadler RB. Is the utility of prostate-specific antigen velocity for prostate cancer detection affected by age? BJU Int. 2008;101(7):817–21.

36. Eggener SE, Yossepowitch O, Roehl KA, et al. Relationship of prostate-specific antigen velocity to histologic findings in a prostate cancer screening program. Urology. 2008;71(6):1016–9.

37. Etzioni RD, Howlader N, Shaw PA, et al. Long-term effects of finasteride on prostate specific antigen levels: results from the prostate cancer prevention trial. J Urol. 2005;174(3):877–81.

38. Loeb S, Sutherland DE, D'Amico AV, Roehl KA, Catalona WJ. PSA velocity is associated with Gleason score in radical prostatectomy specimen: marker for prostate cancer aggressiveness. Urology. 2008;72(5):1116–20. Discussion 1120.

39. D'Amico AV, Renshaw AA, Sussman B, Chen MH. Pretreatment PSA velocity and risk of death from prostate cancer following external beam radiation therapy. JAMA. 2005;294(4):440–7.

40. Sengupta S, Myers RP, Slezak JM, et al. Preoperative prostate specific antigen doubling time and velocity are strong and independent predictors of outcomes following radical prostatectomy. J Urol. 2005;174(6): 2191–6.

41. Carter HB, Ferrucci L, Kettermann A, et al. Detection of life-threatening prostate cancer with prostate-

specific antigen velocity during a window of curability. J Natl Cancer Inst. 2006;98(21):1521–7.

42. Klotz L. Active surveillance for prostate cancer: for whom? J Clin Oncol. 2005;23(32):8165–9.

43. Ross AE, Loeb S, Landis P, et al. Prostate-specific antigen kinetics during follow-up are an unreliable trigger for intervention in a prostate cancer surveillance program. J Clin Oncol. 2010;28(17):2810–6.

44. Loeb S, Kettermann A, Ferrucci L, et al. PSA doubling time versus PSA velocity to predict high-risk prostate cancer: data from the Baltimore Longitudinal Study of Aging. Eur Urol. 2008;54(5):1073–80.

45. Vickers AJ, Savage C, O'Brien MF, Lilja H. Systematic review of pretreatment prostate-specific antigen velocity and doubling time as predictors for prostate cancer. J Clin Oncol. 2009;27(3):398–403.

46. Ward JF, Moul JW. Treating the biochemical recurrence of prostate cancer after definitive primary therapy. Clin Prostate Cancer. 2005;4(1):38–44.

47. Pound CR, Partin AW, Eisenberger MA, et al. Natural history of progression after PSA elevation following radical prostatectomy. JAMA. 1999; 281(17):1591–7.

48. Ward JF, Blute ML, Slezak J, Bergstralh EJ, Zincke H. The long-term clinical impact of biochemical recurrence of prostate cancer 5 or more years after radical prostatectomy. J Urol. 2003;170(5): 1872–6.

49. D'Amico AV, Moul JW, Carroll PR, et al. Surrogate end point for prostate cancer-specific mortality after radical prostatectomy or radiation therapy. J Natl Cancer Inst. 2003;95(18):1376–83.

50. Freedland SJ, Humphreys EB, Mangold LA, et al. Risk of prostate cancer-specific mortality following biochemical recurrence after radical prostatectomy. JAMA. 2005;294(4):433–9.

51. Stephenson AJ, Shariat SF, Zelefsky MJ, et al. Salvage radiotherapy for recurrent prostate cancer after radical prostatectomy. JAMA. 2004;291(11):1325–32.

52. D'Amico AV, Chen MH, Roehl KA, Catalona WJ. Identifying patients at risk for significant versus clinically insignificant postoperative prostate-specific antigen failure. J Clin Oncol. 2005;23(22):4975–9.

Percent Free PSA

5

Kenneth G. Nepple, Gurdarshan S. Sandhu, and Adam S. Kibel

Introduction

The introduction of PSA in 1987 [1] as a serum marker for prostate cancer and its subsequent development as a screening test for early detection [2] dramatically altered the diagnosis and management of this disease. PSA correlated directly with prostate cancer risk and, therefore, was a relatively sensitive test to identify men at risk. However, it became rapidly apparent that PSA had a limited specificity. Numerous nonmalignant processes, such as benign prostatic hyperplasia (BPH) and infection, also resulted in PSA elevations [3].

The inherent limitations of total PSA prompted focused efforts to improve the test characteristics of PSA screening. The inability to differentiate benign from malignant sources of PSA elevation is a particular concern in men with moderate PSA elevation because prostate cancer is only detected in approximately 25% of men with a PSA of 4–10 ng/mL and a normal rectal exam [4], which by definition means that up to 75% of prostate biopsies are negative and, therefore, theoretically

unnecessary. There is obvious utility in avoiding unnecessary prostate biopsy, as each prostate biopsy carries with it discomfort along with the risks of bleeding and infection. Infection has become a particular concern because of the development of fluoroquinolone-resistant bacteria and increasing rate of hospitalization after prostate biopsy [5].

In an effort to decrease the biopsy rate and improve the test characteristics of PSA, more cancer-specific isoforms of PSA were identified. Percent free PSA was one of the first developed specifically to differentiate benign from malignant PSA elevations. In this chapter, we will review the characteristics of percent free PSA, examine the studies that established the use of percent free PSA, review the use of percent free PSA in the contemporary era, and discuss limitations of percent free PSA that have limited its widespread utilization.

Definition of Percent Free PSA

In the early 1990s, work from Stenman et al. [6] and Christensson et al. [7] discovered that serum PSA exists both as a form bound to plasma proteins and as a free form that is unbound. Of PSA that is bound, the majority is complexed to alpha-1-antichymotrypsin (protease inhibitor) and a minority to alpha 2-macroglobulin. Stenman and colleagues quickly established the potential clinical relevance of free PSA when they determined that the proportion of the serum PSA bound

K.G. Nepple, M.D. • G.S. Sandhu, M.D.
Division of Urologic Surgery, Washington University
School of Medicine, St. Louis, MO, USA

A.S. Kibel, M.D. (✉)
Division of Urology, Brigham and Women's Hospital,
Dana Farber Cancer Institute, 75 Francis Street, Boston,
MA 02115, USA
e-mail: akibel@partners.org

J.S. Jones (ed.), *Prostate Cancer Diagnosis: PSA, Biopsy and Beyond*, Current Clinical Urology,
DOI 10.1007/978-1-62703-188-2_5, © Springer Science+Business Media New York 2013

to alpha 1-antichymotrypsin was higher in patients with prostatic cancer than in those with benign hyperplasia [6]. The association between bound PSA and cancer was also identified microscopically, as Bjork et al. identified that production of alpha 1-antichymotrypsin was seen in prostate cancer to a greater extent than benign prostate tissue [8].

With the identification that increased bound serum PSA was associated with an increased risk of prostate cancer, it became apparent that an increased percent free PSA was associated with a lower risk of prostate cancer. The percent free PSA is computed by dividing the measure free PSA by the total serum PSA. It is much more difficult to measure the bound percentage than the free percentage, so using percent free PSA was most achievable. Furthermore, an assay to measure complexed PSA never achieved widespread use and is no longer available.

Numerous studies have demonstrated that percent free PSA is decreased in men with prostate cancer, or taken conversely that men with a higher percent free PSA are less likely to have prostate cancer.

- Higher percent free PSA→Lower risk of prostate cancer
- Lower percent free PSA→Higher risk of prostate cancer

Using Percent Free PSA in Prostate Cancer Screening

Catalona et al. conducted the initial evaluation of percent free PSA. In their study, median percent free PSA was lower in men with cancer (9.2%) compared to the median percent free PSA in men without cancer (18.8%) and in doing so demonstrated that free PSA might improve specificity for detecting prostate cancer over PSA alone [9]. In a subsequent multi-institutional evaluation of percent free PSA in 773 men, Catalona et al. [4] established a significant relationship between percent free PSA and the probability of cancer on prostate biopsy. In this prospective blinded analysis of men undergoing a primary biopsy for an elevated PSA of between 4 and 10 ng/mL, if the

Table 5.1 Probability of prostate cancer in men with PSA 4–10 ng/mL from Ref. [4]

Percent free PSA (%)	Probability of prostate cancer (%)
0–10	56
10–15	28
15–20	20
20–25	16
>25	8

percent free PSA was greater than 25%, then the likelihood of a positive biopsy was 8% compared to a likelihood of 56% if the percent free PSA was less than 10% (Table 5.1). Using an abnormal cutoff of less than 25%, free PSA detected 95% of prostate cancers while avoiding 20% of unnecessary prostate biopsies. FDA approval was granted in 1998 for the percent free PSA test for prostate cancer detection in men aged 50 years and older with PSA levels between 4 and 10 ng/mL [10].

Subsequently, multiple additional studies have evaluated the usefulness of percent free PSA in prostate cancer screening. Most studies have followed a similar format where a population of men has PSA and free PSA measured and then undergo prostate biopsy. Nearly all published reports have demonstrated that percent free PSA is better at predicting the likelihood of a positive biopsy. Study conclusions outcomes have differed somewhat with respect to two factors: how sizable is the improvement and what value should trigger a biopsy. The size of improvement is quantified as an increase in the AUC (area under the curve) of a ROC (receiver operating characteristic) curve, which is a graphical representation of sensitivity and specificity. A larger area under the curve indicates an improved test. This data are then used by the researcher to determine the appropriate balance between a desire for increased sensitivity (identifying prostate cancers that are present) and specificity (avoiding unnecessary prostate biopsies).

Lee et al. [11] performed a meta-analysis in 2006 of 41 studies evaluating percent free PSA in 19,643 men with histopathologically verified diagnosis. In the cohort of patients who had PSA values between 4 and 10 ng/mL, cancer was diagnosed on biopsy in 39%. AUC analysis demonstrated that percent free PSA outperformed PSA alone. The AUC for percent free PSA when PSA was 4–10 ng/mL was 0.68., compared to 0.53 for total PSA, with a range of 0.40–0.75 in reported studies [11]. When using a cut point percent free PSA of 20%, the sensitivity was 94% with a specificity of 13%. In contrast, using a cut point percent free PSA of 10% in this group would result in a sensitivity of 40% but an improved specificity of 72%.

Therefore, for the individual patient, the level at which an abnormal percent free PSA warrants a prostate biopsy balances the potential failure to diagnosis cancer against the risk of performing an unnecessary biopsy. Catalona et al. suggested a percent free PSA cut point of 25% which in their study obtained a sensitivity of 95% and a specificity of 20% [4], which translates to identifying 95% of the cancers while avoiding 20% of the unnecessary biopsies. This use of a relatively high value of percent free PSA is driven by a desire not to miss prostate cancers but unfortunately only modestly reduces the number of unnecessary biopsies. It is important to recognize that the majority of men evaluated with free PSA will be recommended to undergo a prostate biopsy and that then number of cancer missed will be very low but still quantifiable. For example, if 100 men with PSA of 4–10 ng/mL were evaluated, approximately 83 out of 100 men would undergo a biopsy because of free PSA less than 25%. While in the 17 men with free PSA greater than 25%, prostate cancer would be missed in two men.

Percent free PSA has been validated in men of different ethnicities. Catalona et al. [12] found that percent free PSA with a cutoff of 25% free PSA obtained a sensitivity of 95% in African Americans and Caucasians while unnecessary biopsies were avoided in 17% and 20%, respectively. In another study of 137 African American men, percent free PSA was found to perform better than PSA in prostate cancer detection [13].

Kobori et al. [14] examined the utility of percent free PSA in a cohort of 27,730 Japanese men. From 2000 to 2005, men aged 55–69 years underwent prostate cancer screening including both free PSA and total PSA. Patients were referred to a urologist for a PSA above 2.1 ng/mL

from 2000 to 2002. Subsequently, from 2003 to 2005, patients with an elevated PSA of 2.1–10 ng/mL were not further referred if the free to total PSA ratio was >22%. The rate of urology clinic referral decreased after this change was implemented, while the cancer detection rate increased from 13.5% to 22.7% after this staged evaluation was instituted. This demonstrates that the system-wide use of free PSA can increase the yield of prostate biopsies and avoid unnecessary prostate biopsies. However, a limitation of this evaluation was the potential for missing a rare clinically significant prostate cancer in those men who did not undergo prostate biopsy.

Percent Free PSA in Men with Prior Negative Biopsy

In routine clinical practice, percent free PSA is frequently used in patients with prior negative biopsy. The utility of percent free PSA in this patient population was evaluated in patients undergoing biopsy as part of the REDUCE trial. The REDUCE trial was a prostate cancer risk reduction study which evaluated the usefulness of dutasteride in 6,729 men with a moderately elevated PSA and a prior negative prostate biopsy at baseline [15]. As part of the trial, percent free PSA and the novel marker urinary PCA3 were evaluated prospectively in the men in the placebo arm [16]. In evaluating biopsy outcome, the AUC was higher for percent free PSA compared to serum PSA alone (0.637 vs. 0.612). However, PCA3 outperformed not only PSA but also percent free PSA [16]. This is consistent with a second recent study that also found that free PSA underperformed compared to urinary PCA3 in the screening population [17].

Use of Percent Free PSA to Detect High-Risk Prostate Cancer

A potential use of percent free PSA is discriminating clinically indolent prostate cancer from the more biologically aggressive counterpart. This is particularly relevant in contemporary populations because of concerns regarding overdiagnosis and overtreatment of prostate cancer and the need for biomarkers that allow better discrimination of clinical risk. Unfortunately, the literature supporting the use of percent free PSA in this regard is not uniform with studies both supporting and not supporting percent free PSA as a marker of aggressive disease.

Shariat et al. [18] examined 402 patients treated with radical prostatectomy with a total PSA less than 10 ng/mL at the time of diagnosis. They found that in contrast to PSA, a lower percent free PSA preoperatively was associated with pathologically aggressive prostate carcinoma defined as extracapsular extension (ECE), seminal vesicle invasion (SVI), positive surgical margin status, higher final Gleason sum, lymphovascular invasion, and perineural invasion. Furthermore, preoperative multivariate logistic regression analyses adjusting for total PSA, clinical stage, and Gleason sum revealed that lower percent free PSA was independently associated with ECE ($p < 0.001$), SVI ($p < 0.001$), and lymphovascular invasion ($p < 0.001$).

Similarly, Steuber et al. [19] found that on univariate regression analysis, lower percent free PSA was a predictor of ECE ($p = 0.016$), SVI ($p = 0.005$) and biochemical recurrence following radical prostatectomy ($p < 0.0005$) in a cohort of 867 patients. These results are similar to Wenske et al. [20] who reported on 1,356 patients treated with radical prostatectomy, of which 146 patients developed biochemical recurrence. Multivariate logistic regression analysis revealed that higher biopsy Gleason score ($p < 0.0005$), higher total PSA ($p < 0.0005$), and lower percent free PSA ($p = 0.001$) were predictive of biochemical recurrence.

Other groups have failed to demonstrate that percent free PSA predicts pathologic outcomes or PSA failure. Erdem et al. [21] and Graefen et al. [22] both demonstrated no significant correlation between percent free PSA and adverse pathologic features or biochemical failure following radical prostatectomy. These findings raise the possibility that while percent free PSA might help identify patients who would benefit from initial therapy, it could not be used to independently identify patients at increased risk of failure and therefore is of limited ability to guild therapy.

Integrating Percent Free PSA with Other Clinical Variables

Clinical decision making based solely on an elevated PSA can result in a large number of unnecessary biopsies, with one group estimating that annually over 750,000 men in the USA undergo an unnecessary biopsy [23]. The integration of other biomarkers and clinical variables into models and nomograms improves the predictive value of PSA and thus potentially allows a reduction in unnecessary biopsies. Groups have begun to integrate percent free PSA into similar predictive models.

Vickers et al. [23] reported on the improved predictive accuracy of a model for predicting a positive biopsy by integrating three biomarkers—percent free PSA, intact PSA (a single chain, form of free PSA that has not been internally cleaved), and human kallikrein-related peptidase 2 (hk2) (a serine protease sharing 80% sequence homology with PSA)—to a base model incorporating patient age, digital rectal exam (DRE), total PSA in a cohort of 740 Swedish men. The AUC of the base model (0.724) was improved by the addition of each individual biomarker. In particular, the addition of percent free PSA to the base model improved the AUC to 0.779 in a statistically significant manner ($p = 0.025$). The full model incorporating all three additional biomarkers into the base model improved the accuracy of the model (AUC = 0.836, $p < 0.0005$). Using the full model and a strategy of biopsying men with a 20% or higher chance of having prostate cancer, this group found that 57% of men would have been spared biopsy at the cost of missing 16% of low-grade (Gleason score < 7) and 8% of high-grade (Gleason score ≥ 7) cancers.

This group has subsequently validated their results in the Rotterdam arm of the European Randomized Study of Screening for Prostate Cancer (ERSPC), with a significant improvement in the AUC for the full model (0.78) compared

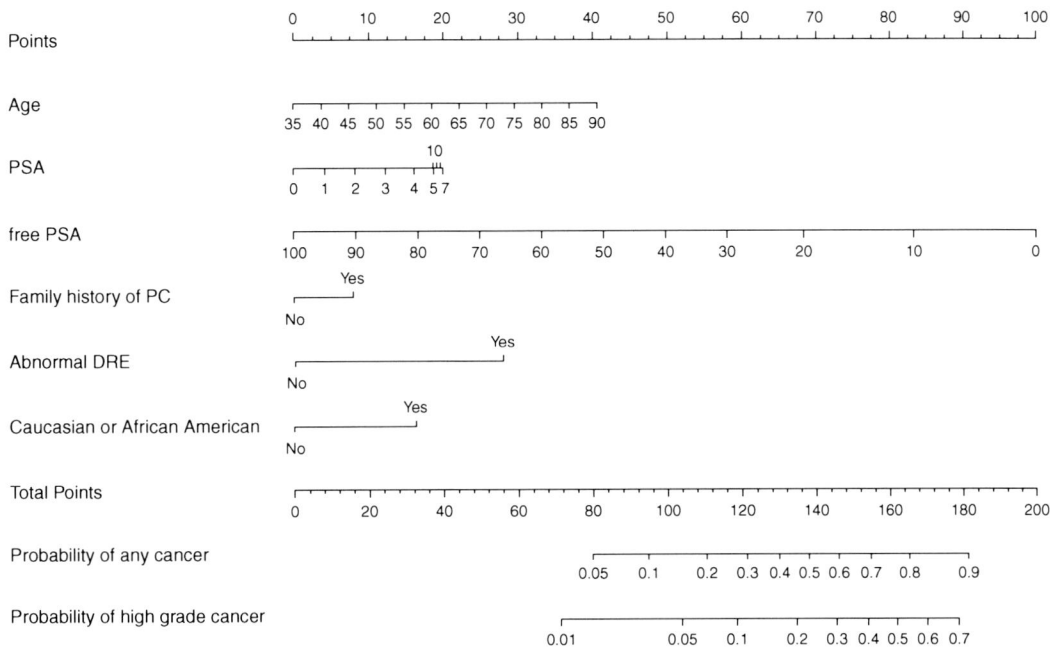

Fig. 5.1 Nomogram for prediction of prostate cancer at prostate biopsy (Used with permission from Zaytoun et al.)

with the base model (0.70) ($p<0.001$). This was a population of previously unscreened men undergoing biopsy as a result of an elevated PSA (≥ 3 ng/mL). Employing a similar biopsy strategy as above, 513 fewer biopsies for every 1,000 men would be performed, at the cost of missing 66 cancers, 12 being Gleason score ≥ 7 [24]. In another study of 1,241 men who had previously undergone prior PSA screening, statistical models were developed incorporating biomarkers studied by Vickers et al. (free PSA, hk2, and intact PSA) into a model based on clinical factors (total PSA, DRE, and patient age) were developed for a cohort. The addition of the three biomarkers to the base model demonstrated significantly better predictive accuracy based on AUC analysis than the base model itself ($p<0.005$) [25], thereby supporting the use of these models in screened and unscreened populations.

Nomograms that integrate standard clinical and pathologic variable with markers have been developed and can be readily applied to clinical practice. These quantify the combined contribution of several risk factors and provide a predicted probability of a positive biopsy for an individual. Several nomograms have demonstrated improved predictive accuracy with the incorporation of free PSA over baseline nomograms. Karakiewicz et al. [26] developed a nomogram incorporating age, DRE, percent free PSA, and total PSA. The nomogram incorporating percent free PSA was developed on a cohort of 1,762 men from Hamburg-Eppendorf, Germany, and then externally validated on a group of 522 men from Montreal, Canada. Importantly, the predictive AUC was increased from 0.69 (95% CI 0.68–0.72) to 0.77 (95% CI 0.72–0.81) with the addition of percent free PSA. Despite having limited input variables and easy clinical use, a limitation of this nomogram is the fact that a sextant biopsy scheme was used. In addition, it is important to note that the PSA range (0–50 ng/mL) was substantially higher than is commonly used in practice today.

Zaytoun et al. [27] developed a nomogram incorporating six readily available clinical variables: age, family history of prostate cancer, total PSA, percent free PSA, race, and DRE findings (Fig. 5.1). All 1,551 men in the study had a

PSA ≤ 10 ng/mL and a prostate biopsy of 8–14 cores, more closely reflecting common, modern practice. The AUC incorporating all variables for predicting prostate cancer was 0.73 and 0.71 for predicting high-grade prostate cancer (Gleason ≥ 7). The percent free PSA was found to add significant predictive accuracy to the model.

Factors that Alter the Measurement of Percent Free PSA

The fact that free PSA correlates strongly with prostate carcinoma does not mean that levels are not influenced by other factors. Clinicians using this test should be aware of some of these factors to assist with interpretation of results. Sokoll evaluated the stability of total and free PSA after blood draw and reported that free PSA was less stable than total PSA. With storage at room temperature or refrigerated (4 °C), the free PSA decreased and led to aberrantly low values. They recommended that specimens that are not analyzed the same day be stored frozen at −20 °C. The assay used is also important for interpretation. Stephan et al. [28] reported that the values of both PSA and free PSA for the new standardized WHO calibrated assays resulted in values that were approximately 25% lower than the traditionally calibrated Hybritech PSA and fPSA assays; however, the percent free PSA was unaffected.

While total serum PSA levels are not altered on hemodialysis or peritoneal dialysis, percent free PSA is higher on hemodialysis or peritoneal dialysis [29], and the recommendation has been made to not utilize percent free PSA in this patient population. Both total PSA and free PSA increase with age and correlate directly with age; however, total and free PSA increase in a nearly identical fashion so that the percent free PSA does not change with age [30]. Strenuous exercise, specifically, cycling may lead to temporary increases in free PSA [31]. Percent free PSA also does not appear to be influenced by race [12], alpha blockers, or 5-alpha reductase inhibitors [32, 33].

Guidelines and Recommendations for the Use of Percent Free PSA

Practice guidelines are being developed by health care organizations, to assist with integration of tests and treatments into urologic care. A review of the current guidelines unfortunately does not provide a clear message as to integration of percent free PSA in practice.

American Urological Association (AUA)

The 2009 AUA Prostate-Specific Antigen Best Practice Statement [34] advised that percent free PSA should be taken into account with multiple other factors (total PSA, DRE results, patient age, PSA velocity, PSA density, family history, ethnicity, prior biopsy history, medical comorbidities) when deciding to proceed with a prostate biopsy. It is also stated that optimal cut points for percent free PSA "are not known with certainty at present."

National Comprehensive Cancer Network (NCCN)

The NCCN clinical practice guidelines for prostate cancer early detection [35] stated that "free PSA is not generally used in deciding whether or not to perform an initial biopsy." They explicitly recommend a biopsy for men with PSA 4–10 ng/mL or "percent free PSA in selected patients where the risk of biopsy and/or diagnosis and treatment is outweighed by comorbid conditions." The NCCN recommendations for cut points were to perform a biopsy for percent free PSA ≤ 10%, consider biopsy for percent free PSA 10–25%, and consider deferring biopsy for percent free PSA > 25%.

The NCCN also commented on the use of free PSA in the follow-up of patients. They state to consider percent free PSA at 6–12-month follow-up for men with PSA 2.6–4 ng/mL in whom an initial prostate biopsy is not performed or in men with an initial negative prostate biopsy. In contrast to the use of free PSA, PSA density was not incorporated into the guidelines as it was felt to have little additional benefit over other tests [36].

European Association of Urology (EAU)

The published EAU guidelines on prostate cancer [37] note that the percent free PSA is the most extensively investigated and most widely used method to discriminate BPH from prostate cancer but recommended caution in the use of percent free PSA due to the influence of preanalytic and clinical factors. They also concluded that percent free PSA was of no clinical utility when total PSA was >10 ng/mL.

Why Percent Free PSA Is Not Often Utilized

Despite the extensive prior research focus on percent free PSA and the readily available access to testing at most laboratories, the utilization of percent free PSA testing is not widespread. The use of percent free PSA hinges on the desire to reduce unnecessary prostate biopsies. While percent free PSA provides a modest improvement compared to PSA alone in deciding on whether to perform a prostate biopsy, the accuracy is far from perfect. In the majority (approximately 85–90%) of patients, the percent free PSA will be in the worrisome range (<10%) or potentially concerning range (10–25%). Unfortunately, the minority of men who have a favorable percent free PSA value (>25%) are often not reassured by the test. While the favorable percent free PSA value of >25% has been associated with only an 8% probability of prostate cancer, in our experience, patients are often not reassured by this percentage. Part of this concern may be due to the patient perception that this represents a high risk of prostate cancer, when in fact it is probably similar to the risk in a patient with a "normal" PSA. In men biopsied as part of the placebo arm in the PCPT trial in men

with PSA levels <0.5, 0.6–1.0, 1.1–2.0, 2.1–3.0, and 3.1–4.0 ng/mL, prostate cancer was detected in 6.6%, 10.1%, 17.0%, 23.9%, and 26.9%, respectively [38]. Thus, the risk of prostate cancer in the most favorable percent free PSA category potentially places the patient's prostate cancer risk as lower than expected in the general population.

In addition to patient concerns, urologist concerns also play a role. Much of the prior study of percent free PSA was based on a "gray area" of doubt in the management of men with PSA values between 4 and 10 ng/mL. However, since that time, there has been a general trend of less acceptance of those PSA values, with the thought that even PSA values in the 2.5–4 ng/mL range should be considered abnormal, especially in younger men. Along with the willingness to biopsy men at lower PSA values likely comes an unwillingness to not pursue biopsy in the 4.0–10 ng/mL range. In addition, a concern may also exist from a medical-legal standpoint that a patient who is not biopsied for an elevated PSA may presently have or go on to develop an aggressive prostate cancer.

The evidence in support of percent free PSA is predominantly for PSA values between 4 and 10 ng/mL. Values over 10 ng/mL clearly warrant biopsy as the risk of prostate cancer is greater than 50%. The data for PSA values between 2.6 and 4.0, which have been advocated by some as a trigger for biopsy, is less conclusive. An evaluation from Roehl et al. [39] using percent free PSA reported an area under the curve of 0.585. A percent free PSA cutoff value of 25% resulted in 85% sensitivity, but the specificity was only 9%. They concluded that percent free PSA was less robust in the lower PSA range and did not recommend use. By contrast, Lee et al. found percent free PSA to maintain its predictive value to be even higher in patients with PSA levels less than 4.0 [40]. Lastly, while there is substantial evidence that percent free PSA helps to discriminate between BPH and prostate cancer, the ability to distinguish chronic prostatitis from prostate cancer is less clear. When Jung et al. [41] evaluated patients with chronic asymptomatic prostatitis, they reported that percent free PSA was not different in men with chronic prostatitis compared to those diagnosed with prostate cancer. However, the study was not definitive as evaluation was by sextant biopsy and the sample size was small.

As a result of the above concerns, free PSA is frequently relegated to evaluation of patients with medical comorbidity to provide reassurance that a prostate biopsy is not needed. In this era of the increasing discussion of the overdiagnosis of prostate cancer [42], the interest remains to properly identify which men need prostate biopsy and who can avoid unnecessary prostate biopsy. Percent free PSA could provide the information needed to defer or avoid biopsy in many patients.

Conclusion

Percent Free PSA is a useful adjunct in patients with PSA between 4 and 10 ng/mL. At the current time, it is underutilized. Increased use, particularly if integrated with other markers of disease risk, could improve sensitivity and specificity of prostate cancer screening and therefore maintain the diagnosis rate while sparing many men an unnecessary biopsy.

Editorial Commentary:
The authors observe that the adoption of percent free PSA remains surprisingly limited due to a number of reasons; the most common one seems to be that its value is often in the indeterminate range. This resistance seems illogical in light of the fact that total PSA is far less predictive of prostate cancer than is percent free PSA. This certainly hasn't slowed use of total PSA in most countries.

Furthermore, most interest in percent free PSA has involved the potential to reduce unnecessary biopsies. Recognizing that many patients won't allow a high percent free PSA to dissuade them from biopsy, it is often overlooked that a very low percent free PSA is extremely likely to indicate underlying prostate cancer. For the patient and urologist not sure whether to proceed to biopsy—or repeat biopsy—a percent free PSA below approximately 12–13% suggests that the decision should almost always be made to perform biopsy. Such patients are highly likely to have undiagnosed prostate cancer, and knowing this is perhaps the most important information gained from percent free PSA.

–J. Stephen Jones

References

1. Stamey TA, Yang N, Hay AR, McNeal JE, Freiha FS, Redwine E. Prostate-specific antigen as a serum marker for adenocarcinoma of the prostate. N Engl J Med. 1987;317(15):909–16.
2. Catalona WJ, Smith DS, Ratliff TL, et al. Measurement of prostate-specific antigen in serum as a screening test for prostate cancer. N Engl J Med. 1991;324(17):1156–61.
3. Nadler RB, Humphrey PA, Smith DS, Catalona WJ, Ratliff TL. Effect of inflammation and benign prostatic hyperplasia on elevated serum prostate specific antigen levels. J Urol. 1995;154(2 Pt 1):407–13.
4. Catalona WJ, Partin AW, Slawin KM, et al. Use of the percentage of free prostate-specific antigen to enhance differentiation of prostate cancer from benign prostatic disease: a prospective multicenter clinical trial. JAMA. 1998;279(19):1542–7.
5. Nam RK, Saskin R, Lee Y, et al. Increasing hospital admission rates for urological complications after transrectal ultrasound guided prostate biopsy. J Urol. 2010;183(3):963–8.
6. Stenman UH, Leinonen J, Alfthan H, Rannikko S, Tuhkanen K, Alfthan O. A complex between prostate-specific antigen and alpha 1-antichymotrypsin is the major form of prostate-specific antigen in serum of patients with prostatic cancer: assay of the complex improves clinical sensitivity for cancer. Cancer Res. 1991;51(1):222–6.
7. Christensson A, Laurell CB, Lilja H. Enzymatic activity of prostate-specific antigen and its reactions with extracellular serine proteinase inhibitors. Eur J Biochem. 1990;194(3):755–63.
8. Bjork T, Bjartell A, Abrahamsson PA, Hulkko S, di Sant'Agnese A, Lilja H. Alpha 1-antichymotrypsin production in PSA-producing cells is common in prostate cancer but rare in benign prostatic hyperplasia. Urology. 1994;43(4):427–34.
9. Catalona WJ, Smith DS, Wolfert RL, et al. Evaluation of percentage of free serum prostate-specific antigen to improve specificity of prostate cancer screening. JAMA. 1995;274(15):1214–20.
10. Food And Drug Administration. Premarket approvals. http://www.fda.gov/MedicalDevices/Productsand MedicalProcedures/DeviceApprovalsandClearances/ PMAApprovals/ucm115142.htm (1998). Accessed 1 June, 2011
11. Lee R, Localio AR, Armstrong K, Malkowicz SB, Schwartz JS. A meta-analysis of the performance characteristics of the free prostate-specific antigen test. Urology. 2006;67(4):762–8.

12. Catalona WJ, Partin AW, Slawin KM, et al. Percentage of free PSA in black versus white men for detection and staging of prostate cancer: a prospective multicenter clinical trial. Urology. 2000;55(3):372–6.

13. Martin BJ, Finlay JA, Sterling K, et al. Early detection of prostate cancer in African-American men through use of multiple biomarkers: human kallikrein 2 (hK2), prostate-specific antigen (PSA), and free PSA (fPSA). Prostate Cancer Prostatic Dis. 2004;7(2):132–7.

14. Kobori Y, Kitagawa Y, Mizokami A, Komatsu K, Namiki M. Free-to-total prostate-specific antigen (PSA) ratio contributes to an increased rate of prostate cancer detection in a Japanese population screened using a PSA level of 2.1–10.0 ng/ml as a criterion. Int J Clin Oncol. 2008;13(3):229–32.

15. Andriole GL, Bostwick DG, Brawley OW, et al. Effect of dutasteride on the risk of prostate cancer. N Engl J Med. 2010;362(13):1192–202.

16. Aubin SM, Reid J, Sarno MJ, et al. PCA3 molecular urine test for predicting repeat prostate biopsy outcome in populations at risk: validation in the placebo arm of the dutasteride REDUCE trial. J Urol. 2010;184(5):1947–52.

17. de la Taille A, Irani J, Graefen M, et al. Clinical evaluation of the PCA3 assay in guiding initial biopsy decisions. J Urol. 2011;185(6):2119–25.

18. Shariat SF, Abdel-Aziz KF, Roehrborn CG, Lotan Y. Pre-operative percent free PSA predicts clinical outcomes in patients treated with radical prostatectomy with total PSA levels below 10 ng/ml. Eur Urol. 2006;49(2):293–302.

19. Steuber T, Vickers AJ, Serio AM, et al. Comparison of free and total forms of serum human kallikrein 2 and prostate-specific antigen for prediction of locally advanced and recurrent prostate cancer. Clin Chem. 2007;53(2):233–40.

20. Wenske S, Korets R, Cronin AM, et al. Evaluation of molecular forms of prostate-specific antigen and human kallikrein 2 in predicting biochemical failure after radical prostatectomy. Int J Cancer. 2009;124(3):659–63.

21. Erdem E, Atsu N, Akbal C, Bilen CY, Ergen A, Ozen H. The free-to-total serum prostatic specific antigen ratio as a predictor of the pathological features of prostate cancer. Int Urol Nephrol. 2002;34(4):519–23.

22. Graefen M, Karakiewicz PI, Cagiannos I, et al. Percent free prostate specific antigen is not an independent predictor of organ confinement or prostate specific antigen recurrence in unscreened patients with localized prostate cancer treated with radical prostatectomy. J Urol. 2002;167(3):1306–9.

23. Vickers AJ, Cronin AM, Aus G, et al. A panel of kallikrein markers can reduce unnecessary biopsy for prostate cancer: data from the European Randomized Study of prostate cancer screening in Goteborg, Sweden. BMC Med. 2008;6:19.

24. Vickers A, Cronin A, Roobol M, et al. Reducing unnecessary biopsy during prostate cancer screening using a four-kallikrein panel: an independent replication. J Clin Oncol. 2010;28(15):2493–8.

25. Vickers AJ, Cronin AM, Aus G, et al. Impact of recent screening on predicting the outcome of prostate cancer biopsy in men with elevated prostate-specific antigen: data from the European Randomized Study of prostate cancer screening in Gothenburg, Sweden. Cancer. 2010;116(11):2612–20.

26. Karakiewicz PI, Benayoun S, Kattan MW, et al. Development and validation of a nomogram predicting the outcome of prostate biopsy based on patient age, digital rectal examination and serum prostate specific antigen. J Urol. 2005;173(6):1930–4.

27. Zaytoun OM, Kattan MW, Moussa AS, Li J, Yu C, Jones JS. Development of improved nomogram for prediction of outcome of initial prostate biopsy using readily available clinical information. Urology. 2011; 78(2):392–8.

28. Stephan C, Kopke T, Semjonow A, et al. Discordant total and free prostate-specific antigen (PSA) assays: does calibration with WHO reference materials diminish the problem? Clin Chem Lab Med. 2009;47(11): 1325–31.

29. Bruun L, Bjork T, Lilja H, Becker C, Gustafsson O, Christensson A. Percent-free prostate specific antigen is elevated in men on haemodialysis or peritoneal dialysis treatment. Nephrol Dial Transplant. 2003; 18(3):598–603.

30. Oesterling JE, Jacobsen SJ, Klee GG, et al. Free, complexed and total serum prostate specific antigen: the establishment of appropriate reference ranges for their concentrations and ratios. J Urol. 1995;154(3) : 1090–5.

31. Kindermann W, Lehmann V, Herrmann M, Loch T. Influencing of the PSA concentration in serum by physical exercise (especially bicycle riding). Urologe A. 2011;50(2):188–96.

32. Keetch DW, Andriole GL, Ratliff TL, Catalona WJ. Comparison of percent free prostate-specific antigen levels in men with benign prostatic hyperplasia treated with finasteride, terazosin, or watchful waiting. Urology. 1997;50(6):901–5.

33. Pannek J, Marks LS, Pearson JD, et al. Influence of finasteride on free and total serum prostate specific antigen levels in men with benign prostatic hyperplasia. J Urol. 1998;159(2):449–53.

34. Greene KL, Albertsen PC, Babaian RJ, et al. Prostate specific antigen best practice statement: 2009 update. J Urol. 2009;182(5):2232–41.

35. Kawachi MH, Bahnson RR, Barry M, et al. NCCN clinical practice guidelines in oncology: prostate cancer early detection. J Natl Compr Canc Netw. 2010;8(2):240–62.

36. Catalona WJ, Southwick PC, Slawin KM, et al. Comparison of percent free PSA, PSA density, and age-specific PSA cutoffs for prostate cancer detection and staging. Urology. 2000;56(2):255–60.

37. Heidenreich A, Bellmunt J, Bolla M, et al. EAU guidelines on prostate cancer. Part 1: screening, diagnosis, and treatment of clinically localised disease. Eur Urol. 2011;59(1):61–71.

38. Thompson IM, Pauler DK, Goodman PJ, et al. Prevalence of prostate cancer among men with a prostate-specific antigen level < or =4.0 ng per milliliter. N Engl J Med. 2004;350(22):2239–46. May 27.

39. Roehl KA, Antenor JA, Catalona WJ. Robustness of free prostate specific antigen measurements to reduce unnecessary biopsies in the 2.6 to 4.0 ng./ml. range. J Urol. 2002;168(3):922–5.

40. Lee BH, Moussa AH, Li J, Fareed K, Jones JS. Percentage of free prostate-specific antigen: implications in modern extended scheme prostate biopsy. Urology. 2011;77(4):899–903.

41. Jung K, Meyer A, Lein M, Rudolph B, Schnorr D, Loening SA. Ratio of free-to-total prostate specific antigen in serum cannot distinguish patients with prostate cancer from those with chronic inflammation of the prostate. J Urol. 1998;159(5): 1595–8.

42. Welch HG, Black WC. Overdiagnosis in cancer. J Natl Cancer Inst. 2010;102(9):605–13.

PCA3 and Other Urinary Markers

6

Benjamin Challacombe, John Fitzpatrick, and Roger Kirby

Introduction

With worldwide increasing diagnosis of localised prostate cancer, primarily due to the sensitive but nonspecific PSA test, urologists have dedicated huge resources to identifying urinary biomarkers for prostate cancer diagnosis. Due to the intimate relationship between the prostate and the evacuation of urine through it, a urinary marker is far more appealing than a serum biomarker. Markers would be easy to collect and may not require an invasive procedure if present in sufficient quantities in the urine naturally. Over the last decade, a range of potential urinary markers have been proposed for this role, and this chapter examines their current and potential use in clinical practice.

Prostate Cancer Urinary Cytology

George Papanicolaou, who is considered the father of cytology, described the presence of prostate cancer cells in voided urine samples as far back as 1958 [1]. Although present in relatively advanced and high-grade disease, the overall pick-up rate is low [2] with cells being scarce and difficult to collect and store. There has been considerable discussion over the origin of prostate cells in the urine with the aim of isolating a robust urinary marker for prostate cancer. Robust identification of prostate cancer cells by traditional urine cytology has been hampered by the low proportion of prostate cancer cells present and by high false-negative rates. Modern PCR-based molecular methods can detect much lower numbers of malignant cells compared with conventional histological or cytological examination and may hold the key to future urinary analysis for prostate cancer.

Prostate Cancer Antigen 3 (PCA3)

Introduction

PCA3 is probably the best known and main urinary biomarker for prostate cancer in clinical use at the current time. A collaboration of investigators at Saint Radboud University in Nijmegen in the Netherlands and Johns Hopkins University, Baltimore, Bussemakers et al. [3] identified the

B. Challacombe, B.Sc., M.S., FRCS (✉)
Guy's and St Thomas' Hospitals NHS Foundation Trust,
London Bridge Hospital, London Bridge Urology,
Emblem House, 27 Tooley Street, London, SE1 2PR, UK
e-mail: benchallacombe@doctors.net.uk

J. Fitzpatrick, M.Ch., FRCSI, FC Urol (SA),
FRCSGlas, FRCS
Department of Surgery, The Mater Misericordiae
Hospital, University College, Dublin, Ireland

R. Kirby, M.A., M.D., FRCS, FEBU
The Prostate Centre, London, UK

J.S. Jones (ed.), *Prostate Cancer Diagnosis: PSA, Biopsy and Beyond*, Current Clinical Urology,
DOI 10.1007/978-1-62703-188-2_6, © Springer Science+Business Media New York 2013

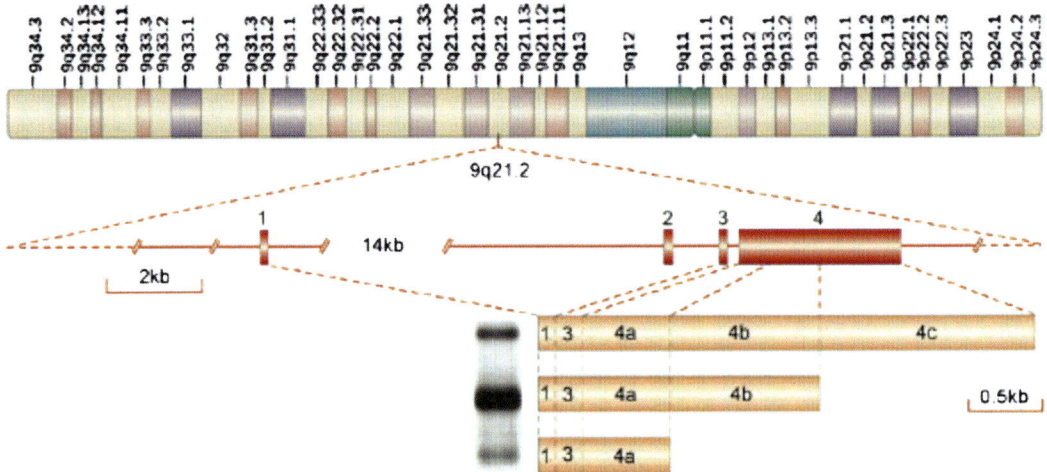

Fig. 6.1 The PCA3 gene. It is located at chromosome 9q21–22, consists of four exons, with exon 2 often omitted by alternative splicing (Reprinted with permission from Nature Publishing Group: Hessels et al., Nature Reviews Urology, copyright 2009 [5])

DD3 gene (subsequently called the PCA3 gene) as a potential marker in the late 1990s. This gene is highly over-expressed in prostate cancer. There is a strong association between PCA3 mRNA over-expression and malignant transformation of prostate epithelium which indicated its potential as a diagnostic biomarker. PCA3 has a lower sensitivity but a higher specificity and a better positive and negative predictive value than PSA. It is available internationally but is significantly more expensive than a PSA assay in many countries. It requires an 'attentive' digital rectal examination (DRE) prior to collection and is measured in the first part of the voided specimen. It is unrelated to prostate size.

PCA3 History and Development

Prostate cancer antigen 3 which is usually referred to as PCA3 (and occasionally as DD3) was first mentioned in 1998 by Jack Schalken, from Nijmegen in The Netherlands, as having potential as a new prostate cancer biomarker [4]. In 1999 via a differential display analysis, which is a method to compare mRNA expression levels between benign and malignant tissue, DD3/PCA3 was more formally described. The PCA3 gene is located on chromosome 9q21–22 (Fig. 6.1) and

was originally described as consisting of four exons with alternative polyadenylation at three different positions in exon 4 [3].

PCA3 had a high level of expression in prostate tumours and was over-expressed in 95% of 56 human radical prostatectomy specimens examined when compared to neighbouring benign tissues. As confirmation using Northern blot analysis, normal prostate and benign prostatic hyperplasia (BPH) tissue from the same subjects expressed little to no PCA3. Further analyses showed undetectable levels of expression in other normal tissues from all major organs. In addition, no expression could be detected in tumours from breast, cervix, endometrium, ovary or testis and cancer cell lines from bladder, breast, kidney and ovaries [4].

In 2002, Shalken's group in the Netherlands reported a different method for the accurate quantification of PCA3 using real-time quantitative reverse transcription-PCR [6]. They described PCA3 as a gene containing non-coding messenger RNA which is over-expressed in prostate cancer. At that stage, it was unclear whether the best clinical application for PCA3 was in the analysis of prostate needle biopsies or other human fluids such as blood, ejaculate, urine or prostate massage fluid. The following year, using a quantitative time-resolved fluorescence (TRF) RT-PCR to detect PCA3 mRNA in centrifuged urine sediments, this group described a 66-fold up-regulation of PCA3 median when compared to benign prostate tissue [7]. This was found in more than 95% of prostate cancer samples analysed. In a cohort of 108 men with a serum PSA value >3 ng/ml, PCA3 had a test sensitivity and specificity of 67% and 83%, respectively, using a predetermined PCA3-PSA cut-off of 200×10^3, and a negative predictive value of 90%. The authors felt that the main role of this molecular urinary test was in reducing the amount of unnecessary primary prostate biopsies.

The initial reverse-transcriptase polymerase chain reaction PCA3 urine test was quite intensive and time-consuming to perform and has now been translated successfully into the quicker and easier transcription-mediated amplification (TMA)-based PCA3 test. The Nijmegen pilot was validated in a larger Dutch multicenter study using this method with similar results [8].

The next advance was the development of an isothermally amplified version of the PCA3 test which was released by DiagnoCure Incorporated. It used nucleic acid sequence-based amplification (NASBA) technology and real-time fluorescence detection in nucleic acid extracts from post-DRE urine sediments. Using this NASBA assay on 201 patients, PCA3 was shown to have a PCA3 sensitivity of 82% and specificity of 76% compared to 87% and 16% for PSA [9]. PCA3 had an area under the curve (AUC) of 81%. A combined study on 517 patients improved the specificity to 89%, whilst the sensitivity dropped to 66% [10]. Importantly the ability of PCA3 to predict prostate cancer was consistent across the usual diagnostic PSA range with no difference seen between those with serum PSA values that were in groups of <4 ng/mL, 4–10 ng/mL and >10 ng/mL.

The final stage in the development came in 2006 with the production of a commercially available urine PCA3 test. Groskopf et al. presented a prototype adaptation of the test to measure PCA3 in whole voided urine samples mixed with an equal volume of a stabilising buffer. This semiautomated, quantitative PCA3 test was developed by Gen-Probe Incorporated (San Diego, CA, United States) using specific target capture, transcription-mediated amplification (TMA) and detection with chemiluminescent DNA probes [11]. This importantly removed the need for urine centrifugation and RNA extraction and allowed the entire process to be performed in a single tube. The stability of the assay was evaluated in archived urine specimens stored at either 4 °C or 30 °C. The PCA3-to-PSA ratio at 4 °C remained within a 20% range of the initial values after 2 weeks indicating good stability when cooled. In contrast at 30 °C, a significant degradation of PCA3 reflected the test's instability at room temperature. The assay measures PCA3 mRNA, which is highly upregulated in neoplastic prostate tissue, simultaneously with prostate-specific antigen (PSA) mRNA, which is not upregulated in prostate cancer and used to normalise for the amount of prostate-specific RNA in the molecular test sample. Thus, a ratio of PCA3 to PSA mRNA is calculated to detect prostate cancer cells in a 'background' of normal prostate cells that express low levels of PCA3. In the commercial Gen-Probe assay, the PCA3/PSA mRNA ratio is multiplied by 1,000 to yield a score, referred to as the PCA3 score, with a clinical cut-off level of 35. Similar to other gene-based tests, the PCA3 assay is comparable in cost and complexity. Samples must be sent to an accredited laboratory experienced in performing molecular testing, and PCA3 scores are reported to the urologist.

Sample collection and specimen stability are robust. Informative rates (percentage of urine samples yielding accurately quantifiable mRNAs for assay) are >95% [12], and the assays have good reproducibility with intra- and interassay coefficients of variation of <13% and <12%, respectively, and total variation of <20% for the PCA3 score [13].

Preliminary Clinical Studies

In Groskopf's primary study using the Gen-Probe TMA technique, the PCA3 score demonstrated a sensitivity of 69%, specificity of 79% and an area under the curve (AUC) of 0.746 (95% CI: 0.574–0.918) [11]. Larger follow-up studies of

North American and European men confirmed that PCA3 performance was independent of serum PSA level and, in contrast to serum PSA, PCA3 was unaffected by prostate size [12, 14, 15].

A key finding of several studies was that the quantitative PCA3 score correlated with the risk of a positive biopsy [12, 14, 16]. Overall, the informative rate of the third-generation PCA3 assay (Gen-Probe, PROGENSA®) was significantly improved over the previously reported 79% by Tinzl et al. [10] and is reported to range from 94% to 100%. The Gen-Probe PCA3 assay was cleared for use in Europe in 2006 under the name PROGENSA® PCA3, and since then, several studies have validated the performance of the this assay with comparable results% ([10], reviewed in [17]). The US Food and Drug Administration approval process is currently still ongoing, whilst in Europe, the CE approved test is licenced to assist clinicians in counselling regarding prostate cancer risk and for confirming the indications for primary and repeat biopsy. Royalties of 16% of cumulative sales of PCA3 kits are still paid to DiagnoCure who produced the previous assay technique.

Clinical Use

Determining a PCA3 score is useful in different clinical scenarios. The score can be used to increase confidence in an initial biopsy decision where the serum tPSA results are uncertain (2.5–10 ng/mL) or close to the age-specific PSA cut-off values. Secondly, PCA3 testing can be used to increase confidence in a re-biopsy decision, wherein the DRE and serum tPSA results are suspicious and/or family history and other factors indicate an increased risk of prostate cancer [13]. There is significant current interest in the ability of PCA3 to predict low-risk versus aggressive disease [18]. Thus, the availability of a PCA3 score alone or combined with existing methods might better guide biopsy decision-making than current methods and might be useful as an indicator of clinical stage and disease significance.

A practical point is that a DRE is required/recommended prior to collection of urine for the PCA3 test. The DRE is presumed to increase the cellular load in the voided urine by the release of prostate cells into the prostatic urethra. It is done to optimise the test, but there is a good chance (around 80%) that sufficient cells will still be released without a DRE [13]. Due to the use of urine sediments from the earlier RT-PCR and NASBA techniques, a prostatic massage was initially recommended, but this is not currently thought necessary. Currently for the PROGENSA® PCA3 assay, the first voided specimen of urine is collected after an 'attentive' DRE consisting of exactly three strokes, with firm pressure to depress the prostate surface for 7 mm, applied from the base to the apex and from the lateral to the median line for each lobe involving three strokes per lobes is recommended to ensure standardisation the collection procedure. In fact, it has been shown that prostate massage to provide extra prostatic secretions does not increase the clinical sensitivity or specificity compared to DRE [19].

Early Detection Using PCA3

The use of PSA testing/screening for prostate cancer leads to a high number of unnecessary biopsies. The use of the PCA3 test to try and reduce the number of negative biopsies is a key goal for this marker. A variety of studies have now shown an improved predictive value for prostate cancer using PCA3 when compared to PSA [12, 14]. Marks et al. [16] studied 226 men with a previous negative prostate biopsy but with evidence of a serum total PSA (tPSA) level persistently above 2.5 ng/mL. Applying receiver-operating characteristic (ROC) curve analysis to PCA3 and serum tPSA results obtained after a re-biopsy of these men yielded a significantly higher AUC for PCA3 than for serum tPSA (0.68 vs. 0.52; $p=0.008$) indicating its superiority as a marker. 35 was used as the most balanced PCA3 score cut-off and this resulted in a sensitivity, specificity and odds ratio of 58%, 72% and 3.6%, respectively. Gen-Probe quotes that men with a PCA3 score ≥ 35 have a 62% probability of a positive biopsy. Disappointingly in this study, there was no difference between aggressive and nonaggressive prostate cancers (Gleason <7 and Gleason ≥7).

The studies from Deras and Haese [12, 14] confirmed these findings in cohorts of European and American men undergoing first repeat biopsies with AUC of 0.68 and 0.65, respectively. Although conflicting with regard to the association with cancer aggressiveness, both these studies showed that when PCA3 was used in combination with previously established biopsy risk factors such as age, PSA, DRE, prostate volume and percent free PSA (%fPSA), the diagnostic accuracy was improved in multivariable regression models. A subsequent subgroup analysis (n=301) of the European multicenter study confirmed PCA3's univariable superiority over %fPSA as a predictor of outcome following repeat biopsy (AUC 0.69 vs. 0.57) [20]. The authors proposed that men with a low free/total ratio and also a low PCA3 score could be spared from unnecessary second biopsy.

In Groskopf's study [11], PCA3 and tPSA were compared in 70 men who had a prostate biopsy based on pre-existing risk factors, with 52 apparently healthy men with no known risk factors. At a PCA3 score threshold of 50, the sensitivity was 69% and the specificity 79%. In comparison for serum tPSA at the established threshold of 2.5 ng/mL and with sensitivity held constant at 69%, the specificity for tPSA was lower at 60%. These results were confirmed using a time-resolved fluorescence-based variant of the PCA3 test by van Gils et al. [19]. In their multicenter study of 583 men with a serum tPSA level of 3–15 ng/mL, the AUC for predicting a positive biopsy was higher for PCA3 than for serum tPSA (0.66 vs. 0.57). There was also a correlation of increasing PCA3 score with increasing probability of positive repeat biopsy.

The Association with Prostate Volume and Tumour Volume/Aggressiveness

An association of a marker with prostate volume regardless of the presence or absence of prostate cancer is an undesirable characteristic, as it indicates nonspecificity of the marker. We know that serum tPSA shows this association, permitting its use in the assessment of BPH, but PCA3 seems not to as illustrated by a lack of correlation with prostate volume in a large study by Deras et al. [14]. In this, the associations of both tPSA and PCA3 with prostate volume were evaluated in 570 men scheduled for initial or repeat prostate biopsy. Serum tPSA values increased significantly ($p < 0.001$) as prostate volume increased, whereas PCA3 scores were unaffected ($p = 0.54$).

The association of a marker such as PCA3 with tumour aggressiveness is clearly highly desirable to identify important cancers posing the most significant risk to life. Nakanishi's group [21] found an impressive correlation of PCA3 with tumour volume and Gleason grading (tumour aggressiveness) in an analysis of urine collections before prostatectomy in 96 men with biopsy-confirmed prostate cancer. The PCA3 score increased linearly and significantly with increasing tumour volume ($R = 0.27$, $p = 0.008$), and there was a significant difference ($p = 0.007$) when comparing PCA3 scores for individuals with low-volume (<0.5 cc) and low-grade tumours (Gleason ≤6) with PCA3 scores in the subpopulation with 'significant cancers' (men with combinations of high dominant tumour volumes and Gleason scores). It did not appear linked to other pathological features such as tumour stage.

Haese's work has also [12] supported these findings in a multicenter, multinational European study where 463 men with one or more previous negative biopsies were re-biopsied after a DRE and urine collections for PCA3; in total, 28% of men had a positive repeat biopsy (128 cancers). The subsequent detected cancers were classified as indolent if they were stage T1c, had a PSA density of <0.15 ng/mL, a Gleason score at biopsy of ≤6, and had ≤33% positive cores (a standardised minimum of 10 peripheral zone cores were acquired). The higher the PCA3 score, the greater the probability of a positive repeat biopsy, and median PCA3 scores were higher in significant compared to indolent cancers (42.1 vs. 21.4, $p = 0.006$). PCA3 scores were also higher for patients with a biopsy Gleason score above 6 ($p = 0.040$) and for patients with stage T2 vs. T1c cancer ($p = 0.005$). Reassuringly in this study, the

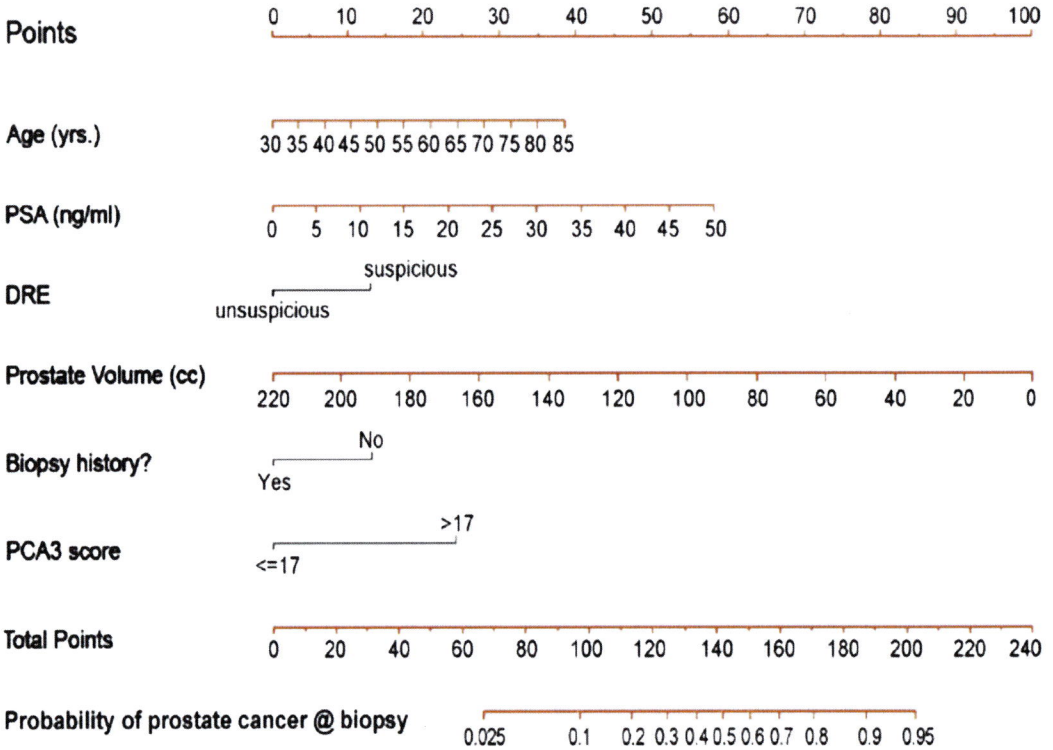

Fig. 6.2 The PCA3 biopsy nomogram. This recently externally validated nomogram combines established biopsy risk factors such as age, digital rectal examination (DRE), total serum prostate-specific antigen (PSA), pros- tate volume and history of previous biopsy together with PCA3 score to predict cancer on prostate initial and repeat biopsy (Reprinted with permission from Elsevier: Chun et al., European Urology, copyright 2009 [22])

PCA3 score was not affected by age, number of previous negative biopsies or total prostate vol- ume (Fig. 6.2).

Current and Emerging Roles of PCA3

The use of PCA3 in combination with serum PSA and other clinical information seems to enhance the diagnostic accuracy of prostate cancer detec- tion and may enable physicians to make more informed decisions with patients at risk for pros- tate cancer. In order to evaluate this, Deras et al. [12] evaluated urinary PCA3 and serum tPSA in both univariate and multivariate logistic regres- sion models. The predictive probability relative to biopsy outcome was determined. For tPSA alone, PCA3 alone and the combination of tPSA + PCA3, the AUCs from ROC were 0.547, 0.686 and 0.752, respectively. The increase in

AUC in the multivariate model was highly significant ($p < 0.001$), showing the synergistic power of employing both methods.

In the Haese study [12], a multivariate logistic regression model for predicting prostate cancer at repeat biopsy was used, and the PCA3 score was an independent predictor ($p = 0.006$) of outcome after adjusting for age, serum tPSA, %fPSA, DRE and prostate volume. Including PCA3 in the base model containing the other terms improved the accuracy of the model by 4.2%, which was significant ($p < 0.001$). The PCA3 score was also the most informative univariate predictor in this study.

When PCA3 was incorporated into the Prostate Cancer Prevention Trial risk calculator (PCPT-RC), it improved the diagnostic accuracy compared with the established biopsy risk factors (AUC 0.65 vs. 0.70) [23]. Although it was not possible to measure directly the urinary

PCA3 scores in the PCPT study population, a multi-institutional collaboration by Chun et al. applied stringent statistical criteria and demonstrated in a large mixed biopsy patient cohort from Europe and North America ($n = 809$) that PCA3 was an independent predictor of prostate cancer, and its addition to established risk factors (age, PSA, DRE, prostate volume and biopsy history) improved predictive values [24]. The most significant increase in predictive value was seen using a PCA3 cut-off value of 17. The AUC for the PCPT calculator incorporating PCA3 was 0.703, which was statistically superior to the PCPT calculator without PCA3 (AUC 0.618, $p < 0.025$). Both the updated PCPT calculator and PCA3 alone were also superior to serum tPSA alone (see Fig. 6.2).

Another large source of data for the use of PCA3 came from The Reduction by Dutasteride of Prostate Cancer Events (REDUCE) trial. This was designed to evaluate the use of dutasteride for the chemoprevention of prostate cancer [22]. This was a 4-year, randomised, placebo-controlled trial evaluating the effect of the 5α-reductase inhibitor dutasteride on prostate cancer risk in men with a total serum PSA ranging from 2.5 to 10 ng/mL and a previous negative biopsy. The placebo arm was made up of more than 4,000 patients, and a large cohort of them (1,140 subjects) provided urine samples for PCA3 analysis prior to TRUS biopsies at year 2 and year 4 [25]. Consistent with previous studies using the TMA PCA3 assay, a large proportion of the specimens (94%, N = 1072) contained sufficient RNA for PCA3 analysis confirming the practical use of the marker without a preceding DRE. The PCA3 score was found to correlate with the percent of biopsy-positive men; the greater the PCA3 score, the greater the probability of a positive biopsy. PCA3 score was also correlated with biopsy Gleason score ($p = 0.0017$). At low PCA3 scores of <5, 6% (7/116) of men were biopsy positive, whereas at higher scores >100, 57% (28/49) were biopsy positive. Using the standard cut-off of 35, the clinical performance of PCA3 in this study was similar to previous studies: sensitivity was 48%, and specificity was 79%. In comparison to serum PSA, the PCA3 score again performed significantly better ($p = 0.008$) with an AUC for PCA3 score of 0.693 (95% CI, 0.649–0.736) compared to 0.612 (95% CI, 0.570–0.655) for serum PSA. In addition, the PCA3 score was statistically significantly higher in men with a positive follow-up biopsy vs. a negative biopsy (median PCA3 score 50.4 vs. 28.2), which is consistent with the median PCA3 scores in the previous European repeat biopsy study [12]. This reinforces the hypothesis that a high PCA3 score in men with a current negative repeat biopsy may predict a future positive repeat biopsy. PCA3 may be detecting cancers that were missed by TRUS biopsy (such as anterior tumours), or PCA3 may alternatively be related to precancerous states that subsequently progress. In clinical practice, this would mean that in men with a negative biopsy but a high PCA3 score close follow-up is needed with a low threshold for repeat trans-rectal or trans-perineal biopsy.

A predictive model incorporating PCA3, serum PSA, % free PSA and other clinical information significantly improved diagnostic accuracy (AUC = 0.753) compared to the model excluding PCA3 (AUC = 0.717, $p = 0.0009$) [15]. This is consistent with other studies that have incorporated PCA3 into statistical models and nomograms [13, 16, 26]. Another suggestive finding from the REDUCE study placebo arm was that year 2 PCA3 scores seemed predictive of year 4 biopsy outcome with an AUC of 0.634 ($p = 0.0002$). These data suggest that prostate cancers that were missed by biopsy at year 2 were in fact detected by PCA3. A trans-rectal needle biopsy samples only a small proportion of the total prostate gland and is not a perfect method to diagnose cancer. In some cases, a false-positive PCA3 may be a true positive if the cancer remained undetected on biopsy. Altogether, data from the placebo arm of the REDUCE trial validated the clinical performance of PCA3.

The Rotterdam group has recently looked at the performance of PCA3 as a first-line diagnostic test using participants from the Rotterdam section of the European randomised study of screening for prostate cancer [27]. They performed sextant biopsies on 721 men aged

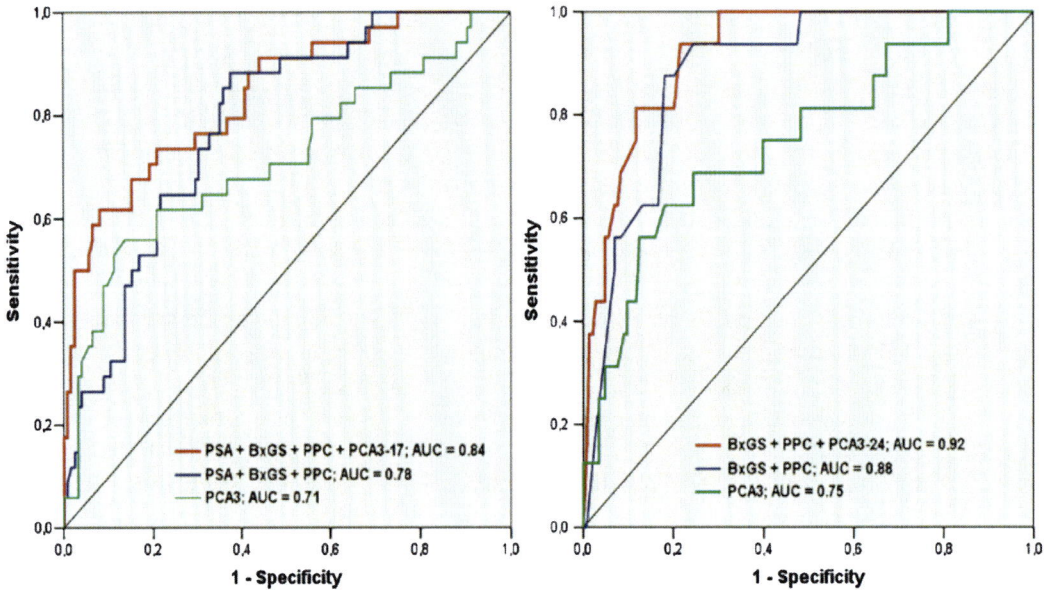

Fig. 6.3 Prediction of small-volume and insignificant prostate cancer with preoperative prostate cancer antigen 3 (PCA3). Receiver-operating characteristic curve analyses and area under the curve (AUC) for predicting (**a**) tumour volume <0.5 ml and (**b**) pathologically confirmed insignificant prostate cancer. *BxGS* biopsy Gleason score, *PPC* percentage of positive cores, *PSA* prostate-specific antigen (Reprinted by permission from Elsevier: Auprich et al. [26]. European Urology, copyright 2011)

63–75 years who had a PCA3 score ≥10. There was a 16% cancer detection rate (122 cancers), and the correlation between PSA and PCA3 was poor (Spearman rank correlation: $p=0.14$; $p<0.0001$). They concluded that PCA3 as a first-line screening test performed better then PSA in performance characteristics and identification of serious disease in this prescreened population. The same group have also evaluated the performance of PCA3 in this cohort when the PCA3 value was very high (>100) and compared them to men with a PCA3 <100 [28]. They found that more cases of prostate cancer (30.0% vs. 18.8%) were detected in re-biopsied men with initial PCA3 scores ≥100 than in men with PCA3 scores <100 but could not explain why many men had excessively high PCA3 scores in spite of the absence of biopsy-detectable prostate cancer. This remains an important unanswered question in the use of PCA3 at present.

A European collaboration two multicenter open-label, prospective studies have evaluated the clinical utility of the PCA3 assay (after DRE) in guiding initial and repeat biopsy decisions [29]. Thirty-four percent of 1,009 men had a positive biopsy, and PCA3 scores were statistically significantly lower in men with lower Gleason grade, clinical stage and tumour volume (<33% core involvement at biopsy and pathological score at radical prostatectomy). They recommended a PCA3 score threshold of 20 (as opposed to the usual 35) as the cut-off that may have the highest utility for selecting men with clinically insignificant prostate cancer in whom active surveillance may be an appropriate management option. A cut-off threshold of 50 was viewed as useful in identifying men at risk of significant prostate cancer who may be suitable for radical prostatectomy, and authors recommended including PCA3 in the prostate cancer assessment strategy. There is also new evidence that similarly to PSA, age-specific PCA3 values should be considered as PCA3 score increases with age, independent of prostate cancer presence [30] and this should be considered when men undergo evaluation for prostate cancer (Fig. 6.3).

Conclusions PCA3

The discovery and evaluation of PCA3 has shown that the marker supplements PSA in diagnosis and is insensitive to the nonspecific factors that can affect circulating PSA levels such as inflammation/prostatitis [31]. Several analyses have shown it to be superior to PSA for primary prostate cancer diagnosis, when compared directly. The addition of PCA3 to the urologist's diagnostic tools will not result in a complete state of certainty; however, diagnostic sensitivity, specificity and the predictive value are incrementally improved by its inclusion whether independently or as part of the diagnostic algorithm. In turn, biopsy, repeat biopsy [32] and further management decisions might be better informed. It has the potential to improve the overall level of patient care by reducing numbers of unpleasant unnecessary biopsies and targeting those men more likely to be positive. At present, the use of PCA3 is limited by a only recent FDA approval (Feb 2012). FDA approval in the USA and concerns about cost in European public health-care systems. For example, in the UK it is not generally available in the public health system and costs circa £300 ($475, €350). It is still probably best analysed following a DRE, and although it consistently has improved specificity when compared to PSA, it has a poorer specificity.

Engrailed-2 (En2)

Following the development of PCA3, many groups have continued the search for another urinary biomarker for prostate cancer diagnosis that is superior in sensitivity. The HOX genes are a group of homeodomain-containing transcription factors that determine the early identity of cells and tissues in early embryonic development and are subsequently re-expressed in cancer. It has been shown that dysregulation of HOX genes occurs in most common cancers, with evidence that targeting HOX/PBX binding has therapeutic value. Engrailed-2 (En2) is a transcriptional repressor and a member of this group which shows a very high degree of functional conservation during development. In addition to a developmental role, En2 has recently been shown to be a potential oncogene in breast cancer [33], as forcing its expression in the non-malignant mammary cells induces a malignant phenotype including increased cell proliferation and a loss of contact dependence. En2 has been shown to be expressed in, and secreted by, prostate cancer but not normal prostatic tissue making it a good potential diagnostic marker. The presence of EN2 protein in urine is therefore currently being evaluated as a diagnostic biomarker for PC.

One group evaluated EN2 levels in men presenting with lower urinary tract symptoms and looked at the subgroups that went onto a subsequent diagnosis of prostate cancer [34]. Having investigated EN2 expression in prostate cancer cell lines and prostate cancer tissue using semi-quantitative RT-PCR and immunohistochemistry, they showed that EN2 was expressed and secreted by PC cell lines and PC tissue but not by normal prostate tissue or stroma. EN2 protein was then measured by ELISA in urine from men with PC ($n=82$) and controls ($n=102$). The presence of EN2 in urine was highly predictive of prostate cancer, with a sensitivity of 66% and a specificity of 88.2%, without the requirement for preceding DRE. There was no correlation with PSA levels. They concluded that urinary EN2 is a highly specific and sensitive candidate biomarker of prostate cancer. This chapter was picked up by many of the health-related media, generating significant interest, and we now await further validation of this exciting work including the examination of the radical prostatectomy and active surveillance cohorts.

Other Markers

GSTP1

Aberrant DNA methylation is a hallmark of carcinogenesis, and GSTP1 hypermethylation is the most common molecular alteration in human prostate cancer. GSTP1 is a member of a large family of glutathione transferases that function to protect cells from oxidative insult; thus, the biological rationale for selecting this marker is its role in preventing damage to cells by neutralising free radicals. Several studies have shown a high sensitivity for this marker to detect the presence of both prostatic intraepithelial neoplasia and prostate cancer, an ability to distinguish these from BPH and a prevalence of methylation in the range of 60–80% in prostate cancer [35]. GSTP1 hypermethylation was evaluated in urine collected following prostatic massage and in core needle biopsies from 100 men referred for diagnostic biopsy. In this pilot, methylation of GSTP1 in the urine specimens had 75% sensitivity and 98% specificity for prostate cancer leading the authors to recommend its potential as a urinary biomarker. Importantly there is no correlation between GSTP1 methylation status and PSA levels, making GSTP1 a potential early and independent marker for the disease.

Transmembrane-Serine Protease Gene (TMPRSS2) and the v-ets Erythroblastosis Virus E26 Oncogene (ERG): TMPRSS2:ERG

TMPRSS2:ERG is the fusion of two genes, TMPRSS2 and ERG, and is found in around half of prostate tumours found through PSA screening [36]. This common recurrent chromosomal aberration in prostate cancer has been evaluated as a urinary biomarker in combination with PCA3 [37]. In this study, the sensitivity was improved to 73%, whilst the specificity dropped to a disappointing 63% compared to the specificity of TMPRSS2:ERG alone of 93%. If two other proteins are also combined (golgi membrane protein 1 (GOLM1), serine peptidase inhibitor, Kazal type 1 (SPINK1)), the AUC increases to a more impressive 0.758 [38], and it may be as part of a battery of tests, including PCA3, that these emerging urinary biomarkers will be at their most predictive. As many of the most recent markers are continuing to evolve, considerable efforts in validation remain to be performed to clearly identify the ideal panel of urinary biomarkers.

Editorial Commentary:

With the limitations of serum PSA as a diagnostic marker becoming progressively evident, there is an explosion of new candidate markers. The logic of a urinary source for this is intuitive based on the unique anatomical relationship of the prostate and urinary flow.

PCA3 is the most mature urinary marker to date as the authors demonstrate. Recognising that some patients with high PCA3 values in the face of a negative biopsy probably actually have prostate cancer that has simply eluded biopsy, so its specificity may be even higher than that calculated based on a negative biopsy rate. Thus, its primary role may be in identifying the patient in need of biopsy or further investigation when the clinical indication otherwise may not be clear. In essence, if the PCA3 value is very high, there is a substantial likelihood of unrecognised prostate cancer, and further investigation is usually in order.

References

1. Foot NC, Papanicolaou GN, Holmquist ND, Seybolt JF. Exfoliative cytology of urinary sediments; a review of 2, 829 cases. Cancer. 1958;11(1):127–37.
2. Krishnan B, Truong LD. Prostatic adenocarcinoma diagnosed by urinary cytology. Am J Clin Pathol. 2000;113(1):29–34.
3. Bussemakers MJ, van Bokhoven A, Verhaegh GW, Smit FP, Karthaus HF, Schalken JA, Debruyne FM, Ru N, Isaacs WB. DD3: a new prostate-specific gene, highly overexpressed in prostate cancer. Cancer Res. 1999;59(23):5975–9.
4. Schalken J. Molecular diagnostics and therapy of prostate cancer: new avenues. Eur Urol. 1998;34 (Suppl 3):3–6.
5. Hessels D, Schalken JA. The use of PCA3 in the diagnosis of prostate cancer. Nat Rev Urol. 2009;6(5):255–61.
6. de Kok JB, Verhaegh GW, Roelofs RW, et al. DD3(PCA3), a very sensitive and specific marker to detect prostate tumors. Cancer Res. 2002;62(9):2695–8.
7. Hessels D, Klein Gunnewiek JM, et al. DD3(PCA3)-based molecular urine analysis for the diagnosis of prostate cancer. Eur Urol. 2003;44(1):8–15.
8. van Gils MP, Hessels D, van Hooij O, et al. The time-resolved fluorescence based PCA3 test on urinary sediments after digital rectal examination; a Dutch multicenter validation of the diagnostic performance. Clin Cancer Res. 2007;13(3):939–43.
9. Fradet Y, Saad F, Aprikian A, et al. UPM3, a new molecular urine test for the detection of prostate cancer. Urology. 2004;64(2):311–5.
10. Tinzl M, Marberger M, Horvath S, Chypre C. DD3PCA3 RNA analysis in urine – a new perspective for detecting prostate cancer. Eur Urol. 2004;46(2):182–6.

11. Groskopf J, Aubin SM, Deras IL, et al. APTIMA PCA3 molecular urine test: development of a method to aid in the diagnosis of prostate cancer. Clin Chem. 2006;52(6):1089–95.

12. Haese A, de la Taille A, van Poppel H, et al. Clinical utility of the PCA3 urine assay in European men scheduled for repeat biopsy. Eur Urol. 2008;54(5):1081–8.

13. Sokoll LJ, Ellis W, Lange P, et al. A multicenter evaluation of the PCA3 molecular urine test: preanalytical effects, analytical performance, and diagnostic accuracy. Clin Chim Acta. 2008;389(1–2):1–6.

14. Deras IL, Aubin SM, Blase A, et al. PCA3: a molecular urine assay for predicting prostate biopsy outcome. J Urol. 2008;179(4):1587–92.

15. Schilling D, Hennenlotter J, Munz M, Bokeler U, Sievert KD, Stenzl A. Interpretation of the prostate cancer gene 3 in reference to the individual clinical background: implications for daily practice. Urol Int. 2010;85(2):159–65.

16. Marks LS, Fradet Y, Deras IL, et al. PCA3 molecular urine assay for prostate cancer in men undergoing repeat biopsy. Urology. 2007;69(3):532–5.

17. Kirby RS, Fitzpatrick JM, Irani J. Prostate cancer diagnosis in the new millennium: strengths and weaknesses of prostate-specific antigen and the discovery and clinical evaluation of prostate cancer gene 3 (PCA3). BJU Int. 2009;103(4):441–5.

18. Auprich M, Chun FK, Ward JF, et al. Critical assessment of preoperative urinary prostate cancer antigen 3 on the accuracy of prostate cancer staging. Eur Urol. 2011;59(1):96–105.

19. van Gils MP, Cornel EB, Hessels D, et al. Molecular PCA3 diagnostics on prostatic fluid. Prostate. 2007;67(8):881–7.

20. Ploussard G, Haese A, van Poppel H, et al. The prostate cancer gene 3 (PCA3) urine test in men with previous negative biopsies: does free-to-total prostate-specific antigen ratio influence the performance of the PCA3 score in predicting positive biopsies? BJU Int. 2010;106(8):1143–7.

21. Nakanishi H, Groskopf J, Fritsche HA, et al. PCA3 molecular urine assay correlates with prostate cancer tumor volume: implication in selecting candidates for active surveillance. J Urol. 2008;179(5):1804–9.

22. Andriole G, Bostwick D, Brawley O, REDUCE Study Group. Chemoprevention of prostate cancer in men at high risk: rationale and design of the reduction by dutasteride of prostate cancer events (REDUCE) trial. J Urol. 2004;172(4 Pt 1):1314–7.

23. Ankerst DP, Groskopf J, Day JR, et al. Predicting prostate cancer risk through incorporation of prostate cancer gene 3. J Urol. 2008;180(4):1303–8.

24. Chun FK, de la Taille A, van Poppel H, et al. Prostate cancer gene 3 (PCA3): development and internal validation of a novel biopsy nomogram. Eur Urol. 2009;56(4):659–67.

25. Aubin SM, Reid J, Sarno MJ, et al. PCA3 molecular urine test for predicting repeat prostate biopsy outcome in populations at risk: validation in the placebo arm of the dutasteride REDUCE trial. J Urol. 2010;184(5):1947–52.

26. Auprich M, Haese A, Walz J, Pummer K, de la Taille A, Graefen M, et al. External validation of urinary PCA3-based nomograms to individually predict prostate biopsy outcome. Eur Urol. 2010;58(5):727–32.

27. Roobol MJ, Schröder FH, van Leeuwen P, et al. Performance of the prostate cancer antigen 3 (PCA3) gene and prostate-specific antigen in prescreened men: exploring the value of PCA3 for a first-line diagnostic test. Eur Urol. 2010;58(4):475–81.

28. Roobol MJ, Schröder FH, van Leenders GL, et al. Performance of prostate cancer antigen 3 (PCA3) and prostate-specific antigen in prescreened men: reproducibility and detection characteristics for prostate cancer patients with high PCA3 scores (≥100). Eur Urol. 2010;58(4):893–9.

29. van Poppel H, Haese A, Graefen M, et al. The relationship between Prostate CAncer gene 3 (PCA3) and prostate cancer significance. BJU Int. 2012;109:360–6.

30. Klatte T, Waldert M, de Martino M, Schatzl G, Mannhalter C, Remzi M. Age-specific PCA3 score reference values for diagnosis of prostate cancer. World J Urol. 2012;30:405–10.

31. Vlaeminck-Guillem V, Bandel M, Cottancin M, Rodriguez-Lafrasse C, Bohbot JM, Sednaoui P. Chronic prostatitis does not influence urinary PCA3 score. Prostate. 2012;72:549–54.

32. Remzi M, Haese A, Van Poppel H, et al. Follow-up of men with an elevated PCA3 score and a negative biopsy: does an elevated PCA3 score indeed predict the presence of prostate cancer? BJU Int. 2010;106(8):1138–42.

33. Martin NL, Saba-El-Leil MK, Sadekova S, Meloche S, Sauvageau G. EN-2 is a candidate oncogene in human breast cancer. Oncogene. 2005;24(46):6890–901.

34. Morgan R, Boxall A, Bhatt A, et al. Engrailed-2 (EN2): a tumor specific urinary biomarker for the early diagnosis of prostate cancer. Clin Cancer Res. 2011;17(5):1090–8.

35. Woodson K, O'Reilly KJ, Hanson JC, Nelson D, Walk EL, Tangrea JA. The usefulness of the detection of GSTP1 methylation in urine as a biomarker in the diagnosis of prostate cancer. J Urol. 2008;179(2):508–11.

36. Tomlins SA, Aubin SM, Siddiqui J, et al. Urine TMPRSS2:ERG fusion transcript stratifies prostate cancer risk in men with elevated serum PSA. Sci Transl Med. 2011;3(94):94ra72.

37. Hessels D, Smit FP, Verhaegh GW, Witjes JA, Cornel EB, Schalken JA. Detection of TMPRSS2-ERG fusion transcripts and prostate cancer antigen 3 in urinary sediments may improve diagnosis of prostate cancer. Clin Cancer Res. 2007;13(17):5103–8.

38. Laxman B, Morris DS, Yu J, et al. A first-generation multiplex biomarker analysis of urine for the early detection of prostate cancer. Cancer Res. 2008;68(3):645–9.

[13, 14]. A variable that is statistically significant in a multivariable model might not improve the model's predictive accuracy. P-value and odds/hazard ratio do not meaningfully describe a biomarker's ability to classify patients. For a biomarker to be potentially clinically useful, it is necessary to show that adding the biomarker to an existing model based on the most important clinical and pathologic factors improves the predictive accuracy (discrimination and calibration) of the model [2, 13, 15–18].

One major issue with model development is the need for appropriate validation. When one develops a model incorporating a biomarker, a set of patients is used to develop the model. By definition, the model is most accurate in predicting the outcome for this set of patients. Therefore biomarker-based models need to be validated on data not used to develop it. There are two general types of validation: internal validation on the original dataset and external validation on an independent dataset (preferred) [2, 6]. External validation on a different dataset evaluates whether the risk prediction tool can be generalized to wider populations than the original dataset. Biomarkers that provide a continuous score provide potentially more useful information than cut points since risk levels are not truly discrete but a continuum of risk [4, 19]. Finally, methods that incorporate clinical consequences such as decision curve analysis are crucial to the evaluation of biomarkers [14, 18, 20]. This type of analysis allows insight into the consequences of using a biomarker in the clinic. Several methods are available including decision curve analysis, which combines simplicity with efficient computations [21–24]. Decision analytic evaluation should be performed during later stages of research before clinical implementation of the biomarker.

PSA Molecular Isoforms

Enhancing the diagnostic accuracy of total PSA (tPSA), particularly specificity, is critical, since higher specificity would reduce the number of biopsies performed in men not affected by PCa.

Several different strategies have been investigated, including the use of age-specific tPSA cutoffs, tPSA density, tPSA density of the transition zone, tPSA velocity, and the measurement of various molecular forms of PSA [25–28]. Prostate-specific antigen exists in free and complexed forms in serum. Improvements in measuring PSA isoforms have allowed the measurement of free PSA (fPSA) and its ratio to tPSA [29–31]. Of the fPSA portion, there are three distinct cleavage isoforms: proPSA, BPH-associated PSA (BPSA), and intact free PSA [32]. The precursor of PSA is a 261 amino acid pre-pro-protein. Subsequent processing by human kallikrein 2 (hK2) and other proteases produces the active 237 amino acid mature PSA [32]. Complexed PSA is a measure of how much PSA in serum is bound to α2-macroglobulin, α1-protease inhibitor, or α1-antichymotrypsin. Currently, there is no commercially available assay which specifically measures the complexes of α2-macroglobulin with PSA.

The FDA has approved the use of percent fPSA [i.e., (fPSA/tPSA) × 100] as an adjunct to tPSA in men with a serum tPSA concentration between 4 and 10 ng/mL. A higher percent fPSA (%fPSA) value indicates a lower probability of finding PCa on biopsy and raises the likelihood that the elevation in tPSA is due to the presence of BPH [33, 34]. In a multicenter, prospective trial, Catalona et al. reported that when a %fPSA of <25% is used for triggering a sextant prostate biopsy, it yielded a 95% sensitivity for PCa detection and increased the specificity by 20% over PSA alone [33]. In response to the realization that sextant biopsies misclassify up to one-third of patients who have PCa as without cancer, a more recent evaluation of the utility of percent free PSA in patients undergoing extended 10- or 12-core biopsy has suggested a lower diagnostic efficiency of %fPSA [35]. A meta-analysis of 41 studies examining fPSA in patients with tPSA between 4 and 10 ng/mL found that a test cutoff of 20% would lead to 94% sensitivity and 13% specificity and that likelihood ratios exceeded 2.0 only at %fPSA of 7% or less [36], suggesting that %fPSA only improves clinical information at extreme values.

While most investigators agree that %fPSA can improve the diagnostic performance of tPSA between 4 and 10 ng/mL, the most appropriate %fPSA cutoff value remains debatable.

The utility of fPSA has also been examined in the tPSA≤4 ng/mL range. Catalona et al. determined that with a %fPSA cutoff of less or equal to 27%, they were able to obtain a sensitivity of 90% and avoid 18% of unnecessary biopsies in men over the age of 50 with a tPSA of 2.6–4.0 ng/mL, with 83% of these cancers being clinically significant [37]. Rowe et al. used a %fPSA cutoff of 20% in patients age 50–65 with tPSA 1.1–3.99 ng/mL and found PCa in 11.3% of the patients biopsied [38]. Pepe et al. used %fPSA thresholds of 15% for patients with tPSA≤2.5 ng/mL and 20% for patients with tPSA between 2.6 and 4 ng/mL and found PCa in 25.6% and 27.4% of the patients, respectively [39]. These studies suggest that %fPSA can help detect PCa in patients with tPSA below 4 ng/mL but the optimal cutoff threshold remains to be determined.

Data on the usefulness of fPSA to predict clinical outcomes is also inconclusive. Graefen and coworkers [40] failed to detect an independent association of preoperative free PSA with biochemical failure in 581 unscreened patients who underwent radical prostatectomy for clinically localized PCa [40]. In contrast, Shariat and colleagues found that lower preoperative serum fPSA is an independent predictor of advanced pathologic features, biochemical progression, and patterns of aggressive disease progression in 402 consecutive men treated with radical prostatectomy for clinically localized PCa who had tPSA levels less than 10 ng/mL [30].

ProPSA

Studies have shown that higher levels of proPSA are associated with PCa. In men with PSA levels between 6.0 and 24.0 ng/ml, the [−2]proPSA fraction was found to be significantly higher in men with PCa [32, 41]. Moreover, authors demonstrated the utility of the proPSA to fPSA ratio for screening patients with PSA levels between 2.5 and 4.0 ng/mL and between 4.0 and 10.0 ng/

mL [42]. Elevated proPSA to fPSA ratios have also been associated with pathologic features of aggressive disease and decreased biochemical disease-free survival after radical prostatectomy [43, 44]. A new automated tool using the [−2] proPSA assay with a %fPSA-based artificial neural network was capable of detecting PCa and the PCa subgroup with more aggressive features with higher accuracy than tPSA or %fPSA alone [45]. In a prospective cohort of men enrolled into active surveillance for PCa, serum and tissue levels of proPSA at diagnosis were associated with the need for subsequent treatment [46]. The authors hypothesized that the increase in the ratio of serum proPSA to %fPSA might be driven by increased proPSA production from "premalignant" cells. In a prospective multicenter cancer detection study, the addition of %[−2]proPSA (defined as [−2]proPSA/10/fPSA) to a logistic regression model including clinical and demographic factors, PSA, and fPSA improved the model's diagnostic accuracy, particularly in the clinically significant 2–10 ng/mL PSA range [47]. In addition, the authors observed that [−2]proPSA may be associated with more aggressive features of PCa [47], suggesting a role for proPSA as a staging and prognostic biomarker.

Molecular forms of PSA may differ in their in vitro stability properties. Therefore, information about the pre-analytical conditions is essential for proper clinical interpretation. For proper measurement of [−2]proPSA, blood samples should be centrifuged within 3 h of blood draw. Serum may be stored at room temperature or refrigerated (+4 °C) for a maximum of 48 h and should be frozen if stored for a longer period. However, two freeze-thaw cycles have no effect on [−2]proPSA stability [48].

BPSA

BPH-associated PSA (BPSA) is formed by the internal cleavage of PSA between Lys182 and Ser183. BPSA is expressed in nodular hyperplasia limited to the transition zone of men with BPH. BPSA can be detected in semen, blood, and prostate, and its levels correlate with transition zone volume and obstructive voiding symptoms [32, 49]. BPSA seems to be a promising marker of BPH since a direct association between its secretion and the volume of the transition zone has been shown to exist [49]. As such, BPSA is a better predictor of prostate enlargement than total and free PSA [50]. In addition, BPSA is not affected by age and is significantly higher in the presence of BPH symptoms. Adjusting the level of fPSA for BPSA resulted in 13–17% improvement in specificity compared to fPSA alone, while maintaining a sensitivity of 90–95% in PCa diagnosis [51].

Intact and Nicked PSA

Intact PSA includes both mature and proPSA single-chain PSA, whereas nicked PSA is PSA that has been internally cleaved between Lys145 and Lys146. The level of intact PSA and ratio of nicked to tPSA have shown potential for improving the discrimination of PCa from BPH [52, 53]. Similar to fPSA, intact PSA levels degrade with freezing, storage, and thawing [52]. The increasing amount of information on these PSA-related markers, together with the clinical parameters, calls for further assessment and integration into diagnostic and prognostic instruments that could serve the daily practice of early detection and screening for PCa.

Emerging Blood-Based Prostate Cancer Biomarkers

Human Kallikrein 2 (hK2)

Human kallikrein-related peptidase 2 is a secreted serine protease from the same gene family as PSA [54]. They share 80% sequence homology and are both primarily expressed in the prostate gland [54]. Despite these structural similarities, hK2 and tPSA differ in their enzymatic activities. The levels of hK2 in prostate tissue, plasma, semen, and serum are less than 2% that of tPSA, although hK2 mRNA transcript expression represents half that of total PSA. Similar to tPSA, serum hK2 is

present in two forms in the blood: one bound to various protease inhibitors and the other (preponderant) free in the circulation. Several studies have shown that, when used in conjunction with free and total PSA, serum hK2 could improve the discrimination of men with PCa from men without cancer [55–57]. It has also been suggested that hK2 could predict poor differentiation, extracapsular extension, and biochemical recurrence in patients treated with radical prostatectomy [58–60]. However, this finding has not been validated by other authors [61]. The usefulness of hK2 for the preoperative staging of localized PCa, therefore, remains controversial. The addition of hK2 to three other kallikreins (total, free, and intact PSA) improved the prediction of prostate biopsy results in men with elevated tPSA (increase of predictive accuracy from 68% to 72% to ~83%) [17]. Considering the risk of PCa at 20%, the number of biopsies would have been reduced by half, missing 3 out of 40 high-grade tumors [17]. This shows that if hK2 is to be used in PCa management, it can only be useful in a panel of biomarkers.

Urokinase Plasminogen Activator (uPA)

The urokinase plasminogen activation axis represents a potential target for PCa markers by being involved in various phases of tumor development and progression through degradation of the extracellular matrix. The serum protease uPA may play a role in cancer progression by binding to the uPA receptor (uPAR) and consequently converting plasminogen to plasmin, which activates proteases related to the degradation of extracellular matrix proteins [62]. Immunohistochemical staining of radical prostatectomy specimens revealed that overexpression of both uPA and its inhibitor (PAI-1) was associated with aggressive PCa recurrence [63]. In patients with a tPSA level above 2 ng/mL, soluble uPAR and fPSA measured in serum before prostate biopsy improved the regression model accuracy for prediction of PCa [64]. Steuber et al. have shown that uPAR fragments were significant predictors of PCa on biopsy specimens of patients with an elevated PSA [64].

Both uPA and uPAR might also have prognostic value. Elevated circulating levels of uPA and uPAR have been linked to PCa stage and bone metastases [63, 65–67]. In a study of 429 patients treated with radical prostatectomy, preoperative plasma uPA was a strong predictor of biochemical recurrence. Both preoperative uPA and uPAR were associated with features of aggressive biochemical recurrence, such as development of distant metastasis and fast PSA doubling time, suggesting an association with occult metastatic disease at the time of local therapy. Moreover, elevation of plasma uPA and uPAR levels in PCa patients seemed to be partly caused by local release from the prostate. Larger multi-institutional studies are under way to validate the potential role of uPA and uPAR as markers of early metastatic PCa.

Transforming Growth Factor-Beta 1 (TGF-β1) and Interleukin-6 (IL-6)

Transforming growth factor-beta 1 is a growth factor involved in the regulation of several cellular mechanisms including proliferation, immune response, differentiation, and angiogenesis [68]. TGF-β1 has been shown to promote cell progression in PCa models, and its local expression has been associated with higher tumor grade, tumor invasion, and metastasis in PCa patients [69–71]. Several studies have shown that increased levels of circulating TGF-β1 were associated with cancer progression, occult and documented metastasis, and biochemical progression in PCa patients [70, 72, 73].

Interleukin-6 is a cytokine with variable effects on immune and hematopoietic mechanisms. *In vitro* and *in vivo* studies have shown that both IL-6 and its receptor (IL-6R) were expressed in PCa [74, 75]. Several authors reported that elevated serum levels of IL-6 and/or IL-6R were associated with metastatic and hormone refractory disease and suggested that IL-6 could predict progression and survival of PCa patients [76–78].

Based on these findings, Kattan and associates developed and internally validated a prognostic model that incorporates plasma TGF-β1 and IL-6R into a standard nomogram for prediction of biochemical recurrence following radical prostatectomy [15]. This combination of serum markers and classical clinical parameters improved the predictive accuracy by a statistically and prognostically substantial margin (increase in predictive accuracy from 75% to 84%). However, before a biomarker can become useful in daily clinical management, it needs to be externally validated in an independent cohort of patients (Fig. 7.1) [2, 6]. Therefore, in a multi-institutional dataset of 423 patients treated with radical prostatectomy, Shariat et al. confirmed that plasma levels of TGF-β1 and IL-6R considerably enhanced the accuracy of the standard preoperative nomogram for the prediction of biochemical recurrence (accuracy of clinical features plus biomarkers 87.9% vs. 71.1% for clinical features alone; $p < 0.001$). Such prognostic models refine our ability to identify patients at a high risk of biochemical recurrence after radical prostatectomy that may benefit from inclusion into perioperative clinical trials and other intensified follow-up protocols.

Endoglin

Endoglin, or CD 105, is a transmembrane glycoprotein that is typically expressed by human vascular endothelial cells. Functionally, it is a cell-surface coreceptor for TGF-β1 and -β3 [79], which modulates cellular responses to TGF-β in the early steps of endothelial cell proliferation. Its critical role in angiogenesis has prompted investigators to evaluate the role of endoglin in cancer progression and metastasis. In PCa, endoglin is preferentially found on new, immature blood vessels, and immunohistochemical analysis supports an association between endoglin expression and disease progression [80]. Urine levels of endoglin may distinguish patients with PCa and may help in the staging of the disease [81]. In addition, preoperative plasma endoglin levels were found to be associated with metastasis to regional lymph nodes [82], as well as established features of biologically aggressive PCa such as higher pathologic Gleason sum and biochemical recurrence following radical prostatectomy [83]. Use of preoperative plasma endoglin could help decide whether and how extensively to perform a lymphadenectomy, as well as preoperative identification of patients at risk for disease progression. This would help select patients for neoadjuvant and/or adjuvant therapy or enrollment into clinical trials. Moreover, endoglin may be valuable as a surrogate biomarker for occult metastatic disease in patients with presumed organ-confined disease. Further investigation is needed to validate endoglin as a useful biomarker in men with PCa and to elucidate the mechanistic role of this biomarker in the progression of PCa.

Prostate Cancer Specific Autoantibodies and α-Methylacyl-CoA Racemase (AMACR)

Autoantibodies, such as those detected in autoimmune and infectious diseases, can be produced by cancer patients in response to tumor-associated antigens overexpressed in cancerous cells. α-Methylacyl-CoA racemase is an enzyme involved in fat metabolism, which has a strong expression in PCa tissues [84]. Immunostaining, using monoclonal antibodies to AMACR, is often used for the diagnosis of PCa, given its high diagnostic accuracy (sensitivity of 97% and specificity of 92%) [85]. A humoral response to tumor-related autoantibodies can be detected in the serum through amplification with high affinity antibodies and T cells. Autoantibodies to AMACR have been detected in the blood of PCa patients, and a recent study showed that they could help distinguish cancerous from healthy patients with more accuracy than PSA [86, 87]. Other autoantibodies to antigens expressed in PCa (Huntington-interacting protein 1, protasomes) have also been detected, and it has been reported that their combination could improve the screening performance, reaching a specificity of 97% [88]. Using a so-called "immunomics" technique, Wang et al. analyzed the overall humoral response against specific tumoral antigens in PCa and were able to identify multiple antigens [89]. With this panel

of autoantibodies, they could detect PCa with a sensitivity of 81.6% and a specificity of 88.2%, which was more accurate than PSA alone. Prior et al. found that combining AMACR, MMP-2, and methylation of GSTP1/RASSF1A with PSA led to a significant improvement in PCa detection over PSA alone with specificities up to 96.6% [90]. Additional studies are needed to validate the potential prognostic value of autoantibodies and AMACR in PCa.

Combination of Multiple Biomarkers for Improved Cancer Detection and/or Prognostication

In the course of validating new biomarkers for PCa, a model combining the new biomarker with PSA is often used and shown to be superior to PSA alone. By combining a panel of biomarkers with varied individual sensitivities and specificities, it is possible to create a model with improved predictive accuracy. Multiple biomarkers are more likely to capture the complex biological potential of the heterogeneous prostate cancer population. For example, Cao et al. combined PCA3, TMPRSS2-ERG, Annexin A3, and sarcosine into a multimodality biomarker panel that outperforms any single biomarker that functions robustly in patients with PSA 4–10 ng/mL [91]. Additional studies are required to optimize and validate this panel. A biomarker may reflect disruption of a biochemical pathway by a particular mechanism. Given the complexity of the molecular abnormalities associated with PCa, it is improbable that a single marker can accurately segregate tumors of similar clinicopathologic phenotypes into distinct prognostic categories. Therefore, combinations of independent, yet complementary markers, may provide a more accurate prediction of outcomes compared to a single marker [27]. The future of cancer profiling relies on the combination of a panel of complimentary biomarkers that can give accurate molecular staging and indicate the likelihood of aggressive behavior [7, 11, 20, 92].

The group of Vickers and Lilja has developed a statistical model that predicts prostate biopsy outcomes based on age, digital rectal exam (DRE), and a panel of four kallikrein markers— tPSA, fPSA, intact PSA, and hK2. Using data from the randomized prostate cancer screening trial in Göteborg, Sweden [one center of the European Randomized Study of Prostate Cancer Screening (ERSPC)], they estimated that, for every 1,000 previously unscreened men with elevated total PSA, use of the model to determine biopsy would reduce biopsy rates by 573, while missing only a small number of cancers (31 out of 152 low-grade cancers and 3 out of 40 high-grade cancers) [17]. These findings were subsequently replicated in independent cohorts, reducing the number of biopsies by 50% and recommending against biopsy primarily in men with low-grade cancer [93, 94]. These findings have also been verified in men who recently have undergone previous screening, with resultant improvements in predictive accuracy [95, 96]. Gupta et al. demonstrated that the panel of four kallikrein markers can predict the outcome of prostate biopsy in men who had previously undergone prostate biopsy during previous screening [97]. This model, in addition to age and DRE, substantially improved the predictive accuracy of a base model (comprising of total PSA, age, and DRE), for both low- and high-grade cancers.

Shariat et al. found that the addition of a panel comprised of preoperative plasma levels of TGF-β1, soluble IL-6R, IL-6, endoglin, vascular endothelial growth factor (VEGF), and vascular cell adhesion molecule-1 (VCAM-1 or CD 106) [67, 68, 70, 82, 83, 98–100] improved the predictive accuracy of the Kattan preoperative nomogram [10] by 15.0% (i.e., 71.6–86.6%) [7, 20]. This increase substantially exceeds accuracy gains obtained from the consideration of detailed pathologic descriptors of PCa at radical prostatectomy. Svatek et al. confirmed the strong predictive value of *pre*operative levels of the candidate biomarkers after adjusting for the effect of postoperative features [92]. The addition of *pre*operative levels of the candidate biomarkers improved the accuracy of the base model (i.e., tPSA, surgical margin status, extracapsular extension, seminal vesicles invasion, lymph node involvement, and pathologic Gleason sum) for prediction of

biochemical recurrence by a statistically and prognostically significant margin (79–86%, $p < 0.001$). Predictive tools integrating biomarker levels could constitute the new standard for counseling patients regarding their risk of recurrence following curative therapy and for designing clinical trials to test neoadjuvant and/or adjuvant treatment strategies in high-risk patients. However, while prediction of biochemical recurrence is important, prediction of response to therapy as well as metastasis and survival is more important for the management of PCa patients [101].

Conclusion

In the PSA era of PCa diagnosis, PCa screening remains controversial due to the risk of overdiagnosis, overtreatment, and the inability to differentiate aggressive tumors. Therefore, new biomarkers are greatly needed to improve the sensitivity and specificity of PCa diagnosis. A substantial amount of effort and funding has been and continues to be invested in the search for new biomarkers and nomograms to improve PCa diagnosis and prognostication by a clinically significant margin. A panel including multiple biomarkers utilizing blood-based, protein-based, gene-based, and/or urine-based modalities in combination with multiple forms of PSA may be necessary to obtain optimal predictive accuracy for PCa diagnosis and prognostication.

Editorial Commentary:

It seems like barely a week goes by when a representative or scientific liaison of some company approaches me regarding new or improved biomarkers or prediction methodologies. The consistent finding is that they seem to all passionately believe that they bring immense value by providing the clinician with more information. Although that concept is intuitively appealing, it has become clear that, "no, I don't need more information—I need actionable information." Despite impressive statistics suggesting a value to the role of the markers discussed in this chapter and other technologies on the horizon, so far none of these candidates has delivered significant value to the clinician or patient, so none has developed broad acceptance in the diagnostic toolbox.

Nevertheless, further work in this arena is undeniably worthwhile based on inadequacy of the king of all markers—PSA. A number of investigators are performing exciting work in this arena, and we are hopeful that this will change soon. Concepts such as the use of panels as described, plus further investigation to define markers that can truly predict—not just give "more information"—are one of the more open fields of discovery at this point in time.

–J. Stephen Jones

References

1. Schroder FH, et al. Screening and prostate-cancer mortality in a randomized European study. N Engl J Med. 2009;360(13):1320–8.

2. Shariat SF, et al. Beyond prostate-specific antigen: new serologic biomarkers for improved diagnosis and management of prostate cancer. Rev Urol. 2004;6(2): 58–72.

3. Shariat SF, Karakiewicz PI. Perspectives on prostate cancer biomarkers. Eur Urol. 2008;54(1):8–10.

4. Shariat SF, et al. Tumor markers in prostate cancer I: blood-based markers. Acta Oncol. 2011;50 (Suppl 1): 61–75.

5. Atkinson AJ, et al. Biomarkers and surrogate endpoints: preferred definitions and conceptual framework. Clin Pharmacol Ther. 2001;69(3):89–95.

6. Bensalah K, Montorsi F, Shariat SF. Challenges of cancer biomarker profiling. Eur Urol. 2007;52(6): 1601–9.

7. Bensalah K, et al. New circulating biomarkers for prostate cancer. Prostate Cancer Prostatic Dis. 2008;11(2):112–20.

8. Verma M, Srivastava S. New cancer biomarkers deriving from NCI early detection research. Recent Results Cancer Res. 2003;163:72–84. discussion 264–6.

9. Winget MD, et al. Development of common data elements: the experience of and recommendations from the early detection research network. Int J Med Inform. 2003;70(1):41–8.

10. Shariat SF, et al. An updated catalog of prostate cancer predictive tools. Cancer. 2008;113(11):3075–99.

11. Shariat SF, et al. New blood-based biomarkers for the diagnosis, staging and prognosis of prostate cancer. BJU Int. 2008;101(6):675–83.

12. Shariat SF, et al. Plasminogen activation inhibitor-1 improves the predictive accuracy of prostate cancer nomograms. J Urol. 2007;178(4 Pt 1):1229–36. discussion 1236–7.

13. Kattan MW. Judging new markers by their ability to improve predictive accuracy. J Natl Cancer Inst. 2003;95(9):634–5.

14. Vickers AJ, Kattan MW, Daniel S. Method for evaluating prediction models that apply the results of randomized trials to individual patients. Trials. 2007; 8:14.

15. Kattan MW, et al. The addition of interleukin-6 soluble receptor and transforming growth factor beta1 improves a preoperative nomogram for predicting biochemical progression in patients with clinically localized prostate cancer. J Clin Oncol. 2003;21(19): 3573–9.

16. Shariat SF, et al. Improved prediction of disease relapse after radical prostatectomy through a panel of preoperative blood-based biomarkers. Clin Cancer Res. 2008;14(12):3785–91.

17. Vickers AJ, et al. A panel of kallikrein markers can reduce unnecessary biopsy for prostate cancer: data from the European Randomized Study of prostate cancer screening in Goteborg, Sweden. BMC Med. 2008;6:19.

18. Vickers AJ, et al. Systematic review of statistical methods used in molecular marker studies in cancer. Cancer. 2008;112(8):1862–8.

19. Thompson IM, et al. Operating characteristics of prostate-specific antigen in men with an initial PSA level of 3.0 ng/ml or lower. JAMA. 2005;294(1): 66–70.

20. Shariat SF, et al. Multiple biomarkers improve prediction of bladder cancer recurrence and mortality in patients undergoing cystectomy. Cancer. 2008;112(2): 315–25.

21. Vickers AJ, Elkin EB. Decision curve analysis: a novel method for evaluating prediction models. Med Decis Making. 2006;26(6):565–74.

22. Vickers AJ, et al. Extensions to decision curve analysis, a novel method for evaluating diagnostic tests, prediction models and molecular markers. BMC Med Inform Decis Mak. 2008;8:53.

23. Vickers AJ. Decision analysis for the evaluation of diagnostic tests, prediction models and molecular markers. Am Stat. 2008;62(4):314–20.

24. Elkin EB, Vickers AJ, Kattan MW. Primer: using decision analysis to improve clinical decision making in urology. Nat Clin Pract Urol. 2006;3(8): 439–48.

25. Lilja H, Ulmert D, Vickers AJ. Prostate-specific antigen and prostate cancer: prediction, detection and monitoring. Nat Rev Cancer. 2008;8(4):268–78.

26. Schroder FH, et al. Early detection of prostate cancer in 2007. Part 1: PSA and PSA kinetics. Eur Urol. 2008;53(3):468–77.

27. Shariat SF, Karam JA, Roehrborn CG. Blood biomarkers for prostate cancer detection and prognosis. Future Oncol. 2007;3(4):449–61.

28. Shariat SF, et al. Inventory of prostate cancer predictive tools. Curr Opin Urol. 2008;18(3):279–96.

29. Lilja H. Significance of different molecular forms of serum PSA. The free, noncomplexed form of PSA

versus that complexed to alpha 1-antichymotrypsin (Review). Urol Clin North Am. 1993;20(4):681–6.

30. Shariat SF, et al. Pre-operative percent free PSA predicts clinical outcomes in patients treated with radical prostatectomy with total PSA levels below 10 ng/ml. Eur Urol. 2006;49(2):293–302.

31. Catalona WJ, et al. Comparison of percent free PSA, PSA density, and age-specific PSA cutoffs for prostate cancer detection and staging. Urology. 2000;56(2): 255–60.

32. Mikolajczyk SD, et al. Free prostate-specific antigen in serum is becoming more complex. Urology. 2002;59(6):797–802.

33. Catalona WJ, et al. Use of the percentage of free prostate-specific antigen to enhance differentiation of prostate cancer from benign prostatic disease: a prospective multicenter clinical trial. JAMA. 1998;279(19):1542–7.

34. Woodrum DL, et al. Interpretation of free prostate specific antigen clinical research studies for the detection of prostate cancer. J Urol. 1998;159(1):5–12.

35. Canto EI, et al. Effects of systematic 12-core biopsy on the performance of percent free prostate specific antigen for prostate cancer detection. J Urol. 2004;172(3):900–4.

36. Lee R, et al. A meta-analysis of the performance characteristics of the free prostate-specific antigen test. Urology. 2006;67(4):762–8.

37. Catalona WJ, Smith DS, Ornstein DK. Prostate cancer detection in men with serum PSA concentrations of 2.6 to 4.0 ng/mL and benign prostate examination. Enhancement of specificity with free PSA measurements. JAMA. 1997;277(18):1452–5.

38. Rowe EW, et al. Prostate cancer detection in men with a 'normal' total prostate-specific antigen (PSA) level using percentage free PSA: a prospective screening study. BJU Int. 2005;95(9):1249–52.

39. Pepe P, et al. Prevalence and clinical significance of prostate cancer among 12,682 men with normal digital rectal examination, low PSA levels (< or =4 ng/ml) and percent free PSA cutoff values of 15 and 20%. Urol Int. 2007;78(4):308–12.

40. Graefen M, et al. Percent free prostate specific antigen is not an independent predictor of organ confinement or prostate specific antigen recurrence in unscreened patients with localized prostate cancer treated with radical prostatectomy. J Urol. 2002; 167(3):1306–9.

41. Mikolajczyk SD, et al. A truncated precursor form of prostate-specific antigen is a more specific serum marker of prostate cancer. Cancer Res. 2001;61(18): 6958–63.

42. Sokoll LJ, et al. Proenzyme psa for the early detection of prostate cancer in the 2.5–4.0 ng/ml total psa range: preliminary analysis. Urology. 2003;61(2): 274–6.

43. Catalona WJ, et al. Serum pro-prostate specific antigen preferentially detects aggressive prostate cancers in men with 2 to 4 ng/ml prostate specific antigen. J Urol. 2004;171(6 Pt 1):2239–44.

44. Catalona WJ, et al. Serum pro prostate specific antigen improves cancer detection compared to free and complexed prostate specific antigen in men with prostate specific antigen 2 to 4 ng/ml. J Urol. 2003;170(6 Pt 1):2181–5.

45. Stephan C, et al. A [−2]proPSA-based artificial neural network significantly improves differentiation between prostate cancer and benign prostatic diseases. Prostate. 2009;69(2):198–207.

46. Makarov DV, et al. Pro-prostate-specific antigen measurements in serum and tissue are associated with treatment necessity among men enrolled in expectant management for prostate cancer. Clin Cancer Res. 2009;15(23):7316–21.

47. Sokoll LJ, et al. A prospective, multicenter, National Cancer Institute early detection research network study of [−2]proPSA: improving prostate cancer detection and correlating with cancer aggressiveness. Cancer Epidemiol Biomarkers Prev. 2010;19(5): 1193–200.

48. Semjonow A, et al. Pre-analytical in-vitro stability of [−2]proPSA in blood and serum. Clin Biochem. 2010;43(10–11):926–8.

49. Mikolajczyk SD, et al. "BPSA," a specific molecular form of free prostate-specific antigen, is found predominantly in the transition zone of patients with nodular benign prostatic hyperplasia. Urology. 2000;55(1):41–5.

50. Canto EI, et al. Serum BPSA outperforms both total PSA and free PSA as a predictor of prostatic enlargement in men without prostate cancer. Urology. 2004;63(5):905–10. discussion 910–1.

51. Stephan C, et al. Benign prostatic hyperplasia-associated free prostate-specific antigen improves detection of prostate cancer in an artificial neural network. Urology. 2009;74(4):873–7.

52. Nurmikko P, et al. Discrimination of prostate cancer from benign disease by plasma measurement of intact, free prostate-specific antigen lacking an internal cleavage site at Lys145-Lys146. Clin Chem. 2001;47(8):1415–23.

53. Steuber T, et al. Association of free-prostate specific antigen subfractions and human glandular kallikrein 2 with volume of benign and malignant prostatic tissue. Prostate. 2005;63(1):13–8.

54. Yousef GM, Diamandis EP. The new human tissue kallikrein gene family: structure, function, and association to disease. Endocr Rev. 2001;22(2): 184–204.

55. Nam RK, et al. Serum human glandular kallikrein-2 protease levels predict the presence of prostate cancer among men with elevated prostate-specific antigen. J Clin Oncol. 2000;18(5):1036–42.

56. Becker C, et al. Clinical value of human glandular kallikrein 2 and free and total prostate-specific antigen in serum from a population of men with prostate-specific antigen levels 3.0 ng/mL or greater. Urology. 2000;55(5):694–9.

57. Becker C, et al. Discrimination of men with prostate cancer from those with benign disease by

measurements of human glandular kallikrein 2 (HK2) in serum. J Urol. 2000;163(1):311–6.

58. Haese A, et al. Human glandular kallikrein 2 levels in serum for discrimination of pathologically organ-confined from locally-advanced prostate cancer in total PSA-levels below 10 ng/ml. Prostate. 2001;49(2): 101–9.

59. Kwiatkowski MK, et al. In prostatism patients the ratio of human glandular kallikrein to free PSA improves the discrimination between prostate cancer and benign hyperplasia within the diagnostic "gray zone" of total PSA 4 to 10 ng/mL. Urology. 1998;52(3):360–5.

60. Recker F, et al. The importance of human glandular kallikrein and its correlation with different prostate specific antigen serum forms in the detection of prostate carcinoma. Cancer. 1998;83(12):2540–7.

61. Kurek R, et al. Prognostic value of combined "triple"-reverse transcription-PCR analysis for prostate-specific antigen, human kallikrein 2, and prostate-specific membrane antigen mRNA in peripheral blood and lymph nodes of prostate cancer patients. Clin Cancer Res. 2004;10(17):5808–14.

62. Duffy MJ. Urokinase-type plasminogen activator: a potent marker of metastatic potential in human cancers. Biochem Soc Trans. 2002;30(2):207–10.

63. Gupta A, et al. Predictive value of the differential expression of the urokinase plasminogen activation axis in radical prostatectomy patients. Eur Urol. 2009;55(5):1124–33.

64. Steuber T, et al. Free PSA isoforms and intact and cleaved forms of urokinase plasminogen activator receptor in serum improve selection of patients for prostate cancer biopsy. Int J Cancer. 2007;120(7): 1499–504.

65. Hienert G, et al. Urokinase-type plasminogen activator as a marker for the formation of distant metastases in prostatic carcinomas. J Urol. 1988;140(6): 1466–9.

66. Miyake H, et al. Elevation of serum levels of urokinase-type plasminogen activator and its receptor is associated with disease progression and prognosis in patients with prostate cancer. Prostate. 1999;39(2): 123–9.

67. Shariat SF, et al. Association of the circulating levels of the urokinase system of plasminogen activation with the presence of prostate cancer and invasion, progression, and metastasis. J Clin Oncol. 2007;25(4):349–55.

68. Shariat SF, et al. Preoperative plasma levels of transforming growth factor beta(1) (TGF-beta(1)) strongly predict progression in patients undergoing radical prostatectomy. J Clin Oncol. 2001;19(11): 2856–64.

69. Truong LD, et al. Association of transforming growth factor-beta 1 with prostate cancer: an immunohistochemical study. Hum Pathol. 1993;24(1):4–9.

70. Shariat SF, et al. Association of pre- and postoperative plasma levels of transforming growth factor beta(1) and interleukin 6 and its soluble receptor

with prostate cancer progression. Clin Cancer Res. 2004;10(6): 1992–9.

71. Shariat SF, et al. Tissue expression of transforming growth factor-beta1 and its receptors: correlation with pathologic features and biochemical progression in patients undergoing radical prostatectomy. Urology. 2004;63(6):1191–7.

72. Shariat SF, et al. Preoperative plasma levels of transforming growth factor beta(1) strongly predict clinical outcome in patients with bladder carcinoma. Cancer. 2001;92(12):2985–92.

73. Ivanovic V, et al. Elevated plasma levels of TGF-beta 1 in patients with invasive prostate cancer. Nat Med. 1995;1(4):282–4.

74. Hobisch A, et al. Interleukin-6 regulates prostate-specific protein expression in prostate carcinoma cells by activation of the androgen receptor. Cancer Res. 1998;58(20):4640–5.

75. Giri D, Ozen M, Ittmann M. Interleukin-6 is an autocrine growth factor in human prostate cancer. Am J Pathol. 2001;159(6):2159–65.

76. Michalaki V, et al. Serum levels of IL-6 and TNF-alpha correlate with clinicopathological features and patient survival in patients with prostate cancer. Br J Cancer. 2004;90(12):2312–6.

77. Nakashima J, et al. Serum interleukin 6 as a prognostic factor in patients with prostate cancer. Clin Cancer Res. 2000;6(7):2702–6.

78. Stark JR, et al. Circulating prediagnostic interleukin-6 and C-reactive protein and prostate cancer incidence and mortality. Int J Cancer. 2009;124(11):2683–9.

79. Cheifetz S, et al. Endoglin is a component of the transforming growth factor-beta receptor system in human endothelial cells. J Biol Chem. 1992;267(27): 19027–30.

80. Wikstrom P, et al. Endoglin (CD105) is expressed on immature blood vessels and is a marker for survival in prostate cancer. Prostate. 2002;51(4):268–75.

81. Fujita K, et al. Endoglin (CD105) as a urinary and serum marker of prostate cancer. Int J Cancer. 2009;124(3):664–9.

82. Karam JA, et al. Use of preoperative plasma endoglin for prediction of lymph node metastasis in patients with clinically localized prostate cancer. Clin Cancer Res. 2008;14(5):1418–22.

83. Svatek RS, et al. Preoperative plasma endoglin levels predict biochemical progression after radical prostatectomy. Clin Cancer Res. 2008;14(11):3362–6.

84. Rubin MA, et al. Alpha-Methylacyl coenzyme A racemase as a tissue biomarker for prostate cancer. JAMA. 2002;287(13):1662–70.

85. Jiang Z, et al. Alpha-methylacyl-CoA racemase: a multi-institutional study of a new prostate cancer marker. Histopathology. 2004;45(3):218–25.

86. Sreekumar A, et al. Humoral immune response to alpha-methylacyl-CoA racemase and prostate cancer. J Natl Cancer Inst. 2004;96(11):834–43.

87. Cardillo MR, et al. Can p503s, p504s and p510s gene expression in peripheral-blood be useful as a

marker of prostatic cancer? BMC Cancer. 2005;
5:111.

88. Bradley SV, et al. Serum antibodies to huntingtin interacting protein-1: a new blood test for prostate cancer. Cancer Res. 2005;65(10):4126–33.

89. Wang X, et al. Autoantibody signatures in prostate cancer. N Engl J Med. 2005;353(12):1224–35.

90. Prior C, et al. Use of a combination of biomarkers in serum and urine to improve detection of prostate cancer. World J Urol. 2010;28(6):681–6.

91. Cao DL, et al. A multiplex model of combining gene-based, protein-based, and metabolite-based with positive and negative markers in urine for the early diagnosis of prostate cancer. Prostate. 2011;71(7): 700–10.

92. Svatek RS, et al. Pre-treatment biomarker levels improve the accuracy of post-prostatectomy nomogram for prediction of biochemical recurrence. Prostate. 2009;69(8):886–94.

93. Vickers A, et al. Reducing unnecessary biopsy during prostate cancer screening using a four-kallikrein panel: an independent replication. J Clin Oncol. 2010;28(15):2493–8.

94. Benchikh A, et al. A panel of kallikrein markers can predict outcome of prostate biopsy following clinical work-up: an independent validation study from the European Randomized Study of prostate cancer screening, France. BMC Cancer. 2010;10:635.

95. Vickers AJ, et al. Impact of recent screening on predicting the outcome of prostate cancer biopsy in men with elevated prostate-specific antigen: data from the European Randomized Study of prostate cancer screening in Gothenburg, Sweden. Cancer. 2010; 116(11):2612–20.

96. Vickers AJ, et al. A four-kallikrein panel predicts prostate cancer in men with recent screening: data from the European Randomized Study of screening for prostate cancer, Rotterdam. Clin Cancer Res. 2010;16(12):3232–9.

97. Gupta A, et al. A four-kallikrein panel for the prediction of repeat prostate biopsy: data from the European Randomized Study of prostate cancer screening in Rotterdam, Netherlands. Br J Cancer. 2010;103(5): 708–14

98. Shariat SF, et al. Plasma levels of interleukin-6 and its soluble receptor are associated with prostate cancer progression and metastasis. Urology. 2001;58(6): 1008–15.

99. Shariat SF, et al. Association of preoperative plasma levels of vascular endothelial growth factor and soluble vascular cell adhesion molecule-1 with lymph node status and biochemical progression after radical prostatectomy. J Clin Oncol. 2004;22(9):1655–63.

100. Shariat SF, et al. External validation of a biomarker-based preoperative nomogram predicts biochemical recurrence after radical prostatectomy. J Clin Oncol. 2008;26(9):1526–31.

101. Shariat SF, et al. Detection of clinically significant, occult prostate cancer metastases in lymph nodes using a splice variant-specific rt-PCR assay for human glandular kallikrein. J Clin Oncol. 2003; 21(7):1223–31.

Prediction Models in Prostate Cancer Diagnosis

8

Carvell T. Nguyen and Michael W. Kattan

Introduction

The contemporary management of prostate cancer has been based upon early detection and treatment of disease when it is still organ-confined and presumably more amenable to cure. Indeed, of the many advances in the field of prostate cancer over the last few decades (e.g., nerve-sparing prostatectomy, brachytherapy, conformal radiation), none have arguably had a greater impact on outcomes than early detection through PSA screening. A significant downward stage migration has been observed, with the vast majority of patients now diagnosed with organ-confined disease [1]. This has been associated with an increased rate of cure with definitive treatment as well as a reduction in the risk of cancer-specific mortality [1, 2].

Yet, despite the substantial increase in prostate cancer detection with current screening regimens, there is still no test, including PSA or any of its variants, that predicts cancer with perfect accuracy. In the PSA era, physicians have traditionally relied on a PSA cutoff and their own clinical judgment for decision-making regarding the need for prostate biopsy. This method of decision-making is inherently biased and inaccurate, leading to over- or underestimation of the positive biopsy rate and either unnecessary biopsies or missed disease, respectively.

To address the suboptimal predictive accuracy of screening regimens based on PSA alone, researchers have developed statistical models, such as the Prostate Cancer Prevention Trial (PCPT) risk calculator, to provide more accurate estimates of the risk of cancer in an individual patient. Furthermore, there is the hope that such decision aids may provide better insight into the tumor biology of prostate cancer, which can be quite variable between individual patients and difficult to foresee based on just one clinical factor (e.g., PSA).

Indeed, given that the majority of men diagnosed with prostate cancer will not die of their disease [3], there is concern that screening has led to overdetection and overtreatment of men with indolent disease who are being exposed to unnecessary morbidity and healthcare costs. Therefore, more accurate prediction of the risk and aggressiveness of cancer has profound medical, ethical, and economic implications.

C.T. Nguyen, M.D., Ph.D.
Urologic Oncology, Glickman Urological & Kidney Institute, Cleveland Clinic, 9500 Euclid Ave Q10, Cleveland, OH 44195, USA
e-mail: nguyenc@ccf.org

M.W. Kattan, Ph.D. (✉)
Department of Quantitative Health Sciences, Cleveland Clinic, 9500 Euclid Avenue, JJN3-01, Cleveland, OH 44195, USA
e-mail: kattanm@ccf.org

J.S. Jones (ed.), *Prostate Cancer Diagnosis: PSA, Biopsy and Beyond*, Current Clinical Urology,
DOI 10.1007/978-1-62703-188-2_8, © Springer Science+Business Media New York 2013

Rationale for Formal Prediction Tools in Diagnosing Prostate Cancer

Predicting any clinical endpoint using only clinical judgment or a single clinical variable is flawed because such simple methods of risk estimation cannot account for the complex tumor biology of prostate cancer. In fact, despite substantially improving early detection of cancer, PSA screening alone demonstrates a relatively low accuracy for predicting disease, ranging from 52% to 60% [4–7]. The sensitivity and specificity of PSA testing is approximately 70% and 90%, respectively, if the traditional cutoff of 4.0 is utilized [8]. Although superior to DRE and TRUS, such performance characteristics will lead to a significant number of false-negatives and false-positives, attributes that are not ideal for any screening test.

The suboptimal accuracy of PSA testing is likely related to the dichotomous cutoff system that has been used to define "normal" levels of PSA and the threshold at which a prostate biopsy should be performed. Such a system fails to account for the fact that PSA is a continuous variable rather than a categorical one. Data from the Prostate Cancer Prevention Trial (PCPT) showed that a significant number of men (~15%) with PSA levels below the traditional threshold of 4.0 ng/mL can have prostate cancer; for example, nearly 7% of men with a PSA<0.5 ng/mL were diagnosed with cancer [7]. Based on such data, the investigators concluded that PSA levels demonstrate a continuous spectrum of prostate cancer risk for which there is no lower limit below which a man's risk of prostate cancer is zero. Moreover, there is no PSA level with sufficient sensitivity and specificity that can be used as a reliable cutoff for diagnosing cancer.

There are also several confounding factors that can affect PSA levels independently of malignancy, thereby reducing its specificity as a screening tool. These include genetic and racial variations in PSA production, drug-induced changes (e.g., with finasteride), and patient-specific factors such as body mass index [9, 10].

Variations on PSA-Based Screening

Investigators have evaluated the performance of screening tests that utilize more sophisticated PSA-related parameters, hoping to improve upon the diagnostic accuracy of standard PSA testing. As mentioned, simple PSA cutoffs demonstrate suboptimal specificity for detecting prostate cancer. One reason may be the normal increase in PSA levels that occurs with age such that many older men can present with elevated PSA levels without harboring prostate cancer. There is evidence that using age-adjusted PSA levels reduces overdetection and false-positives but at the potential cost of inducing unnecessary biopsies in younger men and missing cancers in older men [11].

PSA velocity has also been evaluated as an alternative screening test, but the data are equivocal regarding its predictive capability. Various methods for determining a significant PSA velocity have been evaluated, including percentage increases as well as actual rates. Smith and Catalona reported that a PSA velocity cutoff of 0.75 ng/mL/year maximized the sensitivity and specificity for predicting cancer in men with normal PSA levels [12]. Other investigators have reported that increasing PSA velocity is associated with increased PPV and specificity for cancer on biopsy [13, 14]. However, this appears to come at the cost of reduced overall sensitivity [14]. Furthermore, multivariate analyses including PSA velocity with other prebiopsy variables, such as age, PSA, prostate volume, and DRE findings, have not found it to be an independent predictor of disease [7, 14].

Traditional PSA testing measures total PSA levels in the blood, which consists of both free and complexed forms of the protein. Assays are available that can detect the free form of PSA, while complexed PSA is calculated by subtracting free PSA from total PSA. Fractionated PSA (complexed or free) has demonstrated a low specificity for prostate cancer [15], making it unsuitable as a standalone screening assay. Investigators have also evaluated the utility of combining fractionated PSA with total PSA.

Hoffman and colleagues performed a meta-analysis assessing the accuracy of free-to-total PSA ratio in predicting prostate cancer, finding that there was no percent free PSA level that optimized both sensitivity and specificity of PSA screening .[16]. However, lower percent free PSA has been linked with more aggressive prostate cancer (e.g., associated with a larger tumor volume and a higher risk of extraprostatic spread) [17] and may have utility in the identification of patients more likely to progress and, therefore, benefit from intervention.

PSA density, which is calculated by dividing serum PSA by prostate volume (derived from a TRUS examination), has been compared to standard PSA testing but has not been shown to be independently predictive of prostate cancer [18, 19]. PSA density of the transition zone alone has also been studied and may have greater utility than total PSA density. One study showed that it had the highest predictive accuracy for prostate cancer of any PSA variant [20], while other data suggested that it may be useful in adjusting for benign causes of elevated PSA (e.g., BPH) [21]

Prediction Models as Alternatives to PSA and Its Derivatives

Taken together, the data on PSA as a dichotomous marker or any of its variants indicate inadequate predictive accuracy, resulting in either unnecessary prostate biopsies or missing disease altogether. In order to make an informed decision about the necessity of prostate biopsy, patients require unbiased, reliable predictions regarding their individual risk of cancer. Formal decision aids, such as risk groupings, probability tables, and nomograms, incorporate multiple predictive variables in a statistical model that generate more accurate estimates than single variables or physicians can [22].

The key factors that measure accuracy and quality of any prediction model include discrimination and calibration. Discrimination is the ability to predict which patients will or will not demonstrate the outcome of interest. It is often expressed in terms of the concordance index, which is essentially the area under the receiver operating characteristic (ROC) curve. The concordance index is the probability that, given two randomly selected patients, the patient with the worse outcome is, in fact, predicted to have a worse outcome. Calibration is a measure of how closely the predicted risk generated by the model approximates observed rates of the endpoint of interest. A prediction tool that is perfectly calibrated should demonstrate a 1:1 relationship between predicted and actual outcomes, resulting in a calibration plot with a 45° slope. Utilizing these criteria, comparative studies suggest that nomograms predict outcomes more accurately than any other method of risk estimation, including risk groupings, neural networks, or probability tables [23–29]. Moreover, nomograms have been shown to surpass clinical experts at outcomes prediction [22, 30].

The greater accuracy of nomograms can be explained by several reasons. First, they incorporate patient-specific values and generate risk estimates that are tailored to the individual. In contrast, other types of prediction models often depend on average values derived from heterogeneous populations that may not be similar to an individual patient. For example, the predictive capability of risk groupings is based on the assumption that all patients within a given risk group are equal, when, in fact, such groups can be quite dissimilar. Such heterogeneity blunts the predictive value of risk assignments and likely explains why risk groupings predict less accurately than nomograms (Fig. 8.1) [26, 29]. Moreover, a patient presumably cares about his individual prognosis and not about the outcome of a group that may not even be representative of his specific clinical situation.

Second, nomograms are based upon comprehensive statistical models (e.g., a multiple regression equation) that analyze multiple variables simultaneously, allowing a greater number of predictors to be considered. Models with more prognostic factors are more likely to reflect the complexity of a disease like prostate cancer and, therefore, predict outcomes more accurately.

CaPSURE Heterogeneity within Risk Groups

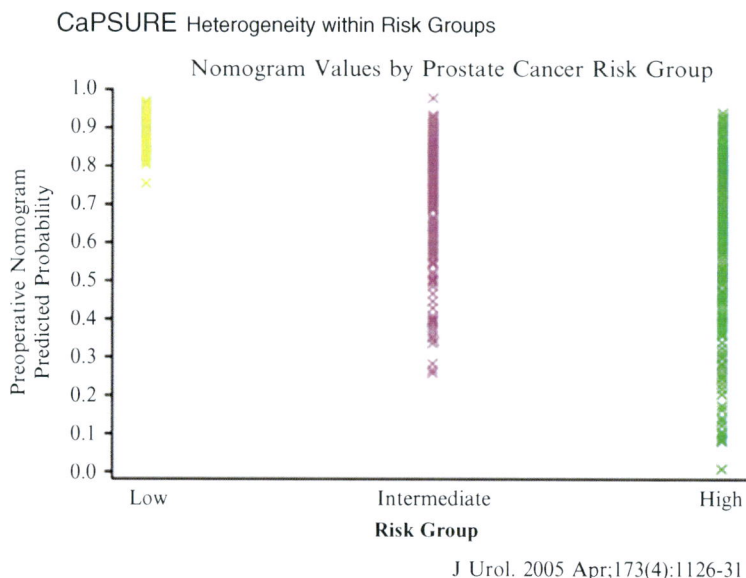

Nomogram Values by Prostate Cancer Risk Group

J Urol. 2005 Apr;173(4):1126-31

Fig. 8.1 Demonstration of the heterogeneity within risk groups when compared against the outcomes predicted by a preoperative nomogram for prostate cancer

Moreover, continuous variables can be kept continuous in a nomogram, whereas other prediction models, like risk groupings or probability tables, require creation of cut points that are often arbitrary with little prognostic basis. Categorizing a continuous variable, such as PSA level, blunts its prognostic value and lowers the overall accuracy of the model [31].

Finally, the complex statistical model behind a nomogram can be presented in a simple graphical format that avoids complex calculations (Fig. 8.2). Nomograms typically consist of sets of axes, each of which represents a predictive variable. Each variable is represented by a scale, with each value of that variable assigned a specific number of points according to its prognostic significance. In a final pair of axes, the total point value from all the variables is converted to the probability of reaching the endpoint. In addition, many nomograms, including the PCPT and Sunnybrook nomograms reviewed in this chapter, are now available as online software presented in a "fill in the blank" format that further facilitates everyday use. These online tools utilize the same statistical models that underlie the original nomograms.

Considered together, these advantages explain why nomograms have become widespread in general medical practice and have been adopted with particular enthusiasm by the urologic oncology community. The natural history of prostate cancer can be divided into a series of clinical states from diagnosis to death from prostate cancer (or death from competing causes) (Fig. 8.3) [32]. Many nomograms have been developed and validated for use in most of the prostate cancer clinical states. Although the pretreatment and posttreatment clinical states are the well represented among current nomograms, a growing number of nomograms are being published for use in pre-diagnosis patient counseling.

Nomograms for Prostate Cancer Diagnosis

A number of nomograms have been developed to predict the probability of cancer prior to biopsy and have consistently demonstrated greater accuracy than other methods of estimation (Table 8.1) [7, 33–38]. Such decision aids can be very helpful in formulating screening regimens as well as active surveillance protocols. By identifying patients at high risk of disease, unnecessary biopsies, and their attendant morbidity, can be avoided.

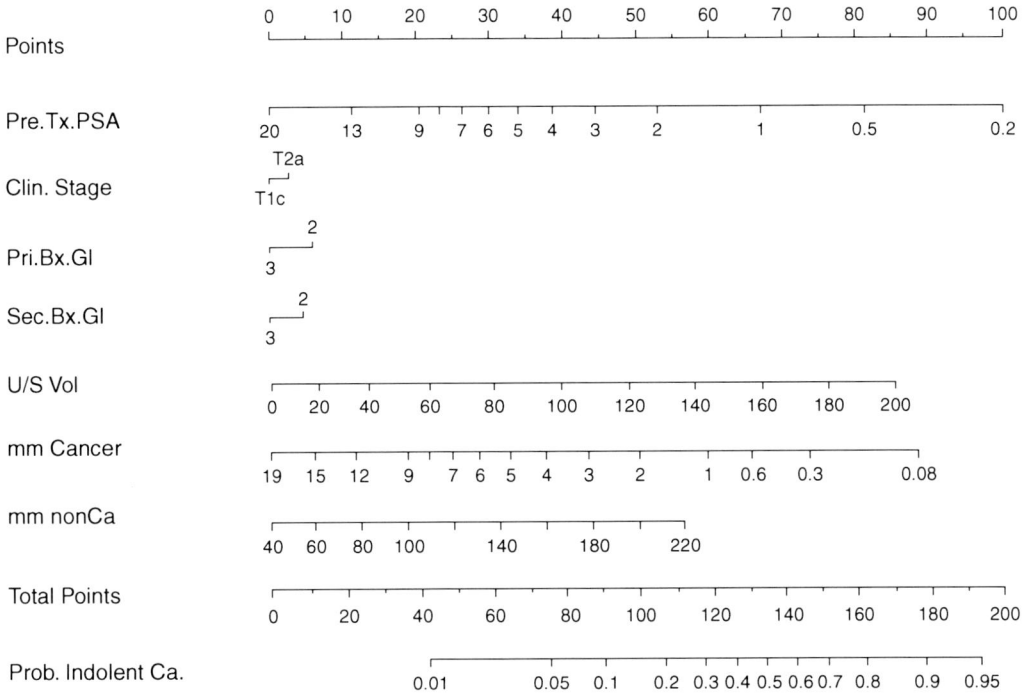

Instructions for Physician: Locate the Patient's PSA on the **PreTx PSA axis**. Draw a line straight upwards to the **Points** axis to determine how many points towards having an indolent cancer the patient receives for his PSA. Repeat this process for the remaining axes, each time drawing straight upward to the **Points** axis. Sum the points achieved for each predictor and locate this sum on the **Total Points** axis. Draw a line straight down to find the patient's probability of having indolent cancer.

Instruction to Patient: "Mr.X, if we had 100 men exactly like you, we would expect <predicted probability from nomogram * 100 > to have indolent cancer."

Fig. 8.2 Nomogram predicting the presence of indolent prostate cancer (pathological Gleason score ≤ 3 + 3, cancer volume < 0.5 cc, organ-confined) based on pretreatment PSA level (Pre.Tx.PSA), clinical stage (Clin.Stage), primary (Pri.Bx.Gl) and secondary (Sec.Bx.Gl) biopsy Gleason grade, prostate volume by ultrasound (U/S Vol), length of cancer (mm) in biopsy specimens (mm cancer), and length of noncancer (mm) in biopsy specimens (mm nonCa)

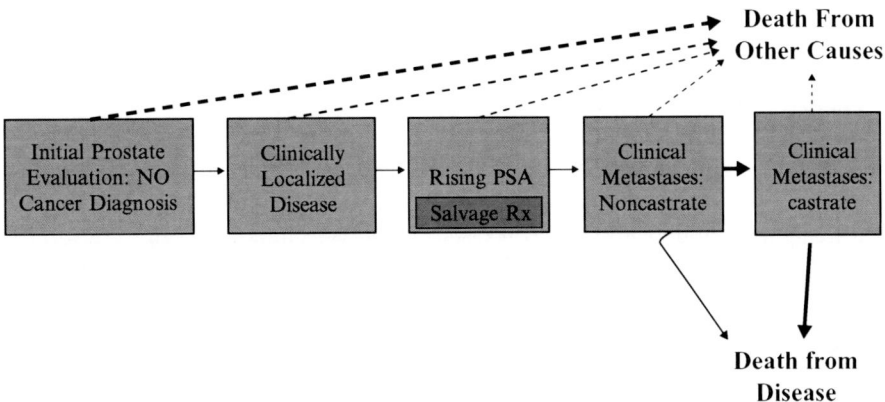

Fig. 8.3 Clinical states model of prostate cancer progression [32]. *Dashed line arrows* indicate pathways from a clinical state to a non-prostate cancer-related mortality; *solid line arrows* indicate pathways from a clinical state to a prostate cancer-related mortality

Table 8.1 Nomograms for prostate cancer diagnosis

Nomogram	Outcome predicted	CI	Variables
Yanke et al. 2005	Probability of cancer at repeat biopsy	0.71	Age, DRE findings, # previous negative cores, previous HGPIN and/or ASAP, PSA, PSA slope, and family history of prostate cancer
Karakiewicz et al. 2005	Probability of cancer at initial sextant biopsy	0.71	Age, DRE findings, PSA, % free PSA
Walz et al. 2006	Probability of cancer at saturation biopsy after previously negative biopsy	0.72	Age, % free PSA, prostate volume, TZ volume
Chun et al. 2007	Probability of cancer at initial extended biopsy	0.73–0.77	Age, DRE findings, PSA, % free PSA, density of cores
Chun et al. 2007	Probability of cancer at repeat extended biopsy	0.77	Age, DRE, PSA, % free PSA, # previous biopsy sessions, prostate volume
Walz et al. 2008	Probability of cancer at biopsy	0.69	DRE findings, % free PSA
Roobol et al. 2009	Probability of cancer at biopsy	NA	PSA, prostate volume, DRE, TRUS findings

CI concordance index, *DRE* digital rectal examination, *PSA* prostate-specific antigen, *TZ* transition zone, *HGPIN* high-grade prostatic intraepithelial neoplasia, *ASAP* atypical small acinar proliferation, *TRUS* transrectal ultrasound

The Prostate Cancer Prevention Trial (PCPT) risk calculator was one of the first nomograms to see widespread clinical use. Data from the PCPT demonstrated that PSA is actually associated with a continuum of prostate cancer risk for which there is no lower limit or "normal" cutoff. Along with the identification of other factors that significantly affect the risk of prostate cancer, these findings prompted the development of a continuous multivariable risk calculator designed to provide individualized estimates of cancer risk and determine the need for a biopsy. The nomogram was developed by Thompson and colleagues using data from the 5,519 men in the placebo arm of the PCPT trial who underwent biopsy for abnormal DRE, PSA>4 ng/mL, or trial's end. Besides PSA, the investigators incorporated age, ethnicity, family history, DRE findings, and previous history of negative biopsy to estimate the risk of overall as well as high-grade prostate cancer. Using the original study cohort as internal validation, the nomogram demonstrated concordance indices of 70.2% and 69.8% for overall and high-grade cancer, respectively.

Due to its accessibility as an online tool with simple "plug and play" operation, the nomogram has seen widespread clinical use despite the fact that this level of discrimination is only incrementally better than that associated with the use of PSA alone, indicating that the other clinical factors in the nomogram added very little predictive value. The PCPT risk calculator has been validated on external datasets, demonstrating comparable accuracy. For example, investigators from the San Antonio Center of Biomarkers of Risk for Prostate Cancer (SABOR) and Johns Hopkins reported concordance indices of 65.5% and 66.7%, respectively, for detection of overall cancer on biopsy using the risk calculator on their patient cohorts [4, 6]. When compared against PSA levels alone, the SABOR group found no significant improvement in predictive accuracy with the nomogram, while Hernandez and colleagues at Johns Hopkins reported a modest increase in performance with the risk calculator (61.9% vs. 66.7%, $p < 0.001$) in 1,108 men.

The largest external validation of the PCPT nomogram was performed by the Cleveland Clinic using a dataset of 3,482 men [5]. They reported concordance indices of only 57% and 60% for overall and high-grade prostate cancer, respectively, although both were still superior to the prediction accuracy of PSA testing alone in their series (52.2% and 55.5% for all cancer and high-grade cancer, respectively). Furthermore, the nomogram demonstrated regression to the mean calibration problems in their validation cohort, underestimating the actual incidence of prostate cancer at low predicted risks and overestimating at higher predicted risks [5].

Such data suggest that the PCPT nomogram may not be completely generalizable to contemporary populations of men being screened for prostate cancer using current extended biopsy techniques. The reduced accuracy of the calculator in the Cleveland Clinic study may be due to several limitations that characterized the original PCPT cohort. For example, the PCPT study cohort demonstrated homogeneous demographics not representative of the general male population within the USA, with only 4.4% of the men categorized as nonwhite (compared to 14.7% nonwhite in the Cleveland Clinic cohort). Furthermore, most men in the PCPT study underwent sextant biopsies, which have been shown to detect fewer cancers than modern extended biopsy schemes (e.g., at least 10 cores) [39–41]. These observations emphasize the need to continuously validate and/or reconstruct multivariable models as clinical practice evolves. The original PCPT dataset was derived from men screened in an earlier era marked by the now antiquated sextant biopsy technique, theoretically underestimating the true risk of cancer in a modern population undergoing extended biopsy. In addition, the PCPT occurred earlier in the "PSA era" when undiagnosed prostate cancer was theoretically higher in the general population.

A Canadian study from the Sunnybrook Health Sciences Center, including 3,108 men who underwent biopsy, was the basis of another nomogram designed to estimate individual risk of prostate cancer [42]. Predictive factors in the Sunnybrook nomogram include PSA, free-to-total PSA ratio, DRE findings, age, family history, ethnicity, and urinary symptoms. As with the PCPT nomogram, models were constructed to calculate the risk of over- and high-grade cancer, demonstrating concordance indices of 0.74 and 0.77, respectively. As with other diagnostic prediction tools, the Sunnybrook nomogram predicted cancer with slightly greater accuracy than PSA alone, which was associated with CIs of 0.62 and 0.69 for any and high-grade prostate cancer, respectively. As with the PCPT, the patient dataset was not as ethnically diverse as the general population, with Caucasians, Asians, and blacks making up 82%, 9%, and 9% of the cohort, respectively. Unlike

the PCPT nomogram, this nomogram has not yet been validated on any external patient cohorts. As such, its applicability and predictive accuracy in other patient populations remains undefined.

The European male population is also represented among available diagnostic nomograms. For example, using data from 1,850 men screened and biopsied in the Rotterdam section of the European Randomised Study of Screening for Prostate Cancer (ERSSPC), Roobol and colleagues developed a nomogram that predicts the chances of a positive initial biopsy using PSA, prostate volume, DRE, and transrectal ultrasound findings [35]. Compared to PSA alone, this nomogram increased the accuracy of cancer detection and decreased the number of unnecessary prostate biopsies by a third. Using a cutoff of 12.5% for the probability of having a positive biopsy, the positive predictive value of this model was 38%.

One advantage of this nomogram compared to its American and Canadian counterparts is its incorporation of prostate volume which has been found to be predictive of cancer [43] and may also adjust for the impact of benign prostatic hypertrophy on the predictive value of PSA. There are also data that indicate significant sampling errors in patients with larger gland volumes [44]. A major limitation of this nomogram is the lack of measurement of discrimination (e.g., using AUC or concordance index), making it difficult to compare its accuracy with that of other nomograms. In addition, the nomogram does not differentiate between low- and high-risk cancers, raising the possibility of overdiagnosis of biologically indolent disease. Finally, it has not been externally validated, and the patients were biopsied using antiquated sextant protocols, which are inadequate for cancer detection, again suggesting the question of how generalizable such a nomogram is to the general male population.

Besides calculating an individual's risk of cancer and determining the need for biopsy, nomograms can also aid biopsy planning and determine the optimal number of cores to be taken. The Vienna nomogram was developed to determine the minimum number of cores required to detect cancers with at least 90% certainty as a function of patient age and gland volume [45, 46]. In building the model, the investigators found that the standard sextant biopsy was inadequate for cancer detection in most cases, particularly in younger men or those with larger glands. Only in men older than 70 years of age was a sextant biopsy indicated in order to avoid overdiagnosis and overtreatment [46].

Additional diagnostic nomograms and their predictive factors are summarized in Table 8.1. Comparative studies will be needed to validate these diagnostic nomograms and confirm that they are more useful than PSA alone for cancer detection. However, they do represent the first steps toward a potentially more discriminating, responsible, and cost-effective approach to screening.

Limitations of Nomograms

Nomograms currently offer the most accurate means of predicting cancer prior to biopsy, but they do have limitations that must be considered when using their risk estimates in patient counseling and decision-making. For example, there are no data demonstrating that use of nomogram-generated predictions has improved patient outcomes in prostate cancer. Clinicians should also be aware that existing nomograms do not predict with perfect accuracy. Despite improving upon the accuracy of PSA testing alone, no published diagnostic nomogram has reported a concordance index of 0.80 or above.

Important, current diagnostic nomograms may not be generalizable to all patients being screened for prostate cancer. Most published nomograms are constructed and validated using patients treated at single academic centers, whose demographics and outcomes may be very different from those of patients treated at community hospitals. Even among academic centers, there can be institutional disparities in the quality and availability of medical care as well as nonuniformity in the way in which data are collected and interpreted. Moreover, such disparities make it difficult to compare the relative accuracy of rival nomograms not constructed on a neutral data set,

that is, not compared in a head-to-head analysis [47]. As such, the concordance indices listed in Table 8.1 for the various prediction models are for reference only and are not meant to be used as an indicator of one model's superiority or inferiority relative to any other model.

The exponential growth of new prostate cancer nomograms over the last decade poses another problem for their use in clinical practice. Although diagnostic nomograms represent only a small proportion of the total number of prostate cancer nomograms, there are still multiple alternative models to consider, and there is a lack of head-to-head studies comparing alternative nomograms that predict the same endpoint. Using published criteria to determine the accuracy and quality of alternative nomograms [48], a clinician can determine which is the preferred model for prostate cancer diagnosis.

Another potential criticism of using nomograms in clinical practice pertains to whether the average patient has the literacy or numeracy required to comprehend the data from these statistical models. As mentioned, nomograms are presented in a simple graphical format that avoids complex calculations and does not require the patient to understand the complex mathematics and statistics that govern nomograms. Indeed, there are data to suggest that the majority of people, regardless of educational level, are able to understand and interpret tabular data for comparative purposes [49].

Considering all of these potential limitations, nomogram predictions should not be the only factor in determining whether a patient should undergo prostate biopsy. Such a decision does indeed benefit from the more accurate risk estimates provided by nomograms but also should be based upon published data, physician judgment and experience, as well as patient preference.

Future Directions

Because no currently available nomogram predicts with perfect accuracy, there is a need to continuously improve and validate current models as well as develop new nomograms. Knowledge of the criteria that determine the quality and utility of a nomogram can provide direction for improvement. The quality of a nomogram is dependent not only upon its predictive accuracy but also on the methods utilized to construct the model. Ideally, the patient cohort on whom the nomogram was constructed should be representative of the general population of patients to whom the model will be applied. The nomogram should be based on a sufficient number of cases that also include a large proportion that reach the endpoint of interest. The nomograms described in this chapter were based on study populations with skewed demographics and, if not already performed, should be subjected to external validation using large patient cohorts from other institutions. This can adjust for bias due to small sample size of the internal dataset as well as that due to regional differences in patient demographics.

Identification and incorporation of additional predictive markers can also improve accuracy in predicting an endpoint. For example, novel biomarkers that correlate with the presence of prostate cancer, such as PCA3, may increase the accuracy of diagnostic nomograms [50]. A nomogram should also incorporate clinical factors that are reliable, routinely employed in the clinical setting, and easy to obtain. A nomogram that utilizes parameters that require specialized or expensive assays or cumbersome procedures may be impractical for general use. Lastly, the generalizability of a nomogram can also be reduced if the datasets have a large proportion of missing information or if data were incorrectly recorded and/or entered into the database.

The performance of current diagnostic nomograms may therefore be improved by updating the model on a more contemporary population that reflects current demographics and clinical practice patterns, incorporating additional predictive variables (e.g., novel biomarkers), and ensuring high-quality and uniform data collection and entry methods. However, even with increased predictive accuracy, current PSA-based screening tools still lack the ability to consistently distinguish the minority of patients who have aggressive tumors from those whose disease will remain organ-confined and nonlethal. Novel biomarkers and prognostic factors that can predict the natural history of a given patient's cancer (i.e., be specific for high-grade cancer) are required to prevent the overdiagnosis and overtreatment of clinically insignificant disease. The future of prostate cancer screening will be based upon individualized risk estimation afforded by more powerful multivariable nomograms that incorporate such predictive factors, allowing rational and judicious application of biopsy and/or definitive therapy.

Conclusions

Predictive models, such as the PCPT and Sunnybrook nomograms, currently offer the best means of estimating prostate cancer risk in the individual patient and can help determine the need for prostate biopsy as well as the optimal number of cores needed to detect disease. However, these nomograms do not have perfect accuracy, and they may not be generalizable to every man being screened for cancer. Their performance may be improved by updating the model on a more contemporary population that reflects current demographics and clinical practice patterns, incorporating additional clinical variables (e.g., novel biomarkers) with improved predictive abilities, and standardizing data collection methods between institutions. It should be emphasized that diagnostic nomograms do not make treatment recommendations, are not surrogates for physician expertise, nor do they provide definitive information on the risk of indolent versus aggressive disease. Thus, the contemporary role of diagnostic nomograms is to provide patients with the best estimates of their personal risk of cancer, which combined with physician expertise and patient input, can then form the basis for truly informed decision-making.

Editorial Commentary:
Dr. Kattan essentially created the field of prediction modeling in prostate cancer, and we continue to work toward the "ultimate biopsy decision guide." These models are used on a daily basis in most urological centers.

It has become easy to create nomograms, and there has been a proliferation of "me, too" models. What remains anything other than easy is linking the numbers to real patients and real decisions. The patient does not care what the CI or AUC is – he cares whether he has cancer or not. Unfortunately, patients (and their physicians) rarely recognize that the prediction model may or may not be based on patients that are representative of their own risks. This has led to misinterpretation, as evidenced by the finding mentioned above that predictions from different eras or study trial models such as PCPT do not predict well for patients in a clinical setting where contemporary patients are evaluated using modern diagnostic strategies. Thus, one should use a different prediction model to plan a clinical trial than one should use to evaluate patients in daily clinical practice.

The second challenge to this field is to transform the models from predictions to decisions. This will require inputs beyond clinical data, such as the patient's goals (desire to prioritize cure vs. tolerance of side effect risk) plus accurate outcomes data, ideally specific to the person who will perform the treatment. Defining the patient's goals is readily achievable, but we simply do not have accurate and verifiable outcomes data that will reflect an individual patient's risk of having both favorable and unfavorable outcomes under the care of a specific treating physician. Until we have that – which honestly may never occur – the key is to follow the authors' advice to incorporate current and future prediction models into well-considered clinical decisions for each individual patient.

–J. Stephen Jones

References

1. Catalona WJ, Smith DS, Ratliff TL, Basler JW. Detection of organ-confined prostate cancer is increased through prostate-specific antigen-based screening. JAMA. 1993;270(8):948–54.
2. Horner MJ, Ries LAG, Krapcho M, Neyman N, Aminou R, Howlader N, Altekruse SF, Feuer EJ, Huang L, Mariotto A, Miller BA, Lewis DR, Eisner MP, Stinchcomb DG, Edwards BK, editors. SEER cancer statistics review, 1975–2006. Bethesda: National Cancer Institute; 2009.
3. Bill-Axelson A, Holmberg L, Ruutu M, Haggman M, Andersson SO, Bratell S, et al. Radical prostatectomy versus watchful waiting in early prostate cancer. N Engl J Med. 2005;352(19):1977–84. May 12.
4. Hernandez DJ, Han M, Humphreys EB, Mangold LA, Taneja SS, Childs SJ, et al. Predicting the outcome of prostate biopsy: comparison of a novel logistic regression-based model, the prostate cancer risk calculator, and prostate-specific antigen level alone. BJU Int. 2009;103(5):609–14.
5. Nguyen CT, Yu C, Moussa A, Kattan MW, Jones JS. Performance of prostate cancer prevention trial risk calculator in a contemporary cohort screened for prostate cancer and diagnosed by extended prostate biopsy. J Urol. 2010;183(2):529–33.
6. Parekh DJ, Ankerst DP, Higgins BA, Hernandez J, Canby-Hagino E, Brand T, et al. External validation of the Prostate Cancer Prevention Trial risk calculator in a screened population. Urology. 2006;68(6):1152–5.
7. Thompson IM, Ankerst DP, Chi C, Goodman PJ, Tangen CM, Lucia MS, et al. Assessing prostate cancer risk: results from the Prostate Cancer Prevention Trial. J Natl Cancer Inst. 2006;98(8):529–34. Apr 19.
8. Partin AW, Oesterling JE. The clinical usefulness of prostate specific antigen: update 1994. J Urol. 1994;152(5 Pt 1):1358–68.
9. Ahn JO, Ku JH. Relationship between serum prostate-specific antigen levels and body mass index in healthy younger men. Urology. 2006;68(3):570–4.
10. Chia SE, Lau WK, Chin CM, Tan J, Ho SH, Lee J, et al. Effect of ageing and body mass index on prostate-specific antigen levels among Chinese men in Singapore from a community-based study. BJU Int. 2009;103(11):1487–91.
11. Etzioni R, Cha R, Cowen ME. Serial prostate specific antigen screening for prostate cancer: a computer model evaluates competing strategies. J Urol. 1999;162(3 Pt 1):741–8.
12. Smith DS, Catalona WJ. Rate of change in serum prostate specific antigen levels as a method for prostate cancer detection. J Urol. 1994;152(4):1163–7.
13. Berger AP, Deibl M, Strasak A, Bektic J, Pelzer AE, Klocker H, et al. Large-scale study of clinical impact of PSA velocity: long-term PSA kinetics as method of differentiating men with from those without prostate cancer. Urology. 2007;69(1):134–8.
14. Wolters T, Roobol MJ, Bangma CH, Schroder FH. Is prostate-specific antigen velocity selective for clinically significant prostate cancer in screening? European Randomized Study of screening for prostate cancer (Rotterdam). Eur Urol. 2009;55(2):385–92.
15. Brawer MK, Meyer GE, Letran JL, Bankson DD, Morris DL, Yeung KK, et al. Measurement of complexed PSA improves specificity for early detection of prostate cancer. Urology. 1998;52(3):372–8.
16. Hoffman RM, Clanon DL, Littenberg B, Frank JJ, Peirce JC. Using the free-to-total prostate-specific

antigen ratio to detect prostate cancer in men with nonspecific elevations of prostate-specific antigen levels. J Gen Intern Med. 2000;15(10):739–48.

17. Arcangeli CG, Humphrey PA, Smith DS, Harmon TJ, Shepherd DL, Keetch DW, et al. Percentage of free serum prostate-specific antigen as a predictor of pathologic features of prostate cancer in a screening population. Urology. 1998;51(4):558–64. discussion 64–5.

18. Babaian RJ, Kojima M, Ramirez EI, Johnston D. Comparative analysis of prostate specific antigen and its indexes in the detection of prostate cancer. J Urol. 1996;156(2 Pt 1):432–7.

19. Bangma CH, Grobbee DE, Schroder FH. Volume adjustment for intermediate prostate-specific antigen values in a screening population. Eur J Cancer. 1995;31A(1):12–4.

20. Djavan B, Remzi M, Zlotta AR, Seitz C, Wolfram R, Hruby S, et al. Combination and multivariate analysis of PSA-based parameters for prostate cancer prediction. Tech Urol. 1999;5(2):71–6.

21. Horninger W, Reissigl A, Klocker H, Rogatsch H, Fink K, Strasser H, et al. Improvement of specificity in PSA-based screening by using PSA-transition zone density and percent free PSA in addition to total PSA levels. Prostate. 1998;37(3):133–7. discussion 8–9.

22. Ross PL, Gerigk C, Gonen M, Yossepowitch O, Cagiannos I, Sogani PC, et al. Comparisons of nomograms and urologists' predictions in prostate cancer. Semin Urol Oncol. 2002;20(2):82–8.

23. Terrin N, Schmid CH, Griffith JL, D'Agostino RB, Selker HP. External validity of predictive models: a comparison of logistic regression, classification trees, and neural networks. J Clin Epidemiol. 2003;56(8):721–9.

24. Shariat SF, Karakiewicz PI, Palapattu GS, Amiel GE, Lotan Y, Rogers CG, et al. Nomograms provide improved accuracy for predicting survival after radical cystectomy. Clin Cancer Res. 2006;12(22):6663–76. Nov 15.

25. Sargent DJ. Comparison of artificial neural networks with other statistical approaches: results from medical data sets. Cancer. 2001;91(8 Suppl):1636–42. Apr 15.

26. Kattan MW, Zelefsky MJ, Kupelian PA, Scardino PT, Fuks Z, Leibel SA. Pretreatment nomogram for predicting the outcome of three-dimensional conformal radiotherapy in prostate cancer. J Clin Oncol. 2000;18(19):3352–9. Oct 1.

27. D'Amico AV, Whittington R, Malkowicz SB, Schultz D, Schnall M, Tomaszewski JE, et al. A multivariate analysis of clinical and pathological factors that predict for prostate specific antigen failure after radical prostatectomy for prostate cancer. J Urol. 1995;154(1):131–8.

28. Chun FK, Karakiewicz PI, Briganti A, Walz J, Kattan MW, Huland H, et al. A critical appraisal of logistic regression-based nomograms, artificial neural networks, classification and regression-tree models, look-up tables and risk-group stratification models for prostate cancer. BJU Int. 2007;99(4):794–800.

29. Graefen M, Karakiewicz PI, Cagiannos I, Hammerer PG, Haese A, Palisaar J, et al. A validation of two preoperative nomograms predicting recurrence following radical prostatectomy in a cohort of European men. Urol Oncol. 2002;7(4):141–6.

30. Kattan MW, Potters L, Blasko JC, Beyer DC, Fearn P, Cavanagh W, et al. Pretreatment nomogram for predicting freedom from recurrence after permanent prostate brachytherapy in prostate cancer. Urology. 2001;58(3):393–9.

31. Kattan MW. Nomograms are superior to staging and risk grouping systems for identifying high-risk patients: preoperative application in prostate cancer. Curr Opin Urol. 2003;13(2):111–6.

32. Scher HI, Heller G. Clinical states in prostate cancer: toward a dynamic model of disease progression. Urology. 2000;55(3):323–7.

33. Chun FK, Briganti A, Graefen M, Porter C, Montorsi F, Haese A, et al. Development and external validation of an extended repeat biopsy nomogram. J Urol. 2007;177(2):510–5.

34. Karakiewicz PI, Benayoun S, Kattan MW, Perrotte P, Valiquette L, Scardino PT, et al. Development and validation of a nomogram predicting the outcome of prostate biopsy based on patient age, digital rectal examination and serum prostate specific antigen. J Urol. 2005;173(6):1930–4.

35. Roobol MJ, Steyerberg EW, Kranse R, Wolters T, van den Bergh RC, Bangma CH, Schröder FH. A risk-based strategy improves prostate-specific antigen-driven detection of prostate cancer. Eur Urol. 2010; 57(1):79–85. http://www.ncbi.nlm.nih.gov/pubmed/19733959

36. Walz J, Graefen M, Chun FK, Erbersdobler A, Haese A, Steuber T, et al. High incidence of prostate cancer detected by saturation biopsy after previous negative biopsy series. Eur Urol. 2006;50(3):498–505.

37. Walz J, Haese A, Scattoni V, Steuber T, Chun FK, Briganti A, et al. Percent free prostate-specific antigen (PSA) is an accurate predictor of prostate cancer risk in men with serum PSA 2.5 ng/mL and lower. Cancer. 2008;113(10):2695–703.

38. Yanke BV, Gonen M, Scardino PT, Kattan MW. Validation of a nomogram for predicting positive repeat biopsy for prostate cancer. J Urol. 2005; 173(2):421–4.

39. Applewhite JC, Matlaga BR, McCullough DL. Results of the 5 region prostate biopsy method: the repeat biopsy population. J Urol. 2002;168(2):500–3.

40. Epstein JI, Walsh PC, Carter HB. Importance of posterolateral needle biopsies in the detection of prostate cancer. Urology. 2001;57(6):1112–6.

41. Gore JL, Shariat SF, Miles BJ, Kadmon D, Jiang N, Wheeler TM, et al. Optimal combinations of systematic sextant and laterally directed biopsies for the detection of prostate cancer. J Urol. 2001;165(5):1554–9.

42. Nam RK, Toi A, Klotz LH, Trachtenberg J, Jewett MA, Appu S, et al. Assessing individual risk for prostate cancer. J Clin Oncol. 2007;25(24):3582–8. Aug 20.

43. Kranse R, Beemsterboer P, Rietbergen J, Habbema D, Hugosson J, Schroder FH. Predictors for biopsy

outcome in the European Randomized Study of screening for prostate cancer (Rotterdam region). Prostate. 1999;39(4):316–22. Jun 1.

44. Uzzo RG, Wei JT, Waldbaum RS, Perlmutter AP, Byrne JC, Vaughan Jr ED. The influence of prostate size on cancer detection. Urology. 1995;46(6):831–6.

45. Djavan B, Zlotta AR, Byttebier G, Shariat S, Omar M, Schulman CC, et al. Prostate specific antigen density of the transition zone for early detection of prostate cancer. J Urol. 1998;160(2):411–8. discussion 8–9.

46. Vashi AR, Wojno KJ, Gillespie B, Oesterling JE. A model for the number of cores per prostate biopsy based on patient age and prostate gland volume. J Urol. 1998;159(3):920–4.

47. Kattan MW. Factors affecting the accuracy of prediction models limit the comparison of rival prediction models when applied to separate data sets. Eur Urol. 2011;59(4):566–7.

48. Kattan MW. Should I use this nomogram? BJU Int. 2008;102(4):421–2.

49. Schwartz LM, Woloshin S, Welch HG. The drug facts box providing consumers with simple tabular data on drug benefit and harm. Med Decis Making. 2007;27(5):655–62.

50. Marks LS, Fradet Y, Deras IL, Blase A, Mathis J, Aubin SM, et al. PCA3 molecular urine assay for prostate cancer in men undergoing repeat biopsy. Urology. 2007;69(3):532–5.

Is There a Role for Medications to Reduce the Need for Prostate Biopsy?

9

Kiran Gollapudi and William J. Aronson

Introduction

The widespread use of prostate-specific antigen (PSA) screening has led to an increased incidence of prostate cancer, and the majority of prostate cancer cases are now detected at an early stage [1]. PSA can be elevated due to a number of non-cancer-related conditions including benign prostatic hyperplasia (BPH), inflammation, infection, and trauma. Also, the PSA value fluctuates, and an elevated PSA can normalize on subsequent measurements [2]. The lack of PSA specificity becomes especially apparent when evaluating patients with a mildly elevated PSA. Only 25–35% of men undergoing prostate biopsy in the PSA "gray zone" of 4–10 ng/ml are found to have prostate cancer, leaving behind a significant portion of patients who undergo potentially unnecessary biopsy [3, 4]. Though prostate biopsy is generally safe, it is an invasive procedure invoking patient anxiety and can be associated with complications such as pain, bleeding, sepsis, and possibly impotence [5–7]. Furthermore, infectious complications from prostate biopsy are increasing in prevalence due to fluoroquinolone

resistance [8]. Hence, the challenge facing the referring physician or urologist is to determine the most appropriate candidates for prostate biopsy among patients who present with an abnormal PSA.

Prostatitis and BPH are two conditions that commonly affect patients who are screened for prostate cancer and can cause an elevated PSA [9–12]. By medically treating these confounding conditions, can we increase the specificity of PSA and limit unnecessary procedures? To rule out subclinical prostatitis, some physicians initially prescribe empiric antibiotics to men with an elevated PSA. A significant decrease in PSA after antibiotic therapy is thought to represent treated prostatitis, and biopsy is avoided or delayed. The results of the Prostate Cancer Prevention Trial (PCPT) and Reduction by Dutasteride of Prostate Cancer Events (REDUCE) trial suggest that the use of 5-alpha reductase inhibitors (5ARIs) may reduce the number of biopsies by both preventing prostate cancer incidence and by improving PSA sensitivity by reducing the confounding effect of BPH [13–15]. Both topics are a matter of significant debate. The use of any pharmacologic strategy to reduce the number of prostate biopsies must have a favorable benefit-risk ratio by safely decreasing the number of procedures without compromising the detection of significant tumors as well as by having limited drug side effects. In this chapter, we will discuss the controversies surrounding the use of antibiotics and 5ARIs to reduce the indications for prostate biopsy.

K. Gollapudi, M.D. • W.J. Aronson, M.D. (✉)
Department of Urology, School of Medicine,
University of California-Los Angeles,
Box 951738, Los Angeles, CA 90095-1738, USA
e-mail: waronson@ucla.edu

J.S. Jones (ed.), *Prostate Cancer Diagnosis: PSA, Biopsy and Beyond*, Current Clinical Urology,
DOI 10.1007/978-1-62703-188-2_9, © Springer Science+Business Media New York 2013

Prostatitis

It is estimated that approximately 2–10% of men will be diagnosed with prostatitis during their lifetime [16]. The National Institutes of Health (NIH) classifies prostatitis into one of four categories: category I – acute bacterial prostatitis, category II – chronic bacterial prostatitis, category III – chronic nonbacterial prostatitis/chronic pelvic pain syndrome (CP/CPPS IIIA – inflammatory, IIIB – noninflammatory), and category IV – asymptomatic inflammatory prostatitis [17]. Of these cases, the majority (90%) are nonbacterial in origin. In this section, we will discuss how each of these categories of prostatitis can affect PSA levels and if antibiotic therapy can reduce the need for prostate biopsy.

Acute and Chronic Bacterial Prostatitis (Category I and II)

A documented bacterial infection exists in both category I and category II prostatitis. Therefore, appropriate antibiotic treatment is necessary. Both types have been shown to increase PSA, and these elevated PSA values decrease after treatment [9, 18, 19]. In secondary analysis of a randomized trial comparing levofloxacin to ciprofloxacin for the treatment of chronic bacterial prostatitis, Schaeffer et al. showed that the mean PSA of all patients decreased significantly from 3.03 to 2.05 ng/ml ($p < 0.0001$) after treatment [19]. In patients who initially presented with a PSA>4 ng/ml, the PSA decreased from 8.33 to 5.36 ng/ml ($p < 0.0001$). Though there was no placebo group for comparison, both antibiotic regimens decreased PSA similarly. Thus, in men that present with an elevated PSA and evidence of category I or II prostatitis, appropriate antibiotic therapy is warranted to eradicate the offending organism. After the PSA nadirs, if it remains elevated, then the risks and benefits of prostate needle biopsy should be discussed as per usual clinical practice.

Chronic Prostatitis/Chronic Pelvic Pain Syndrome (Category III)

Category III CP/CPPS is a common diagnosis that can significantly impair quality of life. It is defined as urologic pain and discomfort associated with urinary and/or sexual symptoms lasting for 3 of the previous 6 months. The inflammatory subtype IIIA is characterized by the presence of leukocytes in expressed prostatic secretions (EPS) [17]. CP/CPPS is a diagnosis of exclusion, and treatment focuses on symptomatic relief. A recent meta-analysis of 23 randomized controlled trials revealed that antibiotics, alphablockers, and anti-inflammatory medications can improve symptoms when compared to placebo [20]. The greatest benefit was seen with combination of antibiotics and alpha-blockers. To our knowledge, only one study has examined the effect of CP/CPPS on PSA. Nadler et al. compared 421 men enrolled in the Chronic Prostatitis Cohort Study with 121 age-matched controls [21]. The total PSA was significantly elevated in CP/CPPS patients compared to controls (1.97 vs. 1.72 ng/ml, $p = 0.03$); however, both values were below either a 2.5- or 4-ng/ml threshold for prompting prostate biopsy. A total of 10% and 7% of patients had a PSA>4 ng/ml in the prostatitis and control groups, respectively ($p = 0.03$). The data in the literature are insufficient to draw firm conclusions regarding the role for antibiotics (or alpha-blockers or anti-inflammatory medications) to lower the PSA and reduce the need for prostate biopsy in patients with category III prostatitis. In our clinical practice, if patients are symptomatic with category III prostatitis and have an elevated PSA, we first treat the prostatitis prior to performing a prostate biopsy. The rationale for this approach is twofold. First, it is possible that these patients have an occult, undetected infection, and we may possibly be able to avoid biopsy-induced sepsis if we treat prior to the prostate biopsy. In addition, in our experience, patients tolerate the prostate biopsy procedure better if we treat the chronic prostatitis symptoms prior to the biopsy. If the PSA remains elevated after treatment, then we discuss the option of undergoing prostate biopsy.

Asymptomatic Prostatitis (Category IV)

Significant controversy exists regarding the role of antibiotics for lowering PSA levels and reducing the need for prostate biopsy in cases of asymptomatic prostatitis. Numerous studies have shown a relationship between category IV prostatitis and elevated PSA. Category IV prostatitis is diagnosed either by the presence of leukocytes in EPS or incidentally on pathologic prostate specimens of asymptomatic men. In a PSA screening population, Nadler et al. reported significantly higher rates of acute and chronic inflammation in benign prostate biopsy specimens from men with a PSA>4 ng/ml compared to those with a PSA<4 ng/ml [11]. Biopsies were indicated due to abnormal DRE findings, and all the men in both groups had multiple previous negative biopsies leading the authors to conclude that inflammation was a significant factor in contributing to an elevated PSA in these patients. Carver et al. randomly selected 300 patients out of 717 men undergoing an annual prostate cancer screening program to determine the prevalence of category IV prostatitis as defined by having more than 10 white blood cells per high-power field in EPS. Of 227 evaluable patients, they found category IV inflammatory prostatitis in 32.2% of patients and found that these men had significantly higher PSA values (2.3 vs. 1.4; $p<0.0004$) as compared to men without prostatitis [22]. Simardi et al. prospectively studied 80 patients with no urinary symptoms undergoing prostate biopsy [23]. Patients with a negative biopsy were stratified into three groups based on the percentage of cores with inflammation present: less than 20%, 20–50%, and greater than 50%. The mean PSA values were 4.96, 7.40, and 8.03 ng/ml ($p=0.02$), respectively. Thus, inflammation in the prostate in asymptomatic men is associated with elevated PSA levels.

Several groups have prospectively demonstrated that empiric antibiotic therapy in patients with asymptomatic prostatitis can decrease PSA levels. Whether this decrease translates into a reduced need for prostate biopsy is less certain. Potts screened 122 asymptomatic men for category IV prostatitis that presented for urological evaluation with an elevated PSA>4 ng/ml [24]. Category IV prostatitis, diagnosed by the presence of leukocytes in EPS or postprostatic massage urine, was found in 51/122 (42%) men. Patients with prostatitis were treated for 4 weeks with trimethoprim-sulfamethoxazole or a quinolone antibiotic, and those without prostatitis underwent immediate biopsy. After treatment, 22/51 (42%) patients had normal PSA levels and were felt to no longer have an indication for biopsy. Cancer was diagnosed in 9/29 (31%) men who were diagnosed with category IV prostatitis and whose PSA did not normalize after antibiotic treatment. Given that 18% (22/122) of patients avoided biopsy as a result of antibiotic usage, the authors advocated screening for asymptomatic prostatitis. Similarly, Bulbul et al. and Bozeman et al. demonstrated that 25/48 (52%) and 44/95 (46%) patients avoided biopsy because of normalized PSA levels after antibiotic treatment, respectively [25, 26]. These groups argued that the specificity of PSA was increased after antibiotic therapy. However, since patients whose PSA decreased to less than 4 ng/ml were not biopsied, their cancer status is unknown, and it is unclear if normalization of a PSA to less than 4 ng/ml justified biopsy deferral.

Several studies have examined the incidence of prostate cancer in asymptomatic individuals whose PSA normalized after antibiotic treatment. Kaygisz et al. studied 48 patients with PSA levels between 4 and 10 ng/ml [27]. Patients were stratified by EPS status, and all patients received 3 weeks of ofloxacin regardless of a diagnosis of asymptomatic prostatitis. The PSA significantly decreased in the entire cohort from 6.53 to 4.56 ng/ml ($p<0.05$), and there was no difference in PSA change between EPS positive and negative patients. Among 10 patients that had a PSA less than 4 ng/ml after treatment, none had cancer on biopsy. Prostate cancer was detected in 10.8% of patients with a PSA between 4 and 10 ng/ml. Serreta et al. examined 99 asymptomatic patients (not evaluated for category IV prostatitis) with

PSA levels between 4 and 20 ng/ml [28]. Patients were treated with 3 weeks of ciprofloxacin and all patients underwent a prostate biopsy. A total of 59 patients had a PSA decrease, and 8 had PSA levels drop below 4 ng/ml. A total of 28 (28.3%) patients were found to have cancer; however, no patients with a 70% or greater decrease in PSA or with a PSA<4 ng/ml were found to have cancer. On the other hand, Baltaci et al. evaluated 100 asymptomatic patients (not evaluated for category IV prostatitis) with a PSA between 4 and 10 ng/ml who were treated with 20 days of ofloxacin [29]. A total of 5/17 patients whose PSA was less than 4 ng/ml after treatment were found to have cancer. Similarly, Kim et al. found that prostate cancer was detected in post-treatment biopsy in 13.3% (2/15), 13.6% (3/22), and 26.5% (13/49) of patients with PSA levels of less than 2.5, between 2.5 and 4.0, and above 4.0 ng/ml [30]. Taken together, these studies suggest that significant reductions in PSA levels after antibiotic therapy and conversion of PSA levels to low normal levels translate to a lower risk of prostate cancer on prostate biopsy, though these conclusions are limited by small sample sizes in the clinical trials. In addition, these trials did not include groups receiving placebo.

Data from prospective randomized studies do not support the widespread use of empiric antibiotics to decrease PSA levels in asymptomatic men with an elevated PSA. In a three-arm randomized controlled study, Ugurlu et al. evaluated 216 asymptomatic men with PSA values between 2.5 and 10.0 ng/ml and normal DRE [31]. All men were screened for category IV prostatitis based on the presence of leukocytes in EPS. Men were separated into EPS positive and negative groups and randomized to receive levofloxacin 500 mg daily, naproxen sodium controlled release 750 mg daily, or no medication for 3 weeks. All patients underwent a biopsy at the end of treatment. Only men who had category IV prostatitis and received antibiotics had a significant decrease in PSA (5.2–4.0 ng/ml; $p<0.0001$). A total of 26/216 (12%) of patients were found to have cancer, and there was no significant difference in the cancer detection rate between groups. Of 24 patients with a PSA less than 2.5 ng/ml after

treatment or observation, none had prostate cancer on biopsy. Though the study is limited by the lack of a placebo group, the authors conclude that if antibiotic therapy is to be prescribed, it should be limited to men with evidence of category IV prostatitis. In a randomized placebo-controlled double-blind study, Stopiglia et al. examined 98 patients with category IV prostatitis [32]. Asymptomatic men with a PSA between 2.5 and 10.0 ng/ml, normal DRE, and diagnosis of category IV prostatitis on EPS or postprostatic massage urine specimens were randomized to 4 weeks of ciprofloxacin 500 mg twice daily or placebo. In the placebo group, 29/49 (59.18%) patients had a decrease in prostate-specific antigen and 9/29 (31%) had cancer on biopsy, while in the antibiotic group, there were 26/49 (53%) patients with a decrease in prostate-specific antigen and 7/26 (27%) with prostate cancer. There was no significant difference between groups. Of note, 8/19 (3/10 placebo and 5/9 antibiotic group) patients with a normalized PSA less than 2.5 ng/ml were found to have cancer. Thus, in this placebo-controlled trial, there was no difference in the decrease seen in PSA levels between the antibiotic and placebo group.

Should Antibiotics Be Prescribed to Men with Asymptomatic Prostatitis Presenting with an Elevated PSA to Reduce Need for Prostate Biopsy?

Based on the lack of level I data, this question remains unresolved. A recent point/counterpoint article in the Journal of Urology further confirmed that this debate is ongoing [33]. Multiple studies have demonstrated that asymptomatic inflammatory prostatitis is associated with an elevated PSA, and antibiotic therapy appears to lower PSA levels in these men, though one placebo-controlled trial did not confirm this finding. Furthermore, if the PSA level normalizes after antibiotic therapy, especially to levels below 2.5 ng/ml, the risk of prostate cancer appears to be significantly reduced. However, given the normal fluctuation of PSA values, there is a significant likelihood that PSA levels will normalize on subsequent testing without antibiotic therapy [2, 34]. In a retrospective analysis of 972 men in the Polyp Prevention Trial, Eastham et al. showed that between 21% and 37% of men without cancer will have an elevated PSA over multiple tests, and between 40% and 55% will normalize with subsequent testing. On follow-up tests, 65–83% of men will continue to have a normal PSA. The downside of widespread use of antibiotic therapy for lowering PSA levels is significant and includes an increased incidence of antibiotic-resistant bacteria in the community and a higher risk of sepsis following prostate biopsy by antibiotic-resistant bacteria. Based on the lack of level I data supporting the use of antibiotics to lower PSA levels and reduce the need for prostate biopsy, we recommend the conduct of further prospective randomized trials to evaluate this important issue. Ultimately, the decision of whether or not to prescribe antibiotics to lower the PSA is left to the clinical judgment of the urologist and an informed discussion with the patient. Based on the literature, if the PSA remains elevated after repeat testing, it appears prudent to test for category IV prostatitis by evaluating for postprostate massage WBC's prior to offering the option of a course of antibiotics.

5-Alpha Reductase Inhibitors

It is well documented that prostate volume is directly correlated with PSA in healthy men without prostate cancer [35]. BPH is a common finding on prostate biopsy when PSA is elevated and biopsy is negative for cancer [11]. Dihydrotestosterone (DHT), the principle prostatic androgen, is responsible for normal development and growth of the prostate as well as for development of BPH. DHT also influences the secretory function of prostatic epithelial cells which produce PSA [36]. Testosterone is converted to DHT by the enzyme 5-alpha reductase. The 5ARI finasteride selectively inhibits the type 2 isoenzyme of 5-alpha reductase, while dutasteride inhibits both type 1 and type 2 isoforms. 5ARIs are effective treatments for men with an enlarged prostate and reduce PSA levels by approximately 50% [36]. There is also some evidence to suggest that 5ARIs

may be effective for the symptomatic treatment of CP/CPPS [37]. In addition, two large randomized placebo-controlled trials have reported that finasteride and dutasteride can reduce the incidence of prostate cancer by 22–25% [13, 15]. Thus, 5ARIs have the potential to reduce the need for prostate biopsy by reducing the risk of prostate cancer. In addition, use of 5ARIs may improve the specificity of PSA for detecting prostate cancer by suppressing BPH-derived PSA [14, 38]. Does the evidence support either one of these approaches? If so, do the benefits of 5ARIs outweigh the risks of therapy?

5ARIs and Prostate Cancer Prevention

The PCPT was conducted to determine if finasteride could reduce the risk of prostate cancer in healthy men [13]. A total of 18,882 men with a normal DRE and PSA of 3.0 ng/ml or less were randomized to receive either finasteride 5 mg daily or placebo for 7 years. Prostate cancer was diagnosed in 803/4,368 (18.4%) men treated with finasteride and in 1,147/4,692 (24.4%) men who received placebo. This resulted in a statistically significant 24.8% relative risk reduction in the prevalence of prostate cancer. While more than 97% of all tumors were clinically localized at diagnosis and a majority had a Gleason score 6 or less, there were significantly more high-grade (Gleason 7–10) tumors in the finasteride group compared to placebo (6.4% vs. 5.1%; odds ratio 1.27, $p = 0.005$). A number of subsequent studies have argued that the increased incidence of high-grade cancer was likely secondary to detection bias due to improved sampling density in the finasteride group [39, 40]. The results of the PCPT thus demonstrated that finasteride could reduce the risk of prostate cancer in healthy men treated for 7 years; however, finasteride was also associated with an increased risk of diagnosis of high-grade prostate cancer that could possibly be explained by detection bias.

While the PCPT evaluated low-risk healthy men, the REDUCE trial was designed to test if dutasteride could decrease the risk of prostate cancer in men who are at higher risk for developing prostate cancer [15]. The men in the REDUCE trial had a PSA between 2.5 and 10.0 ng/ml and had a negative biopsy within 6 months of enrollment. A total of 8,231 patients were randomized to receive dutasteride 0.5 mg daily or placebo for 4 years. Of 6,729 evaluable patients, 659/3,305 (19.9%) patients in the dutasteride group and 858/3,424 (25.1%) men in the placebo group were diagnosed with prostate cancer. This represented a 22.8% relative risk reduction. Whereas the original publication on REDUCE did not find a significant difference in the risk of poorly differentiated prostate cancer between the groups, regrading of the prostate biopsy tissue by a blinded pathologist and reanalysis of the data demonstrated a significant absolute increase of 0.5% representing a relative risk of 2.06 of Gleason 8–10 tumors in the dutasteride arm versus the placebo arm [41].

Given that 5ARIs reduce the risk of prostate cancer, would their use for prostate cancer prevention result in a reduced need for prostate biopsy? Or would patients placed on 5ARIs for prevention be observed more vigilantly and be more likely to undergo a prostate biopsy in clinical practice? The answers to these questions are unknown. In addition, given that 5ARIs are not FDA approved for prostate cancer prevention and were also given a black box warning by the FDA for increased risk of high-grade prostate cancer, use of 5ARIs for prevention and reducing the risk of prostate biopsy is not a viable strategy at the present time.

Can 5ARIs Improve PSA Performance?

The use of 5ARIs is associated with a decrease in serum PSA levels. While the rate and level of PSA decrease varies between individuals, 5ARIs reduce serum PSA on average by 50% by 6–12 months of treatment [36]. In the PCPT trial, serum PSA levels were shown to continue to decrease with increased duration of treatment and were corrected by a factor 2.3 rather than 2.0 after year 4 of treatment. Given the changes in PSA induced by 5ARI therapy, several groups have studied the usefulness of PSA in this patient population for prostate cancer screening. Thompson et al. evaluated the sensitivity of PSA

between the finasteride and placebo groups in the PCPT at a given specificity for various predefined PSA cutoffs [14]. The area under the receiver operating curve (AUC) for the detection of prostate cancer was greater in the finasteride group than placebo group (0.757 vs. 0.681, $p < 0.001$). The sensitivity of PSA was greater in the finasteride arm at all given specificity values and PSA cutoffs. Similar analysis of the REDUCE trial revealed that the optimal PSA cutoff for sensitivity and specificity was between 2.0 and 3.0 ng/ml in the dutasteride arm and between 6.0 and 7.0 ng/ml in the placebo group [38]. While the sensitivity in the placebo arm was slightly higher, the specificity was significantly lower for the detection of prostate cancer. The initial decrease in PSA was not predictive of prostate cancer in men treated with dutasteride; however, any increase in PSA from month 6 to final PSA was a stronger indicator of high-grade prostate cancer in the dutasteride group than the placebo group. Although the data is intriguing with regard to improved utility of PSA or PSA velocity for prostate cancer detection in men on 5ARIs, there are no established guidelines, and level 1 evidence does not exist to support the use of 5ARIs for this purpose. Likewise, given the side effects of 5ARIs and the recent black box warning, we would not recommend using the 5ARIs for purposes of improving the utility of PSA for detection and reducing the need for prostate biopsy.

Editorial Commentary:
Medical management – antibiotics, 5ARIs, or otherwise – to reduce the need for prostate biopsy is intuitively appealing. Nevertheless, no matter what PSA changes occur based on treatment, the clinician is still faced with the same question: should I perform biopsy? As the authors note, it is uncommon for medical manipulations to make clear which patients have prostate cancer. Furthermore, most studies have a significant verification bias because patients whose PSA values normalize often do not undergo biopsy. Knowing the limitations of PSA overall, it is not at all clear whether its return to lower levels is truly meaningful, and there is a high likelihood that this only delays biopsy in many such men.

More significant is the recent emergence of bacterial resistance in most biopsy series. Administering antibiotics in the prebiopsy setting may increase resistance, creating unnecessary risk to the patient. Therefore, we recommend antibiotics for only two indications – treatment of infection or procedural prophylaxis.

References

1. Cooperberg MR, et al. Time trends in clinical risk stratification for prostate cancer: implications for outcomes (data from CaPSURE). J Urol. 2003;170(6 Pt 2):S21–5. discussion S26–7.
2. Eastham JA, et al. Variation of serum prostate-specific antigen levels: an evaluation of year-to-year fluctuations. JAMA. 2003;289(20):2695–700.
3. Brawer MK, et al. Screening for prostatic carcinoma with prostate specific antigen: results of the second year. J Urol. 1993;150(1):106–9.
4. Catalona WJ, et al. Comparison of digital rectal examination and serum prostate specific antigen in the early detection of prostate cancer: results of a multicenter clinical trial of 6,630 men. J Urol. 1994;151(5):1283–90.
5. Aus G, et al. Infection after transrectal core biopsies of the prostate–risk factors and antibiotic prophylaxis. Br J Urol. 1996;77(6):851–5.
6. Rietbergen JB, et al. Complications of transrectal ultrasound-guided systematic sextant biopsies of the prostate: evaluation of complication rates and risk factors within a population-based screening program. Urology. 1997;49(6):875–80.
7. Fujita K, et al. Serial prostate biopsies are associated with an increased risk of erectile dysfunction in men with prostate cancer on active surveillance. J Urol. 2009;182(6):2664–9.
8. Feliciano J, et al. The incidence of fluoroquinolone resistant infections after prostate biopsy–are fluoroquinolones still effective prophylaxis? J Urol. 2008;179(3):952–5. discussion 955.
9. Dalton DL. Elevated serum prostate-specific antigen due to acute bacterial prostatitis. Urology. 1989; 33(6):465.
10. Palou J, Morote J. Elevated serum PSA and acute bacterial prostatitis. Urology. 1990;35(4):373.
11. Nadler RB, et al. Effect of inflammation and benign prostatic hyperplasia on elevated serum prostate specific antigen levels. J Urol. 1995;154(2 Pt 1):407–13.
12. Tchetgen MB, Oesterling JE. The effect of prostatitis, urinary retention, ejaculation, and ambulation on the serum prostate-specific antigen concentration. Urol Clin North Am. 1997;24(2):283–91.
13. Thompson IM, et al. The influence of finasteride on the development of prostate cancer. N Engl J Med. 2003;349(3):215–24.

14. Thompson IM, et al. Effect of finasteride on the sensitivity of PSA for detecting prostate cancer. J Natl Cancer Inst. 2006;98(16):1128–33.
15. Andriole GL, et al. Effect of dutasteride on the risk of prostate cancer. N Engl J Med. 2010;362(13): 1192–202.
16. Habermacher GM, Chason JT, Schaeffer AJ. Prostatitis/chronic pelvic pain syndrome. Annu Rev Med. 2006;57:195–206.
17. Krieger JN, Nyberg Jr L, Nickel JC. NIH consensus definition and classification of prostatitis. JAMA. 1999;282(3):236–7.
18. Neal Jr DE, et al. Prostate specific antigen and prostatitis. I. Effect of prostatitis on serum PSA in the human and nonhuman primate. Prostate. 1992;20(2):105–11.
19. Schaeffer AJ, et al. Treatment of chronic bacterial prostatitis with levofloxacin and ciprofloxacin lowers serum prostate specific antigen. J Urol. 2005;174(1):161–4.
20. Anothaisintawee T, et al. Management of chronic prostatitis/chronic pelvic pain syndrome: a systematic review and network meta-analysis. JAMA. 2011; 305(1):78–86.
21. Nadler RB, et al. Prostate-specific antigen test in diagnostic evaluation of chronic prostatitis/chronic pelvic pain syndrome. Urology. 2006;67(2):337–42.
22. Carver BS, et al. The prevalence of men with National Institutes of Health category IV prostatitis and association with serum prostate specific antigen. J Urol. 2003;169(2):589–91.
23. Simardi LH, et al. Influence of asymptomatic histologic prostatitis on serum prostate-specific antigen: a prospective study. Urology. 2004;64(6):1098–101.
24. Potts JM. Prospective identification of National Institutes of Health category IV prostatitis in men with elevated prostate specific antigen. J Urol. 2000;164(5):1550–3.
25. Bulbul MA, et al. The effect of antibiotics on elevated serum prostate specific antigen in patients with urinary symptoms and negative digital rectal examination: a pilot study. J Med Liban. 2002;50(1–2):23–5.
26. Bozeman CB, et al. Treatment of chronic prostatitis lowers serum prostate specific antigen. J Urol. 2002;167(4):1723–6.
27. Kaygisiz O, et al. Effects of antibacterial therapy on PSA change in the presence and absence of prostatic inflammation in patients with PSA levels between 4 and 10 ng/ml. Prostate Cancer Prostatic Dis. 2006;9(3): 235–8.
28. Serretta V, et al. PSA reduction (after antibiotics) permits to avoid or postpone prostate biopsy in selected patients. Prostate Cancer Prostatic Dis. 2008;11(2): 148–52.
29. Baltaci S, et al. Effectiveness of antibiotics given to asymptomatic men for an increased prostate specific antigen. J Urol. 2009;181(1):128–32.
30. Kim YJ, et al. Prostate cancer can be detected even in patients with decreased PSA less than 2.5 ng/ml after treatment of chronic prostatitis. Korean J Urol. 2011;52(7):457–60.

31. Ugurlu O, et al. Impacts of antibiotic and anti-inflammatory therapies on serum prostate-specific antigen levels in the presence of prostatic inflammation: a prospective randomized controlled trial. Urol Int. 2010;84(2):185–90.

32. Stopiglia RM, et al. Prostate specific antigen decrease and prostate cancer diagnosis: antibiotic versus placebo prospective randomized clinical trial. J Urol. 2010;183(3):940–4.

33. Loeb S. Use of empiric antibiotics in the setting of an increased prostate specific antigen: pro. J Urol. 2011;186(1):17–9.

34. Ornstein DK, et al. Biological variation of total, free and percent free serum prostate specific antigen levels in screening volunteers. J Urol. 1997;157(6): 2179–82.

35. Roehrborn CG, et al. Serum prostate-specific antigen as a predictor of prostate volume in men with benign prostatic hyperplasia. Urology. 1999;53(3):581–9.

36. Marks LS, et al. The interpretation of serum prostate specific antigen in men receiving 5alpha-reductase inhibitors: a review and clinical recommendations. J Urol. 2006;176(3):868–74.

37. Nickel JC, et al. Dutasteride reduces prostatitis symptoms compared with placebo in men enrolled in the REDUCE study. J Urol. 2011;186(4):1313–8.

38. Andriole GL, et al. The effect of dutasteride on the usefulness of prostate specific antigen for the diagnosis of high grade and clinically relevant prostate cancer in men with a previous negative biopsy: results from the REDUCE study. J Urol. 2011;185(1): 126–31.

39. Cohen YC, et al. Detection bias due to the effect of finasteride on prostate volume: a modeling approach for analysis of the Prostate Cancer Prevention Trial. J Natl Cancer Inst. 2007;99(18):1366–74.

40. Redman MW, et al. Finasteride does not increase the risk of high-grade prostate cancer: a bias-adjusted modeling approach. Cancer Prev Res (Phila). 2008;1(3):174–81.

41. Theoret MR, et al. The risks and benefits of 5 alpha-reductase inhibitors for prostate-cancer prevention. N Engl J Med. 2011;365(2):97–9.

Indications for Initial Biopsy: Is the PSA Threshold ERA Over?

10

Christopher L. Amling and Jeffrey C. La Rochelle

Introduction

Traditionally, men have been selected for prostate biopsy based on a specific PSA threshold. Recent studies show that prostate cancer can be found at all PSA levels, and at autopsy, many men have histological evidence of prostate cancer that was of no clinical significance. These findings and the low specificity of total PSA level in discriminating cancer from benign disease have spurred debate about how best to select men for initial biopsy. Lower PSA thresholds, particularly in younger men, are advocated by some. PSA velocity measures may assist in the identification of those most likely to harbor cancer and may be a marker of more aggressive disease. With the development of numerous nomograms to predict the probability of a positive biopsy or the likelihood of high-grade cancer, a more individualized approach may be used. While nearly all nomograms show a greater predictive accuracy than PSA alone, there are several limitations to these tools that must be taken into consideration. This chapter will outline the arguments for and against using a PSA threshold or PSA velocity measure alone and explore the use of predictive nomograms to select men for initial prostate biopsy.

Background

Since the importance of PSA as a tumor marker was first established in the late 1970s, it has become the primary measure prompting recommendation for initial prostate biopsy [1]. Despite the well-established value of this marker in prostate cancer screening and diagnosis, it has several shortcomings. Although PSA is prostate specific, it is not prostate cancer specific. An elevated PSA level can be associated with other conditions including benign prostatic hyperplasia, prostatic infection, and chronic inflammation. In addition, it has now been clearly established that prostate cancer can be detected at PSA levels previously thought to be normal. Recent studies demonstrate that in men with unsuspicious digital rectal examination findings and PSA level less than 4 ng/ml, as many as 15–23% will be found to have cancer upon biopsy, and 15–21% of these cancers are found to be high grade (Gleason score ≥ 7) [2, 3]. The prevalence of prostate cancer at "normal" PSA levels and the low specificity of PSA testing have complicated the decision to proceed with initial prostate biopsy and renewed debate about the wisdom of recommending biopsy at a specific PSA threshold.

The decision to proceed with prostate biopsy is further complicated by the knowledge that many men harbor prostate cancer which may be of no

C.L. Amling, M.D., FACS (✉) • J.C. La Rochelle, M.D.
Department of Urology, Oregon Health & Science University, 3303 SW Bond Avenue, Mail Code CH10U, Portland, OR 97239, USA
e-mail: amling@ohsu.edu

J.S. Jones (ed.), *Prostate Cancer Diagnosis: PSA, Biopsy and Beyond*, Current Clinical Urology,
DOI 10.1007/978-1-62703-188-2_10, © Springer Science+Business Media New York 2013

clinical significance. While the definition of a clinically significant cancer varies, a significant number of men undergoing radical prostatectomy may be found to have clinically insignificant disease. The high prevalence of indolent disease is also supported by autopsy studies [4–7]. Based on 292 autopsies of men over age 50 years performed at John Hopkins Hospital in the 1930s, Rich et al. reported a 14% incidence of occult prostate cancer [4]. In 1954, Franks performed a more systematic analysis of the prostate noting that 38% of men older than 50 years had microscopic evidence of disease [5]. Sakr et al. performed 152 autopsies on young men after traumatic death (65% African-American) finding histological evidence of prostate cancer in 27% and 34% of men in their 30s and 40s, respectively [6]. In a more recent study examining prostates from healthy organ donors who died suddenly between 1994 and 2007, Yin et al. found incidental prostate cancer in 23% of men aged 50–59 years and in 35% of those aged 60–69 years [7].

The high prevalence of incidental prostate cancer and the imperfections of the PSA test have led some to argue that the era of using PSA to select men for biopsy is over. However, until new more accurate markers are available, total PSA level will remain an important factor in selecting men for prostate biopsy. The more relevant question is whether PSA should be the only factor considered or should other information be factored into the decision for biopsy. Additionally, there are now several readily available predictive nomograms to determine the likelihood of a positive biopsy. The accuracy of these nomograms and the predictive value they add to PSA need to be clarified in light of the potential difficulty in using them in a clinical setting. In this new "beyond PSA" era, these are some of the questions that need to be answered. To address these issues, we will focus on four questions to consider when selecting men for initial prostate biopsy:

1. Should a PSA threshold be used to recommend initial prostate biopsy and if so, what is the most appropriate PSA level?
2. Can PSA velocity be used to assist in selection of men for initial prostate biopsy?
3. When should prostatic inflammation be suspected as contributing to an elevated PSA level?
4. Should currently available nomograms be used to select men for prostate biopsy?

Other chapters in this textbook will examine the role of other markers in prostate cancer detection and the indications for repeat prostate biopsy. We will limit our focus to the use of PSA and other factors currently considered in the decision to proceed with initial prostate biopsy.

Should a PSA Threshold Be Used to Recommend Initial Prostate Biopsy and If So, What Is the Most Appropriate PSA Level?

A PSA level greater than 4 ng/ml has traditionally been used to recommend prostate biopsy despite limited evidence that this threshold represented the optimal balance between the sensitivity and specificity of this test [1]. Following the discovery that PSA was more sensitive than prostatic acid phosphatase (PAP) in the detection of prostate cancer in the late 1980s, there were two important studies in the early 1990s that led to the designation of a PSA level above 4 ng/ml as abnormal [8, 9]. In 1990, Cooner et al. used transrectal ultrasound (TRUS), digital rectal examination (DRE), and PSA in 807 men aged 50–89 to screen them for prostate cancer [8]. A PSA level of 4.0 ng/ml was used as a threshold for recommending prostate biopsy in part due to the PSA assay they used in this trial which reported a normal range of 0–3.9 ng/ml. In 1989, Catalona et al. performed the initial large-scale prostate cancer screening study utilizing PSA and DRE as first-line tests [9]. At initiation of this screening trial, PSA values alone were not considered sufficient to recommend prostate biopsy. Instead, a PSA value > 4 ng/ml prompted evaluation with DRE and TRUS. Findings suspicious for cancer on either DRE or TRUS were then used to trigger prostate biopsy. In 1991 the authors changed the study protocol so that prostate biopsy was recommended for suspicious DRE or a PSA > 4 ng/ml. Although 7 years later the same group suggested that the PSA cutoff

Table 10.1 Age-specific mean and median serum PSA levels for US men aged 40–84 without known prostate cancer[a]

Age group	Estimated mean serum PSA in US men, ng/ml (95% CI)	Estimated median serum PSA in US men, ng/ml (25th, 75th percentile)
40–44	0.84 (0.75–0.92)	0.7 (0.5, 1.1)
45–49	1.00 (0.81–1.20)	0.8 (0.5, 1.1)
50–54	1.59 (1.08–2.09)	0.8 (0.5, 1.4)
55–59	1.30 (1.02–1.57)	0.9 (0.6, 1.4)
60–64	1.49 (1.28–2.70)	1.0 (0.6, 2.0)
65–69	1.89 (1.35–2.44)	1.1 (0.7, 2.0)
70–74	2.27 (1.94–2.79)	1.5 (0.8, 3.0)
75–80	3.66 (2.87–4.43)	2.8 (1.0, 4.6)
80–84	4.04 (3.05–5.03)	2.4 (1.5, 5.2)
Overall	1.56 (1.37–1.74)	0.9 (0.5, 1.4)

Table adapted from Porter et al. [11]
[a]Estimates from the NHANES 2001–2002

value should be lowered to 2.5 ng/ml, the widespread use of 4 ng/ml as a threshold for recommending prostate biopsy was established.

Although a PSA level of 4 ng/ml is still widely used to select men for prostate biopsy, there is evidence that a lower threshold may be more appropriate, especially for younger men. For most men, a PSA level of 4 ng/ml is significantly elevated based upon population statistics for median PSA levels. Loeb et al. studied baseline PSA levels in a group of approximately 14,000 men younger than 60 years of age who participated in a prostate cancer screening study between 1991 and 2001. The median PSA level was 0.7 ng/ml for men aged 40–49 and 0.9 ng/ml for men aged 50–59 years [10]. In a similar study utilizing data from the National Health and Nutrition Examination Survey of 2001–2002, the distribution of serum PSA levels in American men was investigated [11]. This study revealed that most men in the United States have PSA levels less than 4 ng/ml (Table 10.1). Of note, median serum PSA levels in men under age 65 years were < 1 ng/ml, suggesting that use of a PSA threshold of 4 ng/ml may be quite high when considering men of this age for biopsy. These studies clearly document that most men have low PSA levels, especially younger men who typically have less benign prostatic enlargement to confound the PSA level.

Another argument in favor of using a lower PSA threshold is the relatively high prevalence of prostate cancer at PSA levels below 4 ng/ml and the realization that many of these "low PSA" cancers are high grade. The Prostate Cancer Prevention Trial (PCPT) was the first study to document this fact [2]. This chemoprevention study randomly assigned 18,882 men to receive either finasteride or placebo. Men were followed with annual digital rectal examinations (DRE) and PSA measurements. After 7 years on study, men who had not been diagnosed with prostate cancer were asked to undergo an end-of-study biopsy. These men were biopsied at PSA levels of ≤ 4 ng/ml with a normal DRE result, and the vast majority of these biopsies were performed using the sextant technique. Overall, prostate cancer was detected in 15% of men with PSA less than 4 ng/ml, and 15% of these were high-grade tumors (Gleason score ≥ 7). This study showed that there was a continuum of risk correlating directly with PSA level, even at very low PSA ranges. In a more recent study of a referral population utilizing a more extended biopsy scheme, Ahyai et al. also examined the prevalence of prostate cancer in men with PSA levels < 4 ng/ml [3]. Consistent with the PCPT results, PSA levels below this traditional cutoff point were associated with a significant risk of prostate cancer that increased incrementally with increases in PSA level (Fig. 10.1).

When cancers are detected at lower PSA values, they usually have smaller volumes and are more likely to be organ confined, but they are still often clinically significant. Krumholtz et al. evaluated the pathologic characteristics of screen-detected clinical stage T1 prostate cancers in 94 patients undergoing radical prostatectomy, comparing cancers detected in the 2.6–4 ng/ml range to the 4.1–10 ng/ml range [12]. Cancers detected at the 2.6–4 ng/ml PSA range had smaller volumes (1.1 vs. 1.8 cc) and were significantly more likely to be organ-confined (88% vs. 63%). Another study of the same screening population examined progression-free survival as a function of preoperative PSA level in men with clinical T1c prostate cancer undergoing radical prostatectomy [13]. The men with PSA level between 2.6

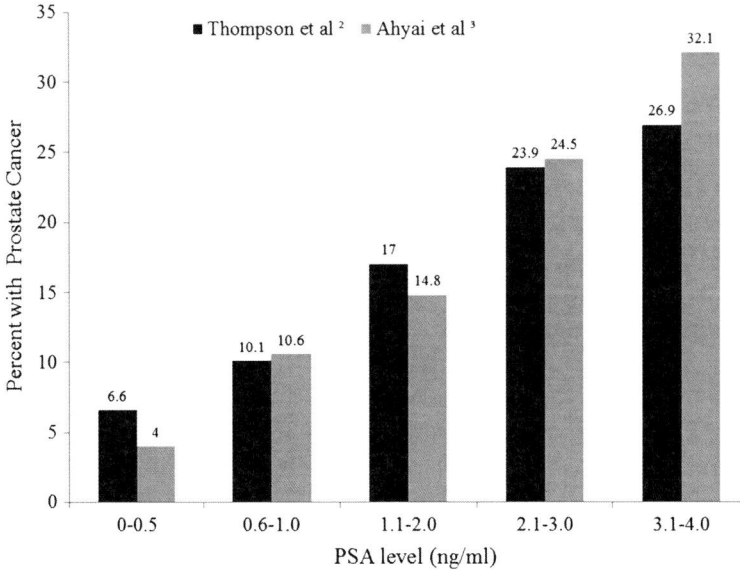

Fig. 10.1 Percentage of men with prostate cancer detected at biopsy by prostate-specific antigen (PSA) level

and 4 ng/ml had an 81% chance of having organ-confined disease compared to 74% in men with PSA between 4.1 and 7 ng/ml. Ten-year progression-free survival was also better in the men with lower preoperative PSA levels. In a study evaluating the pathologic features of cancers detected in the PCPT trial in men who elected to undergo radical prostatectomy, Lucia et al. compared cancers with a preoperative PSA of 2.6–4 ng/ml to those with a PSA of 4–10 ng/ml [14]. A similar number of cancers in these two groups were found to be high grade (Gleason score$\geq$7), and only 18% of cancers in the 2.6–4 ng/ml PSA range met the criteria for insignificant disease. The pathologic characteristics of clinical T1c cancers were similarly compared between preoperative PSA groups 2.6–4 ng/ml and 4.1–6 ng/ml in a series of 2,896 men undergoing radical prostatectomy at Johns Hopkins Hospital [15]. Patients with PSA<4 ng/ml had fewer positive margins, less risk of extraprostatic extension, and less likelihood of having Gleason$\geq$7 disease. Finally, Nadler et al. reported similar pathologic features in men younger than 60 years, aged 60–70 years and older than 70 years with a preoperative PSA level between 2.6 and 4.0 ng/ml [16]. Notably, none of the men over age 70 years were

found to have tumors that were pathologically insignificant.

Despite the potential advantages of using a lower PSA threshold to recommend prostate biopsy, there are obvious disadvantages associated with this approach. First, there is the trade-off between sensitivity and specificity. Use of a higher PSA threshold may result in a delayed cancer diagnosis, which for some cancers may be detrimental, but unnecessary biopsies can be limited. Conversely, a lower threshold will prompt biopsy in many men with indolent cancer, potentially leading to overtreatment and its attendant costs and complications. Schroder et al., using data from the European Randomized Screening of Prostate Cancer (ERSPC) trial, investigated the necessity of detecting all prostate cancers in men with serum PSA levels below 3.0 ng/ml [17]. Comparing biopsy data from the PCPT to outcomes from the ERSPC, the authors concluded that biopsy in men with PSA values less than 3 ng/ml can be safely delayed. The ERSPC prostate cancer screening trial demonstrated that 1,410 men would have to be screened and 48 treated to prevent one cancer death at a follow-up of 9 years [18]. These numbers will certainly decrease with longer follow-up, but a lower PSA threshold inevitably leads to more biopsies and overtreatment of indolent cancer until better markers of tumor aggressiveness are available.

While acknowledging that the use of a specific PSA threshold to select men for prostate biopsy is a balance between the sensitivity and specificity of cancer detection at that level and that lowering the threshold may result in detection of cancers that may not need to be treated, it is nevertheless still widely utilized. What then is the most appropriate threshold to use and should age determine this threshold? Age-specific PSA thresholds were first suggested by Oesterling et al. who studied PSA levels in 471 previously unscreened Minnesota men [19]. Using the 95th percentile of PSA levels as a guide, they proposed age-specific thresholds ranging from 2.5 ng/ml for men in their 40s to 6.5 ng/ml for men in their 70s. Higher PSA thresholds for older men were meant to decrease sensitivity and increase specificity of PSA testing in this group with a more limited life expectancy whose PSA is more likely influenced by benign prostatic hyperplasia. Obviously, the trade-off to applying a higher threshold for older men is that this strategy will miss a number of clinically significant cancers. If the goal of screening and subsequent biopsy is to find the cancers that would benefit from treatment at an earlier point in time, perhaps the same lower PSA threshold (2.5–3.0 ng/ml) should be used in all men with sufficient life expectancy to benefit from curative treatment regardless of age. As the overall life expectancy for American men continues to increase, this strategy certainly seems like a reasonable approach, particularly now that active surveillance is being successfully used to reduce overtreatment of less aggressive disease.

Should PSA Velocity or Other Measures Be Used to Assist in the Decision to Proceed with Initial Prostate Biopsy?

Serum PSA level, at whatever threshold is chosen, is the most valuable marker for detection of prostate cancer, but its usefulness is limited by its low specificity. The rate of change in PSA levels over time, or PSA velocity (PSAV), has been one method investigated to improve the specificity of the standard PSA assay. In the original study of PSAV using the Baltimore Longitudinal Aging Database, Carter et al. showed that a PSA velocity of 0.75 ng/ml or greater was present in 72% of men with prostate cancer, while it was seen in only 5% of men without prostate cancer [20]. Significant differences in PSAV could be detected up to 5 years before the diagnosis of prostate cancer. Berger et al. examined the utility of PSA velocity as a clinical marker to distinguish men who did or did not harbor prostate cancer in 4,800 screened Austrian men followed with biannual PSA for 10 years [21]. Of the 4,272 men who did not develop prostate cancer, the mean PSA velocity was 0.03 ng/ml/year compared to a PSAV of 0.39 ng/ml/year in those who were diagnosed with prostate cancer over this 10-year period . In another study using age and PSAV data available from 13,615 men participating in a large prostate cancer screening trial, median PSAV in the year before diagnosis was 0.6–0.7 ng/ml/year for men with prostate cancer compared to 0–0.01 ng/ml/year in those without prostate cancer [22]. Interestingly, while PSAV was an important predictor of cancer in all age groups, it performed best as a marker of cancer in younger men (40–49 years). A study of 11,861 unscreened men similarly found that PSAV was a better predictor of positive biopsy in younger men [23]. While these and other studies clearly show the value of PSAV as a marker of prostate cancer, its utility as it relates to selection of men for initial prostate biopsy hinges on whether it provides additional predictive information to the use of total PSA level alone. Its use for this purpose is also dependent on being able to accurately determine the PSAV value.

There are several factors that may confound the ability to accurately determine the PSAV. First, it is generally recommended that PSAV be calculated using a series of PSA levels over as long as 1.5–2.0 years. Using several PSA measures over time may increase the accuracy of PSAV by dampening the effect of the natural variability in PSA levels. Some of this variability may be related to specimen handling, laboratory processing, or differences in assay standardization. There is also physiologic variability in PSA that may be related to differences in androgen levels, prostate manipulation, ejaculation, and the presence of benign prostatic conditions. Subclinical prostatitis has been reported to elevate PSA levels and may cause an increase in PSA velocity. In 1997, Ornstein et al. reported on differences in three PSA measurements performed approximately 2 weeks apart in 84 healthy men over 50 years of age [24]. The coefficient of variation was 15% for total PSA and 17% for free PSA. In 11% of men, the coefficient of variation was greater than 30%. For a PSA level of 4 ng/ml, a 15% variability would include PSA levels ranging from 3.4 to 4.6 ng/ml. In 2003, Eastham et al. examined this issue in 972 participants in the Polyp Prevention Trial [25]. Five consecutive blood samples were obtained during a 4-year period and assessed for total and free PSA levels. They showed that the PSA level would ultimately fall below several commonly used thresholds in approximately 40–50% of men who would have been recommended to undergo biopsy. The conclusion of this study was that an isolated PSA level should be confirmed several weeks later prior to making a recommendation for biopsy.

Despite the shortcomings of serial PSA assessment due to physiologic or other variability, it remains a commonly considered variable when serial PSA levels are available. In addition to being a marker for the presence of cancer, PSAV may also predict cancer aggressiveness. D'Amico et al. found that an increase in PSA of more than 2 ng/ml in the year prior to the diagnosis of prostate cancer was associated with a significantly shorter time to death from prostate cancer in both radical prostatectomy and radiotherapy-treated patients [26, 27]. Loeb et al. reported on 1,049 patients from a large community-based screening trial that underwent radical prostatectomy with adequate data on PSAV and Gleason score [28]. The median PSAV was 0.84, 0.97, and 1.39 ng/ml/year in men with Gleason score 6, 7, and 8–10, respectively ($p = 0.05$). A PSAV greater than 2 ng/ml/year was significantly associated with a prostatectomy Gleason score of ≥ 7 on both

univariate and multivariate analysis. In addition, preoperatively PSAV was significantly lower in organ-confined disease ($p = 0.002$). Of note, while PSA doubling time (PSADT) is often used as a trigger for treatment in men on active surveillance and an important marker of more lethal disease after treatment, it may be less accurate than PSAV in prediction of life-threatening prostate cancer prior to diagnosis. In a study of 681 men with serial PSA measurements identified from the BLSA cohort, PSAV in the 5 years prior to diagnosis was significantly higher among men with high-risk or fatal prostate cancer [29]. In contrast, PSADT was not significantly associated with either high-risk or fatal disease.

With regard to selection of men for biopsy, PSA velocity may be particularly useful for those with "normal" PSA levels who may be at higher risk for harboring cancer. It is important to realize that PSA velocity correlates with total PSA level, and as such, lower PSA velocity thresholds should be used to select men for biopsy when total PSA is below 4 ng/ml. Carter et al. investigated the use of PSA velocity at normal PSA levels for detection of potentially life-threatening prostate cancer during the window of curability [30]. Using the Baltimore Longitudinal Study of Aging population, 980 men had PSA velocity determined. The relative risks of prostate cancer death and prostate cancer-specific survival were stratified according to PSA velocity. PSA velocity that was measured 10–15 years before prostate cancer diagnosis when most men had PSA levels below 4 ng/ml was associated with cancer-specific survival 25 years later. Survival was 92% among men with PSA velocity of 0.35 ng/ml/year or less and 54% among men with PSA velocity above 0.35 ng/ml/year. Men with PSA velocity above 0.35 ng/ml/year had a higher relative risk of prostate cancer death as well. This study suggests that a PSA velocity threshold of 0.35 ng/ml may help identify men with life-threatening but curable prostate cancer during the period when their PSA levels were otherwise normal.

Since determination of PSAV may be confounded by inflammation or the physiologic variability of PSA, a method that calculates PSAV at multiple points in time may be a more accurate tumor marker. Carter et al. also introduced the PSA velocity "risk count" concept as a way to potentially identify men at risk for the development of high-risk disease [31]. Using this method, the number of times the PSA velocity exceeded a threshold (PSA velocity risk count) was determined in 717 men over 10–20 years. The probability of high-risk disease increased directly with the risk count with a 1.49 (95% CI, 1.29–1.71) relative risk for the development of high-risk disease using a PSA velocity cut point of 0.4 ng/ml/year. This method of PSA history interpretation could help to identify those men destined to develop high-risk disease who would benefit from diagnosis and treatment of their prostate cancer at PSA levels more likely to be associated with curable disease.

Despite the apparent utility of PSAV in selecting men for biopsy, both the PCPT and the ERSPC prostate cancer screening trials found that PSAV was not an independent predictor of positive biopsy [32, 33]. In the PCPT, predictive factors included PSA, DRE, family history, and prior biopsy findings [32]. Although PSAV predicted the likelihood of a positive biopsy in univariate analysis, in multivariable analysis it was not an independent predictor. Similarly, in the ERSPC prostate cancer screening trial, PSAV that was useful as a univariate predictor of a positive biopsy did not maintain its significance as an independent predictor when analyzed in multivariable analysis [33]. This suggests that PSAV is very closely related to total PSA and may add little to the predictive ability of PSA alone in selecting men for prostate biopsy. It may, however, be useful in determining which men to follow more closely prior to reaching a PSA threshold of concern.

When Should Prostatic Inflammation Be Suspected as Contributing to an Elevated PSA Level?

It is well established that both acute and chronic prostatitis can have significant effects on PSA levels. In a recent study, Candirali et al. examined the relationship between prostatic inflammation and serum PSA level in 150 patients who had a negative prostate biopsy [34]. In this population of men without prostate cancer, they found a significant correlation between the serum PSA level and the extent of inflammation seen in biopsy cores. Prostatitis has been shown to confound PSA velocity as well. In a large PSA screening trial, the effect of prostatitis on PSA velocity was evaluated in 1,851 men who had serial PSA measurements and normal DRE [35]. Although the PSA velocity over the year prior to biopsy predicted prostate cancer, the frequency of histological inflammation was also associated with PSA velocity. While prostate cancer was more common than prostatitis in the lower PSA velocity ranges, at a very high PSA velocity of > 4 ng/ml per year, the likelihood of finding prostatitis was identical to that of finding prostate cancer (13%). Elevated PSA levels induced by inflammation can be lowered after antibiotic treatment. Schaeffer et al. reported that the median PSA level decreased from 8.3 to 5.4 ng/ml in patients with chronic bacterial prostatitis after a 28-day course of a fluoroquinolone [36]. In those whose initial PSA level was > 4 ng/ml, the PSA decreased to < 4 ng/ml after a course of antibiotics in 42% of these patients.

For men with elevated PSA levels in whom prostatitis is suspected clinically, a trial of antibiotic therapy is certainly indicated. Some have suggested that empiric antibiotic therapy should be administered to all patients considering biopsy to eliminate the possibility that subclinical prostatitis could be accounting for their elevated PSA level. Serretta et al. prospectively administered a 3-week course of ciprofloxacin to 99 patients who presented with a PSA level > 4 ng/ml and normal DRE [37]. A repeat PSA was performed after antibiotic therapy, but regardless of interval PSA change, all men underwent prostate biopsy. In this population, 60% of patients had a decrease in PSA after antibiotic therapy. Prostate cancer detection rate was 40% among men with an increasing or stable PSA after antibiotics compared to 20% detection rate among men with a PSA reduction. Furthermore, prostate cancer was not detected in any patient with an initial PSA less than 10 and a > 50% reduction in PSA level in response to antibiotic therapy. Although this study was not randomized, it demonstrated that a large reduction in PSA following antibiotic therapy may help avoid biopsy in selected patients whose PSA elevation was likely due to prostatitis.

Although some PSAs will be lowered with antibiotic administration, it is problematic to advocate empiric antibiotic therapy for all patients with an elevated PSA level. First, a decrease in PSA after antibiotic therapy does not rule out the presence of prostate cancer, even if the PSA decreases to a significantly lower level. Furthermore, a stable or increasing PSA after antibiotic treatment does not necessarily indicate that prostate cancer is present. The indiscriminate use of empiric antibiotics may also lead to the development of resistant organisms, increasing the risk of infectious complications, a greater concern recently with the increasing prevalence of fluoroquinolone-resistant bacteria.

In summary, repeated PSA measurements provide more valid information than a single measurement, and there is considerable evidence that prostatitis can be a significant confounder of the PSA level. An empiric course of antibiotic therapy is certainly reasonable in men with fluctuating PSA values, particularly if they have an exacerbation of their baseline voiding symptoms. However, the indiscriminate use of empiric antibiotic therapy has the potential for associated risks and may not accurately differentiate asymptomatic men who do and do not have prostate cancer. While further study of this issue is necessary, it is reasonable to consider a course of antibiotic therapy in men with a history of prostatitis, an exacerbation of their voiding symptoms, or a fluctuating PSA where subclinical prostatitis is a possibility.

Should Nomograms Be Used to Select Men for Initial Prostate Biopsy?

Nomograms have been utilized in prostate cancer decision making for some time, usually to predict specific pathologic features or clinical outcomes after primary prostate cancer treatment. Nomograms or artificial neural networks can also be used to calculate the probability of a positive prostate biopsy by combining PSA levels with other risk factors in a predictive model [38]. Nomograms to predict prostate biopsy result (positive or negative, a binary outcome) are generally constructed using a multivariable logistic regression analysis. The predictive accuracy of a nomogram is derived using receiver operator characteristic (ROC) area under the curve (AUC) and is expressed as a percentage. Predictive accuracy values range from 50% to 100%, where 50% is equivalent to the flip of a coin and 100% represents perfect prediction. No model is perfect, and predictive accuracy generally ranges from 70% to 80%. The predictive accuracy of a nomogram should ideally be confirmed by testing it in an external cohort (external validation) although internal validation using statistical methods such as bootstrapping may also be used. Artificial neural networks are computer-based systems that attempt to mimic the learning process of neural circuits in the brain. Data (risk factors and outcomes) are fed into the system by a training program that creates a system of weighing these factors. Test cases are run to check the network, and when complete, a validation set is also run. Although comparative studies of nomograms and artificial neural networks suggest that they may differ in their accuracy based on the circumstances of testing, a direct comparison of an artificial neural network and a nomogram to predict prostate cancer on initial biopsy in one study showed that the nomogram was statistically significantly more accurate and was associated with better performance characteristics [39].

The most important question when considering the use of any model to determine the risk of positive biopsy is whether it is more accurate than the use of PSA level alone. Schroder and Kattan recently reviewed available nomograms and artificial neural networks designed to predict the likelihood of a positive prostate biopsy [40]. At the time of that review, there were at least 36 predictive models of this kind available. In addition to total PSA value, these nomograms use additional risk factors such as age, family history, previous biopsy, abnormal DRE, ultrasound findings, prostate volume, and others in the model. With the exception of two studies, all of

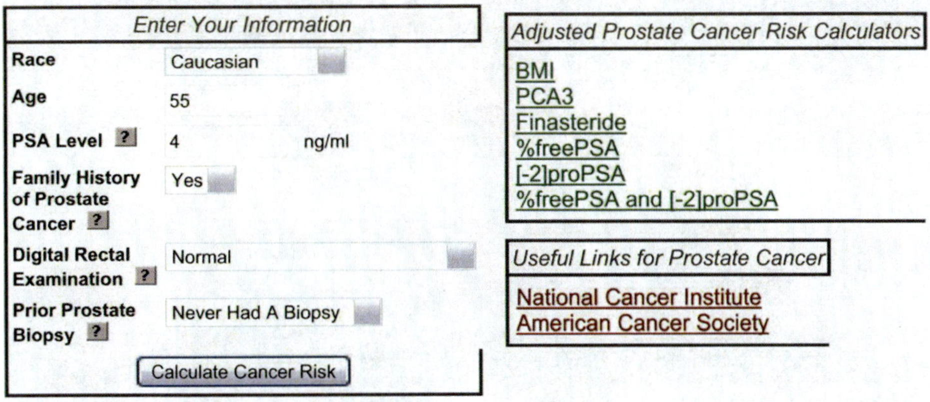

Fig. 10.2 Risk calculator developed from PCPT biopsy information (Image obtained from http://deb.uthscsa.edu/URORiskCalc/Pages/calcs.jsp). Prostate cancer risk calculators adjusted for other factors are also available as listed

the models demonstrated AUC values of ≥0.70, with eight reporting an AUC of ≥0.80. Fourteen studies compared the AUC of the model with the AUC of PSA alone. All of these showed that the model improved predictive accuracy with an increase in AUC ranging from 0.02 to 0.26 compared to PSA alone. Of note, only 16 models underwent external validation, and in 13 of these, the AUC was lower in the comparison population than the model-development population. In addition, the model-development population was shown to strongly influence the prediction of positive biopsy when used in individual patients. The specific risk values generated varied by as much as threefold across the models tested.

One of the smallest incremental benefits in AUC compared to PSA alone was noted in the nomogram developed from the PCPT [41]. In the PCPT, 18,882 men were randomly assigned to receive either finasteride or placebo and were followed with annual digital rectal examinations (DRE) and PSA measurements. After 7 years on study, men who had not been diagnosed with prostate cancer were asked to undergo an end-of-study biopsy. These men were biopsied at PSA levels of ≤4 ng/ml with a normal DRE result. Utilizing the biopsy results of 5,519 men from the placebo group who underwent prostate biopsy, a predictive model of prostate cancer detection was developed. Logistic regression was used to model the risk of prostate cancer and high-grade disease associated with age at biopsy, race, family

history of prostate cancer, PSA level, PSA velocity, DRE result, and previous prostate biopsy. Variables that predicted prostate cancer included higher PSA level, positive family history of prostate cancer, and abnormal digital rectal examination result. Previous negative prostate biopsy was associated with reduced risk. Of note, neither age at biopsy nor PSA velocity contributed independent prognostic information. Higher PSA level, abnormal DRE result, older age at biopsy, and African-American race were predictive for high-grade disease, whereas previous negative prostate biopsy reduced the risk. The PCPT risk calculator (Fig. 10.2, http://deb.uthscsa.edu/URORiskCalc/Pages/calcs.jsp) can be accessed online.

Despite being one of the largest and most systematic studies from which to develop a biopsy nomogram, the improvement in predictive accuracy using the PCPT risk calculator was minimal with an incremental AUC benefit of only 0.02 compared to PSA alone [40]. One potential explanation for this very small benefit may be that this nomogram was derived from a population of men biopsied regardless of PSA level rather than a PSA threshold. Another potential limitation of the PCPT risk calculator is that it was developed from a cohort of men who entered the trial with a PSA of 3.0 ng/ml or less, a normal DRE, and age 55 years or older. Most men presenting for prostate biopsy have an increased PSA level or an abnormal DRE, and many are younger than

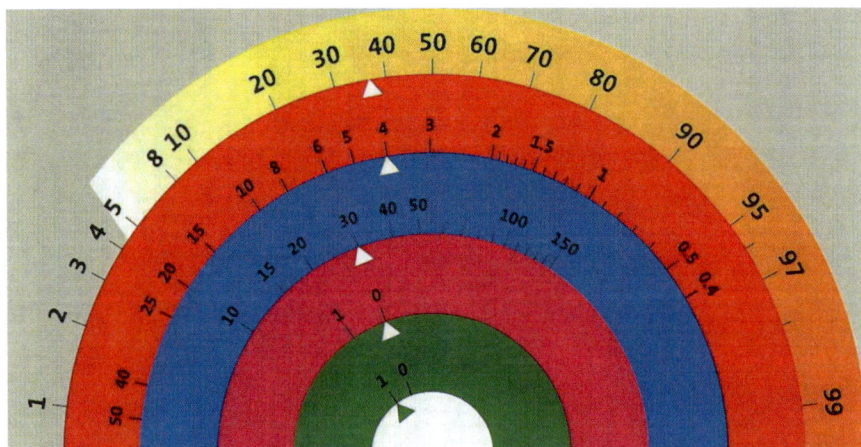

Fig. 10.3 Riskindicator developed from ERSPC biopsy data. This example predicts the risk of prostate cancer in a previously unscreened patient with normal DRE (*pink*) and abnormal TRUS (*green*) with a 30-ml prostate volume (*blue*) and a PSA of 4 ng/ml (*red*). The chance of the patient having a positive biopsy is 37% (Image obtained from SWOP Prostate Cancer Research Foundation [www.prostatecancer-riskcalculator.com])

55 years of age. To validate the PCPT risk calculator, Eyre et al. utilized data from patients undergoing prostate biopsy by 12 urologists at five sites who were enrolled in the Early Detection Research Network (EDRN) study [42]. This analysis revealed that the EDRN and PCPT cohorts were significantly different. Cancer incidence was greater in the EDRN validation cohort (43%) compared to the PCPT cohort (22%). Furthermore, the EDRN participants were younger and more racially diverse than PCPT participants. Prostate cancer severity was worse in the EDRN cohort as well.

A recently developed nomogram using biopsy data from initial and subsequent screening in the ERSPC screening trial aimed to develop a tool that could be used not only to predict the risk of a positive biopsy but to also reduce the risk of unnecessary biopsies [43]. The Riskindicator is a predictive model originally developed in a cohort of 6,288 men from the Rotterdam section of the ERSPC and is available online for public use (Fig. 10.3, www.prostatecancer-riskcalculator. com). In addition to PSA level, this model incorporates digital rectal examination results and transrectal ultrasound findings (prostate volume and the presence or absence of a hypoechoic lesion). In the most recent update of this nomogram, Roobol et al. evaluated the ability of the Riskindicator to predict both initial prostate biopsy results and the relative proportion of potentially "indolent" and "important" cancers that would have been missed using this model [43]. The initial biopsy was triggered by a PSA threshold of 3 ng/ml, and prostate cancer was detected in 29% of men biopsied as a result of initial screening. On receiver operator characteristic analysis, the AUC for the model was 0.77. If a Riskindicator prostate biopsy probability of 12.5% was used as an indication for biopsy, the model would have missed 14% of cancers detected on initial screening although it was estimated that 70% of these missed cancers were potentially indolent. However, the author's definition of indolent cancer (clinical stage $\leq$ T2, PSA $\leq$ 20 ng/ml, primary and secondary Gleason grade $\leq$ 3, $\leq$ 50% positive cores, <20 mm total cancer in biopsy cores and benign tissue in all cores $\geq$ 40 mm) was quite liberal; a much higher number of potentially important tumors would have been missed if more stringent criteria for indolent cancer were used. Another practical disadvantage of the Riskindicator is the inclusion of multiple parameters from TRUS, factors that can only be known after the decision to proceed with biopsy has been made. It may be more appropriate to use the Riskindicator as a model for predicting outcome of repeat biopsy in which case the TRUS parameters from the first biopsy could be incorporated prior to the decision for biopsy has been made.

A recent comparison between the PCPT and ERSPC risk calculators points out the importance of understanding the population tested and the risk factors included in the model before using a nomogram to select for biopsy [44]. Applying these nomograms to virtual patients in this study resulted in significantly discrepant predictions. A 60-year-old, Caucasian man with normal DRE and negative family history with a PSA of 4 ng/ml would have a 35% chance of having a positive initial prostate biopsy according to the PCPT risk calculator. That same man would have a positive biopsy risk of 13% using the ERSPC Riskindicator, almost a threefold lower risk. At a PSA threshold of 10 ng/ml, the corresponding risk levels would be 54% and 39%, respectively, again a significant difference in risk assessment. In general, the PCPT risk calculator indicated a higher likelihood of finding cancer at PSA levels <20 ng/ml, after which the curves crossed and the ERSPC predicted higher risks.

The significant differences in risk estimates between these nomograms are due to important differences in the underlying model design and the populations used to develop them. In the PCPT, there were fewer biopsies in the higher PSA ranges and, in the ERSPC, fewer in the lower ranges. Both risk indicators have incorporated some variables that are absent in the other because they were not found to be independently significant in multivariable analysis. It also appeared that prostate volume (not available in the PCPT) had a larger effect on predictions in comparable PSA ranges than race, age family history, and previous negative biopsy (indicators excluded in the ERSPC). It is clear from this comparison that if the characteristics of the underlying population, including risk factors, are not considered in selecting the appropriate nomogram, significant dissimilarities between

the models will result in grossly discrepant predictions for individual patients.

Both the PCPT and ERSPC risk calculators are based on biopsy results in men undergoing sextant prostate biopsy. This limits their applicability to more contemporary biopsy populations for which extended biopsy schemes are routinely applied. Since the late 1990s, extended biopsy schemes have become the standard of care for initial prostate biopsy. A recent study in which a logistic regression-based model was developed to predict prostate cancer at biopsy found biopsy core number to be an independent predictor of biopsy outcome in multivariable analysis [45]. As such, many clinicians may be reluctant to use nomograms that were developed using the sextant biopsy technique. Some nomograms also incorporate clinical information that is not available prior to initial biopsy such as TRUS-determined prostate size and past biopsy history. These nomograms may be less valuable to the urologist on initial biopsy when these clinical variables are not available and when an extended biopsy scheme is planned.

Two recently reported nomograms based on extended prostate biopsy schemes and readily available clinical information including percent-free PSA may be more applicable to patients undergoing contemporary biopsy [46–48]. The Sunnybrook nomogram, a multi-institutionally derived tool proposed initially in 2007, incorporates PSA, age, family history of prostate cancer, ethnicity, urinary symptoms, percent-free PSA, and digital rectal examination findings [46]. Urinary symptom score was used as a surrogate for prostate size which has been found to be inversely related to prostate cancer detection in previous studies. Of the 3,108 men who underwent prostate biopsy using a 10–12-core biopsy scheme, 42% were found to have prostate cancer. The AUC for detection of all cancers and high-grade cancer was 0.74 and 0.77, respectively. When the performance of the Sunnybrook nomogram was compared to the PCPT risk calculator, the predictive accuracy was higher for the Sunnybrook nomogram for detection of both all cancers and aggressive cancers [47].

Another recent nomogram developed from 1,551 patients undergoing biopsy at Cleveland Clinic, almost all of whom had a 12-core biopsy, reported a positive biopsy rate of 39% [48]. This nomogram incorporated all of the factors used in the Sunnybrook nomogram, except urinary symptoms. The AUC for detection of all cancers was 0.73 and for high-grade cancer was 0.71, a predictive accuracy similar to the Sunnybrook nomogram. It is important to note that although both these nomograms utilized biopsy results from extended biopsy schemes resulting in positive biopsy rates more consistent with contemporary findings, they both include percent-free PSA, a PSA value not always available in those being considered for initial prostate biopsy.

An advantage of a nomogram or risk calculator over a cut-point threshold for determining who to biopsy is the ability of these models to incorporate new markers. An example of this is the recent incorporation of prostate cancer gene 3 (PCA3) into the PCPT risk calculator to improve its diagnostic accuracy [49]. Based on a cohort of 522 men who underwent prostate biopsy with measurements of urinary PCA3, serum PSA, DRE, and biopsy history, this marker was incorporated into the risk assessment. External validation of the updated risk calculator was performed on the cohort of 443 European patients and compared to PCPT risk estimates. Incorporation of PCA3 improved the diagnostic accuracy of the PCPT risk calculator.

Other studies have also explored the possibility of improving the predictive accuracy of nomograms by incorporation of new markers. Vickers et al. investigated the potential role of free PSA, intact-free PSA, and human kallikrein 2 (hK2) in modifying the detection characteristics of total PSA in men biopsied in the first round of the ERSPC screening study in Gothenburg, Sweden [50]. The addition of these three markers improved the AUC for cancer detection from 0.69 to 0.83 and from 0.72 to 0.84 for the two models tested. At a likelihood of 20% for recommending prostate biopsy, 57% of men could have avoided biopsy had these markers been used, and of the cancers missed, only 8% were high grade. A similar study by Jansen et al. utilized the PSA isoforms, p2PSA in conjunction with free PSA in

men biopsied in the Rotterdam section of the ERSPC, showing improved detection compared to total PSA alone [51]. These studies demonstrate that new markers for prostate cancer detection can be readily incorporated into existing or new risk calculators to improve the ability to select men for initial biopsy.

An important question with regard to the use of nomograms in the initial biopsy setting is what risk level should prompt biopsy. The decision to proceed or not with prostate biopsy depends on which threshold probability is used [52]. It has been suggested that threshold probabilities between 10% and 40% should determine the need for prostate biopsy. That is, a risk of 10% for cancer would likely dissuade one from proceeding with biopsy, while a risk of 40% would almost certainly compel one to proceed. However, it is possible that patients and physicians may accept lower or higher risk thresholds as there is no widely agreed-upon risk threshold that should prompt biopsy. While nomograms yield probabilities of a positive biopsy on a continuous scale, the urologist and the patient still must determine the *clinical* significance of this number. The risk threshold selected will have to be individualized, making the use of these nomograms more complex and potentially less practical in the clinic setting. Each nomogram will have different predictive accuracies based on the risk threshold selected. This variability in predictive accuracy, between nomograms and at different threshold probabilities within the same nomogram, may limit their widespread use.

Conclusions and Recommendations

- Most guidelines from professional organizations recommend use of some cutoff PSA threshold to indicate biopsy. With knowledge that prostate cancer exists at all PSA level s and that PSA level represents a continuum of risk, the challenge is selection of a threshold with the most appropriate balance between sensitivity and specificity. To account for increased prostate size in older men (60s and 70s), it seems reasonable to select a higher PSA threshold that may be used to recommend biopsy in these age groups. At the same time, knowing that median PSA levels for young men (40s and 50s) are less than 1 ng/ml, lower PSA thresholds should probably be used to prompt biopsy in these younger men. Using a lower PSA threshold (2.5 ng/ml) regardless of age risks overdiagnosis and the potential for overtreatment. Data from the ERSPC screening trial suggest that it is relatively safe to use a PSA threshold of 3 ng/ml to recommend biopsy in the setting of repeated screening. Since this trial found a prostate cancer mortality advantage, using this threshold for all men would at least be backed by evidence from a randomized trial. An important advantage of using a PSA threshold strategy in selecting men for biopsy is the simple concept that since the majority of men will have PSA levels below this threshold, they can be given the reassuring message that no biopsy is necessary. Also, the simplicity of this strategy makes it likely that cutoff PSA values will continue to be used until better and equally simple alternatives are found.

- PSA velocity should be considered if PSA history is known. However, a lengthy PSA history is not usually available, and there are other potential confounding factors in calculation of PSAV including differences between PSA assays, the biologic variability in PSA, and the impact of prostatitis. Some studies also show that PSAV adds little to total PSA level in predicting a positive biopsy. Despite these limitations, the significant volume of data which suggests that PSAV may be a marker of a more aggressive cancer is hard to ignore. Since an abnormal PSA velocity is a relatively uncommon finding in PSA screening populations, it is hard to make the case that it should replace total PSA level as the primary factor in selection of men for biopsy. Its primary role may be in helping to identify men at lower PSA levels for earlier biopsy, prior to their PSA reaching a threshold at which biopsy might be recommended. It is clear that a PSAV of greater than 0.35–0.40 ng/ml/year at low PSA level (PSA less than 4 ng/ml) should be a cause for concern. At the same time, it seems reasonable to clearly establish

this trend over a long period of time and several PSA measure before recommending biopsy. As noted previously, a PSAV risk count strategy may accomplish this goal.

- It seems unreasonable to recommend repeating every PSA test to confirm it or to advocate a course of antibiotics for everyone found to have an elevated PSA level. However, there are specific clinical situations where this may be appropriate. If a strict PSA threshold is going to be what prompts biopsy and the PSA level is near that threshold, repeating the PSA level may in some cases prove it to be lower, potentially avoiding biopsy. Taking into account the biologic variability of PSA and the knowledge that a slightly lower PSA level only lowers your chance of prostate cancer slightly, this strategy may not make sense in the asymptomatic man. However, for men with a history of prostatitis, a flare in their voiding symptoms, or a fluctuating PSA level, a course of antibiotics for suspected prostatitis is a very reasonable option.

- Nomograms incorporating other factors together with PSA to estimate the probability of a positive prostate biopsy would seem like the ideal and potentially the most accurate way to select men for initial prostate biopsy. Nearly all nomograms show a greater predictive accuracy compared to PSA alone. However, there are several limitations to these tools that must be taken into consideration before they can be used on a regular basis. Since each nomogram is developed from varied populations of men undergoing different PSA testing regimens and specific biopsy strategies, it is important to use a nomogram which most closely represents one's own practice patterns. Nomograms must also be easy to use, incorporating factors that are immediately available when making the biopsy decision. Tools which incorporate factors only known from previous TRUS or ancillary PSA measures that are unavailable will be of little use. Finally, each nomogram will have different predictive accuracies based on the risk threshold selected, and the risk threshold for recommending or proceeding with biopsy may differ significantly between patients. While this individualized approach may appear ideal on the surface, its complexity may make it too cumbersome for routine use in the clinic setting.

Editorial Commentary:

Threshold: a level, point, or value above which something is true or will take place and below which it is not or will not

–Miriam Webster's Dictionary

In an ideal medical world, laboratory tests such as PSA would entail a threshold that—as Webster's would define—would segregate patients with and without prostate cancer by values above and below a meaningful threshold. Unfortunately, in the real medical world in which we all practice, PSA values represent a continuum, and there is not even a clear inflection point at which prostate cancer risk changes enough to create a justifiable threshold for empiric use. Nevertheless, the quandary for an individual patient decision relates to the fact that they don't benefit from knowing where they are on a continuum. For each patient-based decision the outcomes are not continuous, they are categorical—biopsy or no biopsy?

Although the authors demonstrate that it is not a threshold that represents a clear border between cancer and benignity, there is reason to think in terms of PSA values around 2.5 being meaningful to consider biopsy in most healthy men. Around that relatively soft "threshold", they provide guidance on concepts that may move one toward or away from that inevitable yes or no decision. Making that decision through a relationship between doctor and patient is the very essence of personalized medicine.

References

1. Pienta KJ. Critical appraisal of prostate-specific antigen in prostate cancer screening: 20 years later. Urology. 2009;73:11–20.
2. Thompson IM, Pauler DK, Goodman PJ, et al. Prevalence of prostate cancer among men with a prostate-specific antigen level <or =4.0 ng per milliliter. N Engl J Med. 2004;350:2239–46.
3. Ahyai SA, Graefen M, Steuber T, et al. Contemporary prostate cancer prevalence among T1c biopsy-referred men with a prostate-specific antigen level ≤4.0 ng per milliliter. Eur Urol. 2008;53:750–7.
4. Rich AR. On the frequency of occurrence of occult carcinoma of the prostate. J Urol. 1935;33:215–23. Reprinted in Int J Epidemiol 2007; 36:274–77.
5. Franks LM. Latency and progression in tumors: the natural history of prostatic cancer. Lancet. 1956;2:1037–9.
6. Sakr WA, Haas GP, Cassin BF, et al. The frequency of carcinoma and intraepithelial neoplasia of the prostate in young male patients. J Urol. 1993;150:379–85.
7. Yin M, Bastacky S, Chandran U, et al. Prevalence of incidental prostate cancer in the general population: a study of healthy organ donors. J Urol. 2008;179:892–5.
8. Cooner WH, Mosley BR, Rutherford Jr CL, et al. Prostate cancer detection in a clinical urological practice by ultrasonography, digital rectal examination and prostate specific antigen. J Urol. 1990;143:1146–52.
9. Catalona WJ, Smith DS, Ratliff TL, et al. Measurement of prostate-specific antigen in serum as a screening test for prostate cancer. N Engl J Med. 1991;324: 1156–61.
10. Loeb S, Roehl KA, Antenor JV, et al. Baseline prostate-specific antigen compared with median prostate-specific antigen for age group as predictor of prostate cancer risk in men younger than 60 years old. Urology. 2006;67(2):316–20.
11. Porter MP, Stanford JL, Lange PH. The distribution of serum prostate-specific antigen levels among American men: implications for prostate cancer prevalence and screening. Prostate. 2006;66:1044–51.
12. Krumholtz JS, Carvalhal GF, Ramos CG, et al. Prostate-specific antigen cutoff of 2.6 ng/ml for prostate cancer screening is associated with favorable pathologic tumor features. Urology. 2002;60:469–73.
13. Antenor JV, Roehl KA, Eggener SE, et al. Preoperative PSA and progression-free survival after radical prostatectomy for stage T1c disease. Urology. 2005;66: 156–60.
14. Lucia MS, Darke AK, Goodman PJ, et al. Pathologic characteristics of cancers detected in the Prostate Cancer Prevention Trial: implications for prostate cancer detection and chemoprevention. Cancer Prev Res. 2008;1:167–73.
15. Makarov DV, Humphreys EB, Mangold LA, et al. Pathological outcomes and biochemical progression in men with T1c prostate cancer undergoing radical prostatectomy with prostate specific antigen 2.6 to 4.0 vs 4.1 to 6.0 ng/ml. J Urol. 2006;176:554–8.
16. Nadler RB, Loeb S, Roehl KA, et al. Use of 2.6 ng/ml prostate specific antigen prompt for biopsy in men older than 60 years. J Urol. 2005;174:2154–7. discussion 2157.
17. Schröder FH, Bangma CH, Roobol MJ. Is it necessary to detect all prostate cancers in men with serum PSA levels <3.0 ng/ml? A comparison of biopsy results of PCPT and outcome-related information from ERSPC. Eur Urol. 2008;53:901–8.
18. Schröder FH, Hugosson J, Roobol MJ, et al. Screening and prostate-cancer mortality in a randomized European study. N Engl J Med. 2009;360:1320–8.
19. Oesterling JE, Jacobsen SJ, Chute CG, et al. Serum prostate-specific antigen in a community-based population of healthy men. Establishment of age-specific reference ranges. JAMA. 1993;270:860–4.

20. Carter HB, Pearson JD, Metter EJ, et al. Longitudinal evaluation of prostate-specific antigen levels in men with and without prostate disease. JAMA. 1992;267: 2215–20.

21. Berger AP, Deibl M, Strasak A, et al. Large-scale study of clinical impact of PSA velocity: long-term PSA kinetics as method of differentiating men with from those without prostate cancer. Urology. 2007;69: 134–8.

22. Loeb S, Roehl KA, Catalona WJ, et al. Is the utility of prostate-specific antigen velocity for prostate cancer detection affected by age? BJU Int. 2008;101:817–21.

23. Moul JW, Sun L, Hotaling JM, et al. Age adjusted prostate specific antigen and prostate specific antigen velocity cut points in prostate cancer screening. J Urol. 2007;177:499–504.

24. Ornstein DK, Smith DS, Rao GS, et al. Biological variation of total, free, and percent free serum prostate specific antigen levels in screening volunteers. J Urol. 1997;157(6):2179–82.

25. Eastham JA, Riedel E, Scardino PT, et al. Variation of serum prostate-specific antigen levels: an evaluation of year-to-year fluctuations. JAMA. 2003;289(20):2695–700.

26. D'Amico AV, Chen MH, Roehl KA, et al. PSA velocity and the risk of death from prostate cancer after radical prostatectomy. N Engl J Med. 2004;351:125–35.

27. D'Amico AV, Renshaw AA, Sussman B, et al. Pretreatment PSA velocity and risk of death from prostate cancer following external beam radiation therapy. JAMA. 2005;294:440–7.

28. Loeb S, Sutherland DE, D'Amico AV, et al. Preoperative PSA velocity is associated with Gleason score in radical prostatectomy specimen; marker for prostate cancer aggressiveness. Urology. 2008;72:1116–20. discussion 1120.

29. Loeb S, Kettermann A, Ferrucci L, et al. PSA doubling time versus PSA velocity to predict high-risk prostate cancer: data from the Baltimore Longitudinal Study of Aging. Eur Urol. 2008;54:1073–80.

30. Carter HB, Ferrucci L, Kettermann A, et al. Detection of life-threatening prostate cancer with prostate-specific antigen velocity during a window of curability. J Natl Cancer Inst. 2006;98:1521–7.

31. Carter HB, Kettermann A, Ferrucci L, et al. Prostate-specific antigen velocity risk count assessment: a new concept for detection of life-threatening prostate cancer during window of curability. Urology. 2007;70: 685–90.

32. Thompson IM, Ankerst DP, Chen C, et al. Assessing prostate cancer risk: results from the Prostate Cancer Prevention Trial. J Natl Cancer Inst. 2006;98(8): 529–34.

33. Wolters T, Roobol MJ, Bangma CH, et al. Is prostate-specific antigen velocity selective for clinically significant prostate cancer in screening? European Randomized Study for Prostate Cancer. Eur Urol. 2009;55:385–93.

34. Kandirali E, Boran C, Serin E, et al. Association of extent and aggressiveness of inflammation with serum PSA levels and PSA density in asymptomatic patients. Urology. 2007;70(4):743–7.

35. Eggener SE, Yossepowitch O, Roehl KA, et al. Relationship of prostate specific antigen velocity to histological findings in a prostate cancer screening program. Urology. 2008;71:1016–9.

36. Schaeffer AJ, Wu SC, Tennenberg AM, et al. Treatment of chronic bacterial prostatitis with levofloxacin and ciprofloxacin lowers serum prostate specific antigen. J Urol. 2005;174(1):161–4.

37. Serretta V, Catanese A, Daricello G, et al. PSA reduction (after antibiotics) permits to avoid or postpone prostate biopsy in selected patients. Prostate Cancer Prostatic Dis. 2008;11(2):148–52.

38. Chun FK-H, Karakiewicz PI, Briganti A, et al. Prostate cancer nomograms: an update. Eur Urol. 2006;50: 914–26.

39. Chun FK-H, Karakiewicz PI, Briganti A, et al. A critical appraisal of logistic regression-based nomograms, artificial neural networks, classification and regression-tree models, look-up tables and risk-group stratification models for prostate cancer. BJU Int. 2007;99:794–800.

40. Schröder F, Kattan MW. The comparability of models for predicting the risk of a positive prostate biopsy with prostate-specific antigen alone: a systematic review. Eur Urol. 2008;54:274–90.

41. Thompson IM, Ankerst DP, Chi C, et al. Assessing prostate cancer risk: results from the Prostate Cancer Prevention Trial. J Natl Cancer Inst. 2006;98: 529–34.

42. Eyre SJ, Ankerst DP, Wei JT, et al. Validation in a multiple urology practice cohort of the Prostate Cancer Prevention Trial calculator for predicting prostate cancer detection. J Urol. 2009;182: 2653–8.

43. Roobol MJ, Steyerberg EW, Kranse R, et al. A risk-based strategy improves prostate-specific antigen-driven detection of prostate cancer. Eur Urol. 2010;57:79–85.

44. van den Bergh RCN, Roobol MJ, Wolters T, et al. The Prostate Cancer Prevention Trial and European Randomized Study of Screening for Prostate Cancer risk calculators indicating a positive prostate biopsy: a comparison. BJU Int. 2008;102:1068–73.

45. Hernandez DJ, Han M, Humphreys EB, et al. Predicting the outcome of prostate biopsy: comparison of a novel logistic regression-based model, the prostate cancer risk calculator, and prostate-specific antigen level alone. BJU Int. 2008;103:609–14.

46. Nam RK, Toi A, Klotz LH, et al. Assessing individual risk for prostate cancer. J Clin Oncol. 2007;25: 3582–8.

47. Nam RK, Kattan MW, Chin JL, et al. Prospective multi-institutional study evaluating the performance of prostate cancer risk calculators. J Clin Oncol. 2011;29:2959–64.

48. Zaytoun OM, Kattam MW, Moussa AS, et al. Development of improved nomogram for prediction of outcome of initial prostate biopsy using readily available clinical information. Urology 2011;78(2):392–8.

49. Ankerst DP, Groskopf J, Day JR, et al. Predicting prostate cancer risk through incorporation of prostate cancer gene 3. J Urol. 2008;180:1303–8.

50. Vickers AJ, Cronin AM, Aus G, et al. A panel of kallikrein markers can reduce unnecessary biopsy for prostate cancer: data from the European Randomized Study of Prostate Cancer Screening in Goteborg, Sweden. BMC Med. 2008;6:19.

51. Jansen FH, van Schaik RH, Kurstjens J, et al. Prostate-specific antigen (PSA) isoform p2PSA in combination with total PSA and free PSA improves diagnostic accuracy in prostate cancer detection. Eur Urol. 2010;57:921–7.

52. Steyerberg EW, Vickers AJ. Decision curve analysis: a discussion. Med Decis Making. 2008;Jan–Feb: 146–9.

Preparation for Prostate Biopsy

11

Ryan P. Kopp, Christopher J. Kane,
and J. Kellogg Parsons

Introduction

Transrectal ultrasound-guided prostate needle biopsy is considered a safe procedure and is commonly performed in an office setting. However, it carries inherent risks, most notably bleeding and infection. Appropriate patient counseling and preparation mitigates unrealized patient expectations and prevents significant complications associated with prostate biopsy.

Herein, we discuss practical, evidence-based principles of preparation for prostate biopsy, including discontinuation of hematologic agents, bowel preparation, and antibiotic prophylaxis.

Discontinuation of Hematologic Agents

Several medications either directly or indirectly affect bleeding risk through platelet function or proteins within the coagulation cascade that ulti-

R.P. Kopp, M.D. • J.K. Parsons, M.D., MHS
Division of Urology, University of California San Diego Medical Center, 200 W Arbor Drive #8897, San Diego, CA 92020, USA
e-mail: rkopp@ucsd.edu

C.J. Kane, M.D. (✉)
Division of Urology, C. Lowell and JoEllen Parsons Endowed Chair in Urology, University of California San Diego Medical Center, 200 W Arbor Drive #8897, San Diego, CA 92020-8897, USA
e-mail: ckane@ucsd.edu

mately interact with platelets to form a plug and prevent bleeding. Many patients will be taking antiplatelet or anticoagulant agents to prevent significant cardiovascular morbidity and mortality. Historically, prostate needle biopsy was thought unsafe for patients taking these medications and most practitioners would recommend cessation of antiplatelet or anticoagulant therapy prior to biopsy [1]. Recent research, however, has shown that some of these medications may be safe in the periprocedural setting, and the physician must use clinical judgment for each patient to determine if bleeding risks due to these medications outweigh the thromboembolic or cardiovascular risks of holding these medications.

Antiplatelet Therapy: Mechanisms of Action

Platelet aggregation inhibitors include aspirin, nonsteroidal anti-inflammatory drugs (NSAIDs), dipyridamole, and thienopyridines such as clopidogrel (Plavix). These medications target different mechanisms and ultimately lead to platelet inhibition. While some of these medications reversibly bind their targets, others are irreversible inhibitors. Glycoprotein IIb/IIIa inhibitors are not included in this discussion because these medications are primarily used during coronary intervention or for acute coronary syndromes and are not administered orally.

The average life span of circulating platelets is 8–10 days, with approximately 10–15% of circulating platelets replaced daily [2]. After discontinuation of irreversible (aspirin and clopidogrel) platelet inhibitors, functioning platelet counts reach levels required for normal clotting within 4–5 days; in contrast, after discontinuation of reversible inhibitors (NSAIDs), platelets may return to normal functioning levels within 1–2 days [3]. Although dipyridamole leads to reversible effects on platelet aggregation through modulation of adenosine and cGMP, the medication is routinely formulated in combination with the irreversible inhibitor aspirin (Aggrenox). Of note, the selective NSAIDs, COX-2 inhibitors (celecoxib), have negligible effects on COX-1 inhibition and downstream thromboxane A2 levels and consequently do not significantly alter platelet function [4]. Although the mechanisms of action for antiplatelet medications are identical across all patients, the response is not always equivalent; thus, laboratory assessments of platelet function, including bleeding time, and specific assays measuring inhibition by aspirin or clopidogrel may be of value in certain cases [5, 6].

Periprocedural Management of Antiplatelet Therapy

There is limited high-quality prospective evidence to determine the most appropriate management of antiplatelet medications in the periprocedural setting. The urologist must weigh the risk of bleeding resulting from uninterrupted use of antiplatelet agents against the risk of adverse cardiac events secondary to their discontinuation. While it is reasonable to temporarily discontinue NSAIDs prior to prostate biopsy in patients who are not taking them for prevention of cardiovascular disease, recent studies have noted that withdrawal of aspirin or clopidogrel may increase the risk of cardiovascular complications in some patients. At the same time, emerging data suggest that many surgical procedures, including prostate biopsy, may be performed safely during continuation of antiplatelet therapy with limited risk of significant bleeding events.

Aspirin withdrawal may lead to a rebound phenomenon of increased thromboxane A2 activation, resulting in increased platelet aggregation; when this process is coupled with a surgically induced inflammatory state, there is an overall increase in thrombogenic activity [7].

A randomized controlled trial of perioperative aspirin use for elective, high- or intermediate-risk noncardiac surgeries in patients with at least one cardiac risk factor demonstrated that treatment with aspirin resulted in a 7.2% absolute risk reduction [95% confidence interval (CI), 1.3–13%] for postoperative major adverse cardiac events, with a relative risk reduction of 80% (95% CI, 9.2–95%). The number needed to treat to prevent a major adverse cardiac event was 14 (95% CI, 7.6–78) [8]. A meta-analysis of cardiovascular risks after perioperative withdrawal versus bleeding risks with aspirin continuation revealed that aspirin withdrawal may precede up to 10% of acute cardiovascular syndromes; time intervals between discontinuation of aspirin and acute cerebral events, acute coronary syndromes, and acute peripheral arterial syndromes were 14.3 ± 11.3 days, 8.5 ± 3.6 days, and 25.8 ± 18.1 days, respectively [9]. Data on the risk of discontinuing aspirin in these patients for shorter periods of time are lacking.

Furthermore, there is an increasing population prevalence of high-risk patients with coronary stents who are at risk for stent thrombosis and at the highest risk for major adverse cardiac events after discontinuation of aspirin therapy [10]. Continuation of antiplatelet therapy is essential for these patients unless absolutely contraindicated [10–13]. Patients with coronary stents will undergo initial dual antiplatelet therapy with aspirin and thienopyridine (clopidogrel). Practitioners may consider delaying prostate biopsy until completion of mandatory dual antiplatelet treatment depending on the patient's calculated cancer risk and duration of dual antiplatelet therapy, particularly in patients who have undergone coronary stenting within the last month [11–13].

Although there are no specific urological data, previous surveys have demonstrated a lack of consensus opinion among vascular [14] and orthopedic [15] surgeons on management of clopidogrel in the perioperative period. Clopidogrel is a more potent platelet inhibitor compared to aspirin, and consequently there is a lack of data evaluating continuation of therapy during noncardiac surgery [16]. Clopidogrel therapy is usually administered for at least 4 weeks after placement of a bare-metal stent and for 12 months or longer following placement of a drug-eluting stent. The longer duration recommended with drug-eluting stents is due to the elevated risk of delayed in-stent stenosis secondary to endothelialization [10, 13]. Premature discontinuation of clopidogrel therapy results in high cardiac morbidity and mortality [10, 13, 17]. Therefore, it is recommended that elective surgery – and thus prostate biopsy – be postponed when possible until completion of clopidogrel therapy [13, 16].

Competing with cardiovascular complications is the risk of bleeding – some have noted a 1.5-fold increase of bleeding complications for all surgical procedures, although aspirin use only increased the severity of bleeding complications for intracranial surgery and transurethral prostatectomy [9, 18]. Randomized controlled trials of multiple types of surgery [8] and prostate biopsy [19] have not demonstrated significant differences in severe bleeding complications with aspirin use; however, these studies may have been underpowered to determine this outcome, as severe bleeding occurs in < 1% of prostate biopsies [20]. Moreover, reports of baseline bleeding rates from prostate biopsy (rectal bleeding, hematuria, hematospermia) vary widely between studies evaluating aspirin use and prostate biopsy, with bleeding ranges from 2.5% to 81.5% [9, 19, 21]. Although one randomized controlled trial of aspirin and prostate biopsy found no differences in rates of bleeding between those who continued and those who stopped aspirin, the median duration of hematuria and rectal bleeding was significantly greater for patients taking aspirin compared with those who held aspirin (hematuria 6 days vs 2 days, rectal bleeding 3 days vs 1 day) [19]. Further prospective cohort studies of aspirin use and prostate biopsy have not identified significant bleeding complications in patients taking aspirin when compared with patients not taking aspirin, although objective measurement of the amount of bleeding may be difficult [22–24].

The majority of studies on antiplatelet therapy and bleeding risk from prostate biopsy or other surgical procedures focus primarily on low-dose daily aspirin administration. Substantial data on the bleeding risk of high-dose aspirin or other agents such as dipyridamole or thienopyridines (clopidogrel) are not fully matured. Further studies are needed to demonstrate whether continuation of these medications in the procedural setting is safe.

Anticoagulation Therapy

Anticoagulant medications are commonly administered in patients with increased thromboembolic risk secondary to atrial fibrillation, artificial heart valves, hematologic disorders causing hypercoagulable states, or concomitant deep venous thrombosis (DVT). These patients are at increased risk for thromboembolic events including cerebrovascular accident (CVA) or pulmonary embolism (PE) [25–28]. Frequently encountered medications in this class are warfarin and heparin. Warfarin is the only oral agent and is therefore used primarily for chronic disease, while injectable agents are primarily administered for acute disease or while the patient is transitioning off of or on to warfarin, also known as "bridging" therapy.

Anticoagulant medications affect various steps in the coagulation cascade, and therapeutic levels may be monitored through laboratory tests including prothrombin time (PT), international normalized ratio (INR), and partial thromboplastin time (PTT). Warfarin has a relatively long half-life and therefore is routinely held 5–7 days prior to procedures, although medication effects are best monitored through INR [29, 30]. A safe INR of 1.5 is reached in about 4 days after cessation of warfarin in patients with therapeutic levels at baseline [29], and a therapeutic INR of 2.0 is reached in about 3 days after restarting warfarin therapy [30]. Heparins have a shorter half-life and may be monitored through PTT, although this test may be highly variable in patients administered unfractionated heparin. Consequently, low-molecular-weight heparin (LMWH) is increasingly used and in most cases is safe without monitoring [31], but it may be monitored with anti-Xa levels if necessary [32].

Periprocedural Management of Anticoagulation Therapy

Several authors have developed recommendations for periprocedural management of anticoagulation medication, which includes assessment of bleeding risk of the operation and thrombotic risk of the patient [25, 26, 28]. The risk of significant bleeding events from prostate biopsy is relatively low [20], but needle biopsy procedures are not commonly included in discussions of periprocedural bleeding risk from anticoagulation [25, 26, 28].

There are several reasons why withdrawal of anticoagulants may result in thromboembolic events in patients undergoing prostate biopsy. Similar to withdrawal of aspirin therapy, withdrawal of anticoagulation medication also results in a rebound phenomenon of increased thrombin and fibrin formation and may contribute to thrombotic risk [33]. Additionally, patients who have an underlying cancer may exhibit increased thrombin formation, which carries an increased risk of venous thromboembolism [34]. Conversely, approximately 4–8% of patients with preexisting venous thromboembolism may carry an occult malignancy [35, 36]. Furthermore, trauma or tissue damage creates a hypercoagulable state. A large number of patients undergoing surgical procedures have substantially increased risk for venous thromboembolic events [37]; however, this risk appears to be lower for minimally invasive procedures [38] and has not been described for prostate biopsy.

Risks of thromboembolic events depend on the underlying disorder or indication for anticoagulation. Retrospective data of patients with prosthetic heart valves who underwent perioperative bridging anticoagulant therapy demonstrated perioperative thromboembolic events in 1.3–43% of patients, depending on the type and location of valve [28, 39]. These studies were substantially limited by small populations and strict documentation of perioperative coagulation and follow-up. Small prospective studies of perioperative bridging with LMWH demonstrated risk of thromboembolic events around 4% [40, 41]. In general, patients with prosthetic mitral valves appear to be at much higher risk of thromboembolic events compared to patients with prosthetic aortic valves [25, 28], and patients with mechanical valves tend to have higher risk than those with biological valves [25, 42, 43].

Patients with preexisting venous thromboembolism are at high risk for recurrent events, particularly if they recently started anticoagulants, or if they have an underlying chronic coagulation disorder [44]. Chronic atrial fibrillation is associated with a risk of thromboembolic events around 3–7% per year, which is higher if other risk factors are present. Temporary interruption of warfarin results in a perioperative thromboembolic risk of 0.28–0.38%, using interpolated data from high-risk patients [28]; however, more robust clinical data are required to provide better estimates of risk.

In recent years, there have been increasing numbers of investigators attempting to assess the risk of perioperative thromboembolic and bleeding events with anticoagulants. One large prospective trial included nearly 1,300 episodes of warfarin therapy interruption in patients with atrial fibrillation, venous thromboembolism, and mechanical heart valves. Bridging therapy was only used in 8.3% of cases, and 0.7% of patients experienced thromboembolism within 30 days of the procedure. All thromboembolic events occurred without bridging therapy. Clinically significant or major bleeding episodes occurred in 2.3% of patients; 61% of bleeding events occurred with bridging therapy [45]. Another prospective multicenter study of LMWH bridging therapy in 224 patients documented thromboembolism in 3.6% of patients, and 75% of these had warfarin deferred or withdrawn secondary to bleeding. Major bleeding occurred in 6.7% of patients. Five patients (2%) had major bleeding events that occurred after LMWH was restarted [46]. Others have shown that standardization and adherence to strict bridging protocols

Table 11.1 Summary of recommendations for prostate biopsy preparation

Preparation item	Recommendation
Cessation of antiplatelet drugs	• Stop NSAIDs 5–7 days prior
	• Stop aspirin 5–7 days prior
	• Continue aspirin for patients with coronary stents
	• Delay biopsy for patients with coronary stents on dual platelet therapy
	○ Consider laboratory assessment of medication efficacy
	○ Discuss with cardiologist prior to stopping thienopyridine
Cessation of anticoagulants	• Stop anticoagulants 5–7 days prior, or until INR is ≤ 1.5
	• Bridging heparin therapy for high risk of VTE
Enema administration	• Not recommended: enema does not reduce infection or provide significant imaging advantage
Antibiotic prophylaxis	• Single-dose oral antibiotic prior to procedure
	• Fluoroquinolones are antibiotic of choice
	• Fluoroquinolones should be avoided in patients with prior administration or previous documented infection with resistance

may eliminate venous thromboembolism in the periprocedural setting; however, this study of LMWH for periprocedural anticoagulation reported one minor and two major bleeding events in 69 consecutive patients [47].

Periprocedural continuation of oral anticoagulation is always an option; however, even less is known on this subject for most procedure types, and sufficient data are lacking regarding prostate biopsy. One published study of patients who underwent prostate biopsy while on oral anticoagulants documented no increased risk of bleeding complications in 49 patients on anticoagulants who underwent biopsy, compared to 731 controls who were not on anticoagulants; 80% of the anticoagulant group had an INR >2.0. However, these data were obtained by survey 10 days after the procedure, and most patients underwent only 6 core biopsies [48]. Continuation of oral anticoagulants may be safe with other procedures such as cataract surgery [49], dental surgery [50], or cardiac device implantation [51]. Data are conflicting and somewhat lacking for more invasive surgeries. Some have shown safe use of oral anticoagulants in patients undergoing coronary artery bypass graft [52], while others demonstrated that 10% of patients on therapeutic warfarin who underwent colon or rectal abdominal operations required transfusion or reoperation for bleeding [53]. Bleeding risk for prostate biopsy in patients on anticoagulation may lie somewhere between the extremes; however, further prospective evaluation is needed.

Hematologic Agents: Clinical Recommendations

The practitioner must ultimately decide whether to suspend administration of antiplatelet medications prior to prostate biopsy for patients who take these medications to prevent cardiovascular morbidity and mortality. We recommend patients should stop NSAIDs at least 2 days prior to biopsy. Patients without a strong indication for aspirin should stop the medication 5–7 days prior to biopsy. For patients with coronary stents, aspirin should be continued to prevent risk of stent thrombosis. Patients with recent coronary stents on dual platelet therapy may have prostate biopsy delayed until the end of thienopyridine administration. If high-risk prostate cancer is suspected, consider laboratory assay to measure medication efficacy. Discussion with the patient and cardiologist on risks and benefits of biopsy on thienopyridine versus temporary withdrawal of thienopyridine may be necessary. Anticoagulants should be held for 5 days prior to biopsy, or until INR reaches a safe level of 1.5 or less. Patients with a high risk of thromboembolic events should undergo bridging therapy with heparin. Recommendations are summarized in Table 11.1 at the end of this chapter.

Pre-biopsy Enemas

Prescription of an enema for rectal administration prior to prostate biopsy is a common practice among urologists. In theory, passing a needle through a grossly contaminated rectal vault and into the prostate could lead to bacterial seeding of the prostate. Therefore, an argument for pre-biopsy rectal cleansing is to reduce the rate of infection. Evidence exploring this mechanism is weak, as is the evidence documenting the clinical impact of enema administration. In the absence of antibiotic prophylaxis, one study demonstrated higher rates of bacteremia without enema administration. However, the authors noted that those with and those without enemas exhibited similar rates of culture-positive prostate tissue, similar rates of positive swab cultures from biopsy needles, and no differences in clinical infection [54].

The topic of enema administration is controversial, as some have found no advantage [55], while others report reduced rates of infection with rectal preparation [56]. Some practitioners also contend that enema administration provides an improved acoustic window for imaging at the time of biopsy by decreasing the amount of feces in the rectum. Opponents point out that the rectum is normally empty except during defecation [57]; therefore, the enema may actually introduce more feces and air into the rectum and cause interference with ultrasonic transmission [58]. Despite the paucity of high-quality data, most physicians performing biopsy adhere to a policy of pre-biopsy enema administration. A survey of practicing urologists found that 79% of responders routinely prescribed enemas in preparation for prostate biopsy [59]. Furthermore, 27% of responders at teaching centers did not prescribe enemas, while only 9% of community responders did not prescribe enemas. This differential rate among academic and community urologists may be a result of slow diffusion of fairly low-level evidence on enema use and prostate biopsy outcomes.

Multiple studies have assessed post-biopsy infection, using various definitions of infection. The majority of these demonstrate no improvement of infection rates with rectal preparation. One study of 217 patients with bowel preparation and 190 patients without bowel preparation found no difference in prevalence of post-biopsy sepsis between the two groups [60]. Another study of 100 patients randomized to either rectal preparation or no rectal preparation reported 9 positive hemocultures in the rectum cleaning group versus only 2 cases in the control group, which was a significant difference [61]. Other investigators reviewed a cohort of 448 patients, of which 225 received enemas prior to biopsy, and found no differences in clinically significant complications requiring an office visit. Furthermore, no patients who did not receive an enema required hospitalization for infection [55]. More recently, a review of approximately 1,400 patients revealed that a single dose of prophylactic antibiotic is sufficient to prevent both infectious and overall complication rates when compared to 3 days of antibiotic plus a pre-biopsy enema [58]. Based on current evidence, enema administration does not significantly impact infectious complications and therefore does not outweigh the cost and patient discomfort.

Antibiotic Prophylaxis

Transrectal ultrasound-guided prostate biopsy may result in infectious complications ranging in severity from low (asymptomatic bacteriuria) to high (sepsis and possibly death). Infective complications may range from 8% to 25% of patients who are not given antibiotic prophylaxis [62, 63]. Antibiotic administration decreases the prevalence of post-biopsy bacteriuria and urinary tract infection and may result in decreased clinical infection, reduced hospitalizations, and therefore lower health-care cost [62–64]. A recent Cochrane review analyzed 9 trials of antibiotic versus placebo and demonstrated significant benefits of antibiotic prophylaxis to prevent bacteriuria (risk ratio [RR] 0.25, 95% CI 0.15–0.42), bacteremia (RR 0.67, 95% CI 0.49–0.92), fever (RR 0.39, 95% CI 0.23–0.64), urinary tract infection (RR 0.37, 95% CI 0.22–0.62), and hospitalization (RR 0.13, 95% CI 0.03–0.55) [64]. Antibiotic prophylaxis is routinely prescribed prior to prostate biopsy to prevent these complications.

The American Urological Association (AUA) best practice policy statement outlines several general principles of antimicrobial prophylaxis [65]:

> Antimicrobial prophylaxis involves the periprocedural administration of an antibiotic with the goal of reducing post-procedural local and systemic infections; the potential benefit of prophylaxis is related to patient factors, procedural factors, and the potential morbidity of infection. Periprocedural prophylaxis should only be used if the potential benefit outweighs the risks and potential costs of infectious complications. The antibiotic which is administered should be relevant to the bacteria at the operative site, and should be safe, convenient, and cost-effective. Last, the duration of antibiotic prophylaxis should span the time interval when bacterial translocation or infection is likely to occur.

The current recommendation of the AUA is that antimicrobial prophylaxis is indicated in all transrectal prostate biopsies; the agent of choice is a fluoroquinolone, which should be administered no longer than 24 h. Alternative antibiotics are an aminoglycoside plus metronidazole or clindamycin [65]. Tailoring the antibiotic to target relevant bacteria is particularly prudent when considering changing patterns of antibiotic resistance, which will be discussed further in this chapter. Each factor mentioned should be taken into account when planning for prostate biopsy.

The vast majority of practitioners prescribe antibiotic prophylaxis prior to prostate biopsy. However, there is substantial variation among type, timing, and duration of antibiotic administration, and some practitioners do not routinely prescribe prophylaxis [59, 66]. Quinolones are the most commonly prescribed antibiotic prophylaxis [59, 66] and have been the most evaluated in research studies [64]. Quinolones are effective against most intestinal flora causing urinary tract infection, which commonly includes *E. coli*, *Proteus*, *Klebsiella*, and *Enterococcus* [62–65]. Many practitioners prescribe more than one dose of antibiotic; however, multiple studies have shown that a single dose of antibiotic is equally effective at reducing infectious complications [62–64, 67–69]. Patients with pre-procedural bacteriuria are an exception and should undergo treatment prior to the procedure to prevent hematogenous infection [70]. This may include patients with an indwelling catheter or previously diagnosed urinary tract infection.

Quinolone Resistance

As mentioned previously, the antibiotic may need to be tailored to the patient and organ site. There are an increasing number of reports focusing on quinolone-resistant infections after prostate biopsy, usually caused by *E. coli* [58, 71]. An alternative antibiotic therapy may be warranted in higher-risk patients with previous quinolone administration or previous UTI with bacteria resistant to fluoroquinolones due to high rates of *E. coli* with quinolone resistance [71, 72]. An analysis of nearly 1,500 patients who were administered antibiotic prior to prostate biopsy from 2001 to 2010 demonstrated that 50% of infections were due to *E. coli*, and approximately 50% of these were resistant to fluoroquinolone antibiotics [58]. Another large study of nearly 1,300 patients documented higher rates of *E. coli* (89%) in symptomatic patients with positive cultures after biopsy, of which 90% were fluoroquinolone resistant [71]. These and other studies documenting high rates of fluoroquinolone-resistant *E. coli* have led to a recent statement by the AUA that practitioners should consider an alternate agent for prophylaxis in patients at high risk for quinolone-resistant infections.

Orthopedic Patients

Special considerations should be taken for orthopedic patients with total joint replacements. This includes patients with total joint replacement within the previous 2 years and others with risk factors such as previous prosthetic joint infection, immunocompromised state, and other predisposing risk factors according to the American Urological Association advisory statement [73]. Those patients undergoing urologic procedures with increased risk of bacteremia should be administered one of the following recommended antibiotic prophylaxis regimens: a single systemic level dose of a quinolone by mouth 1–2 h prior to procedure or ampicillin 2 g intravenously plus gentamicin 1.5 mg/kg intravenously 30–60 min prior to procedure. Alternatively, vancomycin 1 g intravenously 1–2 h prior to procedure may be administered in those with an allergy to ampicillin.

Special considerations were previously given to patients with valvular heart disease to prevent bacterial endocarditis; however, the AUA removed these recommendations in 2008 based on a report from the American Heart Association [65, 74].

Editorial Commentary:

Perhaps no area of prostate cancer diagnosis entails such diverse practices as patient preparation. The three decisions to be made involve withholding anticoagulation to reduce bleeding, plus efforts to reduce infections including enemas and antibiotics.

Withholding anticoagulants apparently feels safer than continuing them for most urologists, but the authors note that doing so carries significant risk of cardiovascular events in many patients. This is especially notable for patients with drug-eluting stents, in whom there is real risk of sudden death if endothelialization remains incomplete, which can take well over a year in some cases. For those patients, I routinely ask the cardiologist to weigh in on the balance of cardiovascular risk compared to the risk of undiagnosed prostate cancer. We almost always agree that waiting a full year to withhold clopidogrel or similar agents after placement of a drug-eluting stent is the prudent approach, considering that it is reasonable to delay treatment of most prostate cancers (but not all, of course) for up to 1 year based on available data. By contrast, I routinely biopsy patients taking aspirin or NSAIDs and have not recommended cessation regardless of their indication for use for the past decade. The literature has been very clear in support of the safety of doing so. Of course bleeding occurs occasionally, but it has not occurred more commonly in the patients taking aspirin than in the patients who do not. Bleeding risk with clopidogrel, however, is very real, and

we routinely hold it for 2 weeks for those patients in whom decision is made that this is safe to do, again in collaboration with the cardiologist.

Urologists still seem to have a hard time letting go of enemas, even though the literature clearly does not support their use. If readers remain unconvinced, I encourage query of patients, who readily tell us that they truly dislike them.

The final decision regards antibiotic use. This is a rapidly evolving area, with a seeming epidemic of post-biopsy infection and sepsis emerging in the past 3–4 years. Based on our reported findings on this phenomenon (reference 58 in this chapter), we began adding a single dose of aminoglycoside to the single dose of fluoroquinolone in 2010. This significantly reduced, but did not eliminate infection risk. Other authors have advocated rectal wall culture to detect resistance to quinolones or aminoglycosides to direct prophylaxis. Early results have been very intriguing, and I anticipate intense consideration of this or other approaches to address this significant issue.

–J. Stephen Jones

References

1. Connor SE, Wingate JP. Management of patients treated with aspirin or warfarin and evaluation of haemostasis prior to prostatic biopsy: a survey of current practice amongst radiologists and urologists. Clin Radiol. 1999;54(9):598–603.
2. O'Brien JR. Effects of salicylates on human platelets. Lancet. 1968;1(7546):779–83.
3. Mercado DL, Petty BG. Perioperative medication management. Med Clin North Am. 2003;87(1): 41–57.
4. Schnitzer TJ. Cyclooxygenase-2–specific inhibitors: are they safe? Am J Med. 2001;110(1):46S–9.
5. Tello-Montoliu A, Ueno M, Angiolillo DJ. Antiplatelet drug therapy: role of pharmacodynamic and genetic testing. Future Cardiol. 2011;7(3):381–402.
6. Merritt JC, Bhatt DL. The efficacy and safety of perioperative antiplatelet therapy. J Thromb Thrombolysis. 2004;17(1):21–7.
7. Beving H, Zhao C, Albage A, Ivert T. Abnormally high platelet activity after discontinuation of acetylsalicylic acid treatment. Blood Coagul Fibrinolysis. 1996;7(1):80–4.
8. Oscarsson A, Gupta A, Fredrikson M, et al. To continue or discontinue aspirin in the perioperative

period: a randomized, controlled clinical trial. Br J Anaesth. 2010;104(3):305–12.

9. Burger W, Chemnitius JM, Kneissl GD, Rucker G. Low-dose aspirin for secondary cardiovascular prevention – cardiovascular risks after its perioperative withdrawal versus bleeding risks with its continuation – review and meta-analysis. J Intern Med. 2005;257(5):399–414.

10. Serruys PW, Kutryk MJ, Ong AT. Coronary-artery stents. N Engl J Med. 2006;354(5):483–95.

11. Kaluza GL, Joseph J, Lee JR, Raizner ME, Raizner AE. Catastrophic outcomes of noncardiac surgery soon after coronary stenting. J Am Coll Cardiol. 2000;35(5):1288–94.

12. Vicenzi MN, Meislitzer T, Heitzinger B, Halaj M, Fleisher LA, Metzler H. Coronary artery stenting and non-cardiac surgery–a prospective outcome study. Br J Anaesth. 2006;96(6):686–93.

13. Fleisher LA, Beckman JA, Brown KA, et al. ACC/ AHA 2007 guidelines on perioperative cardiovascular evaluation and care for noncardiac surgery: a report of the American College of Cardiology/American Heart Association Task Force on Practice Guidelines (Writing Committee to revise the 2002 guidelines on perioperative cardiovascular evaluation for noncardiac surgery): developed in collaboration with the American Society of Echocardiography, American Society of Nuclear Cardiology, Heart Rhythm Society, Society of Cardiovascular Anesthesiologists, Society for Cardiovascular Angiography and Interventions, Society for Vascular Medicine and Biology, and Society for Vascular Surgery. Circulation. 2007;116(17):e418–99.

14. Smout J, Stansby G. Current practice in the use of antiplatelet agents in the peri-operative period by UK vascular surgeons. Ann R Coll Surg Engl. 2003;85(2):97–101.

15. Joseph JJ, Pillai A, Bramley D. Clopidogrel in orthopaedic\ patients: a review of current practice in Scotland. Thromb J. 2007;5:6.

16. O'Riordan JM, Margey RJ, Blake G, O'Connell PR. Antiplatelet agents in the perioperative period. Arch Surg. 2009;144(1):69–76. discussion 76.

17. Grines CL, Bonow RO, Casey Jr DE, et al. Prevention of premature discontinuation of dual antiplatelet therapy in patients with coronary artery stents: a science advisory from the American Heart Association, American College of Cardiology, Society for Cardiovascular Angiography and Interventions, American College of Surgeons, and American Dental Association, with representation from the American College of Physicians. Circulation. 2007;115(6): 813–8.

18. Thurston AV, Briant SL. Aspirin and post-prostatectomy haemorrhage. Br J Urol. 1993;71(5):574–6.

19. Giannarini G, Mogorovich A, Valent F, et al. Continuing or discontinuing low-dose aspirin before transrectal prostate biopsy: results of a prospective randomized trial. Urology. 2007;70(3):501–5.

20. Ghani KR, Dundas D, Patel U. Bleeding after transrectal ultrasonography-guided prostate biopsy: a study of

7-day morbidity after a six-, eight- and 12-core biopsy protocol. BJU Int. 2004;94(7):1014–20.

21. Halliwell OT, Yadegafar G, Lane C, Dewbury KC. Transrectal ultrasound-guided biopsy of the prostate: aspirin increases the incidence of minor bleeding complications. Clin Radiol. 2008;63(5):557–61.

22. Herget EJ, Saliken JC, Donnelly BJ, Gray RR, Wiseman D, Brunet G. Transrectal ultrasound-guided biopsy of the prostate: relation between ASA use and bleeding complications. Can Assoc Radiol J. 1999;50(3):173–6.

23. Rodriguez LV, Terris MK. Risks and complications of transrectal ultrasound guided prostate needle biopsy: a prospective study and review of the literature. J Urol. 1998;160(6 Pt 1):2115–20.

24. Maan Z, Cutting CW, Patel U, et al. Morbidity of transrectal ultrasonography-guided prostate biopsies in patients after the continued use of low-dose aspirin. BJU Int. 2003;91(9):798–800.

25. Thachil J, Gatt A, Martlew V. Management of surgical patients receiving anticoagulation and antiplatelet agents. Br J Surg. 2008;95(12):1437–48.

26. Kearon C, Hirsh J. Management of anticoagulation before and after elective surgery. N Engl J Med. 1997;336(21):1506–11.

27. Fuster V, Ryden LE, Asinger RW, et al. ACC/AHA/ ESC guidelines for the management of patients with atrial fibrillation: executive summary. A report of the American College of Cardiology/ American Heart Association Task Force on Practice Guidelines and the European Society of Cardiology Committee for Practice Guidelines and Policy Conferences (Committee to develop guidelines for the management of patients with atrial fibrillation): developed in collaboration with the North American Society of Pacing and Electrophysiology. J Am Coll Cardiol. 2001;38(4):1231–66.

28. Douketis JD. Perioperative anticoagulation management in patients who are receiving oral anticoagulant therapy: a practical guide for clinicians. Thromb Res. 2002;108(1):3–13.

29. White RH, McKittrick T, Hutchinson R, Twitchell J. Temporary discontinuation of warfarin therapy: changes in the international normalized ratio. Ann Intern Med. 1995;122(1):40–2.

30. Harrison L, Johnston M, Massicotte MP, Crowther M, Moffat K, Hirsh J. Comparison of 5-mg and 10-mg loading doses in initiation of warfarin therapy. Ann Intern Med. 1997;126(2):133–6.

31. Hirsh J, Warkentin TE, Shaughnessy SG, et al. Heparin and low-molecular-weight heparin: mechanisms of action, pharmacokinetics, dosing, monitoring, efficacy, and safety. Chest. 2001;119(1 Suppl): 64S–94.

32. Rosenberg AF, Zumberg M, Taylor L, LeClaire A, Harris N. The use of anti-Xa assay to monitor intravenous unfractionated heparin therapy. J Pharm Pract. 2010;23(3):210–6.

33. Genewein U, Haeberli A, Straub PW, Beer JH. Rebound after cessation of oral anticoagulant therapy:

the biochemical evidence. Br J Haematol. 1996;92(2): 479–85.

34. Ay C, Dunkler D, Simanek R, et al. Prediction of venous thromboembolism in patients with cancer by measuring thrombin generation: results from the Vienna Cancer and Thrombosis Study. J Clin Oncol. 2011;29(15):2099–103.

35. Oktar GL, Ergul EG, Kiziltepe U. Occult malignancy in patients with venous thromboembolism: risk indicators and a diagnostic screening strategy. Phlebology. 2007;22(2):75–9.

36. Monreal M, Lensing AW, Prins MH, et al. Screening for occult cancer in patients with acute deep vein thrombosis or pulmonary embolism. J Thromb Haemost. 2004;2(6):876–81.

37. Lee CH, Cheng CL, Lin LJ, Tsai LM, Yang YH. Epidemiology and predictors of short-term mortality in symptomatic venous thromboembolism. Circ J. 2011; 75(8):1998–2004.

38. Lindberg F, Bergqvist D, Rasmussen I. Incidence of thromboembolic complications after laparoscopic cholecystectomy: review of the literature. Surg Laparosc Endosc. 1997;7(4):324–31.

39. Carrel TP, Klingenmann W, Mohacsi PJ, Berdat P, Althaus U. Perioperative bleeding and thromboembolic risk during non-cardiac surgery in patients with mechanical prosthetic heart valves: an institutional review. J Heart Valve Dis. 1999;8(4):392–8.

40. Spandorfer JM, Lynch S, Weitz HH, Fertel S, Merli GJ. Use of enoxaparin for the chronically anticoagulated patient before and after procedures. Am J Cardiol. 1999;84(4):478–480, A410.

41. Tinmouth AH, Morrow BH, Cruickshank MK, Moore PM, Kovacs MJ. Dalteparin as periprocedure anticoagulation for patients on warfarin and at high risk of thrombosis. Ann Pharmacother. 2001;35(6):669–74.

42. Russo A, Grigioni F, Avierinos JF, et al. Thromboembolic complications after surgical correction of mitral regurgitation incidence, predictors, and clinical implications. J Am Coll Cardiol. 2008;51(12):1203–11.

43. Salem DN, Stein PD, Al-Ahmad A, et al. Antithrombotic therapy in valvular heart disease–native and prosthetic: the seventh ACCP conference on antithrombotic and thrombolytic therapy. Chest. 2004;126(3 Suppl):457S–82.

44. Heit JA, Mohr DN, Silverstein MD, Petterson TM, O'Fallon WM, Melton 3rd LJ. Predictors of recurrence after deep vein thrombosis and pulmonary embolism: a population-based cohort study. Arch Intern Med. 2000;160(6):761–8.

45. Garcia DA, Regan S, Henault LE, et al. Risk of thromboembolism with short-term interruption of warfarin therapy. Arch Intern Med. 2008;168(1):63–9.

46. Kovacs MJ, Kearon C, Rodger M, et al. Single-arm study of bridging therapy with low-molecular-weight heparin for patients at risk of arterial embolism who require temporary interruption of warfarin. Circulation. 2004;110(12):1658–63.

47. Jaffer AK, Ahmed M, Brotman DJ, et al. Low-molecular-weight-heparins as periprocedural anticoagulation for patients on long-term warfarin therapy: a standardized bridging therapy protocol. J Thromb Thrombolysis. 2005;20(1):11–6.

48. Ihezue CU, Smart J, Dewbury KC, Mehta R, Burgess L. Biopsy of the prostate guided by transrectal ultrasound: relation between warfarin use and incidence of bleeding complications. Clin Radiol. 2005;60(4):459–63. discussion 457–458.

49. Jamula E, Anderson J, Douketis JD. Safety of continuing warfarin therapy during cataract surgery: a systematic review and meta-analysis. Thromb Res. 2009;124(3):292–9.

50. Nematullah A, Alabousi A, Blanas N, Douketis JD, Sutherland SE. Dental surgery for patients on anticoagulant therapy with warfarin: a systematic review and meta-analysis. Tex Dent J. 2009;126(12):1183–93.

51. Li HK, Chen FC, Rea RF, et al. No increased bleeding events with continuation of oral anticoagulation therapy for patients undergoing cardiac device procedure. Pacing Clin Electrophysiol. 2011;34(7):868–74.

52. Airaksinen KE, Biancari F, Karjalainen P, et al. Safety of coronary artery bypass surgery during therapeutic oral anticoagulation. Thromb Res. 2011;128(5): 435–9.

53. Iqbal CW, Cima RR, Pemberton JH. Bleeding and thromboembolic outcomes for patients on oral anticoagulation undergoing elective colon and rectal abdominal operations. J Gastrointest Surg. 2011;15(11): 2016–22.

54. Lindert KA, Kabalin JN, Terris MK. Bacteremia and bacteriuria after transrectal ultrasound guided prostate biopsy. J Urol. 2000;164(1):76–80.

55. Carey JM, Korman HJ. Transrectal ultrasound guided biopsy of the prostate. Do enemas decrease clinically significant complications? J Urol. 2001; 166(1):82–5.

56. Jeon SS, Woo SH, Hyun JH, Choi HY, Chai SE. Bisacodyl rectal preparation can decrease infectious complications of transrectal ultrasound-guided prostate biopsy. Urology. 2003;62(3):461–6.

57. Gordon PH. Anorectal anatomy and physiology. Gastroenterol Clin North Am. 2001;30(1):1–13.

58. Zaytoun OM, Anil T, Moussa AS, Jianbo L, Fareed K, Jones JS. Morbidity of prostate biopsy after simplified versus complex preparation protocols: assessment of risk factors. Urology. 2011;77(4):910–4.

59. Davis M, Sofer M, Kim SS, Soloway MS. The procedure of transrectal ultrasound guided biopsy of the prostate: a survey of patient preparation and biopsy technique. J Urol. 2002;167(2 Pt 1):566–70.

60. Ruddick F, Sanders P, Bicknell SG, Crofts P. Sepsis rates after ultrasound-guided prostate biopsy using a bowel preparation protocol in a community hospital. J Ultrasound Med. 2011;30(2):213–6.

61. Kanjanawongdeengam P, Viseshsindh W, Santanirand P, Prathombutr P, Nilkulwattana S. Reduction in bacteremia rates after rectum sterilization before

transrectal, ultrasound-guided prostate biopsy: a randomized controlled trial. J Med Assoc Thai. 2009;92(12):1621–6.

62. Kapoor DA, Klimberg IW, Malek GH, et al. Single-dose oral ciprofloxacin versus placebo for prophylaxis during transrectal prostate biopsy. Urology. 1998; 52(4):552–8.

63. Aron M, Rajeev TP, Gupta NP. Antibiotic prophylaxis for transrectal needle biopsy of the prostate: a randomized controlled study. BJU Int. 2000;85(6): 682–5.

64. Zani EL, Clark OA, Rodrigues Netto Jr N. Antibiotic prophylaxis for transrectal prostate biopsy. Cochrane Database Syst Rev. 2011;5:CD006576.

65. Wolf JS, Jr., Bennett CJ, Dmochowski RR, Hollenbeck BK, Pearle MS, Schaeffer AJ. Best practice policy statement on urologic surgery antimicrobial prophylaxis. J Urol. Apr 2008;179(4):1379–90.

66. Shandera KC, Thibault GP, Deshon Jr GE. Variability in patient preparation for prostate biopsy among American urologists. Urology. 1998;52(4):644–6.

67. Cam K, Kayikci A, Akman Y, Erol A. Prospective assessment of the efficacy of single dose versus traditional 3-day antimicrobial prophylaxis in 12-core transrectal prostate biopsy. Int J Urol. 2008;15(11): 997–1001.

68. Shandera KC, Thibault GP, Deshon Jr GE. Efficacy of one dose fluoroquinolone before prostate biopsy. Urology. 1998;52(4):641–3.

69. Isen K, Kupeli B, Sinik Z, Sozen S, Bozkirli I. Antibiotic prophylaxis for transrectal biopsy of the prostate: a prospective randomized study of the prophylactic use of single dose oral fluoroquinolone versus trimethoprim-sulfamethoxazole. Int Urol Nephrol. 1999;31(4):491–5.

70. Olson ES, Cookson BD. Do antimicrobials have a role in preventing septicaemia following instrumentation of the urinary tract? J Hosp Infect. 2000;45(2): 85–97.

71. Feliciano J, Teper E, Ferrandino M, et al. The incidence of fluoroquinolone resistant infections after prostate biopsy-are fluoroquinolones still effective prophylaxis? J Urol. 2008;179(3):952–5. discussion 955.

72. Tal R, Livne PM, Lask DM, Baniel J. Empirical management of urinary tract infections complicating transrectal ultrasound guided prostate biopsy. J Urol. 2003;169(5):1762–5.

73. American Urological Association, American Academy of Orthopaedic Surgeons. Antibiotic prophylaxis for urological patients with total joint replacements. J Urol. 2003;169(5):1796–7.

74. Wilson W, Taubert KA, Gewitz M, et al. Prevention of infective endocarditis: guidelines from the American Heart Association: a guideline from the American Heart Association Rheumatic Fever, Endocarditis, and Kawasaki Disease Committee, Council on Cardiovascular Disease in the Young, and the Council on Clinical Cardiology, Council on Cardiovascular Surgery and Anesthesia, and the Quality of Care and Outcomes Research Interdisciplinary Working Group. Circulation. 2007;116(15):1736–54.

Pain Prevention

12

Allison Glass, Sanoj Punnen, and Katsuto Shinohara

Introduction

In 2010, it was estimated that 217, 730 men in the United States were diagnosed with prostate cancer [1]. Although serum prostate-specific antigen (PSA) testing and digital rectal exams (DRE) help identify men at risk for prostate cancer, the gold standard for diagnosis is currently biopsy of the prostate. With recent trends toward PSA screening, there has been an increase in the number of men being diagnosed with prostate cancer and the number of men undergoing biopsy of the prostate. It has been estimated that as many as 800,000 biopsies of the prostate are performed in the United States each year making it one of the most common office procedures for urologists [2].

The number of prostate biopsies for detection of prostate cancer has been increasing. Since the majority of prostate cancer foci are not visible on ultrasonography, Hodge et al. proposed systematic sextant random biopsy in order to improve cancer detection rate in 1989 [3]. Over the years, the development of prostate biopsy has moved from the original 6-core sextant biopsy to more extended protocols, which allow more extensive

A. Glass, B.S. • S. Punnen, M.D.
• K. Shinohara, M.D. (✉)
Department of Urology, Helen Diller Family Comprehensive Cancer Center, University of California, San Francisco, 1600 Divisadero St. A-634, San Francisco, CA 94143-1695, USA
e-mail: kshinohara@urology.ucsf.edu

sampling of the gland. Most contemporary biopsy protocols today attain 12–16 cores with some protocols advocating for 20 plus cores [4]. Furthermore, the development of active surveillance protocols have required men to undergo serial biopsies as frequently as every 6–12 months to detect tumor progression, making prostate biopsy a frequent procedure for men on such surveillance protocols. Local anesthesia prior to biopsy is crucial to improving pain control throughout the procedure. There are many different methods of administering local anesthesia of the prostate, and debate still remains regarding the best site for injection, as well as the ideal type and dosage of anesthetic to use for maximum pain relief. Below, we outline the history behind local anesthesia of the prostate, the different methods used to administer it, and the pros and cons of these approaches.

Although biopsy of the prostate has been considered a fairly well-tolerated procedure, recent studies have suggested that as many as 90% of patients found the procedure painful [5]. A recent study by Irani et al. reported that 6% of patients felt the procedure should be done under general anesthesia and 19% of patients would refuse the procedure without any analgesia [6]. Furthermore, another study found that 16% of biopsies could not be completed due to pain when anesthesia was not used compared to only 2% of procedures that could not be completed when anesthesia was provided. As a result, the American Urological Association, the European Urological Association, and the National Comprehensive Cancer Network

J.S. Jones (ed.), *Prostate Cancer Diagnosis: PSA, Biopsy and Beyond*, Current Clinical Urology,
DOI 10.1007/978-1-62703-188-2_12, © Springer Science+Business Media New York 2013

currently call for the use of analgesia for pain relief during biopsy of the prostate. Despite this, a recent survey suggested that one third of urologists do not provide any anesthesia during the procedure [7].

Currently, there is no consensus on the form or technique used for analgesia; most urologists administer local anesthetic to the prostate prior to biopsy. The most common forms of local anesthesia to the prostate currently include periprostatic nerve block, intrarectal local anesthesia and intraprostatic injection of local anesthetic. In this chapter, we will discuss the development of local anesthesia of the prostate and the various techniques used to administer it.

Anatomy of the Prostate

The average prostate weighs 20–25 g in size in young men and is located just beneath the bladder. It is fixed to the pubic bone anteriorly by the puboprostatic ligaments, cradled laterally by the levators, and directly related to the overlying endopelvic fascia. The prostate is composed of 70% glandular, and 30% fibromuscular stroma and can be divided into 4 main zones. The transitional zone, which makes up 5–10% of the gland, surrounds the urethra and is responsible for prostate enlargement problems. It accounts for approximately 20% of prostate cancers. The central zone accounts for 25% of the gland, surrounds the ejaculatory ducts, and is responsible for approximately 1–5% of cancers. The anterior fibromuscular zone does not contain any glandular components but rather muscle and connective tissue. Finally, the peripheral zone makes up 70% of the gland, covering the posterolateral aspect of the prostate, and accounts for the majority of prostate cancers [8].

Vascular and Lymphatic Supply

The main arterial blood supply to the prostate is through the prostatic artery, which is a branch of the inferior vesical artery. It divides into a urethral artery and a capsular artery. The urethral artery enters the prostatovesical junction posterolaterally and supplies the transition zone, the prostatic urethra, and the periurethral glands. The capsular artery runs posterolateral to the prostate with the cavernous nerves in the neurovascular bundle. It pierces the gland at right angles and sends several small branches to the anterior capsule. Venous drainage of the prostate is abundant through the periprostatic plexus. Lymphatic drainage of the prostate is primarily to the obturator and internal iliac lymph nodes [8].

Innervation of the Prostate

The prostate is thought to have both sympathetic and parasympathetic innervations. Sympathetic fibers come from the gray matter of the last 3 thoracic and first 2 lumbar segments of the spinal cord. They traverse the paravertebral sympathetic chain and reach the pelvic plexus via the superior hypogastric plexus [9]. The parasympathetic fibers originate from the intermediolateral cell column of the second, third, and fourth sacral spinal nerves. They arise as pelvic splanchnic nerves that join the hypogastric nerve and branch from the sacral sympathetic ganglia to form the pelvic plexus [9].

The pelvic plexus sits lateral to the rectum and is perforated by several vessels going to and from various pelvic organs. Its midpoint is at the tips of the seminal vesicles [10]. The caudal portion of the pelvic plexus gives rise to the innervation of the prostate and the cavernous nerves [11]. These nerves pass the tips of the seminal vesicles then lie in the lateral endopelvic fascia near its junction with Denonvilliers' fascia [12]. They join the capsular artery of the prostate and travel along the posterolateral border of the prostate on the surface of the rectum and make up the neurovascular bundle [13].

With respect to the sensory innervations of the prostate, neuronal cell bodies that give rise to sensory afferent fibers are not well known. Studies in cats have suggested that over 90% of primary afferent neurons are located in the sacral dorsal root ganglion. It is thought that 70% of these primary sensory afferents project axons to reach the prostate via the pelvic nerve, while 30% project axons via the pudendal nerve. The remaining 10% of primary afferent neurons are found in autonomic neurons in the sympathetic chain ganglia, inferior mesenteric ganglia, and ganglia in the pelvic plexus [14].

Sources of Pain

During transrectal ultrasound-guided biopsy of the prostate, there are often two sources of pain described by the patient. The first is during insertion of the ultrasound probe into the rectum. This is due to mechanical stretching of the anal canal distal to the dentate line, which is full of sensory fibers [15]. The rectal mucosa above the dentate line has a relatively low sensitivity to pain, and it is believed that the pain during biopsy is not closely related to needle penetration of the rectal wall. In contrast, the prostate capsule and parenchyma are very sensitive to pain, and needle penetration of the capsule can cause pain via nerve stimulation of sensory receptors in the capsule and transmission of pain through the neurovascular bundle [15].

A recent study randomized 150 men to no anesthesia, 10 ml of 2% lidocaine gel intrarectally or a periprostatic injection of 5 ml of 1% lidocaine solution prior to ultrasound-guided biopsy of the prostate [16]. They found that both groups who received anesthesia reported less pain than the group that did not receive anesthesia. The group that received intrarectal lidocaine gel reported the least pain with ultrasound probe insertion, while the group that received periprostatic lidocaine injection reported the least pain with the actual biopsy. This study lends support to the two different sources of pain described during the biopsy procedure. Innovative techniques to anesthetize the prostate during the procedure tend to address both sources of pain to maximize analgesic affect and tolerability of the procedure.

History of Prostate Anesthesia

First Utilization

While transrectal ultrasound (TRUS)-guided prostatic biopsy came of widespread clinical use in the mid-1980s [17], prostate local anesthesia was not common practice until 1996 when Nash et al.

first described the benefit of prostate nerve block during prostate biopsy [18]. Periprostatic block was achieved by single local injection, on each side of the prostate, into the region of the prostatic pedicle at the base of the prostate just lateral to the junction between the prostate and seminal vesicles (Fig. 12.1). The posterolateral area of fat within the notch between the prostate and seminal vesicle is described as the "Mount Everest sign" as it creates a hyperechoic pyramid by fat plane, which can allow for localization of anesthetic placement [19] (Figs. 12.2 and 12.3). Soloway et al. further modified this technique by placing two additional depot injections on each side of the prostate on the lateral aspect [14]. Subsequent studies have demonstrated successful periprostatic infiltration only at the apex at the 4 and 8 o'clock positions [20, 21].

Evolution of Prostatic Analgesia

After successful application of periprostatic nerve block, different forms of analgesia were investigated. In 2000, Issa et al. first described application of intrarectal lidocaine gel during TRUS-guided prostate biopsy [22]. This form of local analgesic was found to be simple, safe, and effective in providing satisfactory anesthesia during this procedure. Furthermore, this technique was found to be more convenient, better tolerated, and less invasive compared to transrectal and transperineal prostate nerve blocks. Subsequent studies have supported the use of intrarectal anesthetic gel for purposes of prostate biopsy [16, 23]. Several researches have successfully improved intrarectal lubricating analgesia by adding topical drugs or compounds [24–27]. Nifedipine blocks slow calcium channels and thus potentially allows for analgesia during probe insertion by way of anal sphincter relaxation [27]. Topical glyceryl trinitrate (GTN) similarly causes smooth muscle relaxation with subsequent decreases in anal sphincter tone. GTN was found to be safe, easy to handle, and effective in pain control during prostatic biopsy [25, 26]. Dimethyl sulfoxide (DMSO) is known to facilitate movement of drugs across cell membranes. It has been shown to be effective for musculoskeletal pain

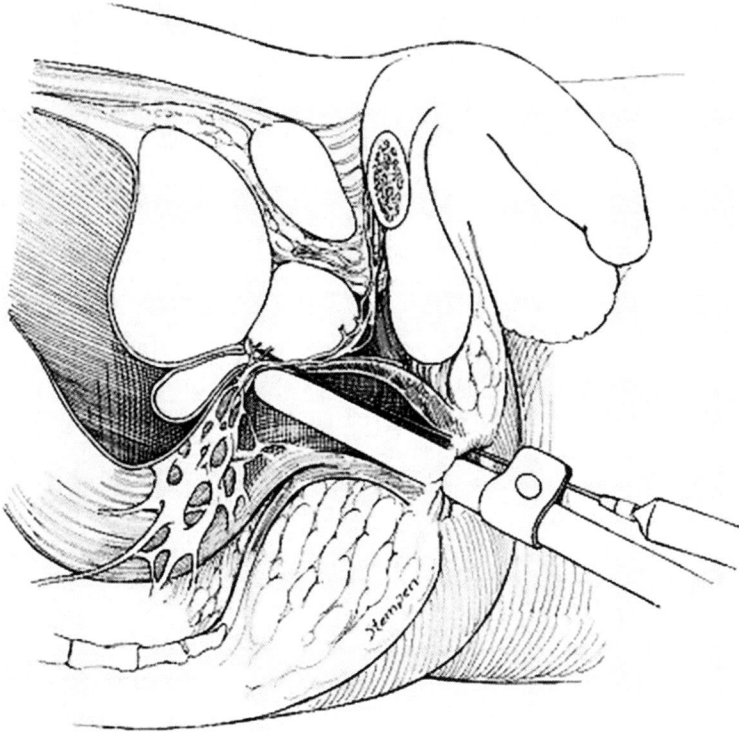

Fig. 12.1 Diagram showing innervations of prostate gland and the location of periprostatic lidocaine injection (From Ref. [18])

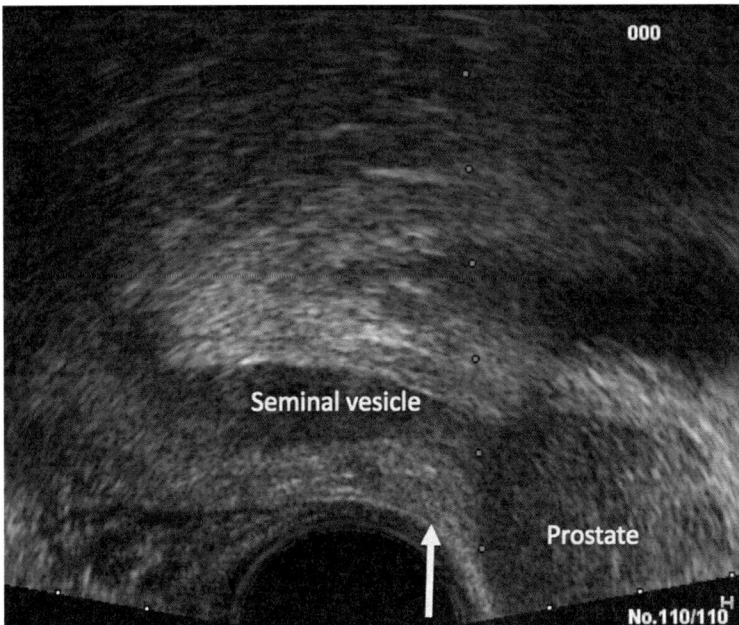

Fig. 12.2 Sagittal section of a prostate gland by transrectal ultrasonography at the lateral aspect of the base showing prostate-seminal vesicle junction and a hyper-echoic triangular shaped fat plane (*arrow*)

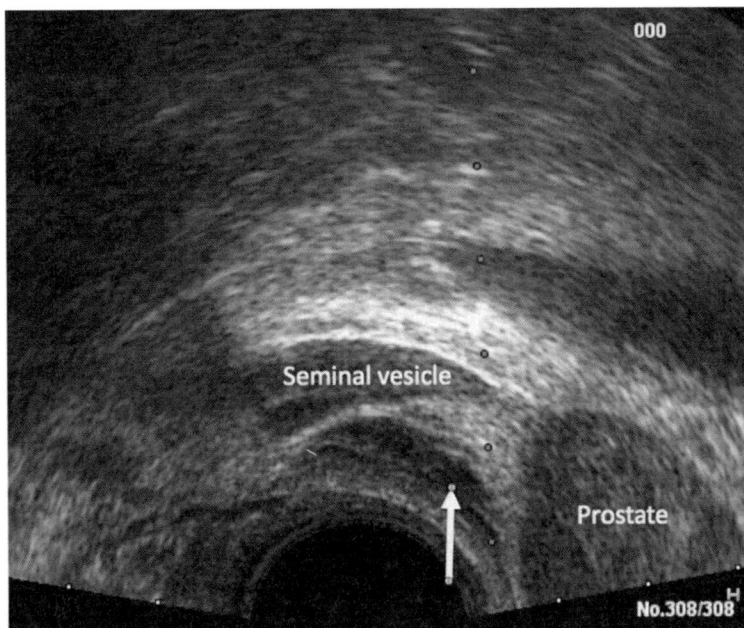

Fig. 12.3 After injection of lidocaine into the fat plane showing a separation of tissue by lidocaine in the *triangle* (*arrow*)

when applied topically and has a potential to reduce rectal discomfort [28]. Recently, more attention has been given to using a combination of these approaches to maximize anesthetic efficiency and pain relief. In 2001, pelvic plexus block during TRUS-guided prostate biopsy was first described. This approach failed to diminish biopsy-associated pain [29]. Alternatively, several studies did demonstrate success with pelvic plexus block under skilled guidance and Doppler ultrasound [30, 31]. Caudal block has also been utilized as an approach to anesthetize the prostate as it provides perianal analgesia and anal sphincter relaxation. However, mixed results have been published regarding its efficacy [32, 33].

Use of Prostatic Analgesia

Local Agents

Periprostatic nerve block has become of widespread use and is the most common form of analgesia for prostatic biopsy [28, 34]. One percent or two percent lidocaine is typically used as it is effective, economical, and safe. Lidocaine also has relatively long duration of action, but it is unclear what the optimal dose, concentration, and location are for maximum pain relief. The most common injection site is the angle between the prostate base and the seminal vesicles bilaterally [28].

Lidocaine gel is the most widely used lubricating agent during prostate biopsy [28]. This form of prostatic analgesia is considered to be safe, easy to handle, and inexpensive. Studies have revealed that this type of anesthetic is effective in controlling pain associated with rectal probe insertion and manipulation [28]. Twenty percent benzocaine gel (Hurricane, Beutlich Lp Pharmaceuticals, Waukegan IL) is a mucosal analgesic frequently used for an oral cavity. Benzocaine gel is a fast-acting mucosal anesthetic, and it can be conveniently applied to the proctocanal at the time of digital rectal examination just prior to the insertion of a rectal ultrasound probe.

Caudal block and pudendal nerve block require the presence of an anesthetist as knowledge and individualization of the anatomy is required as well as need for patient monitoring after drug administration during hospitalization [28].

Systemic Agents

While early strategies for prostatic analgesia during TRUS-guided biopsy typically involved use of local agents, current investigations are evaluating safety and efficacy of combination and systemic therapies. A meta-analysis done by Maccagnano et al. found that pain control seems to be superior with systemic analgesic such as tramadol or combination tramadol, especially with nonsteroidal anti-inflammatory agents [28]. Nitrous oxide, while not widely available in urology outpatient clinics, has shown to be an attractive systemic alternative in several studies [35–37]. Sedoanalgesia with agents such as propofol, fentanyl, or midazolam requires proper monitoring of patients and should be reserved for when extensive or repeat biopsies are needed [17, 28].

Applications Beyond Prostate Biopsy

Use of local prostatic analgesia has successfully extended beyond TRUS-guided prostatic biopsy alone. Local prostatic analgesia has been proven to provide safe and effective pain relief during other minimally invasive procedures of the prostate, including various procedures used to treat symptomatic benign prostatic hypertrophy (BPH). Historically, these procedures are accomplished by way of general and/or regional systemic analgesia. There is now greater recognition of the potential to use local analgesia because of cost-effectiveness and relatively fewer contraindications to local rather than systemic or regional anesthesia.

Periprostatic nerve block has been shown to be effective during transurethral resection of the prostate (TURP) [38–40]. Other minimally invasive treatments for BPH have been performed successfully under local anesthesia with good results including transurethral microwave ablation of the prostate, transurethral needle ablation of the prostate, transurethral ethanol ablation of the prostate, and photoselective laser prostate vaporization [41–45].

Furthermore, studies have shown that periprostatic nerve block can successfully be applied to procedures such as internal urethrotomy, transurethral incision of prostate, and bladder biopsies or fulguration while providing excellent pain relief. Periprostatic nerve block has also been used effectively for other urologic procedures such as the placement of intraprostatic fiducial markers prior to external beam radiotherapy [46, 47]. Local anesthesia of the prostate has also been used for brachytherapy and cryoablation of the prostate with a high degree of patient satisfaction and cost-effectiveness [48, 49].

Technique

Periprostatic Nerve Block

The first description of periprostatic injection was by Nash et al. who described bilateral injections between the base of the prostate and the seminal vesicles [18]. The original study reported a decrease in pain on the side that was injected with local anesthetic compared to the side that was not. This was modified by Soloway and Obek, who proposed two additional injections on each side, with one at the midgland and one at the apex of the prostate [14]. Periprostatic nerve block works by anesthetic blockage of capsular sensory fibers, resulting in less pain, anxiety, and more relaxation of the pelvic muscles, making the procedure more tolerable.

Since its first description by Nash et al., multiple studies have tested the efficacy of periprostatic nerve block. A recent study randomized 90 patients to no anesthesia, periprostatic injection with saline, and periprostatic injection with 1% lidocaine 5 min before biopsy and used a visual analog scale to assess pain [50]. They reported a significant reduction in pain for those men who received periprostatic injection of anesthetic. This study has been supported by many meta-analyses, which have showed a benefit in pain reduction during biopsy with periprostatic injection of local anesthetic compared to placebo or no anesthesia [51–53]. A recent meta-analysis involving 20 studies and 1,685 patients found a significant reduction in pain (weighted mean difference of -2.09, 95% CI -2.44 to -1.75, $p < 0.0001$ on a 10-point scale) when comparing periprostatic nerve block to no anesthesia or placebo [53]. These authors found similar benefits for periprostatic nerve block over no anesthesia or placebo regardless of the site injected.

Studies have also compared the efficacy of periprostatic nerve block to intrarectal anesthetic. Song et al. conducted a placebo-controlled randomized trial where men were given either 20 ml 2% lidocaine gel intrarectally, a periprostatic injection of 5 ml of 2% lidocaine delivered near the junction of the seminal vesicle and base of the prostate, or a periprostatic injection of 5 ml of normal saline injected in a similar location prior to prostate biopsy [54]. They reported a benefit of periprostatic nerve block with lidocaine over placebo injection and intrarectal lidocaine gel. They did not find a benefit for intrarectal lidocaine gel over placebo injection. These results are supported by a meta-analysis of 6 studies with 872 patients comparing periprostatic nerve block to intrarectal local anesthetic [53]. The authors reported a weighted mean difference of −1.53, 95% CI −2.67 to −0.39 ($p = 0.008$), on a 10-point scale in favor of periprostatic nerve block over intrarectal local anesthetic.

Currently, there is much variation reported on the ideal location for injection to provide maximum pain relief throughout the biopsy procedure. The initial description by Nash et al. suggested bilateral injections between the base of the prostate and seminal vesicles [18]. Since then, many studies have advocated for more apical injections [55, 56]. The neurovascular bundles run posterolateral to the prostate gland between the capsule and Denonvilliers' fascia and pierce the capsule at the base and apically at the 4 and 8 o'clock location. It has been suggested that injection at these locations will numb the whole gland [20]. A recent study randomized 60 men to bilateral basal injections and 57 men to a single apical injection and found a significant benefit for men who received a single apical injection ($p = 0.01$) [55]. The other benefit for a single apical injection was less anesthetic required. This was supported by a study involving 386 men, who were randomized to receive no anesthetic, 10 ml of 1% lidocaine at the apical region of the prostate, 5 ml of 1% lidocaine at the bases of the prostate bilaterally, and lastly 4 ml at the apex and 3 ml at the bases bilaterally of 1% lidocaine [56]. The authors

found that 10 ml of apical local anesthetic had the most superior pain relief. However, other studies have not supported this finding. For instance, a study by Philip et al. randomized 143 men to either apical or basal injections and found no significant difference in pain relief between the two ($p = 0.36$). Currently, the location of injection to induce maximal pain relief is still debatable.

Several studies have assessed the most appropriate dosage of local anesthetic for pain relief during the procedure. Ozden et al. randomized 175 men to receive either 2.5, 5, or 10 ml of 1% lidocaine and found that 10 ml of local anesthetic provided significantly better pain relief than lower doses [57]. The authors felt that 2.5 ml of local anesthetic was probably not very effective. It has also been suggested that the use of longer-acting anesthetics, like bupivacaine, in combination with shorter-acting agents can provide longer-lasting analgesia and decrease post biopsy discomfort while acting as fast as shorter-acting agents [58]. There is still much variation among urologists as to the dose, concentration, and type of local anesthetic used.

Intrarectal Local Anesthetic

Another method of providing pain relief during the procedure is to deliver 10–20 ml of intrarectal gel containing local anesthetic before the procedure. This works to anesthetize the sensory fibers in the anal canal below the dentate line and serves mainly to decrease pain during insertion of the ultrasound probe. Intrarectal application of lidocaine jelly prior to biopsy was first described by Issa et al., who demonstrated reduced discomfort and pain during the procedure [22]. This was supported by a study involving 80 men who were randomized to either no anesthesia or perianal or intrarectal local anesthetic. The authors reported that perianal anesthesia might solely be sufficient to decrease the pain during prostate biopsy. A recent meta-analysis involving 5 studies and 466 patients found the intrarectal local anesthetic provided better pain relief than no anesthetic or placebo, but the weighted mean difference between the groups did not reach statistical significance [53]. Other studies have suggested that intrarectal local anesthetic alone is not sufficient for pain relief during the biopsy procedure [59, 60]. Although it works well to reduce the pain associated with probe insertion, it does not address the pain associated with injection of the prostate capsule.

Combination Periprostatic Block and Intrarectal Local Anesthetic

Contemporary protocols have suggested a combination of periprostatic nerve block and intrarectal local anesthetic prior to biopsy of the prostate. This is thought to provide the most efficient relief of pain during the procedure by addressing the two sources of pain individually (probe insertion and injection into prostate capsule). Obek et al. found that the combination of periprostatic block and intrarectal lidocaine worked better than periprostatic block alone in a randomized study of 300 men [61]. This is supported by a study involving 223 men showing that periprostatic nerve block in addition to intrarectal local anesthetic provided superior pain relief compared to periprostatic nerve block and intrarectal placebo [62]. Raber et al., noticed a similar benefit to combined periprostatic nerve block and intrarectal local anesthetic over periprostatic nerve block alone especially with respect to pain during insertion of the ultrasound probe [63]. This lends support to local anesthesia protocols that address both sources of pain during the biopsy procedure. Giannarini et al. reported randomized study of perianal anesthetic cream application and periprostatic nerve block combination. Interestingly in this study, the group with perianal-intrarectal anesthetic cream application had reduced pain score associated with periprostatic block and prostate biopsy. These results suggest large dose of lidocaine-prilocaine (5 g) intrarectal application 30 min prior to the procedure itself can achieve certain anesthetic effect on not only the proctocanal but also the prostate gland [60].

Intraprostatic Injection of Local Anesthetic

The first use of intraprostatic injection was described by Mutaguchi et al. who observed a significant benefit in 71 patients who received intraprostatic injection from 2002 to 2003 compared to 99 patients who received traditional periprostatic injection from 2001 to 2002 [64]. Intraprostatic injection provides local anesthetic to sensory fibers within the parenchyma of the prostate, which have a high sensitivity to pain. Secondly, periprostatic nerve block does not anesthetize the anterior part of the gland, while intraprostatic injection does. A randomized, double-blind, 3-arm parallel-group study compared 243 men randomized to intraprostatic injection of local anesthetic, periprostatic block to the apical region of the prostate, and periprostatic block to the base of the prostate [65]. The authors found that intraprostatic injection provided superior pain relief compared to basal blockade and similar pain relief to apical blockade.

Other studies have suggested that a combination of intraprostatic injection and periprostatic injection of local anesthetic provides superior pain relief than either alone [66–68]. For example, Binggian et al. randomized 300 men to periprostatic and intraprostatic local anesthetic versus periprostatic local anesthetic and intraprostatic saline [66]. They reported significantly less pain in the group that received combined periprostatic and intraprostatic local anesthetic. Cam et al. found a similar benefit with combined intraprostatic and periprostatic blockade over periprostatic blockade alone with no increase in morbidity [67]. Finally, a recent study randomizing 152 patients to either intraprostatic local anesthetic and periprostatic placebo injection, intraprostatic placebo injection and periprostatic local anesthetic, or intraprostatic and periprostatic local anesthetic found a significant benefit in pain relief in men who received combined intraprostatic and periprostatic local anesthetic to just periprostatic or intraprostatic local anesthetic alone [68].

Current Protocol for Local Anesthesia of the Prostate at University of California, San Francisco (UCSF)

Currently, at UCSF, we use a combination of intrarectal local anesthetic, periprostatic nerve block, and intraprostatic injection of anesthetic to provide fast and efficient relief of pain throughout the procedure. We use intrarectal 20% benzocaine cream applied to the proctocanal at the time of the digital rectal examination prior to the ultrasound procedure. Benzocaine is a fast-acting mucosal anesthetic achieving effective pain relief in 30 s to help minimize pain during probe insertion. Currently, a 1% lidocaine 20 cc without sodium bicarbonate nor epinephrine is used. About 4 cc of the solution is injected in the periprostatic fat at the lateral aspect of prostate and seminal vesicle junction bilaterally. The rest of the solution is directly injected into the prostate at three locations in each lobe by inserting 22-G needle all the way to the anterior capsule at the base, the midgland, and the apex, and as the needle is pulled back, about 2 cc of anesthetics is slowly infiltrated in the prostate parenchyma at each location. By doing this, systemic circulation of anesthetics can be avoided and can anesthetize the entire gland including the anterior part.

Complications

There has been comparatively little emphasis placed on evaluation of complications from local prostatic analgesia. Current studies suggest that most forms of local prostatic analgesia are generally safe and well tolerated [69]. The reported complication rate associated with periprostatic nerve block ranges from 2% to 4% [17, 20, 69, 70]. No significant complication differences were found with intraprostatic analgesia injection [64, 67, 68] or topical agents [22, 60, 71]. Of note, reported morbidity is confounded by the fact that many of the complications (i.e., bleeding, infection) can result from the prostatic biopsy itself (i.e., without use of anesthetic).

Pain

A short-lived, mild "stinging" sensation during injection of the periprostatic nerve block has been reported in the current literature [20]. One study found that about a third of patients undergoing TRUS-guided prostate biopsy experienced discomfort upon injection of analgesic [69]. There are no studies that have documented persistent pain from any form of prostatic analgesia.

Bleeding

While bleeding can be associated with TRUS-guided prostatic biopsy [54, 72], no reports of significant bleeding attributed to administration of prostatic analgesia have been reported. One study compared complication rates according to number of injections and found no increase in bleeding with greater number of injections [57]. Obek et al. actually found decrease in incidence of bleeding in patients who received periprostatic nerve block which was explained by improved patient comfort resulting in less movement during the procedure [70].

Infection

As the rectum is highly colonized by bacteria, it was questioned whether periprostatic analgesia was associated with high infection rate [70]. The current literature generally disproves this theory [20, 57, 73]. Conversely, Obek et al. did find the incidence of bacteriuria, high fever, and hospitalization to be higher in the anesthesia group, but none of these findings were statistically significant [70].

Urinary Symptoms

Transient urinary incontinence was reported in 1.5% of patients within first 10 min after injection of anesthetic [69]. It was further recommended that patients undergo pre-procedure micturition. Another study found no change in post biopsy continence after periprostatic local anesthesia [74].

Systemic Toxicity

Systemic toxicity results from accidental intravascular injection of anesthetic agent. Clinically, this can appear as dizziness, visual disturbance, tinnitus, metallic taste, lightheadedness, diaphoresis, or respiratory distress. Reported incidence from periprostatic nerve block ranges from 2% to 4% [17, 20, 70]. Vasovagal syncope was reported in as high as 1% of patients [54]; however, vasovagal responses without the application of anesthetic have been reported as well [69]. In addition to aspiration prior to injection, Seymour et al. suggested the use of color Doppler ultrasound to prevent accidental intravascular injection [20].

Other Considerations

Authors have expressed concern that minute amounts of air are potentially injected during periprostatic analgesia, creating significant image artifacts. Several studies disclaim this. Risk of image artifacts can further be reduced with careful bleeding of the syringe prior to injection and assurance that anesthetic agent is injected outside of the gland [28]. Studies have also reported no difference in intraoperative findings such as fibrosis or loss of places between rectum and prostate [53].

Conclusion

With increasing trends toward PSA screening and more utilization of active surveillance protocols for low-volume minimal-risk disease, the number of prostate biopsies being performed is increasing. Contemporary biopsy protocols are calling for more cores and extended sampling of the peripheral zone compared to the previous sextant description. Although once considered a fairly benign procedure, most patients find biopsy of the prostate to be painful and have expressed a desire to be given some anesthetic for pain relief. Most guidelines now consider anesthesia to be a standard of care when performing biopsy of the prostate as it provides better comfort throughout the procedure and less movement of the patient allowing for better visualization of the prostate during the biopsy. Most urologists provide local anesthesia of the prostate of which the most common type is periprostatic blockade. There is still some debate as to the best site for injection as well as the type and dosage of local anesthetic to use. Contemporary studies have suggested that combined anesthesia with perirectal anesthetic gel application and periprostatic block provides good pain relief by addressing sources of pain from both the rectal probe insertion and the biopsy itself. However, several studies have suggested that any form of local anesthesia is better than no anesthesia and urologists should use whatever method they are comfortable with. To not provide our patients with some form of local anesthetic for pain would be considered beneath most standards of care today.

Editorial Commentary:
The senior author should receive one of urology's highest awards for his seminal work to improve patient tolerance of prostate biopsy. As noted, any form of anesthesia is beneficial, but clearly a periprostatic block is the most critical.

We have recently begun to intentionally inject the rectal wall as the lidocaine needle enters the tissue. Our early observations are that this even further reduces pain during apical biopsy. Furthermore, when taking apical cores, we have described the rectal sensation test, which lightly touches the biopsy needle against the bowel wall as the first step of apical biopsy. Approximately half of patients cannot sense the needle, suggesting that their dentate line is below that point. Firing the needle is then painless. However, for the other half of patients, it is immediately evident that this area is intensely sensitive. This finding indicates that the needle is about to traverse the anus, not rectum. In that scenario, the needle is advanced 2–4 mm more cranially until sensation is no longer present. At that point, the needle is placed through the rectal wall and the probe maneuvered to point the needle back toward apical tissue. Firing in that scenario causes no pain, and apical biopsy is as tolerable as biopsy of the remainder of the gland.

References

1. Jemal A, Siegel R, Xu J, Ward E. Cancer statistics, 2010. CA Cancer J Clin. 2010;60(5):277–300.
2. Halpern E, Strup S. Using gray-scale and color and power Doppler sonography to detect prostatic cancer. AJR Am J Roentgenol. 2000;174:623–7.
3. Hodge KK, McNeal JE, Terris MK, Stamey TA. Random systematic versus directed ultrasound guided transrectal core biopsies of the prostate. J Urol. 1989;142(1):71–4. Discussion 74–75.
4. Rodriguez-Covarrubias F, Gonzalez-Ramirez A, Aguilar-Davidov B, Castillejos-Molina R, Sotomayor M, Feria-Bernal G. Extended sampling at first biopsy improves cancer detection rate: results of a prospective, randomized trial comparing 12 versus 18-core prostate biopsy. J Urol. 2011;185(6):2132–6.
5. Clements R, Aideyan OU, Griffiths GJ, Peeling WB. Side effects and patient acceptability of transrectal biopsy of the prostate. Clin Radiol. 1993;47(2):125–6.
6. Collins GN, Lloyd SN, Hehir M, McKelvie GB. Multiple transrectal ultrasound-guided prostatic biopsies–true morbidity and patient acceptance. Br J Urol. 1993;71(4):460–3.
7. Davis M, Sofer M, Kim SS, Soloway MS. The procedure of transrectal ultrasound guided biopsy of the prostate: a survey of patient preparation and biopsy technique. J Urol. 2002;167(2 Pt 1):566–70.
8. Brooks J. Campbell-Walsh urology/editor-in-chief, Alan J. Wein; editors, Louis R. Kavoussi ... (et al.). 9th ed. Philadelphia: W.B. Saunders; 2007.
9. Benoit G, Merlaud L, Meduri G, et al. Anatomy of the prostatic nerves. Surg Radiol Anat. 1994;16(1):23–9.
10. Schlegel PN, Walsh PC. Neuroanatomical approach to radical cystoprostatectomy with preservation of sexual function. J Urol. 1987;138(6):1402–6.
11. Walsh PC, Lepor H, Eggleston JC. Radical prostatectomy with preservation of sexual function: anatomical and pathological considerations. Prostate. 1983;4(5):473–85.
12. Lepor H, Gregerman M, Crosby R, Mostofi FK, Walsh PC. Precise localization of the autonomic nerves from the pelvic plexus to the corpora cavernosa: a detailed anatomical study of the adult male pelvis. J Urol. 1985;133(2):207–12.
13. Davies MR. Anatomy of the nerve supply of the rectum, bladder, and internal genitalia in anorectal dysgenesis in the male. J Pediatr Surg. 1997;32(4):536–41.
14. Soloway MS, Obek C. Periprostatic local anesthesia before ultrasound guided prostate biopsy. J Urol. 2000;163(1):172–3.
15. Shinohara K. Pain: easing the pain: local anesthesia for prostate biopsy. Nat Rev Urol. 2009;6(7):360–1.
16. Stirling BN, Shockley KF, Carothers GG, Maatman TJ. Comparison of local anesthesia techniques during transrectal ultrasound-guided biopsies. Urology. 2002;60(1):89–92.
17. Aus G, Damber JE, Hugosson J. Prostate biopsy and anaesthesia: an overview. Scand J Urol Nephrol. 2005;39(2):124–9.
18. Nash PA, Bruce JE, Indudhara R, Shinohara K. Transrectal ultrasound guided prostatic nerve blockade eases systematic needle biopsy of the prostate. J Urol. 1996;155(2):607–9.
19. Jones JS, Oder M, Zippe CD. Saturation prostate biopsy with periprostatic block can be performed in office. J Urol. 2002;168(5):2108–10.
20. Seymour H, Perry MJ, Lee-Elliot C, Dundas D, Patel U. Pain after transrectal ultrasonography-guided prostate biopsy: the advantages of periprostatic local anaesthesia. BJU Int. 2001;88(6):540–4.
21. Rodriguez A, Kyriakou G, Leray E, Lobel B, Guille F. Prospective study comparing two methods of anaesthesia for prostate biopsies: apex periprostatic nerve block versus intrarectal lidocaine gel: review of the literature. Eur Urol. 2003;44(2):195–200.
22. Issa MM, Bux S, Chun T, et al. A randomized prospective trial of intrarectal lidocaine for pain control during transrectal prostate biopsy: the Emory University experience. J Urol. 2000;164(2):397–9.
23. Mallick S, Humbert M, Braud F, Fofana M, Blanchet P. Local anesthesia before transrectal ultrasound guided prostate biopsy: comparison of 2 methods in a prospective, randomized clinical trial. J Urol. 2004;171(2 Pt 1):730–3.
24. Demir E, Kilicer M, Bedir S, Kilciler G, Erten K, Ozgok Y. Pain scores and local anesthesia for transrectal ultrasound-guided prostate biopsy in patients with anorectal pathologies. J Endourol. 2007;21(11):1367–9.
25. McCabe JE, Hanchanale VS, Philip J, Javle PM. A randomized controlled trial of topical glyceryl trinitrate before transrectal ultrasonography-guided biopsy of the prostate. BJU Int. 2007;100(3):536–8. Discussion 538–539.
26. Brewster S, Rochester M. A randomized controlled trial of topical glyceryl trinitrate before transrectal ultrasonography-guided biopsy of the prostate. BJU Int. 2007;100(6):1412–3.
27. Cantiello F, Imperatore V, Iannuzzo M, et al. Periprostatic nerve block (PNB) alone vs PNB combined with an anaesthetic-myorelaxant agent cream for prostate biopsy: a prospective, randomized double-arm study. BJU Int. 2009;103(9):1195–8.
28. Maccagnano C, Scattoni V, Roscigno M, et al. Anaesthesia in transrectal prostate biopsy: which is the most effective technique? Urol Int. 2011;87(1):1–13.

29. Wu CL, Carter HB, Naqibuddin M, Fleisher LA. Effect of local anesthetics on patient recovery after transrectal biopsy. Urology. 2001;57(5):925–9.

30. Akpinar H, Tufek I, Atug F, Esen EH, Kural AR. Doppler ultrasonography-guided pelvic plexus block before systematic needle biopsy of the prostate: a prospective randomized study. Urology. 2009;74(2):267–71. e261.

31. Adsan O, Inal G, Ozdogan L, Kaygisiz O, Ugurlu O, Cetinkaya M. Unilateral pudendal nerve blockade for relief of all pain during transrectal ultrasound-guided biopsy of the prostate: a randomized, double-blind, placebo-controlled study. Urology. 2004;64(3):528–31.

32. Horinaga M, Nakashima J, Nakanoma T. Efficacy compared between caudal block and periprostatic local anesthesia for transrectal ultrasound-guided prostate needle biopsy. Urology. 2006;68(2):348–51.

33. Ikuerowo SO, Popoola AA, Olapade-Olaopa EO, et al. Caudal block anesthesia for transrectal prostate biopsy. Int Urol Nephrol. 2010;42(1):19–22.

34. Heidenreich A, Bellmunt J, Bolla M, et al. EAU guidelines on prostate cancer. Part I: screening, diagnosis, and treatment of clinically localised disease. Actas Urol Esp. 2011;35(9):501–14.

35. Masood J, Shah N, Lane T, Andrews H, Simpson P, Barua JM. Nitrous oxide (Entonox) inhalation and tolerance of transrectal ultrasound guided prostate biopsy: a double-blind randomized controlled study. J Urol. 2002;168(1):116–20. Discussion 120.

36. McIntyre IG, Dixon A, Pantelides ML. Entonox analgesia for prostatic biopsy. Prostate Cancer Prostatic Dis. 2003;6(3):235–8.

37. Manikandan R, Srirangam SJ, Brown SC, O'Reilly PH, Collins GN. Nitrous oxide vs periprostatic nerve block with 1% lidocaine during transrectal ultrasound guided biopsy of the prostate: a prospective, randomized, controlled trial. J Urol. 2003;170(5):1881–3. Discussion 1883.

38. Sinha B, Haikel G, Lange PH, Moon TD, Narayan P. Transurethral resection of the prostate with local anesthesia in 100 patients. J Urol. 1986;135(4):719–21.

39. Gorur S, Inanoglu K, Akkurt BC, Candan Y, Kiper AN. Periprostatic nerve blockage reduces postoperative analgesic consumption and pain scores of patients undergoing transurethral prostate resection. Urol Int. 2007;79(4):297–301.

40. Kedia KR. Local anesthesia during interstitial laser coagulation of the prostate. Rev Urol. 2005;7 Suppl 9:S23–8.

41. Bartoletti R, Cai T, Tinacci G, et al. Transperineal microwave thermoablation in patients with obstructive benign prostatic hyperplasia: a phase I clinical study with a new mini-choked microwave applicator. J Endourol. 2008;22(7):1509–17.

42. Zargar Shoshtari MA, Mirzazadeh M, Banai M, Jamshidi M, Mehravaran K. Radiofrequency-induced thermotherapy in benign prostatic hyperplasia. Urol J. 2006;3(1):44–8.

43. El-Husseiny T, Buchholz N. Transurethral ethanol ablation of the prostate for symptomatic benign prostatic hyperplasia: long-term follow-up. J Endourol. 2011;25(3):477–80.

44. Leocadio DE, Frenkl TL, Stein BS. Office based transurethral needle ablation of the prostate with analgesia and local anesthesia. J Urol. 2007;178(5):2052–4. Discussion 2054.

45. Pedersen JM, Romundstad PR, Mjones JG, Arum CJ. 2-year followup pressure flow studies of prostate photoselective vaporization using local anesthesia with sedation. J Urol. 2009;181(4):1794–9.

46. Shinohara K, Roach 3rd M. Technique for implantation of fiducial markers in the prostate. Urology. 2008;71(2):196–200.

47. Linden RA, Weiner PR, Gomella LG, et al. Technique of outpatient placement of intraprostatic fiducial markers before external beam radiotherapy. Urology. 2009;73(4):881–6.

48. Wallner K. Prostate brachytherapy under local anesthesia; lessons from the first 600 patients. Brachytherapy. 2002;1(3):145–8.

49. Cardiovascular and Interventional Radiological Society of Europe. Cryotherapy. Available at: http://www.cirse.org/index.php?pid=114. Accessed 30 Sep 2011.

50. Inal G, Yazici S, Adsan O, Ozturk B, Kosan M, Centinkaya M. Effect of periprostatic nerve blockade before transrectal ultrasound-guided prostate biopsy on patient comfort: a randomized placebo controlled study. Int J Urol. 2004;11(3):148–51.

51. Richman JM, Carter HB, Hanna MN, et al. Efficacy of periprostatic local anesthetic for prostate biopsy analgesia: a meta-analysis. Urology. 2006;67(6):1224–8.

52. Hergan L, Kashefi C, Parsons JK. Local anesthetic reduces pain associated with transrectal ultrasound-guided prostate biopsy: a meta-analysis. Urology. 2007;69(3):520–5.

53. Tiong HY, Liew LC, Samuel M, Consigliere D, Esuvaranathan K. A meta-analysis of local anesthesia for transrectal ultrasound-guided biopsy of the prostate. Prostate Cancer Prostatic Dis. 2007;10(2):127–36.

54. Song SH, Kim JK, Song K, Ahn H, Kim CS. Effectiveness of local anaesthesia techniques in patients undergoing transrectal ultrasound-guided prostate biopsy: a prospective randomized study. Int J Urol. 2006;13(6):707–10.

55. Akan H, Yildiz O, Dalva I, Yucesoy C. Comparison of two periprostatic nerve blockade techniques for transrectal ultrasound-guided prostate biopsy: bilateral basal injection and single apical injection. Urology. 2009;73(1):23–6.

56. Kuppusamy S, Faizal N, Quek KF, Razack AH, Dublin N. The efficacy of periprostatic local anaesthetic infiltration in transrectal ultrasound biopsy of prostate: a prospective randomised control study. World J Urol. 2010;28(6):673–6.

57. Ozden E, Yaman O, Gogus C, Ozgencil E, Soygur T. The optimum doses of and injection locations for periprostatic nerve blockade for transrectal ultrasound guided biopsy of the prostate: a prospective,

randomized, placebo controlled study. J Urol. 2003; 170(6 Pt 1): 2319–22.

58. Lee-Elliott CE, Dundas D, Patel U. Randomized trial of lidocaine vs lidocaine/bupivacaine periprostatic injection on longitudinal pain scores after prostate biopsy. J Urol. 2004;171(1):247–50.

59. Yurdakul T, Taspinar B, Kilic O, Kilinc M, Serarslan A. Topical and long-acting local anesthetic for prostate biopsy: a prospective randomized placebo-controlled study. Urol Int. 2009;83(2):151–4.

60. Giannarini G, Autorino R, Valent F, et al. Combination of perianal-intrarectal lidocaine-prilocaine cream and periprostatic nerve block for pain control during transrectal ultrasound guided prostate biopsy: a randomized, controlled trial. J Urol. 2009;181(2):585–91. Discussion 591–583.

61. Obek C, Ozkan B, Tunc B, Can G, Yalcin V, Solok V. Comparison of 3 different methods of anesthesia before transrectal prostate biopsy: a prospective randomized trial. J Urol. 2004;172(2):502–5.

62. Skriapas K, Konstantinidis C, Samarinas M, Xanthis S, Gekas A. Comparison between lidocaine and glyceryl trinitrate ointment for perianal-intrarectal local anesthesia before transrectal ultrasonography-guided prostate biopsy: a placebo-controlled trial. Urology. 2011;77(4):905–8.

63. Raber M, Scattoni V, Roscigno M, et al. Topical prilocaine-lidocaine cream combined with peripheral nerve block improves pain control in prostatic biopsy: results from a prospective randomized trial. Eur Urol. 2008;53(5):967–73.

64. Mutaguchi K, Shinohara K, Matsubara A, Yasumoto H, Mita K, Usui T. Local anesthesia during 10 core biopsy of the prostate: comparison of 2 methods. J Urol. 2005;173(3):742–5.

65. Ashley RA, Inman BA, Routh JC, et al. Preventing pain during office biopsy of the prostate: a single center, prospective, double-blind, 3-arm, parallel group, randomized clinical trial. Cancer. 2007;110(8):1708–14.

66. Binggian L, Peihuan L, Yudong W, Jinxing W, Zhiyong W. Intraprostatic local anesthesia with periprostatic nerve block for transrectal ultrasound guided prostate biopsy. J Urol. 2009;182(2):479–83.

67. Cam K, Sener M, Kayikci A, Akman Y, Erol A. Combined periprostatic and intraprostatic local anesthesia for prostate biopsy: a double-blind, placebo controlled, randomized trial. J Urol. 2008;180(1): 141–4. Discussion 144–145.

68. Lee HY, Lee HJ, Byun SS, Lee SE, Hong SK, Kim SH. Effect of intraprostatic local anesthesia during transrectal ultrasound guided prostate biopsy: comparison of 3 methods in a randomized, double-blind, placebo controlled trial. J Urol. 2007;178(2):469–72. Discussion 472.

69. Turgut AT, Olcucuoglu E, Kosar P, Geyik PO, Kosar U. Complications and limitations related to periprostatic local anesthesia before TRUS-guided prostate biopsy. J Clin Ultrasound. 2008;36(2):67–71.

70. Obek C, Onal B, Ozkan B, Onder AU, Yalcin V, Solok V. Is periprostatic local anesthesia for transrectal ultrasound guided prostate biopsy associated with increased infectious or hemorrhagic complications? A prospective randomized trial. J Urol. 2002;168(2):558–61.

71. Cormio L, Lorusso F, Selvaggio O, et al. Noninfiltrative anesthesia for transrectal prostate biopsy: a randomized prospective study comparing lidocaine-prilocaine cream and lidocaine-ketorolac gel. Urol Oncol. 2011 (Epub ahead of print)

72. Raaijmakers R, Kirkels WJ, Roobol MJ, Wildhagen MF, Schrder FH. Complication rates and risk factors of 5802 transrectal ultrasound-guided sextant biopsies of the prostate within a population-based screening program. Urology. 2002;60(5):826–30.

73. Taverna G, Maffezzini M, Benetti A, Seveso M, Giusti G, Graziotti P. A single injection of lidocaine as local anesthesia for ultrasound guided needle biopsy of the prostate. J Urol. 2002;167(1):222–3.

74. Addla SK, Adeyoju AA, Wemyss-Holden GD, Neilson D. Local anaesthetic for transrectal ultrasound-guided prostate biopsy: a prospective, randomized, double blind, placebo-controlled study. Eur Urol. 2003;43(5): 441–3.

Principles of Prostate Ultrasound

13

Martha K. Terris and Jason Burnette

Recent epidemiologic studies performed in 2008 demonstrated that prostate cancer still remains the most commonly diagnosed cancer in men, accounting for approximately 25% [1]. Thus, the use of transrectal ultrasound is employed by most urologists predominantly as a tool to accurately direct prostate biopsies, and identification of prostatic abnormalities on sonographic images can be critical in some patients [2]. In general, ultrasound cannot reliably detect prostate cancer; however, it is an inexpensive and portable method for imaging the prostate gland. While ultrasound may not accurately detect prostate cancer, studies by Hambrock et al. have demonstrated that prostate imaging via multimodal 3 Tesla magnetic resonance imaging can accurately detect significant prostate cancer in men with repeat negative biopsies [1].

Many protocols have subsequently been proposed for prostate biopsy. Eskicorapci et al. have proposed a scheme where the number of cores taken were based on prostate volume, with 8 cores from prostates less than 30 cc, 10–12 cores from 30- to 50-cc glands and >12 cores from prostates >50 cc [3]. Nonetheless, repeat negative biopsies have caused much debate in current prostate biopsy protocols. For example, Ploussard et al. demonstrated that extended biopsies in addition to transurethral prostate resection may aid in the diagnosis of prostate cancer in men with a history of two or more negative biopsies with increasing or persistently elevated prostate-specific antigen (PSA) [4].

Conversely, data from Vickers et al. recently evaluated PSA parameters, such as PSA velocity [5]. They found little support for any clinically useful role for PSA velocity in men with a previous negative biopsy. However, the National Comprehensive Cancer Network guidelines promote prostate biopsy if PSA velocity is greater than 0.035 ng/ml. Furthermore, newer studies have indicated a role for using a 24-core scheme when performing repeat biopsies in men with previously undetected cancer. In a study by Novara et al., 143 consecutive patients were evaluated who subsequently underwent 24-core transperineal biopsies of the prostate. They were able to correlate the use of a 24-core scheme with higher detection rates of prostate cancer. It was also deduced that as prostate sizes increased, the detection rate subsequently decreased [6].

Clearly, one of the most challenging dilemmas that urologists face today is repeat biopsy in patients who are at high risk of developing prostate cancer. Patients with atypical small acinar proliferation (ASAP) are recommended to

M.K. Terris, M.D. (✉)
Department of Urology, Georgia Health Sciences University, Charlie Norwood VA Medical Center, 1120 15th Street, Augusta, GA 30912, USA
e-mail: mterris@georgiahealth.edu

J. Burnette, M.D., Ph.D.
Department of Urology, Georgia Health Sciences University, Augusta, GA, USA

J.S. Jones (ed.), *Prostate Cancer Diagnosis: PSA, Biopsy and Beyond*, Current Clinical Urology,
DOI 10.1007/978-1-62703-188-2_13, © Springer Science+Business Media New York 2013

undergo repeat biopsy. PSA density (PSAD), PSA velocity (PSAV), and total prostate volume (TPV) are all significant predictive factors of a diagnosis of prostate cancer in men with an initial diagnosis of ASAP [7]. Thus, numerous groups have developed nomograms for predicting a positive repeat biopsy [8]. Nonetheless, a clinical decision must be made individually for each patient with respect to repeat biopsy or initial biopsy based upon clinical factors.

In this chapter, we will focus on the basic concepts of ultrasound and the physics behind ultrasound imaging. Also, these principles will be applied specifically to imaging of the prostate, which may facilitate transrectal ultrasound (TRUS)-guided prostate biopsy. Clearly, to accurately decipher the pathology conveyed in the areas of shadow and brightness displayed in ultrasound images, an understanding of the physical principles generating these images is essential [9]. Used in combination with extended core biopsies, knowledge of prostate imaging may eventually aid in the diagnosis of prostate cancer.

Basic Concepts

Ultrasound is defined as sound with a frequency too high for the human ear to hear [10, 11]. *Frequency*, or the number of sound waves per second, is measured in *hertz* (Hz). Sound with a frequency over 20 kilohertz (kHz) is outside human hearing range. Transrectal prostate ultrasound is generally performed at very high frequencies of 5–10 megahertz (mHz). By comparison, adult renal imaging is performed at frequencies of 2–3 mHz.

Wavelength is the distance between the onset of one sound wave to the next. In general, as wavelength increases, frequency decreases. The relationship of the wavelength to the frequency defines the *velocity*. Velocity is the speed at which sound waves travel through a particular medium or tissue and is equal to the frequency multiplied by the wavelength. This becomes clinically important when interpreting ultrasound since velocity depends on the medium through which

the ultrasound wave is traveling. The velocity through human soft tissues is approximately 1540 m per second, very similar to the velocity through water. The change in velocity when ultrasound waves encounter air, bone, and other structures accounts for many of the artifacts and landmarks encountered during ultrasound imaging. For example, its velocity in air is 330 m/s, dramatically lower than soft tissue. Therefore, when air is present between the ultrasound probe and the tissue of interest, the image can be distorted or completely obscured. For this reason, a water-density substance, termed a *coupling medium*, is utilized for transmission of the ultrasound waves across the space between the transducer and the body surface, where air pockets frequently occur. This coupling medium is usually a sonographic jelly or lubricant and should be placed between the probe and the rectal surface as well as between the probe and any protective sheaths covering the probe.

Acoustic impedance refers to how resistant a particular structure is to penetration by sound waves [10, 11]. As sound waves progress through tissues of varying impendence characteristics, they decrease in amplitude, a process called *attenuation*. Higher frequencies are attenuated by tissue more than lower frequencies. A key component of successful ultrasound imaging is accurately establishing settings on the ultrasound console to amplify attenuated echoes. This process of amplification is known as *time-gain compensation*. The goal is increasing amplification of more distant sound waves to generate a uniform image rather than an image that is very bright near the transducer and rapidly becomes too dark to distinguish structures progressively further from the transducer. The appropriate time-gain compensation varies with the location being studied, the organ of interest, the distance from the transducer to the area of interest, and the characteristics of the tissue between the transducer and the area of interest. Most ultrasound consoles with a capacity for transrectal prostate ultrasonography include factory-installed default settings for optimal time-gain compensation in prostate imaging.

Ultrasound Transmission

Ultrasound waves are generated by a transducer. The transducer contains the transmitting element, electrodes, and protective face. The transducer, focusing and steering mechanisms, scanning apparatus, and associated wiring for connection to the ultrasound console are housed in an ultrasound *probe* which is shaped for the desired application, such as cylindrical for transrectal ultrasonography. Some authors refer to the entire ultrasound probe as the transducer.

The transmitting element, also referred to as the pulser or crystal, is the component that creates the impulses sent to the transducer to generate sound energy. Transmitters were historically composed of crystals, such as quartz. These were replaced by ferroelectric ceramics. Currently, more durable and flexible piezoelectric polymer materials are being employed.

The focus of the ultrasound delineates the area where the sound waves are most concentrated. In general, with increasing frequency of the ultrasound waves transmitted by the transducer, the focus becomes closer to the transducer. The location and size of the focus (the focal range) can be further optimized by focusing mechanisms within the ultrasound probe. These focusing mechanism may be mechanical, annular, linear array, or electronic. Mechanical focusing is performed by placing an acoustic lens on the surface of the transducer or using a transducer with a concave face. With annular focusing, circular or ringlike elements are used to focus the beam. Rather than focusing a single transmitting element, linear array imaging employs a row of elements producing a broad beam. Electronic focusing also utilizes multiple elements, using a process called *phased array*; the multiple elements are fired sequentially to focus the beam. Most modern transrectal ultrasound probes use electronic, phased array focusing. Unlike mechanical, annular, and linear array probes that can emit ultrasound waves at a fixed frequency and have a fixed focal range, most electronic probes have dynamic, adjustable frequency and focal range.

Array transducers have the ability to be steered as well as focused. As with focusing, the beam is directed by sequentially stimulating certain groups of elements. For example, by alternately stimulating elements in two rows perpendicular to each other, some models allow one to display a transverse or longitudinal image of the prostate without moving the transrectal probe. Those probe models with more sophisticated electronics can display both transverse and longitudinal imaging simultaneously (known as biplane imaging). Some probe models, utilizing mechanical focusing of a single transducer, have a switch that will rotate the transducer at a right angle within the probe to provide both transverse and longitudinal imaging, but simultaneous imaging in two planes is not possible. Annular probes are limited to transverse imaging, whereas linear array and "side-fire" mechanically focused transducers provide only longitudinal images. The "end-fire" mechanically focused probes (currently more commonly used for transvaginal ultrasound) can produce both transverse and longitudinal images by manually rotating the probe 90 ° (clockwise, if the patient is in left lateral decubitus position).

The scanning apparatus in the probe assures that the sound waves are distributed over an adequate area for imaging. Sound waves are emitted from the transducer in a single, very narrow band. To produce a recognizable image in models utilizing a single transducer, the transducer must be mechanically swept across the area of interest producing multiple bands that are combined to form an image. The system for moving the transducer is called mechanical scanner. As the speed at which the scanner sweeps across the imaged area decreases, the resolution increases. Faster scanner speeds are necessary to detect motion. For example, very rapid scanner rates, at the expense of resolution, are necessary in echocardiography, in which detection of cardiac wall motion and valve characteristics during each heart beat is the goal of imaging. In contrast, the stationary prostate affords the luxury of high-resolution, slow scanner rates. Linear and electronic probes do not require scanners since the multiple transmitting elements generate numerous ultrasound bands that are combined to produce an image.

Electronic scanners allow creation of smaller probes as well as the capacity for biplane steering and dynamic focusing described above but are much more expensive than the mechanical and linear array scanners.

Generation of Images

The essential component of diagnostic ultrasound, however, is not the sound wave generated by the transducer, but the sound waves that reflect (or echo) back to the transducer after bouncing off of the tissue of interest [10, 11]. In addition to the transmitting element, the transducer also contains a receiving element to detect returning sound waves. In general, transducers transmit sound only 1% of the scanning time and act as a receiver the other 99% of the time. Through a process called *acoustic-electric conversion*, the transducer transforms the sound energy into electrical energy which is processed by the computer in the ultrasound console to generate an image of minute white dots (*pixels*) corresponding to the returning signals, displayed on a black background to produce an image of assorted shades of gray on the monitor.

When the sound waves travel easily through uniform substances (water, oil, urine, etc.), no echoes are generated. The ultrasound image seen on the screen is, therefore, black. Structures not generating echoes displaying a black appearance are termed *anechoic*. When the sound waves encounter a tissue that reflects the sound, a wave is reflected back to the probe. The ultrasound image is white or gray depending on the intensity of the reflection. Unlike plain radiographs or computerized tomography scans, ultrasound does not detect tissue density. Rather, it detects *sonotransmission* (the passage or reflection of sound). Sonotransmission depends on two principles: the angle of incidence of the sound wave to be reflected and the difference between the acoustic impedance values of adjacent tissues. If the difference is great, a large part of the sound will be reflected back. Tissues with high acoustic impedance such as bone, prostatic calcifications, or brachytherapy implants readily reflect echoes

and, therefore, appear bright white on an ultrasound. A medium such as air, as seen in the bowel, also readily reflects echoes. Thus, the edge of the bowel appears white on an ultrasound. Therefore, substances with widely differing densities (such as air and bone) may both appear bright white on an ultrasound. The range of gray shades generated lends this imaging technique the alternative label "grayscale imaging" which distinguishes it from color Doppler ultrasonography.

The types of echoes that are converted to sonographic images are divided into two broad categories known as specular echoes and scattered echoes. Specular echoes originate from relatively large, regularly shaped objects with smooth surfaces such as the bladder and the outer capsule of the prostate. These echoes are relatively intense and angle dependent. Scattered echoes that originate from relatively small, weakly reflective, irregularly shaped objects are less angle dependent and less intense. The prostatic parenchyma generally reflects scattered echoes.

Resolution describes how well an imaging technique can distinguish two adjacent objects. In ultrasound imaging, resolution is related to the transducer frequency, the scanner rate, and the focusing mechanism. Two types of resolution are considered: lateral resolution and axial resolution. *Lateral resolution* is the ability to resolve objects side by side. Lateral resolution is proportionally affected by the frequency; therefore, the higher the frequency, the greater the lateral resolution. With higher frequency and higher resolution, however, there is a decrease in the ultrasound depth of penetration. *Axial resolution* is the ability to resolve objects that lie one above the other. Axial resolution is inversely proportional to the frequency of the transducer depending on the size of the prostate. The higher the frequency, the lower the axial resolution is in the anterior aspect of large prostates. This state results from the rapid absorption of the ultrasound energy with lower penetration. Lower frequencies can be utilized to increase depth of penetration and image the anterior aspect of large prostates, but there will be a corresponding decrease in the resolution of the peripheral zone of the gland. The most common frequencies utilized for prostate imaging are 7–7.5 mHz, which have optimal resolution approximately 0.5–4 cm from the surface of the transducer. For imaging larger prostates, lower frequency transducers can be employed. For example, a 4-mHz transducer will produce a focal range of approximately 2–6 mHz.

Normal Appearance of the Prostate

The peripheral zone comprises the posterior and caudal portion (the apex) of the gland, is palpable on digital rectal examination, and is the site of origin of the vast majority of prostate cancers (>80%) [12]. The central zone is a small, cone-shaped zone at the cephalad aspect of the prostate (the base) surrounding the ejaculatory ducts; cancers arising from this zone are quite rare [12]. The anatomical distinction between central and peripheral zones is technically difficult to visualize via ultrasound, with both zones normally demonstrating a homogeneous light- to medium-gray area occupying the posterior third of the prostate. The echogenicity of structures within the prostate gland is expressed relative to the

normal medium-gray echogenicity of the peripheral zone (Fig. 13.1). Structures exhibiting the same echogenicity as the normal peripheral zone and central zone are termed *isoechoic*. Structures brighter than this point of reference are termed *hyperechoic*, while darker areas are termed *hypoechoic*. Areas that sonographically appear completely black are referred to as *anechoic*.

The transition zone, located anteriorly on either side of the urethra, can exhibit wide variability in size depending on the degree of benign prostatic hyperplasia (BPH), which arises primarily from this zone. Furthermore, approximately 10–20% of prostate cancers can also arise from this area of the prostate [12]. Relative to the peripheral zone, the anteriorly located transition zone exhibits moderately heterogeneous hypoechogenicity (Fig. 13.2). Hyperplastic nodules in the transition zone can be isoechoic or hyperechoic but are most often hypoechoic. This heterogeneity and hypoechogenicity becomes progressively more prominent with increasing volume of benign hyperplasia and is most likely due to variations in the amount of stromal and glandular elements comprising the hyperplasia. With increased size of the transition

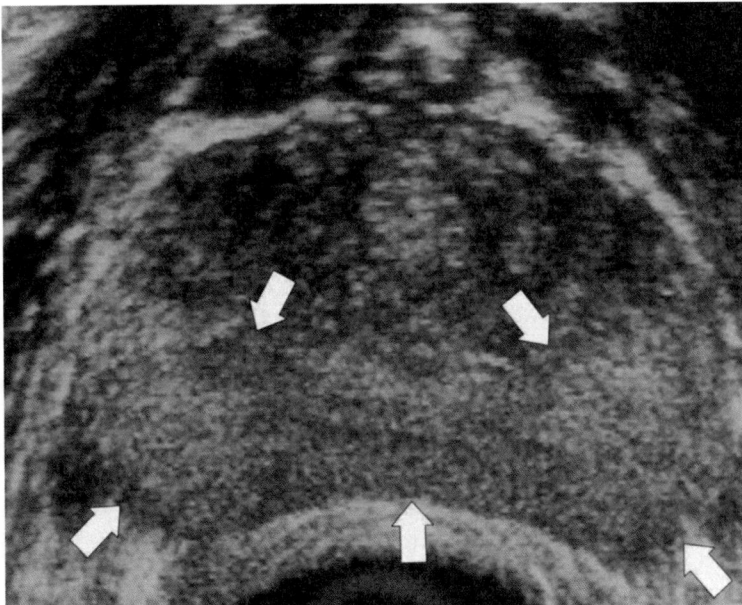

Fig. 13.1 Transverse ultrasound image of a normal prostate with the medium-*gray* peripheral zone delineated by *arrows*

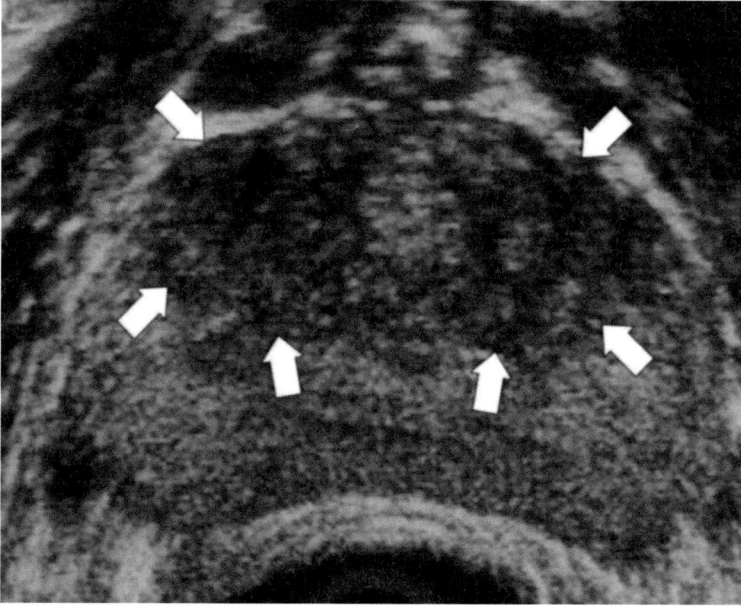

Fig. 13.2 Transverse ultrasound image of a normal prostate with the hypoechoic transition zone delineated by *arrows*

zone, the peripheral and central zones become progressively more compressed.

The boundary between the transition zone and peripheral zone is often sharply demarcated on ultrasound images as a hypoechoic convex line. With increasing BPH, this boundary becomes less convex. This margin often contains corpora amylacea, which are markedly hyperechoic. When these deposits become more calcified and concentrated, they can totally interrupt the ultrasound waves causing posterior shadowing, thus obscuring some or the entire transition zone. The bladder neck and periurethral tissue comprising the preprostatic sphincter is located between the two lobes of the transition zone. This area demonstrates the dramatic hypoechogenicity typical of muscle due to the high concentration of smooth muscle fibers. On transverse images, these muscles form an inverted "Y" on either side of the verumontanum, creating an anatomic landmark termed the Eiffel Tower sign (Fig. 13.3). The lumen of the prostatic urethra should not be visible sonographically unless it has been surgically altered, such as with transurethral resection or by distention during sonography. For example, distending the urethra with a urethral catheter is commonly performed during ultrasonography for

brachytherapy in order to avoid seed placement near the urethra. Distal to the prostatic apex, the periurethral tissue appears as a hypoechoic inverted horseshoe in the transverse plane. In the sagittal plane, this structure appears tubular and can be followed along its course to the external sphincter and proximal bulbar urethra.

The pubic bone demonstrates a hyperechoic margin with dramatic posterior shadowing. The inner margins of the pubic bone can be recognized and compared to the outer margins of the prostate during evaluation for pubic arch interference during prostate brachytherapy.

The thick muscular wall and fluid-filled lumens of the seminal vesicles, vas deferens, and ejaculatory ducts lend these structures a dark-gray echo pattern. Anterior to the seminal vesicles, the muscular bladder wall is dark gray and of variable thickness. Urine within the bladder is anechoic and can aid in delineating the anterior extent of the prostate and the presence of any median lobe.

Due to their predominantly adipose composition, the periprostatic tissues are generally quite echogenic, appearing almost entirely white on ultrasound images. The posterolateral aspect of the prostate margin where the neurovascular

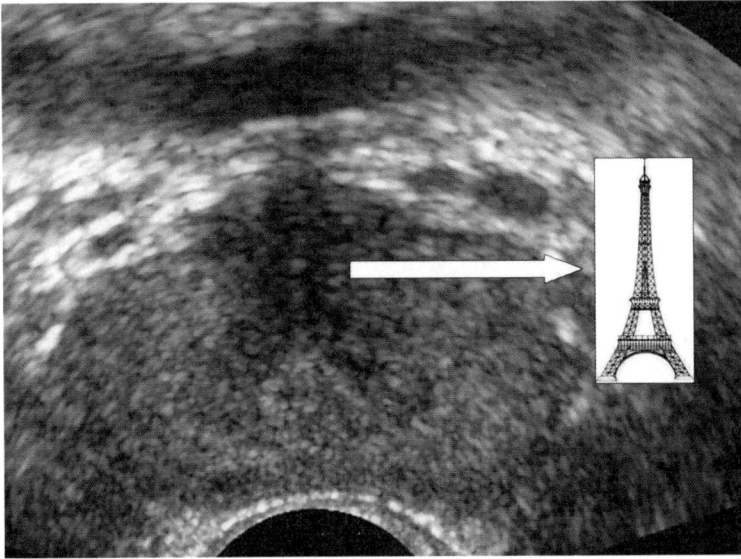

Fig. 13.3 Transverse ultrasound image of the normal prostate at the level of the verumontanum. The periurethral muscle fibers diverge on either side of the verumontanum in a configuration some authors find reminiscent of the Eiffel Tower

structures enter the gland is generally dark gray with areas that are completely anechoic due to the fluid-filled thin-walled veins. With the patient in left lateral decubitus position, the dependent left neurovascular bundle is often more prominent than the right. The anteromedial venous structure of the dorsal vein complex can also be seen as anechoic and somewhat linear structures within the white periprostatic adipose. Since the scanner rate for prostate sonography is slow, flow in these vascular structures is often not readily apparent. Extending toward the rectum from the dramatic anterior shadowing of the pubic bone, just lateral and distal to the prostate apex, is the levator musculature. This muscle has a distinctive hypoechoic appearance with hyperechoic parallel streaks representing the adipose-containing fascia separating the muscle bundles.

Ultrasonography of Prostatic Malignancy

Peripheral zone prostatic adenocarcinomas are typically considered to demonstrate hypoechogenicity on prostate ultrasound [12, 13]. Indeed, an estimated 50–70% of palpable prostate nodules are hypoechoic. However, few nonpalpable peripheral zone cancers show any abnormal echo patterns. The proportion of newly diagnosed tumors characterized by palpable lesions and/or hypoechogenicity has fallen progressively with the stage migration of prostate cancer. Transition zone malignancies are even more commonly isoechoic than peripheral zone cancers. A small number of transition zone tumors will actually demonstrate hyperechogenicity. The elusive nature of prostatic malignancies on ultrasound imaging has stimulated the development of various extended biopsy schemes.

Appearance Following Treatment

External irradiation results in a significant decrease in the calculated volume of the prostate by 6 months after radiotherapy. The rate and degree of reduction correlates significantly with the histologic grade of the tumor (poorly differentiated tumors shrinking most rapidly) and the outcome of treatment but not with stage. The entire prostate is more diffusely hypoechoic, and intraprostatic anatomy is poorly defined. There is often associated thickening of the rectal surface which displaces the prostate anteriorly. Larger hypoechoic cancer foci, particularly those

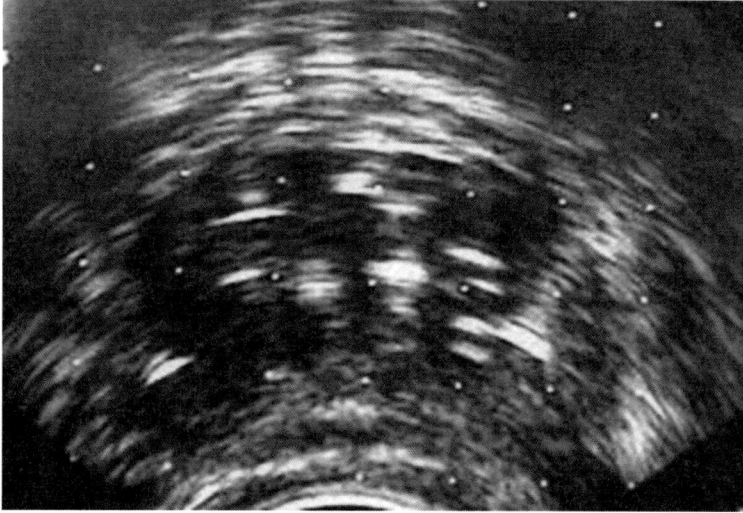

Fig. 13.4 Transverse ultrasound image of the prostate following brachytherapy. Scattered hyperechoic brachytherapy seeds are readily apparent throughout the prostate

that have not responded well to radiation therapy, will show little change in appearance once irradiated, but smaller foci and those responding well to therapy tend to become isoechoic. In general, ultrasound findings are poorly correlated with pathological findings in the irradiated prostate [12–14].

Following brachytherapy, the prostate exhibits many of the same long-term changes in volume and sonographic appearance as with external irradiation. Within the first few weeks after implantation, however, approximately one-third of patients will demonstrate an increase in prostate volume due to post-implant edema. No single parameter, including preimplant prostate volume, preimplant hormonal deprivation, or supplemental external beam radiation therapy, can accurately predict the degree of swelling. The most distinctive characteristic of post-brachytherapy prostate sonography is the appearance of numerous seeds distributed more or less evenly throughout the gland. These seeds are dramatically hyperechoic (Fig. 13.4).

Androgen deprivation therapy results in an approximately 30% decrease in prostate volume in patients with and without prostate cancer. The reduction in volume is greatest in the quartile of men with the largest initial gland volume and least in men with smallest glands. The reduction in volume does not correlate with response of the cancer to therapy. After discontinuation of androgen deprivation, the prostate demonstrates gradual regrowth. Any hypoechoic lesions or sonographically apparent extraprostatic extension will progressively diminish in patients with a favorable biochemical response to hormone therapy.

Artifacts

As explained above, sonographic images are generated with the assumption that sound waves propagate through tissue at a constant velocity and reflect back in a narrow straight line. The velocity and angle of the ultrasound signal is affected by tissue density. Such changes in tissue density (abrupt vs. gradual) ultimately cause deviation of the signal, thus creating artifacts [9, 14].

Refraction, also called dispersion or scatter, is bending of sound waves in fanlike configuration resulting in a curving and elongation of the structure being imaged. A similar phenomenon can be observed when an object partially submerged in water appears to bend. This often manifests as an unnaturally curved appearance of the prostate on ultrasound images (Fig. 13.5).

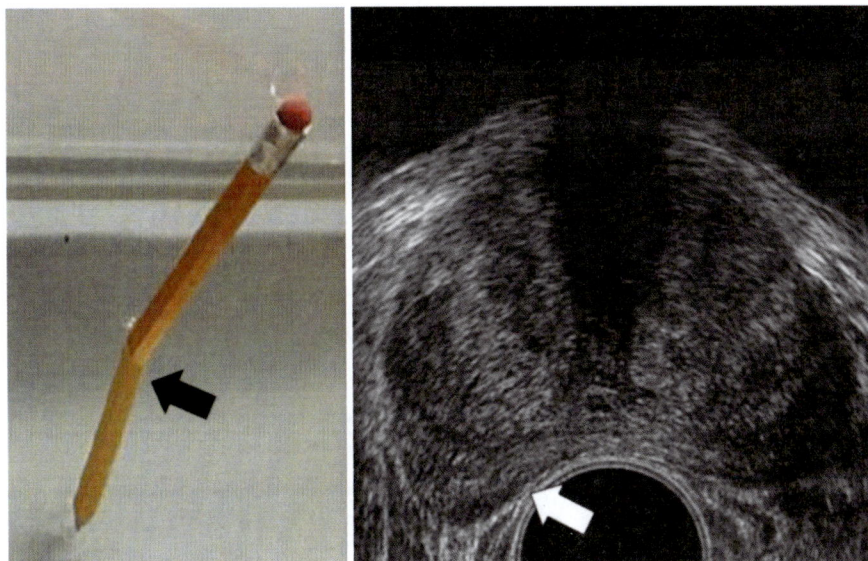

Fig. 13.5 In the left image, refraction of light waves by the change in density from air to water causes the pencil to appear bent (*arrow*). In the right image, the posterolateral aspect of the prostate further from the transducer exhibits an artifactual curved appearance (*arrow*) due to refraction of sound waves

Posterior shadowing results from intense reflectors such as calcifications or air. When structures offer sufficiently high impendence, such that the ultrasound waves are completely interrupted, no sound waves can be transmitted to the structures on the opposite side of the echogenic structure from the transducer. A dark fan will be displayed on the opposite side of the intense reflector, obscuring any pathology located in that area (Fig. 13.6). Note that the term "posterior shadowing" was coined for abdominal imaging, and while still used by convention, it is inaccurate for transrectal prostate imaging. The shadowing resulting from echogenic structures encountered while imaging the prostate transrectally will actually be anterior.

Increased through-enhancement is exhibited with fluid-filled sonolucent structures, such as cysts, and is manifested as hyperechogenicity posterior to the structure (Fig. 13.7). Increased through-enhancement is caused by the ultrasound waves moving rapidly, without reflection through the low-impedance cyst fluid, then abruptly striking the opposite wall of the cyst; the time-gain compensation and higher concentration of sound

waves reaching the opposite wall of the cyst and the tissues beyond it will make these areas appear brighter than the surrounding tissues despite having similar sonotransmission characteristics.

Reverberation is an artifact caused by sound waves striking a very echogenic surface. This signal is ricocheted back and forth between the transducer and the reflector. An image is accurately produced representing the echogenic structure, but subsequent reflections of the signal, each taking twice as long as the prior signal to reach the transducer, are displayed as equally spaced images of the original reflector of decreasing intensity (Fig. 13.8). In TRUS imaging, the intense reflector is usually the rectal wall and results in multiple hyperechoic arches evenly spaced between the rectal wall and the anterior aspect of the image. This can be minimized by assuring that there is copious coupling medium and no air between the probe and the rectum.

Phase cancelation can occur when the signal tangentially strikes a curved structure reflecting it laterally rather than back toward the transducer. Also known as "edge" or "side-lobe" effect, this ultrasound phenomenon was capitalized upon in

Fig. 13.6 While occasionally observed with
calcifications in the prostate,
the best demonstration of
posterior shadowing is seen
on renal ultrasound imaging
in patients with nephrolithia-
sis. The dense stone results in
an intensely hyperechoic
border and shadowing of all
tissues posterior to the stone
(*arrow*)

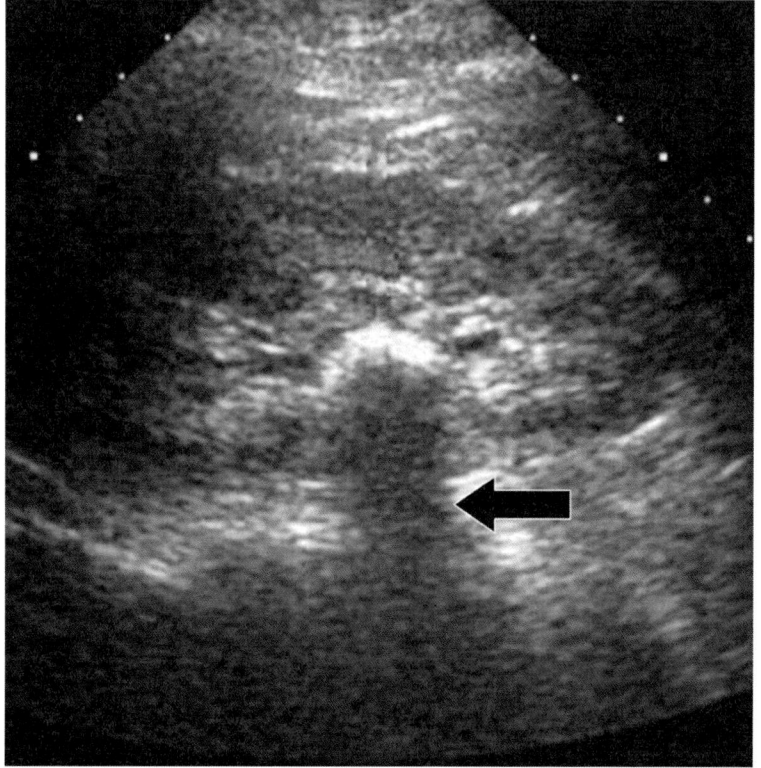

Fig. 13.7 Cystic structures
may occur in the transition
zone in conjunction with
BPH. As seen in this renal
ultrasound with a simple
renal cyst, the tissues
posterior to the cyst appear
hyperechoic due to the
unattenuated sound waves
that passed through the cyst
fluid

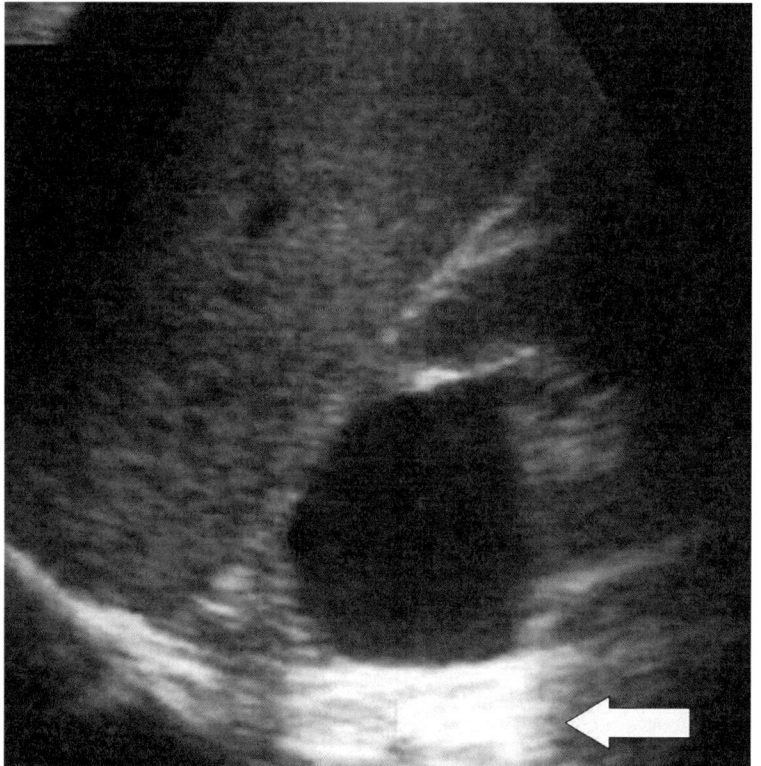

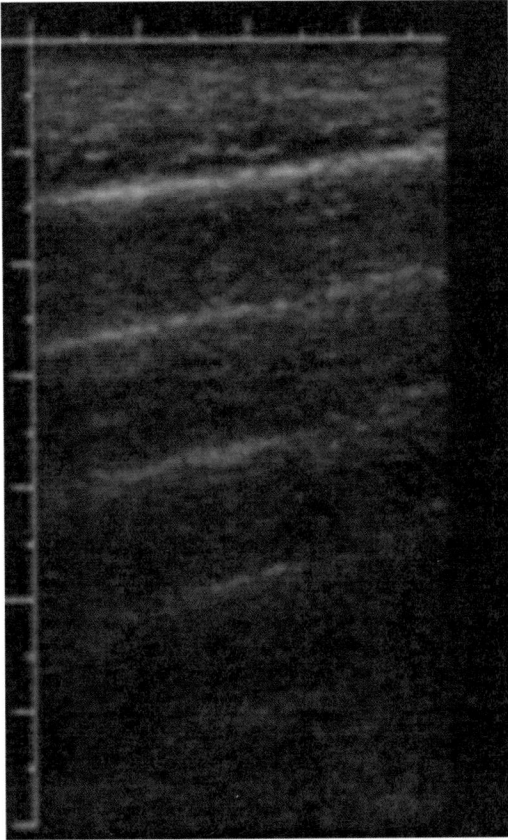

Fig. 13.8 A hyperechoic line, evenly spaced with progressively decreasing intensity, is characteristic of reverberation artifact. These lines can be distinguished from hyperechoic structures by their movement in concert with movement of the ultrasound transducer

the production of stealth aircraft which display acute angles rather than flat surfaces, causing phase cancelation of radar waves (Fig. 13.9). The lack of signal returning to the transducer is misinterpreted as a lack of tissue and displays a black area on the image. In prostate ultrasonography, this artifact is often encountered during scanning of broad prostates. The sound waves striking the curved posterolateral margin of the prostate are scattered resulting in a hypoechoic shadow extending from the edge of the prostate (Fig. 13.10). Similar shadows may also be generated by the posterolateral margin of the transition zone and even the posterolateral aspect of individual BPH nodules resulting in multiple bands of shadowing fanning across the prostate producing an appearance that has been likened to a scallop shell (Fig. 13.11). These shadows can be minimized by centering the probe under the lateral portions of the gland when inspecting this area.

Editorial Commentary:
It is easy to overlook the importance of understanding what really occurs to generate an ultrasound image. Through understanding why structures have specific appearances, we can better understand the prostate and its abnormal conditions. We also emphasize to our residents as well as attendees at our cryotherapy courses that movement to take advantage of the real-time

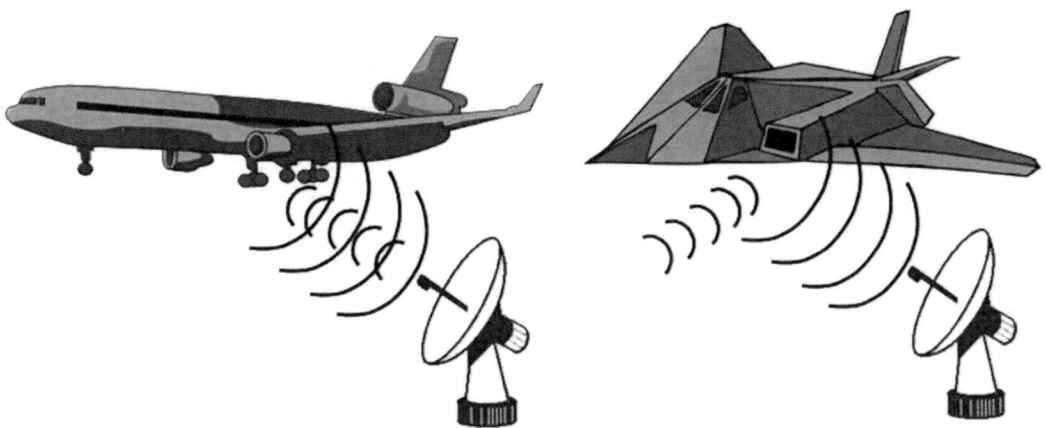

Fig. 13.9 Sound waves employed for radar detection of aircraft are easily reflected by standard construction planes (*left*). Phase cancelation, due to the acute angles of stealth aircraft deflecting echoes away from the receiving unit, prevents detection (*right*)

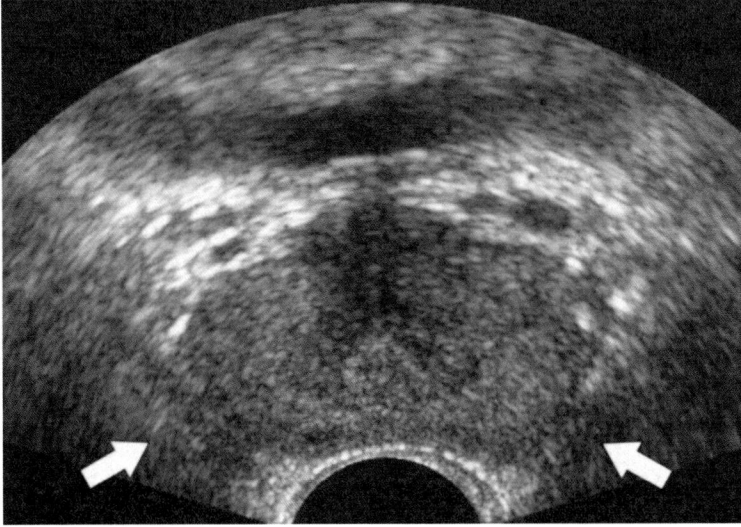

Fig. 13.10 Transverse ultrasound image of the prostate in which the posterolateral edges of the prostate deflected the echoed ultrasound waves away from the transducer resulting in phase cancelation. On images, this appears as a dark band on either side of the gland (*arrows*)

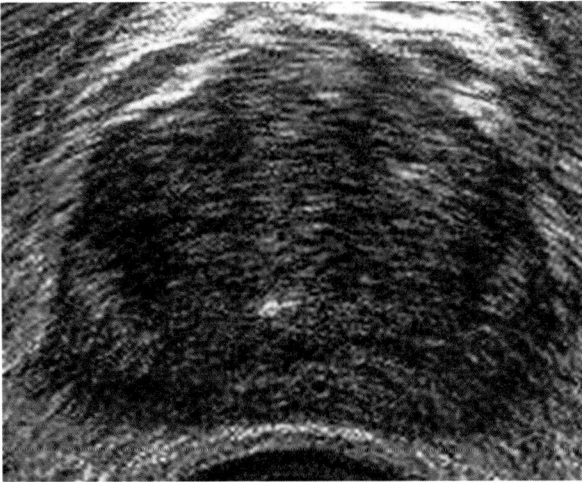

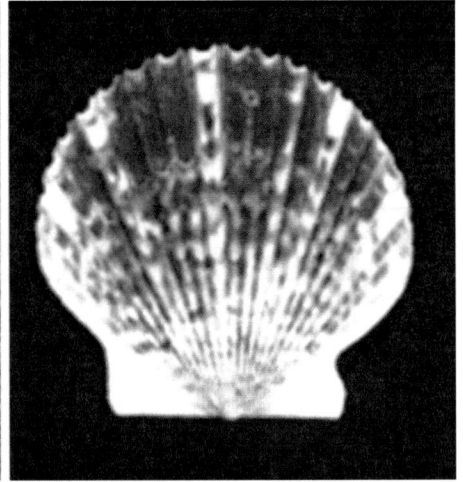

Fig. 13.11 Transverse ultrasound image of a prostate with BPH (*left*) causing multiple hypoechoic bands comparable to a scallop shell (*right*)

nature of ultrasonography greatly improves visualization and is critical for knowing where the needles should be placed for either procedure. For example, it is easy when looking at the two-dimensional sagittal image on the screen to lose track of where the image is from within a three-dimensional structure such as the prostate. By quickly scanning medially and laterally, the location becomes readily apparent. Doing so allows identification of the urethra and lateral borders of the prostate, so tissue is biopsied in an appropriate distribution.

This allows more precise biopsy as well as accurately targeted interventions such as brachytherapy and cryotherapy. As focal therapy for prostate cancer becomes more widely utilized, understanding of ultrasound principles becomes critical to success and safety.

–J. Stephen Jones

References

1. Hambrock T, Somford DM, Hoeks C, Bouwense SA, Huisman H, Yakar D, van Oort IM, Witjes JA, Fütterer JJ, Barentsz JO. Magnetic resonance imaging guided prostate biopsy in men with repeat negative biopsies and increased prostate specific antigen. J Urol. 2010;183(2):520–7.
2. Amiel GE, Slawin KM. Newer modalities of ultrasound imaging and treatment of the prostate. Urol CLin North Am. 2006;33(3):329–37.
3. Eskicorapci SY, Guliyev F, Akdogan B, Dogan HS, Ergen A, Ozen H. Individualization of the biopsy protocol according to the prostate gland volume for prostate cancer detection. J Urol. 2005;173:1536.
4. Ploussard G, Dubosq F, Boublil V, Allory Y, de la Taille A, Vordos D, Hoznek A, Abbou CC, Salomon L. Extensive biopsies and transurethral prostate resection in men with previous negative biopsies and high or increasing prostate specific antigen. J Urol. 2009; 182(4):1342–9.
5. Vickers AJ, Wolters T, Savage CJ, Cronin AM, O'Brien MF, Roobol MJ, Aus G, Scardino PT, Hugosson J, Schroder FH, Lilja H. Prostate specific antigen velocity does not aid prostate cancer detection in men with prior negative biopsy. J Urol. 2010;184(3):907–12.
6. Novara G, Boscolo-Berto R, Lamon C, Fracalanza S, Gardiman M, Artibani W, Ficarra V. Detection rate and factors predictive the presence of prostate cancer in patients undergoing ultrasonography-guided transperineal saturation biopsies of the prostate. BJU Int. 2010;105(9):1242–6.
7. Ryu JH, Kim YB, Lee JK, Kim YJ, Jung TY. Predictive factors of prostate cancer at repeat biopsy in patients with an initial diagnosis of atypical small acinar proliferation of the prostate. Korean J Urol. 2010; 51(11):752–6.
8. Moussa AS, Jones JS, Yu C, Fareed K, Kattan MW. Development and validation of a nomogram for predicting a positive repeat prostate biopsy in patients with a previous negative biopsy session in the era of extended prostate sampling. BJU Int. 2010;106(9):1309–14.
9. Hulsmans FJ, Castelijns JA, Reeders JW, Tytgat GN. Review of artifacts associated with transrectal ultrasound: understanding, recognition, and prevention of misinterpretation. J Clin Ultrasound. 1995;23:483–94.
10. Kossoff G. Basic physics and imaging characteristics of ultrasound. World J Surg. 2000;24:134–42.
11. Kremkau FW. Diagnostic ultrasound: physical principles and exercises. 4th ed. Philadelphia: WB Saunders; 1993.
12. Peterson AC, Terris MK. Urologic imaging without X-rays: ultrasound, MRI, and nuclear medicine. eMedicine.com. 2006. Available at: http://www.eMedicine.com/med/topic/3373.htm
13. Singer EA, Golijanin DJ, Davis RS, Dogra V. What's new in urologic ultrasound? Urol Clin North Am. 2006;33(3):279–86.
14. Terris MK. Prostate ultrasonography. In: Walsh P, Partin, editors. Campbell's urology. 8th ed. Philadelphia: WB Saunders; 2002. p. 3038–54.

Prostate Biopsy Techniques

14

Edouard J. Trabulsi, Arjun Khosla,
and Leonard G. Gomella

Introduction

Early detection of prostate cancer has benefited greatly from the introduction and refinement of systematic *transrectal ultrasound (TRUS)-guided prostate biopsy* techniques as well as increased public awareness about prostate cancer. Widespread PSA-based screening has increased the number of men undergoing early prostate cancer biopsy, with estimates as high as 800,000 prostate biopsies annually in the United States alone [1]. First described by Watanabe et al., TRUS of the prostate expanded to routine clinical use with improvements in ultrasound technology and the introduction of the TRUS-guided systematic sextant biopsy by Hodge et al. [2, 3]. TRUS-guided prostate biopsy is an essential tool in the diagnosis, staging, and management of prostate cancer.

Prostate cancer is pathologically characterized by a loss of glandular architecture as well as increased microvascular and cellular density, allowing for visualization and targeting using ultrasonography. The loss of glandular architecture,

particularly in high-grade cancers, causes a reduction in the acoustically reflective interfaces seen on ultrasound, resulting in a hypoechoic mass that is characteristic of prostate cancer. Prostate cancer is also associated with increased angiogenesis and microvessel density. Enhanced ultrasound techniques, such as color and power Doppler, can be used to assess blood flow patterns within larger vessels in the prostate, while contrast-enhanced ultrasound may be used to demonstrate the microvascular architecture perfusing a malignant neoplasm [4]. In addition, increased cellular density is associated with increased firmness of prostate tissue and decreased tissue elasticity that can be demonstrated by real-time elastography [5]. However, the majority of prostate cancers are not visualized on standard TRUS, and the primary goal of the ultrasound imaging is to direct the needle placement for biopsy.

Transrectal *fine-needle aspiration (FNA)* of palpable abnormalities of the prostate is still advocated in many countries outside the United States because it is less expensive, faster, and easier to perform and results in lower morbidity than any other biopsy technique. This technique should be considered historical, however, with the widespread availability of inexpensive ultrasound machines available to urologists. Considerable concern remains regarding the ability of finger-guided FNA to achieve adequate sensitivity, specificity, and efficacy for prostate cancer detection in the era of ultrasound-guided biopsies. There is also significant controversy in

L.G. Gomella, M.D., FACS (✉)
• E.J. Trabulsi, M.D., FACS • A. Khosla, M.D.
Department of Urology, Kimmel Cancer Center,
Thomas Jefferson University, 1025 Walnut Street,
Philadelphia, PA 19107, USA
e-mail: Leonard.Gomella@Jefferson.edu;
Edouard.Trabulsi@Jefferson

J.S. Jones (ed.), *Prostate Cancer Diagnosis: PSA, Biopsy and Beyond*, Current Clinical Urology,
DOI 10.1007/978-1-62703-188-2_14, © Springer Science+Business Media New York 2013

interpreting the smears, as to whether FNA is as reliable as core biopsy for grading purposes [6, 7].

Due to the high prevalence of prostate cancer and the frequency with which TRUS-guided prostate biopsies are performed, significant efforts have been focused on determining the appropriate indications and refining the techniques by which to image and biopsy the prostate. This chapter evaluates the background, indications, techniques, new technologies, and future considerations for the use of TRUS-guided biopsy in the diagnosis and management of prostate cancer.

Indications and Contraindications

There are several indications for TRUS evaluation of the prostate, which fall into the following general categories: prostate cancer diagnosis and treatment, BPH management and workup, infertility evaluation, and other non-oncologic interventions such as prostatic abscess drainage or aspiration of prostatic or ejaculatory duct cysts. The most common indications for TRUS-guided prostate biopsy include an elevated serum PSA level and/or an abnormality detected on digital rectal exam (DRE) on routine screening. However, screening guidelines and recommendations are rapidly evolving and being continually redefined and are beyond the scope of this chapter [8].

TRUS-guided prostate needle biopsy remains the gold standard for the diagnosis of prostate cancer. There is wide variability amongst urologists with regard to patient preparation and biopsy techniques used when performing TRUS-guided prostate biopsy [9–11]. The evaluation of a patient with an elevated serum PSA commonly includes a TRUS with ultrasound-guided prostate biopsy. Before TRUS improvements and serum PSA testing became widespread, clinicians relied mainly on DRE to establish suspicion of prostate cancer and performed *digitally directed lesional biopsies*. Today, PSA-based screening of asymptomatic men has resulted in the adaptation of systematic TRUS-guided biopsy, which has demonstrated an improved rate of cancer detection, as the standard of care for routine prostate biopsy [3, 12]. However, the presence of focal nodules on DRE will still prompt a biopsy using the TRUS technique, regardless of PSA level.

Prostate biopsy may also be indicated on the basis of the pathologic analysis of previous biopsy specimens. In men who have undergone prostate biopsy and are found to have *high-grade prostatic intraepithelial neoplasia (HGPIN) or atypical small acinar proliferation (ASAP)*, a follow-up biopsy has traditionally been recommended. HGPIN represents a premalignant lesion and carries a 23–35% risk of diagnosing prostate cancer on subsequent biopsy [13, 14]. Contemporary studies, in the era of extended systematic prostate biopsy schema (10–12 cores or greater), have demonstrated a lower prostate cancer detection rate on subsequent biopsy than if a traditional six-core sextant biopsy scheme is utilized, in the range of 22%, calling into question the pathologic significance of HGPIN [15]. The natural history of ASAP is less well defined than that of HGPIN, but if ASAP is present in the initial biopsy specimen, the risk of diagnosing prostate cancer on subsequent biopsy is significantly increased [16, 17]. Thus, irrespective of follow-up PSA values, current recommendations are to re-biopsy all patients with ASAP in their initial biopsy specimen within 3–6 months. HGPIN is more complex and is covered in another chapter.

A variety of tools are available to assist in decision making for prostate biopsy that may be useful to both the patient and clinician [18]. Online risk assessment tools may also be useful in the decision to perform prostate biopsy (available at http://deb.uthscsa.edu/URORiskCalc/Pages/uroriskcalc.jsp and http://www.prostatecancer-riskcalculator.com/) [19, 20].

When evaluating an individual patient for TRUS-guided prostate biopsy, certain conditions would preclude or be considered a contraindication for biopsy, including significant coagulopathy, painful anorectal conditions, severe immunosuppression, and acute prostatitis. These conditions must be treated prior to proceeding with biopsy of the prostate.

Patient Preparation and Positioning

Patients should be informed of the risks and benefits of the procedure and provide informed consent. Traditionally, anticoagulant therapy is stopped 7–10 days before prostate biopsy. For those patients with underlying coagulopathy, prostate biopsy should not be performed until the patient's INR is below 1.5. However, with the increased use of medicated cardiac stents for whom long-term antiplatelet therapy such as aspirin or clopidogrel is necessary, the need to stop anticoagulation has been questioned, with bleeding risks remaining low [21]. According to the European Association of Urology (EAU) guidelines, the use of low-dose aspirin is not a contraindication to prostate biopsy [22].

Administration of *antibiotic prophylaxis* prior to TRUS biopsy is considered standard of care, but there is some debate regarding the type of antibiotic administered as well as the duration of the antibiotic course [23]. Studies have shown that a single-dose fluoroquinolone has a similar efficacy to a 3-day course [24–26]. At our institution, we prescribe a 3-day course of an oral fluoroquinolone and provide the first dose approximately 30–60 min prior to biopsy. If a patient is at risk of developing endocarditis or infection of a prosthesis, we generally administer intravenous ampicillin and gentamicin. If the patient has an allergy to penicillin, vancomycin is administered instead of ampicillin. The patient then completes the 3-day course of fluoroquinolone post-biopsy. The AUA guidelines suggest the short-term use of a fluoroquinolone or TMP-SMX as drugs of choice with the following as acceptable alternatives: an aminoglycoside (or aztreonam substituted for renal insufficiency) with or without ampicillin, a first-/second-generation cephalosporin, or amoxicillin/clavulanate [26].

By using similar protocols, large studies have reported minimal infectious complications, although bacteremia or sepsis still occurs in 0.1–0.5% of patients [27, 28]. The growing emergence of drug-resistant organisms in the community, however, indicates that these guidelines may require modification in the future and that broad-spectrum cephalosporins should be used for the management of post-biopsy infection [29].

Approximately 1 h prior to the procedure, we have patients self-administer a cleansing enema to empty the rectal vault. Although no randomized trial has demonstrated an advantage to using a cleansing enema prior to prostate biopsy, we believe this practice provides an improved ultrasound image while reducing the probability of bacterial infection.

In many centers, patients are placed in the *left lateral decubitus* position with the hips flexed 90°. An arm board is attached parallel to the table, and a pillow between the knees helps maintain this position. The buttocks should be flush with the end of the table to allow manipulation of the probe and biopsy gun without obstruction. However, because patient positioning alters the blood flow distribution of the prostate, we prefer positioning the patient in the *dorsal lithotomy* position when Doppler imaging and contrast-enhanced imaging are used to visualize blood flow patterns [30]. DRE should be performed prior to insertion of the TRUS probe, and any palpable contour abnormalities should be documented, including descriptive identifiers as well as their location on the gland and any concomitant anal pathology.

There is strong evidence demonstrating that periprostatic local anesthetic infiltration near the nerve bundles provides excellent pain control during prostate biopsy [31, 32]. A local prostatic block using 2% lidocaine is administered using a 22-gauge spinal needle through the biopsy channel of the ultrasound probe. Under TRUS guidance, 5 mL of 2% lidocaine is injected on each side of the midline at the junction of the seminal vesicle with the prostate. Other approaches include infiltration of 10 mL of lidocaine starting at the junction of the seminal vesicles and along the lateral aspect of the prostate from base to apex. Direct intraprostatic injection can augment the anesthetic benefit seen with periprostatic injection [33, 34]. Care must be taken, however, to avoid direct intravascular injection because of the risk of systemic lidocaine absorption. Local anesthesia for transperineal biopsies should include infiltration of the skin and subcutaneous tissue of the perineum initially. Ultrasound guidance may then be employed to aid infiltration of deeper tissues along the anticipated biopsy tracts. Post-biopsy analgesia regimens, if used, should avoid the use of aspirin and NSAIDs because of the increased risk of bleeding.

Instrumentation

Grayscale TRUS has become the most common imaging modality for the prostate. Although the role of TRUS is expanding in directing the biopsy of prostate cancer, the role of staging localized prostate cancer using TRUS is very limited [35]. Commercially available endorectal probes include both *side-fire* and *end-fire* models and transmit frequencies of 6–10 MHz. A study of 1,705 patients undergoing prostate biopsy with side-fire and end-fire transrectal probes showed no significant difference in cancer detection rates between the two types of probes, but did demonstrate an improved patient tolerance profile when the side-fire probe was utilized [36]. Most modern ultrasound machines have optimized self-programming for TRUS-guided prostate biopsy. Some newer biplane probes provide simultaneous sagittal and transverse imaging modes. Probes providing a scanning angle approaching 180° allow simultaneous visualization of the entire gland in both the transverse and sagittal planes. Increasing transmit frequency yields increased spatial resolution, at the cost of decreased tissue penetration, which may limit the resolution of the anterior prostate, especially in the setting of BPH. As the frequency of the probe is increased, the portion of the image that is in focus, known as the focal range, is closer to the transducer [37]. The commonly used 7-MHz transducer produces a high-resolution image with a focal range from 1 to 4 cm from the transducer (best for visualization of the peripheral zone, where most cancers arise). Lower-frequency transducers have a focal range from 2 to 8 cm but at a lower resolution. Lower-frequency transducers improve anterior delineation of large glands, increasing the accuracy of volume measurements, but provide poor visualization of internal architecture. The acoustic properties of soft tissue are similar to those of water, but clinically useful ultrasound energy does not propagate through air. For this reason, a water-density substance, termed a coupling medium, is used. The coupling medium, usually sonographic jelly or lubricant, is placed between the probe and the rectal surface. If the probe is covered with a protective condom, the coupling medium is placed between the probe and the condom as well as between the condom and the rectal surface.

The image magnification is adjusted so that most of the prostate is visible without the image being too small to allow detection of abnormalities. In general, the magnification is low during prostate measurements so that the entire gland is seen. During biopsies, magnification is maximal for visualization of needle passage. The ultrasonographer can alter the brightness (or gain) slightly to obtain a better image. The optimal brightness setting results in a medium-gray image of the normal peripheral zone. This gray tone serves as a reference point for judging lesions as hypoechoic, isoechoic, hyperechoic, or anechoic.

Technique

The urologist must be facile in TRUS evaluation of the prostate and have expertise in recognizing normal and abnormal anatomy (see Fig. 14.1). Complete TRUS evaluation of the prostate includes scanning in both the sagittal and transverse planes to obtain a volume calculation. Hypoechoic areas of the prostate should be specifically targeted for biopsy as the likelihood that these areas harbor cancer is higher [38]. A systematic evaluation of the entire prostate, seminal vesicles, and vasa deferentia should be performed together with three-dimensional volume measurement prior to performing any prostate biopsy (see Fig. 14.2). Evaluation should also include assessment of the prostatic capsule for any contour abnormalities as well as evaluation of the rectal mucosa for masses or abnormal thickness.

Patients are typically scanned in the left lateral decubitus position (see section "Patient Preparation and Positioning"). TRUS should be performed in both transverse and sagittal planes. There are two approaches to probe manipulation for transverse imaging. With radial and some

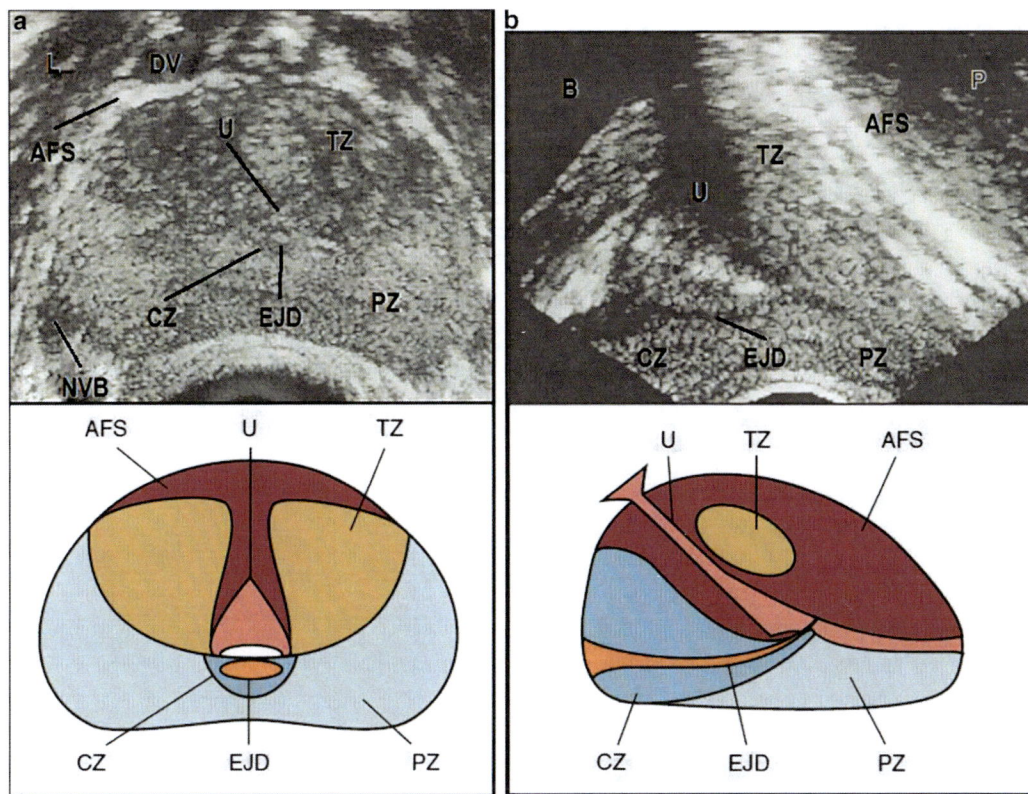

Fig. 14.1 Normal prostate ultrasound images (*top*) with diagrams (*bottom*) at approximately the level of the verumontanum demonstrating zonal anatomy. (**a**) Transverse view. (**b**) Sagittal view. AFS, anterior fibromuscular stroma; B, bladder; CZ, central zone; DV, dorsal vein complex; EJD, ejaculatory ducts; NVB, neurovascular bundle; L, levator muscles; P, prostate; PZ, peripheral zone; TZ, transition zone; U, urethra

biplane probes, advancing the probe cephalad into the rectum images the prostate base, the seminal vesicles, and the bladder neck. Pulling the probe caudally toward the anal sphincter images the prostatic apex and proximal urethra. Transverse imaging with end-fire, side-fire, and some biplane probes is accomplished by angling the handle of the probe right or left using the anal sphincter as a fulcrum. Angling the probe toward the scrotum produces more cephalad images, and angling the probe toward the sacrum produces more caudal images. There are also two approaches to probe manipulation for sagittal imaging. One method is rotation of the probe. Clockwise rotation yields images of the left side of the prostate, and counterclockwise rotation yields images of the right side. Alternatively, sagittal imaging can be accomplished by angling the

probe up or down using the anal sphincter as a fulcrum. In the left lateral decubitus position, angling the handle of the probe down (toward the floor) images the right side of the prostate and angling the handle of the probe up (toward the ceiling) images the left side. Urologists often prefer the angling method because it is similar to the manipulation of a cystoscope and is less uncomfortable for the patient.

Prostate volume can be calculated through a variety of formulas. Volume calculation requires measurement of up to three prostate dimensions. The mature average prostate is between 20 and 25 g and remains relatively constant until about age 50 years, when the gland enlarges in many men [39]. In the axial plane, the transverse and anteroposterior (AP) dimensions are measured at he point of widest transverse diameter. The longitudinal

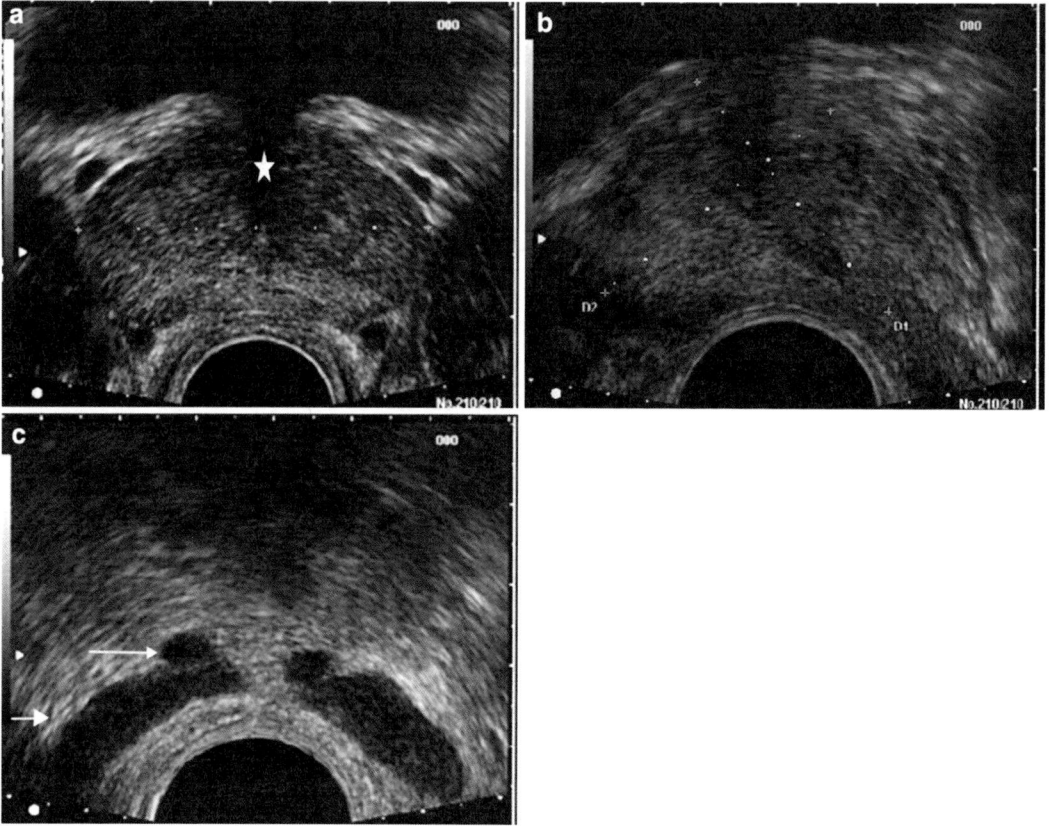

Fig. 14.2 Classic grayscale TRUS imaging of the prostate. (**a**) In the transverse plane with the hypoechoic urethra centrally located (*star*) and *dotted line* representing transverse measurement. (**b**) Midline sagittal view with the hypoechoic urethra running the length of the gland, *D1* represents longitudinal and *D2* anteroposterior measurement. (**c**) Seminal vesicles (*large arrow*) and vasa deferentia (*small arrow*) in the transverse plane

dimension is measured in the sagittal plane just off the midline because the bladder neck may obscure the cephalad extent of the gland. Most formulas assume that the gland conforms to an ideal geometric shape: an ellipse, sphere, or a prolate (egg-shaped) spheroid. Despite the inherent inaccuracies that arise from these geometric assumptions, all formulas reliably estimate gland volume and weight, with correlation coefficients greater than 0.90 with radical prostatectomy specimen weights, since 1 cm^3 equals approximately 1 g of prostate tissue [40]. While most modern ultrasound machines have prostate preset functions to determine prostate volume, an easy formula is that of the volume of a prolate ellipse: height × width × length × ($\pi/6$ or 0.52) to give an accurate prostate volume determination.

When a more accurate determination of gland volume is required, such as during brachytherapy, planimetry may be employed. With the patient in the lithotomy position, the probe is mounted to a stepping device, and serial transverse images are obtained at set intervals (e.g., 3–5 mm) through the entire length of the gland. The surface area of each serial image is determined, and the sum of these measurements is then multiplied by total gland length to yield the prostate volume.

Once gland volume is obtained, one can calculate derivatives such as the PSA density (PSAD = serum PSA/gland volume). An elevated PSAD of the entire gland has been shown to have a sensitivity and specificity of 75% and 44%, respectively, for predicting a positive cancer diagnosis on repeat biopsy [41]. Unfortunately, there is high interoperator and intraoperator variability in PSAD determinations, and similar predictive information can now be obtained using serum free-to-total PSA ratio [42].

A standard protocol or template should be used in documenting the transrectal ultrasound procedure. The template should state the indication, PSA, as well as the findings on digital rectal exam. The technique and position of the patient should also be documented. The machine as well as the probes utilized during the procedure should be described. The anatomy, including the gland size calculation, should be recorded, and any abnormal findings should be noted.

A spring-driven 18-gauge needle core biopsy device or biopsy gun, which can be passed through the needle guide attached to the ultrasound probe, is most often used. Most ultrasound units provide best visualization of the biopsy needle path in the sagittal plane. Images are typically superimposed with a ruled puncture path that corresponds to the needle guide of the TRUS unit. The biopsy gun advances the needle 0.5 cm and samples the subsequent 1.5 cm of tissue with the tip extending 0.5 cm beyond the area sampled [43]. Therefore, when sampling the peripheral zone, the needle tip may be placed 0.5 cm posterior to the prostate capsule before firing. Advancing the needle to or through the capsule can result in sampling more anterior tissue, missing the most common location of cancers. Avoiding adjustment or movement of the probe while the biopsy needle is in contact with the rectal surface, and applying pressure with the probe to compress the rectal mucosa before biopsy, can help avoid rectal bleeding. Pressing the probe against the rectum also minimizes the discomfort of the biopsy needle traversing the rectal mucosa. The biopsy sample is typically placed in 10% formalin or per local protocol. There is no universally accepted method for submission of biopsy samples (e.g., submitted individually or all together in one container). Some pathologists believe strongly that each site should be specially identified because certain locations may be predisposed to cancer "look-alikes" (e.g., Cowper's gland at the apex, seminal vesicles at the base).

At the very least, samples should be segregated into left- and right-sided containers.

All hypoechoic lesions within the peripheral zone should be noted and included in the biopsy material. The lack of a distinct hypoechoic focus does not preclude proceeding with biopsy because 39% of all cancers are isoechoic and up to 1% of tumors may be hyperechoic on conventional grayscale TRUS [44]. Despite the higher prevalence of cancers discovered in prostates with hypoechoic areas, the hypoechoic lesion itself was not associated with increased cancer prevalence compared with biopsy cores from isoechoic areas in a contemporary series of almost 4,000 patients [35]. Prostatic, seminal vesicle, and vas deferens cysts also appear hypoechoic on ultrasound (see Fig. 14.3). Furthermore, other disease processes such as granulomatous prostatitis, prostatic infarct, and lymphoma may all produce hypoechoic lesions [45–47]. Transition zone and BPH nodules are typically hypoechoic as well but may contain isoechoic or even hyperechoic foci. A hyperechoic lesion is malignant in 17–57% of cases, highlighting the need to biopsy these lesions, but recognizing they are not pathognomonic for cancer as once thought [38].

Other TRUS findings that may suggest prostate cancer include lobar asymmetry, capsular bulging, deflection of the junction between the transition zone and peripheral zone, focal loss of the typically bright white periprostatic fat, and any area of increased vascularity.

The original *sextant biopsy scheme* involves taking one core from the base, midgland, and apex of the prostate bilaterally. This method significantly improved cancer detection over digitally directed biopsy of palpable nodules and ultrasound-guided biopsy of specific hypoechoic lesions [3]. Taken in the parasagittal plane, these cores sample a portion of the peripheral zone but also include a significant amount of tissue from the transition zone. Subsequent studies of radical prostatectomy specimens demonstrated that the vast majority of adenocarcinomas arise in the posterolateral peripheral zone, explaining some of the false-negative results of standard sextant biopsy [48, 49].

Fig. 14.3 A hypoechoic midline cystic structure (*arrow*) arising from the ejaculatory duct is shown in the transverse (**a**) and sagittal (**b**) planes and demonstrates through-transmission classic for simple cysts

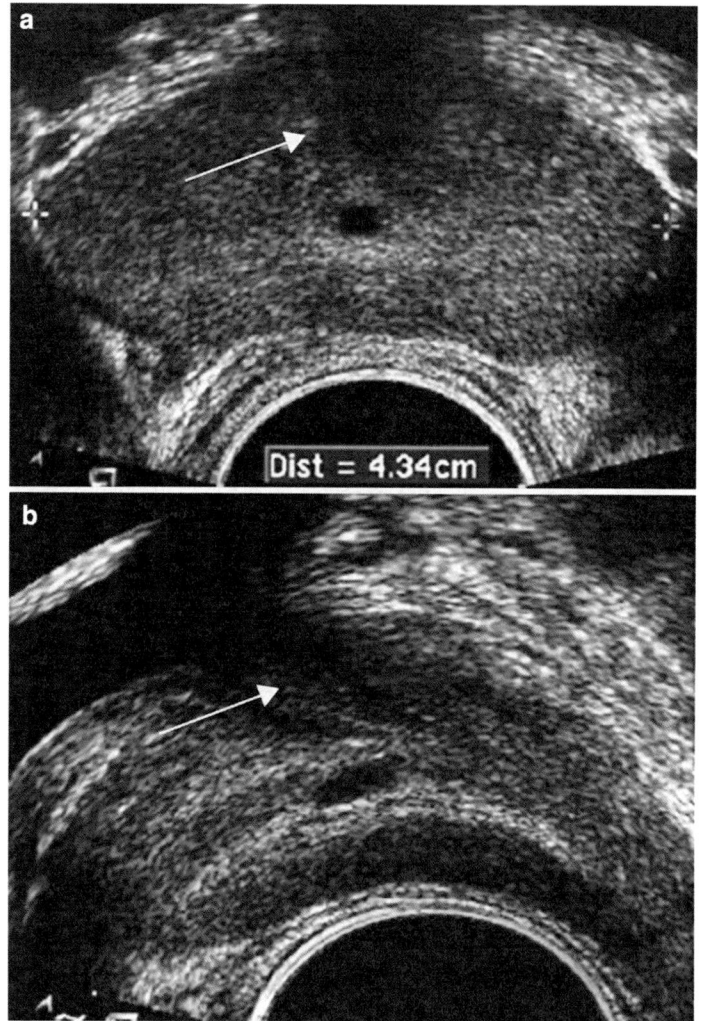

Modifications to the standard sextant biopsy scheme have focused on the importance of *laterally directed cores* [50]. Numerous studies have shown improved cancer detection rates by incorporating additional laterally directed cores into the standard systematic sextant technique, ultimately taking 8–13 cores (see Fig. 14.4) [49, 51–57]. In a prospective study of 483 patients, Presti et al. found that adding laterally directed cores from the base and midgland bilaterally improved cancer detection from 80% with standard sextant to 96% with this 10-core scheme [55]. Presently, six cores are considered inadequate for routine prostate biopsy for cancer detection. The transition zone and seminal vesicles are not routinely sampled because these regions have been shown to have consistently low yields for cancer detection at initial biopsy, but transition zone and anteriorly directed biopsies may occasionally prove necessary to diagnose prostate cancer in those patients with persistently elevated PSA levels and prior negative biopsies [45, 58–61]. Furthermore, there may be a role for transition zone biopsies in men with a gland size greater than 50 cm^3, with an additional yield of 15% cancer detection in these larger prostates [62]. Seminal vesicle biopsy is not routinely performed unless there is a palpable abnormality or, as some suggest, when the PSA value is greater than 30 ng/mL or if brachytherapy is being considered [63].

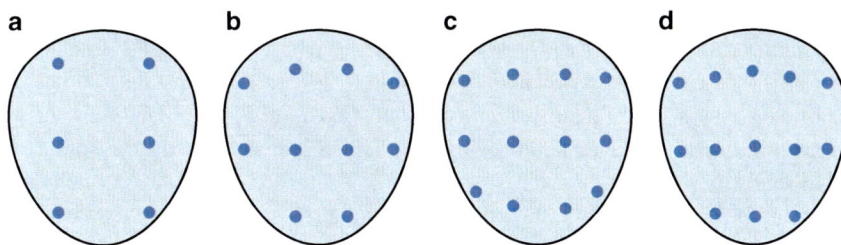

Fig. 14.4 Various reported systematic biopsy schemes. (**a**) Sextant biopsy scheme originally proposed by Hodge and associates (Hodge et al. 1989); (**b**) the 10-core biopsy of Presti and coworkers [55]; (**c**) the 12-core, or double sextant, biopsy; (**d**) the 13-core "5-region biopsy" of Eskew and colleagues [49]. Base is at the *top* of figure; apex is at the *bottom*

Patients often present with a persistently elevated PSA or an abnormal DRE, of clinical concern for prostate cancer, and have undergone multiple negative biopsies despite the well-documented decline in cancer detection with each successive biopsy [42]. Keetch et al. reported an initial positive biopsy rate of 34% in 1,136 men from their PSA-based prostate cancer screening program [64]. Cancer detection rates then fell to 19%, 8%, and 7% on the second, third, and fourth biopsy, respectively. These findings were confirmed by results from the European Prostate Cancer Detection Study, in which, of 1,051 men with PSA values between 4.0 and 10.0 ng/mL, the initial cancer detection rate with sextant biopsy was 22%. Positive cores were then found in only 10%, 5%, and 4% of patients on subsequent biopsies [65].

These diminishing returns coupled with improved cancer detection rates on initial biopsy with extended core protocols have led some researchers to examine "*saturation biopsy*" techniques in this difficult subset of patients. In a study of 57 men with an average of two prior negative sextant biopsies, a cancer detection rate of 30% was obtained with an average of 22.5 cores per patient [66]. Similar protocols have demonstrated improved cancer detection rates [67, 68]. However, a drawback to these techniques is that additional anesthetic requirements often require these saturation biopsies to be performed in a hospital setting, although investigators at the Cleveland Clinic report success with an office-based approach to saturation biopsy [69]. In addition, a saturation biopsy scheme may result in increased detection of clinically insignificant cancers, increased cost, and potential morbidity. In a reassessment of their previous work on saturation biopsy, investigators at the Mayo Clinic performed a large prospective study of standard systematic and saturation biopsy techniques and did not find a significant increase in prostate cancer detection [70].

A study from our institution utilizing intravenous microbubble contrast-enhanced TRUS and a targeted biopsy protocol suggests that equally improved cancer detection rates can be achieved in an outpatient setting with only 10 cores, thereby minimizing the morbidity and costs associated with saturation biopsies [71]. The use of the free and total PSA may also allow classification of patients into low probability or high probability of having prostate cancer and help determine the need for additional prostate biopsy after an initial negative result [72].

Patients who have persistently elevated or rising PSA after several biopsy sessions remain a diagnostic dilemma. Unfortunately, there is no definitive answer of when to stop performing biopsies in a patient who has a high degree of suspicion for undiagnosed prostate cancer. In the European Prostate Cancer Detection study, in over 1,000 men, despite differences in location and multifocality, pathologic and biochemical features of cancers detected on first and second biopsy were similar, suggesting similar biologic behavior. Cancers found on third and fourth biopsies had a lower grade, stage, and cancer volume as compared with cancers on first and repeat biopsies. Morbidity of first and repeat biopsies was similar, whereas third and fourth biopsies had a slightly higher complication rate. The use of a second prostate biopsy in all cases of a negative finding on initial biopsy appears justified. Third and fourth repeat biopsies, however, should only be obtained in selected patients with high suspicion of cancer and/or poor prognostic factors on the first or second biopsy [73].

Transperineal biopsy is most commonly performed in patients who have congenital anorectal malformations or have undergone a previous colorectal operation, making transrectal ultrasound unfeasible. The patient is placed in dorsal lithotomy position. An end-fire ultrasound transducer is utilized. Despite significant limitations in visualization via this technique when compared to TRUS, the prostate can and should be imaged in both the coronal and sagittal planes with calculation of gland volume. Via the transperineal window, focal peripheral zone hypoechoic lesions are difficult to visualize, as are the seminal vesicles. The urethra will appear as a hypoechoic midline structure and may be readily identified by following the corpus spongiosum proximally from the base of the penis. Once the boundaries of the gland have been clearly delineated in the coronal plane, six cores should be taken, three from either side of midline.

The diagnostic yield of routine transperineal ultrasound-guided prostate biopsy in all patients was compared to that of TRUS-guided biopsies in a routine biopsy setting [74]. By utilizing radical prostatectomy specimens with TRUS biopsy-detected prostate cancer, simulated transperineal biopsies were performed and transrectal biopsies were repeated. Significantly, 82.5% of the known tumors were detected with the longitudinal transperineal approach versus 72.5% of cancer detection with repeat transrectal biopsy. The longitudinal orientation of their cores may allow more efficient sampling of the peripheral zone, improving cancer detection. By using this approach in the repeat biopsy setting, Pinkstaff et al. obtained a mean of 21.2 cores in 210 men using a template perineal biopsy [75]. The transperineal approach enhanced identification of transition zone cancers not detected by previous transrectal prostate biopsy in high-risk patients.

Conversely, in a recent Japanese randomized trial comparing transrectal and transperineal techniques for initial prostate biopsy, the cancer detection rate was similar for both, with higher complications noted in the transperineal approach [76]. Therefore, the authors concluded that transrectal prostate biopsy should be the preferred technique for initial prostate biopsy.

Transurethral resection biopsy was once advocated for the diagnosis of transition zone cancers or after negative TRUS sampling. In contemporary series, solitary transition zone cancers, without concomitant peripheral zone tumors, are estimated to occur in less than 5% of prostate cancer patients [77]. In addition, for patients with a persistently elevated PSA after previously negative transrectal biopsies, the diagnostic yield of transurethral resection is low [78]. However, studies have shown that in some patients with an elevated PSA, minor lower urinary tract symptoms, and low suspicion for prostate cancer, transurethral resection has been shown to normalize the PSA level, which was presumably elevated due to bladder outlet obstruction from BPH [79, 80]. With improved TRUS techniques including local anesthesia, the transition zone can be adequately sampled, and the value of transurethral biopsy for the diagnosis of prostate cancer has been questioned for the vast majority of patients [81].

Advanced Ultrasonographic Techniques

In an effort to make the prostate biopsy procedure less random and more targeted, advanced ultrasound techniques have been developed to better identify areas of the prostate more suspicious for cancer. *Color Doppler* imaging is based on the frequency shift in the reflected sound waves from the frequency of insonation and thus depicts the velocity of blood flow in a directionally dependent manner. *Power Doppler* imaging utilizes amplitude shift to detect flow in a velocity and directionally independent manner (see Fig. 14.5) [82]. Patients with detectable color Doppler flow within their dominant tumor at the

Fig. 14.5 Color Doppler
(**a**) TRUS and power Doppler
(**b**) TRUS identify a Gleason
4 + 4 = 8 adenocarcinoma in the
left midgland

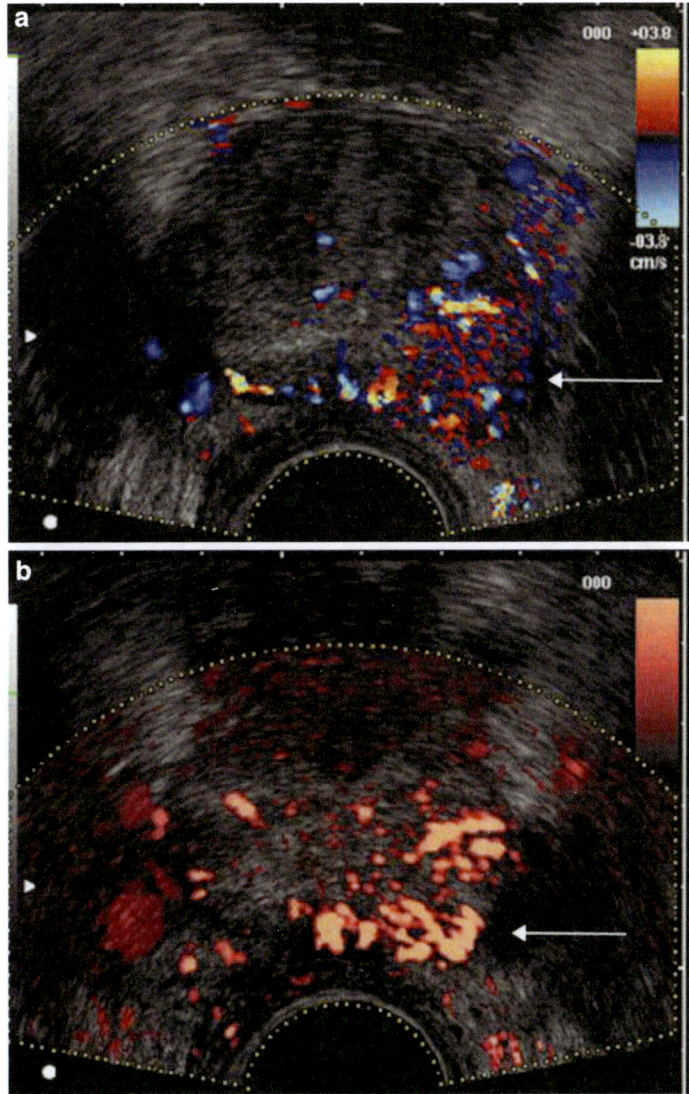

time of TRUS-guided biopsy have a tenfold increased risk for PSA recurrence, higher Gleason grade, increased incidence of seminal vesicle invasion, and lower biochemical disease-free survival rate [83]. However, some benign conditions, such as prostatitis, result in increased blood flow to the prostate, clouding the picture for targeted biopsies using this technique. In 251 patients, Halpern et al. found color Doppler to have a sensitivity and specificity of 14.6% and 93.9%, respectively, in the identification of cancer [1]. Whereas Doppler modes showed an improved

diagnosis versus grayscale TRUS, 45% of cancers still went unidentified by any sonographic modality. Others have shown increased cancer detection rates using Doppler-targeted biopsy strategies, but none is sufficiently accurate to replace systematic biopsy.

Enhancements in the technical aspects of color Doppler TRUS, including the use of contrast agents, may provide the necessary improvements to specifically identify and target cancer sites for biopsy in the future [30, 84–90]. Current unenhanced Doppler modalities are not able to

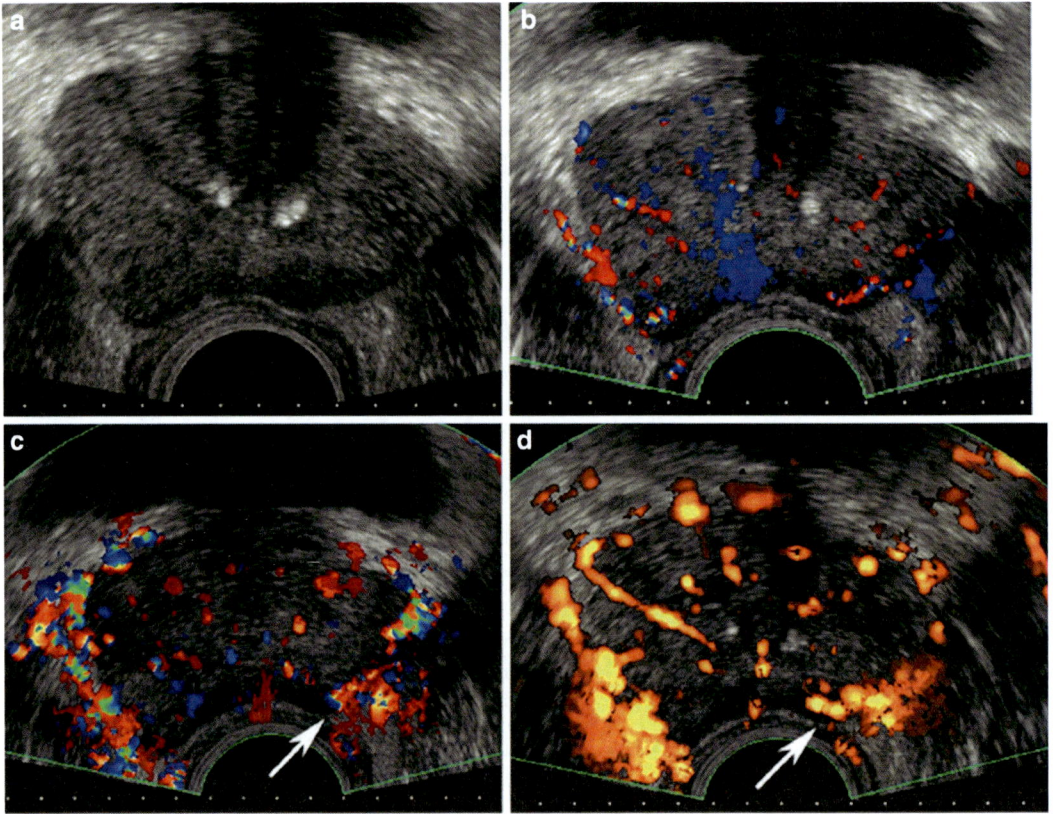

Fig. 14.6 Gleason 6 prostate adenocarcinoma. Transverse images through the midgland of the prostate. (**a**) Conventional gray scale demonstrates a hypoechoic area in the peripheral zone of the left posterior midgland; (**b**) unenhanced color Doppler shows slightly increased flow to the cancerous area; (**c**) contrast medium-enhanced color Doppler shows markedly increased flow (*arrow*) to the cancerous area; (**d**) contrast medium-enhanced power Doppler shows markedly increased flow (*arrow*) to the cancerous area (*lower right*)

identify the microvessels of prostate cancer, which are typically 10–15 μm in diameter. Intravenous *microbubble ultrasound contrast agents*, generally 1–10 μm in size, have been infused systemically during grayscale and TRUS Doppler imaging to amplify flow signals within the microvasculature of prostate tumors, allowing selective visualization of malignant foci in clinical trials (see Fig. 14.6) [91, 92]. Using *contrast medium-enhanced TRUS (CE-TRUS)* for prospective prostate cancer detection, Halpern et al. demonstrated an increase in sensitivity from 38% to 65% versus baseline unenhanced imaging, without significantly altering specificity [93]. Subsequent studies have improved sonographic detection of malignant foci utilizing CE-TRUS

and targeted biopsy of enhancing lesions [71, 94–97]. In a multi-institutional trial involving several European centers, CE-TRUS has been recommended for routine care in prostate biopsy but these agents are no approved for use in the prostate in the U.S. [98].

Grayscale harmonic imaging is method for imaging ultrasound contrast agents that provides better spatial and temporal resolution as compared with color Doppler imaging. A variation on grayscale harmonic imaging is *flash-replenishment* imaging, which utilizes a combination of high-power flash pulses to destroy contrast microbubbles followed by low-power pulses to demonstrate contrast replenishment, providing improved visualization of neovessels that are below the

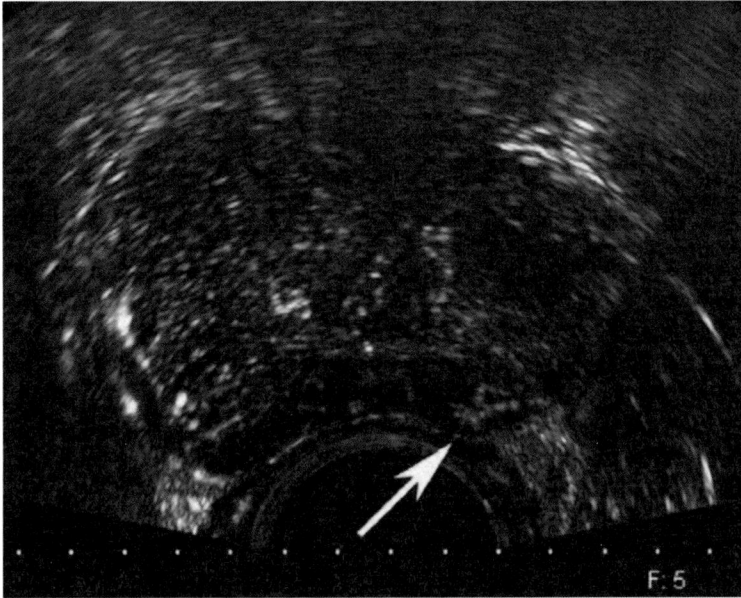

Fig. 14.7 Gleason 6 prostate adenocarcinoma. Transverse image through the midgland of the prostate. Microbubble contrast enhancement with flash replenishment and max- imum-intensity projection reveals an intensely enhancing tangle of blood vessels in the peripheral zone (*arrow*) corresponding to a biopsy-proven cancer

standard resolution of even grayscale ultrasound. Using this technique, we have demonstrated much finer vascular detail for targeting biopsy, and targeted biopsy cores were significantly more likely to be cancerous than random systematic biopsy cores (see Fig. 14.7) [99]. Future develop- ments in these and other imaging modalities that can selectively visualize prostate cancers based on the presence of angioneogenesis may ulti- mately allow more accurate localization of malignancy.

A new sonographic technique known as *elas- tography* may prove to be superior to color Doppler imaging in the identification of malig- nant areas in the prostate [100, 101]. This tech- nique employs real-time sonographic imaging of the prostate at baseline and under varying degrees of compression. The loss of glandular architec- ture and increased cellular density resulting from prostate cancer produces decreased tissue elas- ticity. Through computerized calculations, dif- ferences in displacement between ultrasonic images from baseline and during compression may be visualized, and regions with decreased

tissue elasticity may be tagged as suggestive of malignancy (see Fig. 14.8). In a preliminary study of 404 cases with 151 cases positive for prostate cancer, the malignancy was found in 127 patients (84.1%) with real-time elastography directing the biopsy [5]. A study performed in 2008 showed elastography to have a sensitivity and specificity of 86% and 72%, respectively, in detecting prostate cancer [102]. In contrast to CE-TRUS or Doppler techniques, elastograms provide a less subjective target and thus shows promise in the future of TRUS-guided prostate biopsy.

Endorectal magnetic resonance imaging (MRI) and MR spectroscopy as combined modalities might be able to guide, and therefore limit, the number of iterative biopsies and cores performed on patients [103]. Studies have shown that MRI significantly contributes to DRE and TRUS in localizing cancer within the prostate [103–106]. However, utilization of MRI will require modifications in instrumentation and the technique of biopsy [107]. In addition, these MRI-directed biopsy techniques require expensive equipment that is not widely available for biopsy procedures.

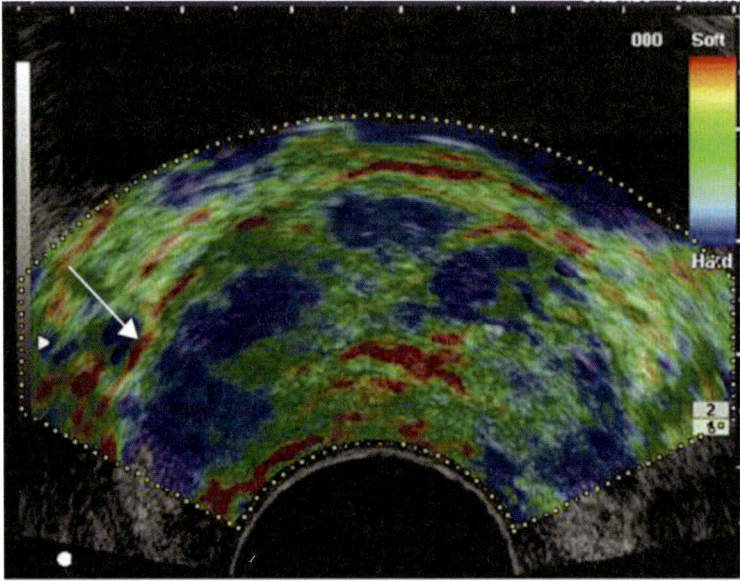

Fig. 14.8 Elastography demonstrates an area of decreased compliance in the right base consistent with an underlying malignancy *(blue near arrow)*. Note color scale in *upper* *right* corner indicating relative tissue "firmness." Targeted biopsy of this region revealed a Gleason $4+4=8$ adenocarcinoma

Conclusion

Transrectal ultrasound-guided prostate biopsy plays a crucial role in the evaluation and management of both benign and malignant diseases of the prostate. The long-term goal of research efforts in TRUS-guided biopsy techniques is to provide a noninvasive method that can detect prostate cancer while eliminating the need for prostate biopsy in patients without clinically significant disease. Transrectal ultrasound is ideally suited to provide an inexpensive, noninvasive modality for characterization of the prostate. Advanced ultrasound techniques such as Doppler, contrast medium-enhanced imaging, elastography, and other developing methods have the potential to further refine the use of TRUS and allow more accurate localization and diagnosis of prostate malignancy. These promising techniques are more targeted and may minimize or eliminate the need for multiple unnecessary biopsies. However, until these approaches are proven superior in the localization of prostate cancer, systematic grayscale TRUS-guided core needle biopsy will continue to be regarded as the "gold standard" for the diagnosis of prostate cancer.

Key Points:
- TRUS-guided biopsy is considered the gold standard for the diagnosis of prostate cancer.
- Digitally directed lesional biopsy has been replaced by systematic TRUS-guided biopsy, which has demonstrated an improved cancer detection rate.
- TRUS-guided biopsy is indicated in patients with elevated PSA and an abnormal DRE or in those patients who demonstrate HGPIN or ASAP on previous biopsy.
- Prior to TRUS-guided biopsy, patients should be counseled on the risks and benefits of the procedure, any coagulopathy should be corrected, perioperative antibiotic prophylaxis as well as a cleansing enema should be administered, patients should be placed in a left lateral decubitus or dorsal lithotomy position, and a prostatic block should be performed for analgesia.
- TRUS probes are available in side-fire and end-fire models that transmit frequencies of 6–10 MHz. TRUS evaluation of the prostate, seminal vesicles, and vasa deferentia should include scanning in both the transverse and

sagittal planes, prostatic volume measurement, and targeting of suspicious lesions.

- Systematic TRUS-guided biopsy should include a minimum of 8–10 prostatic cores. Laterally directed cores increase cancer detection rates. A repeat biopsy is justified if the first biopsy is negative and clinical suspicion remains. Transition zone biopsy is indicated if a patient exhibits a persistently elevated PSA or has a gland size greater than 50 cm^3.
- Transperineal biopsy is an alternative to TRUS for patients with congenital malformations or a history of a previous colorectal operation that makes TRUS more challenging or impossible. Routine transperineal biopsy in the absence of ano-rectal pathology is uncommon.
- Transurethral biopsy for the diagnosis of prostate cancer exhibits a low yield and is, therefore, not advised in most patients.
- Advanced imaging techniques, such as color and power Doppler, contrast medium-enhanced TRUS, flash-replenishment imaging, elastography, and MRI, are being developed to specifically target lesions with an increased likelihood of malignancy, hopefully reducing or eliminating the performance of multiple unnecessary biopsies.

Editorial Commentary:

Ultimately, prostate cancer detection is based on a needle traversing the malignant areas of tissue. A needle can be placed anywhere in the prostate, including transition zone and anterior tissue, especially when using the end-fire probe. We have reported significantly higher cancer detection with the end-fire probe in both the initial and repeat biopsy settings. This becomes most important for large prostate glands and for patients with clinical suspicion following an initial negative biopsy.

References

1. Halpern EJ, Strup SE. Using gray-scale and color and power Doppler sonography to detect prostatic cancer. AJR Am J Roentgenol. 2000;174:623–7.
2. Watanabe H, Kato H, Kato T, Morita M, Tanaka M. Diagnostic application of ultrasonotomography to the prostate. Nihon Hinyokika Gakkai Zasshi. 1968;59:273–9.
3. Hodge KK, McNeal JE, Terris MK, Stamey TA. Random systematic versus directed ultrasound guided transrectal core biopsies of the prostate. J Urol. 1989;142:71–4. Discussion 4–5.
4. Trabulsi EJ, Sackett D, Gomella LG, Halpern EJ. Enhanced transrectal ultrasound modalities in the diagnosis of prostate cancer. Urology. 2010;76:1025–33.
5. Konig K, Scheipers U, Pesavento A, Lorenz A, Ermert H, Senge T. Initial experiences with real-time elastography guided biopsies of the prostate. J Urol. 2005;174:115–7.
6. Perez-Guillermo M, Acosta-Ortega J, Garcia-Solano J. The continuing role of fine-needle aspiration of the prostate gland into the 21st century: a tribute to Torsten Lowhagen. Diagn Cytopathol. 2005;32:315–20.
7. Algaba F, Epstein JI, Aldape HC, et al. Assessment of prostate carcinoma in core needle biopsy–definition of minimal criteria for the diagnosis of cancer in biopsy material. Cancer. 1996;78:376–81.
8. Gomella LG, Liu XS, Trabulsi EJ, et al. Screening for prostate cancer 2011: the current evidence and guidelines controversy. Can J Urol. 2011;18:5875–83.
9. Matlaga BR, Eskew LA, McCullough DL. Prostate biopsy: indications and technique. J Urol. 2003;169:12–9.
10. Davis M, Sofer M, Kim SS, Soloway MS. The procedure of transrectal ultrasound guided biopsy of the prostate: a survey of patient preparation and biopsy technique. J Urol. 2002;167:566–70.
11. Fink KG, Schmid HP, Paras L, Schmeller NT. Prostate biopsy in Central Europe: results of a survey of indication, patient preparation and biopsy technique. Urol Int. 2007;79:60–6.
12. Lippman HR, Ghiatas AA, Sarosdy MF. Systematic transrectal ultrasound guided prostate biopsy after negative digitally directed prostate biopsy. J Urol. 1992;147:827–9.
13. Davidson D, Bostwick DG, Qian J, et al. Prostatic intraepithelial neoplasia is a risk factor for adenocarcinoma: predictive accuracy in needle biopsies. J Urol. 1995;154:1295–9.
14. Kronz JD, Allan CH, Shaikh AA, Epstein JI. Predicting cancer following a diagnosis of high-grade prostatic intraepithelial neoplasia on needle biopsy: data on men with more than one follow-up biopsy. Am J Surg Pathol. 2001;25:1079–85.
15. Montironi R, Mazzucchelli R, Lopez-Beltran A, Scarpelli M, Cheng L. Prostatic intraepithelial neoplasia: its morphological and molecular diagnosis and clinical significance. BJU Int. 2011;108(9):1394–401.
16. Iczkowski KA, Bassler TJ, Schwob VS, et al. Diagnosis of "suspicious for malignancy" in prostate biopsies: predictive value for cancer. Urology. 1998;51:749–57. Discussion 57–8.

17. Ouyang RC, Kenwright DN, Nacey JN, Delahunt B. The presence of atypical small acinar proliferation in prostate needle biopsy is predictive of carcinoma on subsequent biopsy. BJU Int. 2001;87:70–4.

18. Zaytoun OM, Kattan MW, Moussa AS, Li J, Yu C, Jones JS. Development of improved nomogram for prediction of outcome of initial prostate biopsy using readily available clinical information. Urology. 2011;78:392–8.

19. Thompson IM, Ankerst DP, Chi C, et al. Assessing prostate cancer risk: results from the Prostate Cancer Prevention Trial. J Natl Cancer Inst. 2006;98:529–34.

20. van Vugt HA, Roobol MJ, Kranse R, et al. Prediction of prostate cancer in unscreened men: external validation of a risk calculator. Eur J Cancer. 2011;47:903–9.

21. Ihezue CU, Smart J, Dewbury KC, Mehta R, Burgess L. Biopsy of the prostate guided by transrectal ultrasound: relation between warfarin use and incidence of bleeding complications. Clin Radiol. 2005;60:459–63. Discussion 7–8.

22. Giannarini G, Mogorovich A, Valent F, et al. Continuing or discontinuing low-dose aspirin before transrectal prostate biopsy: results of a prospective randomized trial. Urology. 2007;70:501–5.

23. Shandera KC, Thibault GP, Deshon Jr GE. Variability in patient preparation for prostate biopsy among American urologists. Urology. 1998;52:644–6.

24. Kapoor DA, Klimberg IW, Malek GH, et al. Single-dose oral ciprofloxacin versus placebo for prophylaxis during transrectal prostate biopsy. Urology. 1998;52:552–8.

25. Sabbagh R, McCormack M, Peloquin F, et al. A prospective randomized trial of 1-day versus 3-day antibiotic prophylaxis for transrectal ultrasound guided prostate biopsy. Can J Urol. 2004;11:2216–9.

26. Wolf Jr JS, Bennett CJ, Dmochowski RR, Hollenbeck BK, Pearle MS, Schaeffer AJ. Best practice policy statement on urologic surgery antimicrobial prophylaxis. J Urol. 2008;179:1379–90.

27. Djavan B, Waldert M, Zlotta A, et al. Safety and morbidity of first and repeat transrectal ultrasound guided prostate needle biopsies: results of a prospective European prostate cancer detection study. J Urol. 2001;166:856–60.

28. Raaijmakers R, Kirkels WJ, Roobol MJ, Wildhagen MF, Schrder FH. Complication rates and risk factors of 5802 transrectal ultrasound-guided sextant biopsies of the prostate within a population-based screening program. Urology. 2002;60:826–30.

29. Zaytoun OM, Vargo EH, Rajan R, Berglund R, Gordon S, Jones JS. Emergence of fluoroquinolone-resistant *Escherichia coli* as cause of postprostate biopsy infection: implications for prophylaxis and treatment. Urology. 2011;77:1035–41.

30. Halpern EJ, Frauscher F, Forsberg F, et al. High-frequency Doppler US of the prostate: effect of patient position. Radiology. 2002;222:634–9.

31. Berger AP, Frauscher F, Halpern EJ, et al. Periprostatic administration of local anesthesia during transrectal ultrasound-guided biopsy of the prostate: a randomized, double-blind, placebo-controlled study. Urology. 2003;61:585–8.

32. Trucchi A, De Nunzio C, Mariani S, Palleschi G, Miano L, Tubaro A. Local anesthesia reduces pain associated with transrectal prostatic biopsy. A prospective randomized study. Urol Int. 2005;74:209–13.

33. Lee HY, Lee HJ, Byun SS, Lee SE, Hong SK, Kim SH. Effect of intraprostatic local anesthesia during transrectal ultrasound guided prostate biopsy: comparison of 3 methods in a randomized, double-blind, placebo controlled trial. J Urol. 2007;178:469–72. Discussion 72.

34. Cam K, Sener M, Kayikci A, Akman Y, Erol A. Combined periprostatic and intraprostatic local anesthesia for prostate biopsy: a double-blind, placebo controlled, randomized trial. J Urol. 2008;180:141–4. Discussion 4–5.

35. Onur R, Littrup PJ, Pontes JE, Bianco Jr FJ. Contemporary impact of transrectal ultrasound lesions for prostate cancer detection. J Urol. 2004;172:512–4.

36. Raber M, Scattoni V, Gallina A, et al. Does the transrectal ultrasound probe influence prostate cancer detection in patients undergoing an extended prostate biopsy scheme? Results of a large retrospective study. BJU Int. 2011;109(5):672–7.

37. Kossoff G. Basic physics and imaging characteristics of ultrasound. World J Surg. 2000;24:134–42.

38. Frauscher F, Klauser A, Halpern EJ. Advances in ultrasound for the detection of prostate cancer. Ultrasound Q. 2002;18:135–42.

39. Griffiths K. Molecular control of prostate growth. In: Kirby R, editor. Textbook of benign prostatic hyperplasia. Oxford: Isis Medical Media; 1996.

40. Terris MK, Stamey TA. Determination of prostate volume by transrectal ultrasound. J Urol. 1991;145:984–7.

41. Djavan B, Zlotta A, Remzi M, et al. Optimal predictors of prostate cancer on repeat prostate biopsy: a prospective study of 1,051 men. J Urol. 2000;163:1144–8. Discussion 8–9.

42. Djavan B, Remzi M, Marberger M. When to biopsy and when to stop biopsying. Urol Clin North Am. 2003;30:253–62. viii.

43. Kaye KW. Prostate biopsy using automatic gun. Technique for determination of precise biopsy site. Urology. 1989;34:111–2.

44. Shinohara K, Wheeler TM, Scardino PT. The appearance of prostate cancer on transrectal ultrasonography: correlation of imaging and pathological examinations. J Urol. 1989;142:76–82.

45. Terris MK, Macy M, Freiha FS. Transrectal ultrasound appearance of prostatic granulomas secondary to bacillus Calmette-Guerin instillation. J Urol. 1997;158:126–7.

46. Purohit RS, Shinohara K, Meng MV, Carroll PR. Imaging clinically localized prostate cancer. Urol Clin North Am. 2003;30:279–93.

47. Varghese SL, Grossfeld GD. The prostatic gland: malignancies other than adenocarcinomas. Radiol Clin North Am. 2000;38:179–202.

48. McNeal JE, Redwine EA, Freiha FS, Stamey TA. Zonal distribution of prostatic adenocarcinoma. Correlation with histologic pattern and direction of spread. Am J Surg Pathol. 1988;12:897–906.

49. Eskew LA, Bare RL, McCullough DL. Systematic 5 region prostate biopsy is superior to sextant method for diagnosing carcinoma of the prostate. J Urol. 1997;157:199–202. Discussion −3.

50. Terris MK, McNeal JE, Stamey TA. Detection of clinically significant prostate cancer by transrectal ultrasound-guided systematic biopsies. J Urol. 1992;148:829–32.

51. Chang JJ, Shinohara K, Bhargava V, Presti Jr JC. Prospective evaluation of lateral biopsies of the peripheral zone for prostate cancer detection. J Urol. 1998;160:2111–4.

52. Levine MA, Ittman M, Melamed J, Lepor H. Two consecutive sets of transrectal ultrasound guided sextant biopsies of the prostate for the detection of prostate cancer. J Urol. 1998;159:471–5. Discussion 5–6.

53. Babaian RJ. Extended field prostate biopsy enhances cancer detection. Urology. 2000;55:453–6.

54. Brossner C, Madersbacher S, Bayer G, Pycha A, Klingler HC, Maier U. Comparative study of two different TRUS-guided sextant biopsy techniques in detecting prostate cancer in one biopsy session. Eur Urol. 2000;37:65–71.

55. Presti Jr JC, Chang JJ, Bhargava V, Shinohara K. The optimal systematic prostate biopsy scheme should include 8 rather than 6 biopsies: results of a prospective clinical trial. J Urol. 2000;163:163–6. discussion 6–7.

56. Durkan GC, Sheikh N, Johnson P, Hildreth AJ, Greene DR. Improving prostate cancer detection with an extended-core transrectal ultrasonography-guided prostate biopsy protocol. BJU Int. 2002;89:33–9.

57. Fink KG, Hutarew G, Esterbauer B, et al. Evaluation of transition zone and lateral sextant biopsies for prostate cancer detection after initial sextant biopsy. Urology. 2003;61:748–53.

58. Bazinet M, Karakiewicz PI, Aprikian AG, et al. Value of systematic transition zone biopsies in the early detection of prostate cancer. J Urol. 1996;155:605–6.

59. Epstein JI, Walsh PC, Sauvageot J, Carter HB. Use of repeat sextant and transition zone biopsies for assessing extent of prostate cancer. J Urol. 1997;158:1886–90.

60. Mazal PR, Haitel A, Windischberger C, et al. Spatial distribution of prostate cancers undetected on initial needle biopsies. Eur Urol. 2001;39:662–8.

61. Fleshner NE, Fair WR. Indications for transition zone biopsy in the detection of prostatic carcinoma. J Urol. 1997;157:556–8.

62. Chang JJ, Shinohara K, Hovey RM, Montgomery C, Presti Jr JC. Prospective evaluation of systematic sextant transition zone biopsies in large prostates for cancer detection. Urology. 1998;52:89–93.

63. Gohji K, Morisue K, Kizaki T, Fujii A. Correlation of transrectal ultrasound imaging and the results of systematic biopsy with pathological examination of radical prostatectomy specimens. Br J Urol. 1995;75:758–65.

64. Keetch DW, Catalona WJ, Smith DS. Serial prostatic biopsies in men with persistently elevated serum prostate specific antigen values. J Urol. 1994;151:1571–4.

65. Djavan B, Ravery V, Zlotta A, et al. Prospective evaluation of prostate cancer detected on biopsies 1, 2, 3 and 4: when should we stop? J Urol. 2001;166:1679–83.

66. Borboroglu PG, Comer SW, Riffenburgh RH, Amling CL. Extensive repeat transrectal ultrasound guided prostate biopsy in patients with previous benign sextant biopsies. J Urol. 2000;163:158–62.

67. Stewart CS, Leibovich BC, Weaver AL, Lieber MM. Prostate cancer diagnosis using a saturation needle biopsy technique after previous negative sextant biopsies. J Urol. 2001;166:86–91. Discussion −2.

68. Fleshner N, Klotz L. Role of "saturation biopsy" in the detection of prostate cancer among difficult diagnostic cases. Urology. 2002;60:93–7.

69. Zaytoun OM, Moussa AS, Gao T, Fareed K, Jones JS. Office based transrectal saturation biopsy improves prostate cancer detection compared to extended biopsy in the repeat biopsy population. J Urol. 2011;186:850–4.

70. Ashley RA, Inman BA, Routh JC, Mynderse LA, Gettman MT, Blute ML. Reassessing the diagnostic yield of saturation biopsy of the prostate. Eur Urol. 2008;53:976–81.

71. Halpern EJ, Ramey JR, Strup SE, Frauscher F, McCue P, Gomella LG. Detection of prostate carcinoma with contrast-enhanced sonography using intermittent harmonic imaging. Cancer. 2005;104:2373–83.

72. Catalona WJ, Partin AW, Slawin KM, et al. Use of the percentage of free prostate-specific antigen to enhance differentiation of prostate cancer from benign prostatic disease: a prospective multicenter clinical trial. JAMA. 1998;279:1542–7.

73. Djavan B, Milani S, Remzi M. Prostate biopsy: who, how and when. An update. Can J Urol. 2005;12(Suppl 1):44–8. Discussion 99–100.

74. Vis AN, Boerma MO, Ciatto S, Hoedemaeker RF, Schroder FH, van der Kwast TH. Detection of prostate cancer: a comparative study of the diagnostic efficacy of sextant transrectal versus sextant transperineal biopsy. Urology. 2000;56:617–21.

75. Pinkstaff DM, Igel TC, Petrou SP, Broderick GA, Wehle MJ, Young PR. Systematic transperineal ultrasound-guided template biopsy of the prostate: three-year experience. Urology. 2005;65:735–9.

76. Hara R, Jo Y, Fujii T, et al. Optimal approach for prostate cancer detection as initial biopsy: prospective randomized study comparing transperineal versus transrectal systematic 12-core biopsy. Urology. 2008;71:191–5.

77. Pelzer AE, Bektic J, Berger AP, et al. Are transition zone biopsies still necessary to improve prostate cancer detection? Results from the tyrol screening project. Eur Urol. 2005;48:916–21. Discussion 21.

78. Zigeuner R, Schips L, Lipsky K, et al. Detection of prostate cancer by TURP or open surgery in patients with previously negative transrectal prostate biopsies. Urology. 2003;62:883–7.

79. van Renterghem K, Van Koeveringe G, Achten R, Van Kerrebroeck P. Clinical relevance of transurethral resection of the prostate in "asymptomatic" patients with an elevated prostate-specific antigen level. Eur Urol. 2007;52:819–26.

80. van Renterghem K, Van Koeveringe G, Achten R, van Kerrebroeck P. Prospective study of the role of transurethral resection of the prostate in patients with an elevated prostate-specific antigen level, minor lower urinary tract symptoms, and proven bladder outlet obstruction. Eur Urol. 2008;54:1385–92.

81. Bratt O. The difficult case in prostate cancer diagnosis–when is a "diagnostic TURP" indicated? Eur Urol. 2006;49:769–71.

82. Bude RO, Rubin JM. Power Doppler sonography. Radiology. 1996;200:21–3.

83. Ismail M, Petersen RO, Alexander AA, Newschaffer C, Gomella LG. Color Doppler imaging in predicting the biologic behavior of prostate cancer: correlation with disease-free survival. Urology. 1997;50:906–12.

84. Kelly IM, Lees WR, Rickards D. Prostate cancer and the role of color Doppler US. Radiology. 1993;189:153–6.

85. Rifkin MD, Sudakoff GS, Alexander AA. Prostate: techniques, results, and potential applications of color Doppler US scanning. Radiology. 1993;186:509–13.

86. Newman JS, Bree RL, Rubin JM. Prostate cancer: diagnosis with color Doppler sonography with histologic correlation of each biopsy site. Radiology. 1995;195:86–90.

87. Sakarya ME, Arslan H, Unal O, Atilla MK, Aydin S. The role of power Doppler ultrasonography in the diagnosis of prostate cancer: a preliminary study. Br J Urol. 1998;82:386–8.

88. Cornud F, Hamida K, Flam T, et al. Endorectal color Doppler sonography and endorectal MR imaging features of nonpalpable prostate cancer: correlation with radical prostatectomy findings. AJR Am J Roentgenol. 2000;175:1161–8.

89. Okihara K, Kojima M, Nakanouchi T, Okada K, Miki T. Transrectal power Doppler imaging in the detection of prostate cancer. BJU Int. 2000;85:1053–7.

90. Shigeno K, Igawa M, Shiina H, Wada H, Yoneda T. The role of colour Doppler ultrasonography in detecting prostate cancer. BJU Int. 2000;86:229–33.

91. Halpern EJ, Verkh L, Forsberg F, Gomella LG, Mattrey RF, Goldberg BB. Initial experience with contrast-enhanced sonography of the prostate. AJR Am J Roentgenol. 2000;174:1575–80.

92. Ismail M, Gomella LG. Ultrasound for prostate imaging and biopsy. Curr Opin Urol. 2001;11:471–7.

93. Halpern EJ, Rosenberg M, Gomella LG. Prostate cancer: contrast-enhanced us for detection. Radiology. 2001;219:219–25.

94. Frauscher F, Klauser A, Halpern EJ, Horninger W, Bartsch G. Detection of prostate cancer with a microbubble ultrasound contrast agent. Lancet. 2001;357:1849–50.

95. Halpern EJ, Frauscher F, Rosenberg M, Gomella LG. Directed biopsy during contrast-enhanced sonography of the prostate. AJR Am J Roentgenol. 2002;178:915–9.

96. Roy C, Buy X, Lang H, Saussine C, Jacqmin D. Contrast enhanced color Doppler endorectal sonography of prostate: efficiency for detecting peripheral zone tumors and role for biopsy procedure. J Urol. 2003;170:69–72.

97. Heijmink SW, Barentsz JO. Contrast-enhanced versus systematic transrectal ultrasound-guided prostate cancer detection: an overview of techniques and a systematic review. Eur J Radiol. 2007;63:310–6.

98. Wink M, Frauscher F, Cosgrove D, et al. Contrast-enhanced ultrasound and prostate cancer; a multicentre European research coordination project. Eur Urol. 2008;54:982–92.

99. Linden RA, Trabulsi EJ, Forsberg F, Gittens PR, Gomella LG, Halpern EJ. Contrast enhanced ultrasound flash replenishment method for directed prostate biopsies. J Urol. 2007;178:2354–8.

100. Nelson ED, Slotoroff CB, Gomella LG, Halpern EJ. Targeted biopsy of the prostate: the impact of color Doppler imaging and elastography on prostate cancer detection and Gleason score. Urology. 2007;70:1136–40.

101. Sumura M, Shigeno K, Hyuga T, Yoneda T, Shiina H, Igawa M. Initial evaluation of prostate cancer with real-time elastography based on step-section pathologic analysis after radical prostatectomy: a preliminary study. Int J Urol. 2007;14:811–6.

102. Pallwein L, Aigner F, Faschingbauer R, et al. Prostate cancer diagnosis: value of real-time elastography. Abdom Imaging. 2008;33:729–35.

103. Amsellem-Ouazana D, Younes P, Conquy S, et al. Negative prostatic biopsies in patients with a high risk of prostate cancer. Is the combination of endorectal MRI and magnetic resonance spectroscopy imaging (MRSI) a useful tool? A preliminary study. Eur Urol. 2005;47:582–6.

104. Mullerad M, Hricak H, Kuroiwa K, et al. Comparison of endorectal magnetic resonance imaging, guided prostate biopsy and digital rectal examination in the preoperative anatomical localization of prostate cancer. J Urol. 2005;174:2158–63.

105. Yuen JS, Thng CH, Tan PH, et al. Endorectal magnetic resonance imaging and spectroscopy for the detection of tumor foci in men with prior negative transrectal ultrasound prostate biopsy. J Urol. 2004;171:1482–6.

106. Pinto PA, Chung PH, Rastinehad AR, et al. Magnetic resonance imaging/ultrasound fusion guided prostate biopsy improves cancer detection following transrectal ultrasound biopsy and correlates with multiparametric magnetic resonance imaging. J Urol. 2011;186:1281–5.

107. Beyersdorff D, Hamm B. MRI for troubleshooting detection of prostate cancer. Rofo. 2005;177: 788–95.

Transperineal Biopsy

15

Vassilis J. Siomos, E. David Crawford,
and Al B. Barqawi

The Progression of Prostate Biopsy

Medicine and art have always had one thing in common: the concept of reemergence. Open prostatic biopsy was first described in the early twentieth century, and the procedure has progressed to where we are today with transrectal ultrasound (TRUS) biopsy, transperineal (TP) biopsy, and transperineal 3-D mapping biopsy (TP-3DMB). These techniques are perpetually being modified and enhanced, but we are often reminded of their cyclical nature and favorability after each was described.

In the 1930s, Astraldi introduced digitally guided transrectal prostate biopsy. Parry and Fellini described transperineal biopsy with digital rectal guidance in the 1950s. This approach allowed the authors more precise needle control as their finger stabilized the prostate [1]. Infection during biopsy was of concern, and this technique

V.J. Siomos, M.D.
Division of Urology, University of Colorado
Hospital, Denver, CO, USA
e-mail: vassilis.siomos@ucdenver.edu

E.D. Crawford, M.D.
Division of Urology, School of Medicine,
University of Colorado Denver, Denver, CO, USA

A.B. Barqawi, M.D., FRCS (✉)
Department of Surgery/Urology, University of Colorado
Hospital, University of Colorado Denver School of
Medicine, 12631 East 17th Ave., MS C-319, Academic
Office One Bldg., Room L15–5602, Aurora,
CO 80045, USA
e-mail: al.barqawi@ucdenver.edu

attenuated the risk of fecal contamination versus transrectally obtained tissue samples. It was still unclear whether a digital rectal examination (DRE), open, transrectal, or transperineal biopsy, was best. Colby retrospectively reviewed the methods of diagnosis in 100 patients who underwent prostatectomy for presumed cancer. He revealed that there was no difference in prostate cancer (CaP) detection in DRE and needle biopsy and that cancer detection rate was 91% in patients who underwent open biopsy. Thus, he concluded that no patient should undergo a prostatectomy without open biopsy [2].

At this point, the best way to biopsy was not defined; however, the introduction of imaging-directed biopsy in the late 1980s revolutionized prostatic biopsy. Weaver compared DRE-guided biopsy with TRUS biopsy and described a 50% increase in CaP detection with TRUS use. Furthermore, Hodge pioneered the sextant biopsy when he revealed a 9% improved CaP detection versus focal TRUS prostate biopsy [3]. While the focus shifted to when to perform sextant TRUS biopsy based on PSA level, transperineal biopsy was left at the wayside. By the late 1990s, sextant biopsy was still used by 76% American Urologists [4].

Reemergence of Transperineal Prostate Biopsy

As the technique of TP biopsy resurfaced, there have been numerous studies published comparing it with TRUS biopsy. The complication rates between the two modalities have not been shown to be statistically different, but investigators continued to evaluate the number of biopsy cores and location of cores needed for improved diagnosis. Initially, sextant biopsy only detected up to 30% of CaP [5]. There has been much debate on the number of cores needed to best identify CaP and various groups began to revisit the efficacy of transperineal prostate biopsy. Several alternative biopsy schemes included more cores and also targeting the specific zones such as the posterolateral and anterior transition zones. These practices have been shown to almost double the accuracy.

In 2000, Vis et al. evaluated the efficacy of transperineal biopsy using radical prostatectomy specimens to redetect CaP. While this was an ex vivo study, he postulated that transperineal biopsy was at least as effective and possibly more effective in diagnosing CaP in the peripheral zone and base versus TRUS biopsy. This was attributed to the perpendicular angle of the biopsy used in transperineal biopsy [6].

Subsequently, Emiliozzi et al. reviewed the literature of TRUS sextant biopsy with PSA greater than 4.0 ng/mL and found CaP detection ranged from 25% to 46%. This prompted his prospective study using TP biopsy in 141 men with PSA values greater than 4.0 ng/mL. CaP was identified in 51% of the patients with a median Gleason grade of 7. Forty-one percent of the detected cancer was in patients with PSA values between 4 and 10 ng/mL [7]. These findings seemed to indicate that TP biopsy might be superior to TRUS biopsy.

Not satisfied with the CaP detection rates of TRUS biopsy, Emiliozzi led a prospective study comparing TRUS sextant biopsy with transperineal biopsy. The TRUS sextant biopsy that was then assumed to be the standard of care was compared with a fan transperineal approach. The fan approach involved taking three samples of each side of the prostate using the same puncture site. Both techniques were completed in 107 patients with PSA greater than 4.0 ng/mL and a median of 8.2 ng/mL. The overall CaP detection rate was 40%. Thirty-eight percent of CaP discovered occurred via TP biopsy and 32% via

Table 15.1 CaP detection rates in patients undergoing initial TP prostate biopsy (unless otherwise specified) for 4–10 ng/mL PSA

Author	Patients	Cores (mean)	Detection (%)
Emiliozzi 2001	97	12	45
Kojima 2001	541	12	40.8
Emiliozzi 2003	70	6 TP + 6 TR	30
Kawakami 2004	148	14	27
Emiliozzi 2004	72	12	49
Furuno 2004	86	18	49
Ficarra 2005	389	14	42.4
Watanabe 2005	180	14 TP + 12 TR	33.9
Yamamoto 2005	184	12	31

TRUS approach. Of the detected cancers, 95% were found with the transperineal approach and 79% transrectally ($p = 0.012$) [8]. Table 15.1 summarizes similar studies of TP biopsy with some compared to TRUS biopsy [9].

Transperineal Mapping Biopsy

Even though increasing the number of prostate biopsy cores improved accuracy of the biopsy, it was neither precise nor reproducible. Prostate biopsy is operator dependant and no fixed points in the prostate exist to identify the exact location of the cancer focus. TP-MB has been used to assess whether a patient is suitable for whole gland and for focal therapy. Barzell et al. described the use of comparing TP-MB to TRUS biopsy prior to the use of total gland cryotherapy ablation. Of the 80 patients initially deemed appropriate for focal therapy, 43 were found to be unsuitable for focal therapy. In this study, TRUS biopsy yielded a false-negative rate of 47% and negative predictive value of 49% [10]. TP-MB is not only being used to diagnose CaP but also to better classify the disease. TP-MB has been used to confirm findings from initial TR or TP biopsy, assess laterality, but also upgrade or downgrade CaP. Onik and Barzell evaluated 110 patients who had all been diagnosed with low-risk disease on TRUS biopsy. They underwent TP-MB using a 5-mm grid as described by Barqawi et al. Fifty-five percent of these patients were found to have bilateral disease following TP-3DMB. They reported 23% of patient's cancer was upgraded versus initial TRUS biopsy. Of the patients who previously underwent TRUS biopsy, 25% had sextant TRUS biopsies, while >50% had 10 cores or more. There was no statistical difference between these two groups in relation to TP-3DM biopsy regardless of the amount of cores biopsied [11]. In another study, Onik et al. evaluated 180 patients who had been diagnosed with unilateral CaP on TRUS and performed TP-3DM biopsy under similar methods described above. Sixty-one percent of the patients proved to have bilateral disease and 22.7% were upgrade to Gleason 7 or greater. Thirty-six patients had a negative TP-MB versus TRUS [12].

Transperineal Three-Dimensional Mapping Biopsy

We know that the diagnosis of prostate cancer is not binary, but how are we supposed to counsel patients on therapy if detection from biopsy is 40–50% accurate? Why can we not treat prostate cancer like the board game Battleship and identify exactly where the cancer is and use the biopsy map to target it? To address the emerging need for accurate tumor staging, grading, and location of prostate cancer foci within the prostate gland, in 2006, we pioneered a staging transperineal 3D mapping biopsy (TP-3DMB) performed as an outpatient procedure under conscious sedation in the operative suite. The inclusion criteria for this procedure are as follows: (1) patient diagnosed with what appear to be low-risk disease (Gleason score <7, PSA<10 ng/dL and positive cores in less than 50% positive cores, (2) multiple negative TRUS biopsies with persistent elevated PSA, (3) patients electing not to undergo radical treatment as the primary option at the time of initial diagnosis, and (4) patient electing to be on a watchful waiting protocol.

The procedure is performed as an outpatient procedure. Patients receive peri-procedure antibiotics, often levofloxacin, and are given 10 cc of a local anesthetic. Positioning and needle placement is depicted in Fig. 15.1. An ultrasound transducer is placed in the rectum, and a transperineal grid, similar to a brachytherapy grid, with 5-mm spacing is used for biopsy mapping. Two fixing needles are placed and a fiduciary golden marker is placed in a midpoint position between the apex and base, and the coordinates are recorded for patient for future exact organ

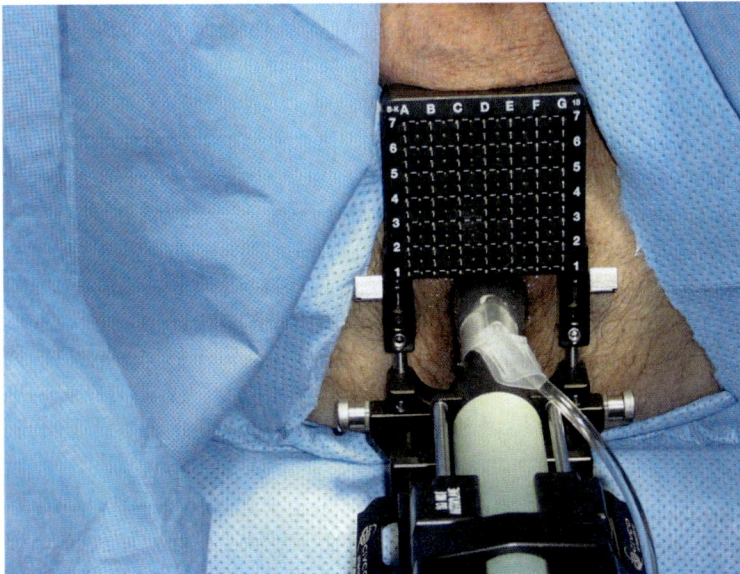

Fig. 15.1 Transperineal 3-D mapping biopsy template with rectal ultrasound probe

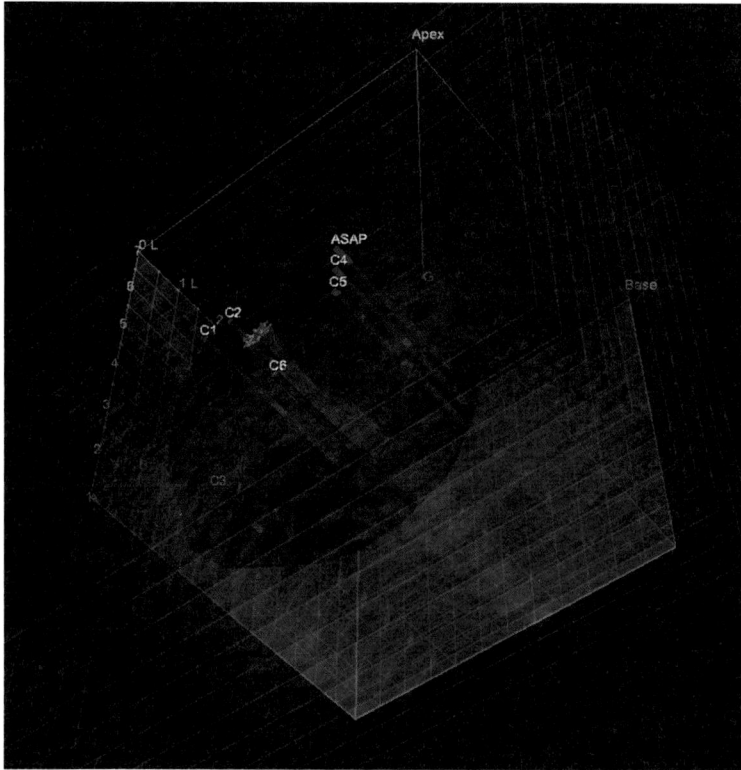

Fig. 15.2 Three-dimensional ultrasound reconstruction of the prostate gland depicting the cancer foci coordinates. The cores are *numbered in blue* with *orange portions* of core indicating the cancer present. Grouped midline *orange bars* demonstrate the prostatic urethra

realignment location. Then, serial imaging of the prostate for reconstruction of the 3D model is done (Fig. 15.2). Systematic biopsies are done in accordance to the 3D imaging using the grid starting from right to left and apex to base. Samples are labeled with the x-y-z coordinate and placed in separate jar and sent to pathology [13].

In 2005, Crawford et al. described the use of a transperineal grid coupled with computer simulation to identify the exact location of CaP cores in cadaveric and T1c radical prostatectomy specimens. The purpose was to identify all possible clinically significant cores and define their exact location. Two different template spacing grids were compared, a 5-mm template and 10-mm template. The 5-mm template for TP-3DM biopsy effectively diagnosed CaP in autopsy and prostatectomy specimens (72 vs. 51) versus method B (52 vs. 32 $p < 0.001$) [14]. TP-3DMB not only can be used for diagnosis and localizing cancer

foci but also has been studied as a modality to measure efficacy of therapy. Barqawi et al. described a cohort of 148 patients with low-grade prostate cancer who received dutasteride for at least 3 months. The patients underwent TP-3DMB and revealed a 24.2% decrease in upstaging with TP-3DM biopsy [13].

Morbidity and Feasibility

Overall, there are no significant complication differences between transrectal biopsy versus transperineal biopsy. When comparing these modalities to TP-3DMB, the only difference that has been described is with regard to urinary retention. The catheter dependency rate is higher than that found with TRUS biopsy. However, there was no long-term catheter dependency past 12 days [15]. In our experience, there have not been any cases of sepsis or severe morbidity. In fact this was significantly lower UTI/urosepsis rate than TRUS biopsies. In isolated number of cases, the sole indication for a transperineal approach was a previous negative TRUS biopsy that was complicated with urosepsis.

Many of the patients in the above studies had more than 50 cores sampled. Evaluating all of the cores adds significant cost burden to the patient; however, it may be less so if a more accurate interpretation of the grade of the cancer is achieved. The cost of TP-3DMB depends on individual physician fees, anesthesia, and histologic interpretation. In light of these costs, the overall difference in cost between the mapping biopsy and the TRUS biopsy can be greatly offset by the number of procedures that can be saved from pretreatment accurate staging and grading.

Histologic Interpretation

Crawford et al. recently described results that TP-3DMB specimens improved correlation with whole-mounted prostatectomy specimens versus TRUS biopsy specimens. Thirty-two men with CaP proven on TRUS biopsy underwent TP-3DM biopsy and subsequent radical prostatectomy. In the evaluation of the whole mount prostatectomy specimen, TP-3DM biopsy had identical Gleason sums in 56% of patients versus 40% in TRUS biopsy samples. Eight percent of cancers were upgraded in TP-3DM samples versus 52% in TRUS [16]. In the same population group, Rove et al. recently proposed an improved method of determining overall Gleason score with TP-3DMB. When using the highest Gleason score from the TP-3 MB cores, 56% had identical scores with whole mount prostatectomy specimens with 8% being upgraded. When using a cumulative sum of all of the cores, 72% were identical and 12% were upgraded [17].

Counseling Patients

Pathology from the initial prostate biopsy is one of the most important factors influencing joint patient and physician decision making in the treatment of prostate cancer. As described in various studies, cancer burden may be significantly worse and the patient may be undertreated. CaP is often upgraded or upstaged following TP-3DMB and after review of the prostate specimen following prostatectomy. For example, a retrospective review of the National Database of the Department of Defense Center for Prostate Disease Research evaluated men diagnosed with low-grade prostate cancer (Gleason 6 or 7) who had a radical prostatectomy to treat their disease. There were 2,249 men in this group. Of these patients, the prostate cancer in 619 (27.5%) was upgraded from Gleason 6 to Gleason 7. To evaluate the importance of the upgrading, the authors evaluated the odds of biochemical recurrence. They found that patients who were upgraded to Gleason 7 behaved similarly to patients who had concordant Gleason 7 [18].

In light of these findings, Barqawi et al. evaluated the role of TP-3DM biopsy in decision making for early stage prostate cancer. The study group performed TP-3DM biopsy on 180 patients, over a 3-year period, who had been diagnosed with early stage prostate cancer and undergone an ultrasound-guided 10- and 12-core biopsies. Thirty-five of these men had a history of negative TRUS biopsies. Of these men, 40 were upstaged and upgraded with TP-3DM biopsy. Only two men were downgraded and downstaged. Of the 35 patients who had previously had negative TRUS biopsies, 24 of them had positive TP-3DMB (Fig. 15.3). Of the patients, 38 underwent radical prostatectomy, 45 whole gland cryotherapy, 60 elected to be enrolled in a targeted focal therapy clinical study, 11 chose radiation, and 44 elected for active surveillance [19].

At this point, there are no definitive indications for TP-3DMB. Patients are often interested in a second opinion or have had several negative TRUS biopsies. Other patients are anxious and would like another assessment of their cancer burden. With the emergence of TFT, patients are undergoing 3D-TP-MB prior to the procedure to identify and reproducibly locate the cancer foci. The "ideal" candidates for TFT remains controversial, but overall patients are classified in the low-risk and low-grade profile group (See Table 15.2).

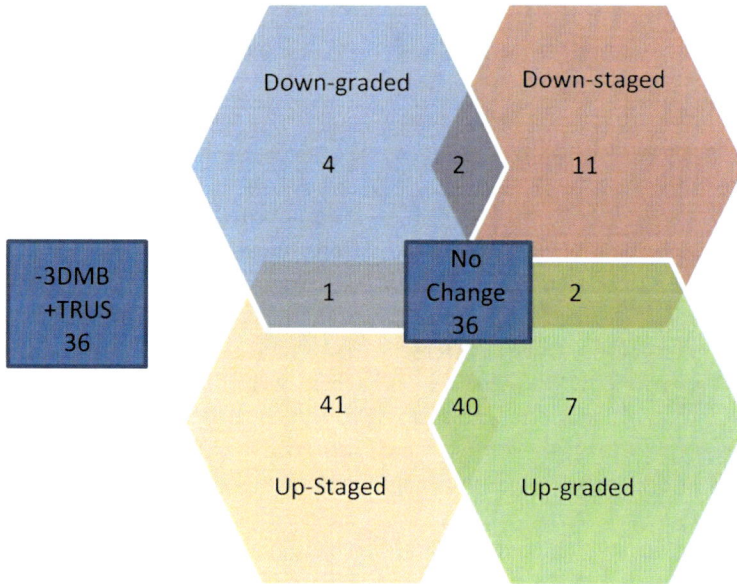

Fig. 15.3 Changes in stage and grade following TP-3DMB after initial TRUS biopsy

Table 15.2 Potential candidates for targeted focal therapy (TFT)

1. Patient undergo a TP-3DMB
2. Patient is counseled regarding all options for the management of his disease and the actual risk of under- or overtreatment
3. Clinical stage: T1N0M0 or T2aN0M0
4. PSA < 10 ng/mL or PSAD < 0.15 ng/mL/g, unless negative imaging studies
5. Gleason score (3 + 4) or less, no more than three adjacent regions for cancer foci
6. Less than 30% of cores positive

In an undertreatment due to an inaccurate prostate biopsy, Gleason score is one of the consequences one must consider when looking at the upgrading statistics. Inaccurately assessing disease at the beginning gives patients a false sense of cancer burden and may prove dangerous especially if patients opt for active surveillance.

Future Direction

The Scandinavian Prostate Cancer Group Study Number 4 investigators recently published their results on the outcomes between patients randomized to radical prostatectomy or watchful waiting. There was a 6.1% absolute risk reduction with prostatectomy in prostate cancer deaths in all patients and 9.4% in patients less than age 65 ($p = 0.01$ and $p = 0.008$). Of note, patients with low-risk cancer (PSA < 10 ng/dL and Gleason <7) did not see a significant risk reduction in death due to prostate cancer, even when categorized with patients less than 65 ($p = 0.14$) [20]. In May 2011, at the American Urological Association, the results from the Prostate Cancer Intervention versus Observation Study (PIVOT) were presented which also compared radical prostatectomy to watchful waiting. The absolute risk reduction in all cause mortality was 2.9% and reduction in mortality due to prostate cancer was 2.7% ($p = 0.22$ and 0.09). Only patients in the high-risk category (PSA > 10 ng/dL) revealed a significant absolute risk reduction of 7.2%, a benefit in prostatectomy ($p = 0.03$) [21].

These studies provide more information about low-grade prostate cancer and the potential for watchful waiting. TP-3DM is an exciting modality that may provide the best overall diagnostic spectrum available and may play a more active role in earlier prostate biopsy, especially in patients with low-grade disease. The ability to localize disease may also provide a therapeutic map available for targeted focal therapy. However, we do not believe that TP-3DMB ultimately should become the gold standard for staging prostate cancer, but will provide more information and potentially aid the emergence of TFT. Promising imaging techniques include using dual transrectal US/MRI 4-D imaging and targeted molecular imaging are on the horizon. Future advancements in imaging modalities will hold the key to improve our decision making in prostate cancer management and minimize under and over treatment.

Editorial Commentary:

It has now become clear that the prostate can be adequately biopsied via either transrectal or transperineal approach. The latter offers access without the risk of coliform bacteria whose emerging resistance is becoming a major public health concern. This can be performed under local anesthetic if using the "fan technique" popularized in Italy, and results have been shown in several publications to be equivalent to transrectal.

Nevertheless, the transperineal approach is uncommon in North America and is more often performed under general anesthesia. Doing so incurs the most significant complication, urinary retention in approximately 10% of cases. The trade-off with apparently lower risk of infectious complications is appealing, but has not become commonplace except in a few centers performing template mapping biopsy. This is explored in a later chapter as well.

References

1. Parry WL, Finelli JF. Biopsy of the prostate. J Urol. 1960;84:643–8.
2. Silletti JP, Gordon GJ, Bueno R, et al. Prostate biopsy: past, present, and future. Urology. 2007;69:413–6.
3. Hodge KK, McNeal JE, Terris MK, et al. Random systematic versus directed ultrasound guided transrectal core biopsies of the prostate. J Urol. 1989;142:71–4.
4. Orozco R, O'Dowd G, Kunnel B, et al. Observations on pathology trends in 62,537 prostate biopsies obtained from urology private practices in the United States. Urology. 1998;51:186.
5. Miller J, Perumalla C, Heap G. Complications of transrectal versus transperineal prostate biopsy. ANZ J Surg. 2005;75:48.
6. Vis AN, Boerma MO, Ciatto S, et al. Detection of prostate cancer: a comparative study of the diagnostic efficacy of sextant transrectal versus sextant transperineal biopsy. Urology. 2000;56:617–21.
7. Emiliozzi P, Longhi S, Scarpone P, et al. The value of a single biopsy with 12 transperineal cores for detecting prostate cancer in patients with elevated prostate specific antigen. J Urol. 2001;166: 845–50.
8. Emiliozzi P, Corsetti A, Tassi B, et al. Best approach for prostate cancer detection: a prospective study on transperineal versus transrectal six-core prostate biopsy. Urology. 2003;61:961–6.
9. Galfano A, Novara G, Iafrate M, et al. Prostate biopsy: the transperineal approach. EAU-EBU Update Ser. 2007;5(6):241–9.
10. Barzell WE, Melamed M. Appropriate patient selection in the focal treatment of prostate cancer: the role of transperineal 3-dimensional pathologic mapping of the prostate – a 4-year experience. Urology. 2007; 70(6 Suppl):27–35.
11. Onik G, Barzell W. Transperineal 3D mapping biopsy of the prostate: an essential tool in selecting patients for focal prostate cancer therapy. Urol Oncol. 2008; 26(5):506–10.
12. Onik G, Miessau M, Bostwick DG. Three-dimensional prostate mapping biopsy has a potentially significant impact on prostate cancer management. J Clin Oncol. 2009;27:4321–6.
13. Barqawi AB, O'Donnell CI, Siomos VJ, et al. The effect of short-term dutasteride intake in early stage prostate cancer: analysis of 148 patients who underwent three-dimensional prostate mapping biopsy. Urology. 2010;76:1067.
14. Crawford ED, Wilson SS, Torkko KC, et al. Clinical staging of prostate cancer: a computer-simulated study of transperineal prostate biopsy. BJU Int. 2005;96:999.
15. Merrick GS, Taubenslag W, Andreini H, Brammer S, Butler WM, et al. The morbidity of transperineal template-guided prostate mapping biopsy. BJU Int. 2008;101:1524–9.
16. Crawford ED, Rove KO, Maroni PD, et al. Transperineal mapping biopsies provide improved histopathological correlation with whole-mounted prostatectomy specimens. Podium presentation. Chicago: American Urologic Association; 2011.
17. Rove KO, Marioni PD, Crawford ED, et al. Improved method of determining overall Gleason score when using transperineal mapping biopsy. Abstract. Accepted South Central Section of the AUA, San Antonio; 2011.
18. Serkin FB, Soderdahl DW, Cullen J, et al. Patient risk stratification using Gleason score concordance and upgrading among men with prostate biopsy Gleason score 6 or 7. Urol Oncol. 2010;28(3):302–7.

19. Barqawi AB, Rove KO, Gholizadeh S, et al. The role of 3-dimensional mapping biopsy in decision making for treatment of apparent early stage prostate cancer. J Urol. 2011;186(1):80–5.

20. Bill-Axelson A, Holmberg L, Ruutu M, et al. Radical prostatectomy versus watchful waiting in early prostate cancer. N Engl J Med. 2005;352:1977–84.

21. Wilt T. The VA/NCI/AHRQ CSP #407: Prostate Cancer Intervention Versus Observation Trial (PIVOT): main results from a randomized trial comparing radical prostatectomy to watchful waiting in men with clinically localized prostate cancer. Plenary session podium presentation. Chicago: American Urologic Association; 2011.

Pathological Implications of Prostate Biopsy

16

David G. Bostwick

The prostate biopsy report provides a wealth of diagnostic and prognostic information for the urologist and patient. Each element of diagnosis should adhere to contemporary standards. All biopsies should report the presence and extent of inflammation, nodular hyperplasia, and important mimics of cancer that may confound diagnosis. When adenocarcinoma is present, the Gleason grade and extent should be reported for each core, as well as other clinically important findings when present, including perineural invasion, extraprostatic extension, cancer subtype if clinically important or unusual, and treatment-alteration effects. Immunohistochemical stains are an invaluable adjunct for diagnosis. In addition, numerous molecular markers that can be performed on biopsy tissue samples are entering clinical practice to provide clinically important prognostic information. Biopsy quality control is addressed in this chapter, including amount of tissue obtained per core and measures of patient identification. This chapter describes the importance of pathologic findings in biopsies, with emphasis on malignancy.

Prostate Biopsy Tissue Sampling

Introduction of the automatic spring-driven narrow-gauge core biopsy gun in the late 1980s began a new era in sampling of the prostate for histological diagnosis. The cores are now intact, with less fragmentation and no compression artifact, unlike previous biopsies (Fig. 16.1).

There is variation between laboratories in the number of serial sections obtained from prostate tissue blocks for routine examination [1, 2]; we routinely obtain 6 sections on each of two slides, yielding a total of 12 sections. The first three sections and last three sections are placed on one slide and submitted for routine hematoxylin and eosin staining; the intervening six sections are placed on another slide and saved for additional stains or special studies such as immunohistochemistry (see below) or digital image analysis for DNA ploidy analysis. In our experience, recutting the block for additional levels is useful in about half of cases, with usually no more than four additional slides before the tissue specimen is exhausted. Based on sampling trajectory techniques, most biopsy specimens consist only of tissue from the peripheral zone, seldom including the central or transition zones.

Table 16.1 describes the known variables that influence the diagnostic yield of prostate biopsies.

D.G. Bostwick, M.D., MBA (✉)
Bostwick Laboratories, 4355 Innslake Drive,
Glen Allen, VA 23060, USA
e-mail: bostwick@bostwicklaboratories.com

J.S. Jones (ed.), *Prostate Cancer Diagnosis: PSA, Biopsy and Beyond*, Current Clinical Urology,
DOI 10.1007/978-1-62703-188-2_16, © Springer Science+Business Media New York 2013

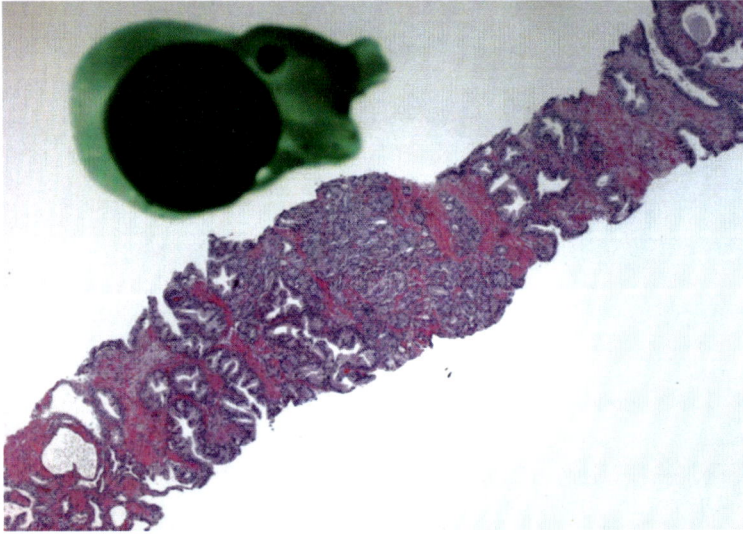

Fig. 16.1 Prostate needle biopsy. Centrally, there is a large adenocarcinoma. The large *green* mark above was placed by dotting pen on the slide to identify the site of the cancer for quality control

Table 16.1 Factors that influence the detection rate of cancer in contemporary prostate needle biopsies

Patient factors
- Patient population (e.g., screening population vs. urologic practice)
- Patient symptoms
- Serum PSA
- Clinical stage
- Patient age
- Patient race
- Prior biopsy findings (e.g., PIN, ASAP)
- Prostate volume
- TRUS and other imaging findings

Physician-controlled factors
- Number of needle cores obtained
- Method of biopsy (e.g., random, ultrasound guided)
- Location of biopsy (e.g., laterally directed biopsies vs. midline)
- Amount of tissue obtained (e.g., biopsy "gun" employed; operator skill)
- Histotechnologist's skill in processing and cutting prostate biopsies
- Number of needle cores embedded per cassette
- Number of tissue cuts obtained per specimen
- Pathologist's skill in prostate biopsy interpretation

Normal Histology

The epithelium of the prostate is composed of three principal cell types: secretory cells, basal cells, and neuroendocrine cells. A fourth cell type that usually requires immunohistochemistry to identify (the transition cell) displays features of both secretory and basal cells and is considered to be in the process of trans-differentiation.

The secretory luminal cells are cuboidal to columnar, with pale to clear cytoplasm, and produce PSA, PAP, PSMA, acidic mucin, and other secretory products.

The basal cells possess the highest proliferative activity of the prostatic epithelium, albeit low, and are thought to contain a subset of stem cells that repopulate the secretory cell layer. Basal cells retain the ability to undergo metaplasia, including squamous differentiation in the setting of infarction and myoepithelial differentiation in sclerosing adenosis. Antibodies against high molecular weight cytokeratin (34βE12) and p63 are frequently used basal cell markers, a property that is exploited immunohistochemically to aid in separating benign acinar processes such as atrophy (that retains a basal cell layer) from adenocarcinoma (that lacks a basal cell layer) (see below) [3].

The neuroendocrine cells are the least common cell type of the prostatic epithelium and are usually not identified in routine hematoxylin and eosin-stained sections except for rare cells with large eosinophilic granules [4, 5]. Although their function is unknown, neuroendocrine cells probably have an endocrine-paracrine regulatory role in growth and development, similar to neuroendocrine cells in other organs, and contain multiple neuropeptides that can modulate cell growth and proliferation [6, 7]. Serotonin and chromogranin are the best immunohistochemical markers of neuroendocrine cells in formalin-fixed sections of the prostate. Neurosecretory cells are considered to be terminally differentiated, with little or no proliferative capability in the normal epithelium.

The seminal vesicle mucosa displays complex papillary folds and irregular convoluted lumens, and the lining cells are predominately secretory, with microvesicular lipid droplets and characteristic lipofuscin pigment granules. The pigment is granular (1–2 μm diameter), abundant, golden brown, and refractile, increasing in amount with age; conversely, lipochrome pigment granules in prostatic epithelium are coarse to fine, generally smaller (0.25–4 μm), scant or variable in amount, and poorly refractile or nonrefractile [8]. These cells express androgen receptors like the prostatic epithelium, but not prostate-specific antigen (PSA) or prostatic acid phosphatase (PAP) [8]. The seminal vesicles begin to shrink in the seventh decade. The tall columnar cells lining the mucosa in young men are slowly replaced by flattened cuboidal cells. With advancing age, the stroma of the seminal vesicles becomes hyalinized and fibrotic. The flattening of the epithelium is accompanied by striking nuclear abnormalities, and highly atypical cells are present in about 75% of seminal vesicles in older men. When encountered in needle biopsies, such "pseudomalignant"

cytological atypia may lead to a mistaken diagnosis of prostatic carcinoma. DNA content analysis reveals aneuploidy in 6.7% of seminal vesicles [9].

Cowper's glands are small, paired bulbomembranous urethral glands that may be mistaken for prostatic carcinoma in biopsy specimens. These glands are composed of lobules of closely packed uniform acini lined by cytologically benign cells with abundant apical mucinous cytoplasm. Nuclei are inconspicuous. There is no PAP or PSA immunoreactivity [10], although one study reported weak clumped PSA immunoreactivity [11]. Carcinoma of Cowper's glands is very rare and is characterized by frank anaplasia of tumor cells [12].

Inflammation

The immune response in the prostate is primarily cell mediated. Lymphocytes are more numerous in the stroma, and T cells represent over 90% of the total number of prostatic lymphocytes present in both stromal and intraepithelial compartments (Fig. 16.2). Stromal T cells are mainly helper/inducer, whereas intraepithelial T cells are mainly cytotoxic/suppressor cells (inverted CD4/CD8 ratio). The inverted CD4/CD8 ratio in the intraepithelial compartment indicates that cytotoxic/suppressor T cells may represent the first line of defense against luminal foreign agents reaching the prostate through the urethra by retrograde flow. There is no significant difference in the number of lymphocytes (either T or B cells, stromal, or intraepithelial) according to patient age, race, or anatomic zone (peripheral, central, or transition zones) [13]. These findings indicate that the regulation of lymphocyte function and distribution is tightly controlled and that there is a relatively constant level of immunosurveillance in the prostate from birth to at least the seventh decade of life. Increased CD4+ T-lymphocyte infiltration within the tumor was stage independent and associated with poor outcome in patients with prostate cancer [14, 15].

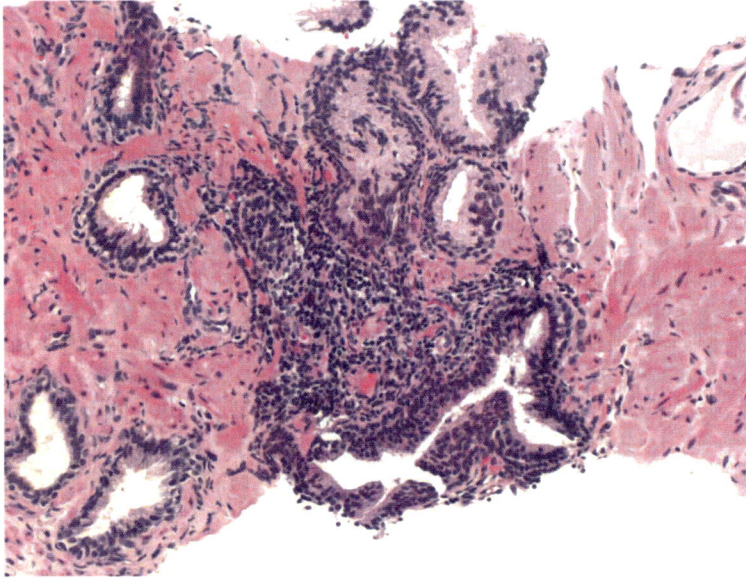

Fig. 16.2 Mild patchy chronic inflammation within the stroma and impinging on the epithelium. These cells are predominantly T cells

Minimal to mild chronic inflammation of the epithelium should probably be considered a normal finding, owing to its universality, similar to the epithelium of the gastrointestinal tract [16]. No difference exists in the extent of inflammation between African-American and white men [17]. When inflammation is acute, severe, extensive, or clinically apparent, the term "prostatitis" is warranted, although there is a wide spectrum of prostatitides, many of which are rare and poorly understood, often with a disconnect between symptoms and histopathologic findings [18].

Contemporary transrectal biopsy of the prostate induces a predictable inflammatory response along a very narrow track [19]. The biopsy track consists of a partially collapsed cavity, often filled with red blood cells, rimmed by mixed acute and chronic inflammation, including lymphocytes, macrophages, and occasional eosinophils. There is a variable amount of hemosiderin pigment, granulation tissue, and fibrosis, usually limited to the edge of the cavity. Venous thrombosis and foreign body giant cell reaction are seen infrequently. Although tumor cells are frequently enmeshed within fibrous connective tissue, they are not seen within the cavity following 18-gauge biopsy [19]. Conversely, cancer cells are occasionally identified in the track following the wider 14-gauge biopsy in men with prostate cancer, particularly with perineal biopsy [20].

Biopsy tracks in prostatectomies obtained 4–6 weeks after biopsy show fewer red blood cells and less acute inflammation than in those obtained earlier, but no other histological differences are noted. There is no evidence of florid granulomatous prostatitis or fibrinoid necrosis that is often seen after transurethral resection.

Inflammation is a significant confounding factor in evaluating serum PSA and the risk of prostate cancer [21]. There was an inverse relationship between inflammation and prostate cancer, at least among men with serum PSA of 10–50 ng/mL [22, 23]. About 31% of patients with elevated serum PSA will have a drop with ciprofloxacin therapy, but the risk of subsequent prostate cancer appears to be independent of this PSA decline [24, 25]. Inflammation within prostate cancer can be significantly decreased with the use of statins [26].

Atrophy

Atrophy is a near-constant microscopic finding in the prostate, consisting of small distorted glands with flattened epithelium, hyperchromatic nuclei,

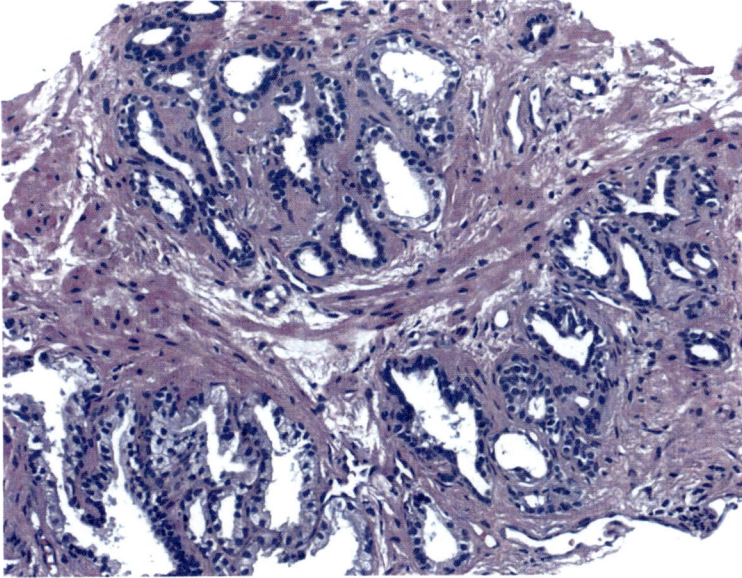

Fig. 16.3 Post-atrophic hyperplasia. The lobular clusters of small distorted acini set in a variably fibrotic stroma comprise a significant histological mimic of adenocarcinoma

and stromal fibrosis. The prevalence and extent increase with advancing age, particularly over the age of 40 years. Billis and colleagues reported that atrophy is an important predictor of serum PSA [27]. Atrophy may be confused with adenocarcinoma due to prominent acinar architectural distortion, but it lacks nuclear and nucleolar enlargement. The nucleus-to-cytoplasmic ratio may be high due to scant cytoplasm, and nuclei are hyperchromatic.

Atrophic acini with proliferative epithelial changes are referred to as post-atrophic hyperplasia (PAH) [28]. PAH is at the extreme end of the morphologic continuum of acinar atrophy that most closely mimics adenocarcinoma (Fig. 16.3). This continuum varies from mild acinar atrophy with a flattened layer of attenuated cells with scant cytoplasm to that of PAH in which the lining cells are low cuboidal with moderate cytoplasm. The morphologic similarity of PAH and carcinoma creates the potential for misdiagnosis and in our experience is the most common misdiagnosis to result in unnecessary prostatectomy [28, 29].

PAH is distinguished from carcinoma by its characteristic lobular architecture, intact or fragmented basal cell layer, inconspicuous or mildly enlarged nucleoli, and adjacent acinar atrophy with stromal fibrosis or smooth muscle atrophy. Nucleolar changes are also useful in separating PAH and carcinoma; mildly enlarged nucleoli may be present in PAH, but only focally, and the majority of cells have micronucleoli.

Proliferative regenerative changes in association with atrophy, referred to as proliferative inflammatory atrophy (PIA), have been postulated to be precancerous. The hypothesis is that cellular injury and regeneration is induced by inflammation and release of reactive oxygen species (oxidative stress) resulting from insult owing to chemicals (e.g., dietary carcinogens), physical factors (e.g., arteriosclerosis-induced ischemia), or bacteria. The regenerating cells are at increased risk of mutation which, in turn, predisposes them to cancerous initiation, promotion, and progression. The clinical implication of this hypothesis is that anti-inflammatory drugs such as statins could potentially block pro-carcinogenic inflammatory processes [30]. Evidence to date is inconclusive as to whether PIA is a precursor of PIN, direct precursor of cancer that bypasses PIN, or simply an epiphenomenon not linked to cancer. In the original description, proliferative inflammatory atrophy included all histopathologic varieties of atrophy, including post-atrophic hyperplasia (PAH) and simple atrophy [31]. However, some studies have included only post-atrophic hyperplasia within the spectrum of PIA. At present, PIA is best considered to be a working hypothesis rather than a specific histopathologic entity, as atrophy may occur with or without inflammation and/or proliferation [32, 33]. What is clear is that any association with cancer requires proliferative changes, and these changes in the setting of atrophy are most often associated with inflammation. Inflammation is often linked with infectious and noninfectious prostatitis, and emerging data indicates a causative role for inflammation in prostate cancer development over time [34, 35]. A recent review concluded that PIA was likely not a precursor of cancer [36], but a rebuttal by others took the opposite stance [37]. Despite the controversy regarding the role of atrophy (or lack thereof), virtually all authors agree that inflammation-induced oxidative stress is the most plausible explanation for initiation of prostatic carcinogenesis.

Metaplasia

Metaplasia may result from a variety of insults to the prostate, including acute inflammation, infarction, radiation therapy, and androgen deprivation therapy. The most common form is squamous metaplasia. The changes may be focal or diffuse, appearing as intraacinar syncytial aggregates of flattened cells with abundant eosinophilic cytoplasm or cohesive aggregates of glycogen-rich clear cells with shrunken hyperchromatic nuclei. Keratinization is unusual except at the edge of infarcts or areas of acute inflammation. Squamous metaplasia commonly involves the prostatic urethra in patients with indwelling catheter.

Nephrogenic metaplasia is an important and unique variant of metaplasia that most often occurs in adult patients in the urinary bladder, renal pelvis, ureter, and urethra; prostatic urethral involvement is rare, and extension into the prostatic parenchyma may create diagnostic confusion with adenocarcinoma. It usually follows instrumentation, urethral catheterization, infection,

or calculi. Patients present with lower urinary tract symptoms, including hematuria, dysuria, obstruction, and urethral mass [38, 39]. Nephrogenic metaplasia appears as an exophytic papillary mass of cystic and solid tubules protruding from the urethral mucosa. The tubules may extend into the underlying prostate as a proliferation of small round to oval tubules, sometimes filled with colloid-like material. The lining consists of flattened or simple cuboidal cells, often with a distinctive hobnail appearance (Fig. 16.4). Nuclei display finely granular uniform chromatin with inconspicuous nucleoli; occasional prominent nucleoli are observed. There is frequently chronic inflammation and edema of the stroma, but no desmoplasia is present. The tubules contain scant or moderate mucin that is positive with alcian blue and PAS stains. The basement membrane is accentuated with PAS stain. Epithelial membrane antigen is positive in the tubular epithelial cells, and high molecular weight keratin 34ßE12 stains many of the basal cells. PSA, PAP, and CEA are negative [39].

There is no direct evidence that links atypical nephrogenic metaplasia to cancer [40]. Some investigators suggested that nephrogenic metaplasia is neither metaplastic nor neoplastic in nature. Nephrogenic metaplasia in renal-transplant recipients is apparently derived from tubular cells of the renal transplants and is not a metaplastic proliferation of the recipient's bladder urothelium [41].

Hyperplasia

Enlargement of the prostate, also known as nodular hyperplasia or benign prostatic hyperplasia (BPH), consists of overgrowth of the epithelium and/or fibromuscular tissue of the transition zone and periurethral area (Table 16.2; Fig. 16.5). Symptoms are caused by interference with muscular sphincteric function and by obstruction of urine flow through the prostatic urethra. Development of nodular hyperplasia includes three pathologic changes: nodule formation, diffuse enlargement of the transition zone and periurethral tissue, and enlargement of nodules.

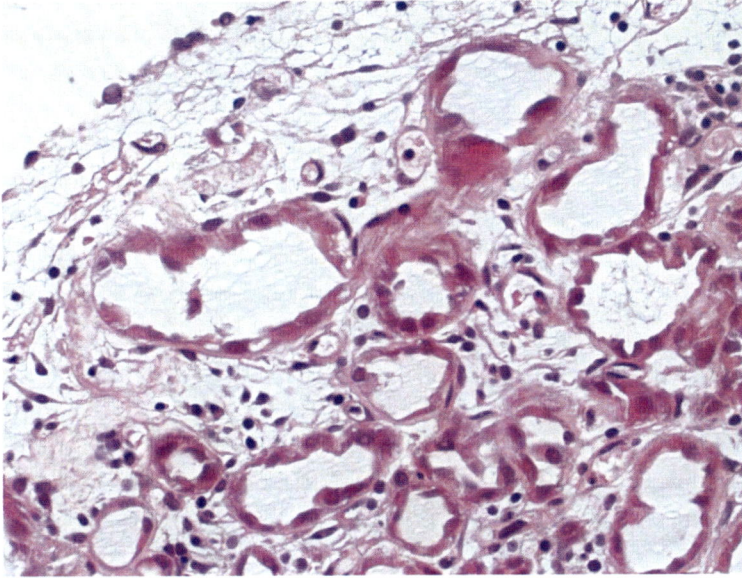

Fig. 16.4 Nephrogenic metaplasia. The irregular subepithelial clusters of tubules are lines by hobnail cells with distinctive eosinophilic cytoplasm

Table 16.2   Histopathologic variants of nodular hyperplasia

Variant	Microscopic features	Usual location
Stromal hyperplasia with atypical giant cells	Stromal nodules in the setting of cellularity and nuclear atypia	Transition zone
Basal cell hyperplasia	Proliferation of basal cells, two or more cells in thickness; may have prominent nucleoli (atypical basal cell hyperplasia) or form a nodule (basal cell adenoma)	Transition zone
Atypical adenomatous hyperplasia	Localized proliferation of small acini in association with BPH nodule which architecturally mimics adenocarcinoma but lacks cytological features of malignancy	Transition zone
Post-atrophic hyperplasia	Atrophic acini with epithelial proliferative changes; easily mistaken for adenocarcinoma due to architectural distortion	All zones
Cribriform hyperplasia	Acini with distinctive cribriform pattern, often with clear cytoplasm; easily mistaken for proliferative acini of the central zone	Transition zone
Sclerosing adenosis	Circumscribed proliferation of small acini in a dense spindle cell stroma without significant atypia; usually solitary and microscopic	Transition zone
Hyperplasia of mesonephric remnants	Rare benign lobular proliferation of colloid-like material in the lumina; may mimic nephrogenic metaplasia focally; acini do not apparently express PSA or PAP	All zones (very rare)
Verumontanum mucosal gland hyperplasia	Small benign acinar proliferation	Verumontanum

In men under 70 years of age, diffuse enlargement predominates; in older men, epithelial proliferation and expansile growth of existing nodules predominates, probably as the result of androgenic and other hormonal stimulation. The proportion of epithelium to stroma increases as symptoms become more severe [42].

Grossly, nodular hyperplasia consists of variably sized nodules that are soft or firm, rubbery, and yellow gray and bulge from the cut surface upon transection. If there is prominent epithelial hyperplasia in addition to stromal hyperplasia, the abundant luminal spaces create soft and grossly spongy nodules that ooze a pale-white

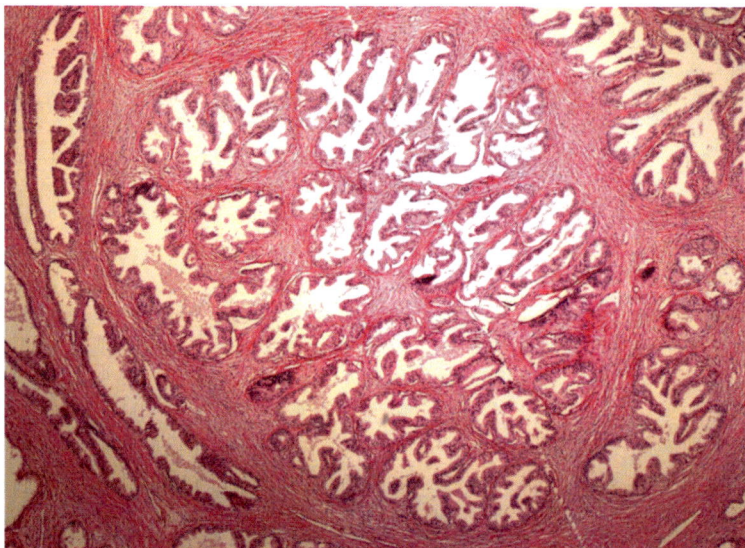

Fig. 16.5 BPH nodule. This circumscribed nodule is predominantly composed of epithelium, the most common form of hyperplasia

watery fluid. If the nodular hyperplasia is predominantly fibromuscular, there may be diffuse enlargement or numerous trabeculations without prominent nodularity. Degenerative changes include calcification and infarction. Nodular hyperplasia usually involves the transition zone, but occasionally nodules arise from the periurethral tissue at the bladder neck. Protrusion of bladder neck nodules into the bladder lumen are referred to as median lobe hyperplasia.

Microscopically, nodular hyperplasia is composed of varying proportions of epithelium and stroma (fibrous connective tissue and smooth muscle). The most common are adenomyofibromatous nodules that contain all elements. The diagnosis of nodular hyperplasia is often used in needle biopsy specimens when only normal benign peripheral zone prostatic tissue is present. The transition zone is infrequently sampled by needle biopsies unless the urologist specifically targets this area or there is massive nodular hyperplasia that compresses the peripheral zone. We require the presence of at least part of a nodule for the diagnosis of nodular hyperplasia in needle biopsies, and this is unusual. Narrow 18-gauge biopsies virtually never contain the entire nodule unless it is very small and fortuitously sampled. Casual use of the term nodular hyperplasia for benign

prostatic tissue may mislead the urologist into believing that a palpable nodule or hypo-echoic focus of concern has been sampled and histologically evaluated. Vascular insufficiency probably accounts for infarction of hyperplastic nodules, seen in up to 20% of resected cases. The center of the nodule undergoes hemorrhagic necrosis, often with reactive changes in the residual epithelium at the periphery, including squamous metaplasia and urothelial metaplasia.

Nodular hyperplasia is not a precursor of cancer, but there are a number of similarities [43]. Both display a parallel increase in prevalence with patient age according to autopsy studies, although cancer lags by 15–20 years. Both require androgens for growth and development, and both may respond to androgen deprivation treatment. Most cancers arise in patients with concomitant nodular hyperplasia, and cancer is found incidentally in a significant number (10%) of transurethral prostatectomy specimens. Nodular hyperplasia may be related to prostate cancer arising in the transition zone, perhaps in association with certain forms of hyperplasia [43, 44]. The pathogenesis of nodular hyperplasia is still poorly understood; it is presumed that there is no single mechanism, but represents a synergistic effect of multiple events within biological communication systems (nervous, endocrine, immune systems) during the aging process of the prostate [45].

In addition to BPH and post-atrophic hyperplasia, other common forms of hyperplasia include basal cell hyperplasia and atypical adenomatous hyperplasia, both of which usually arise in the peripheral zone. Basal cell hyperplasia consists of numerous small to normal-sized, round basophilic acini with several layers of basal cells (glandular architectural type) or solid nests either arranged in a lobular configuration or seldom "infiltrating" the stroma. Basal cell hyperplasia frequently involves only part of an acinus, and sometimes protrudes into the lumen, retaining the overlying secretory cell layer; less commonly, there is symmetric duplication of the basal cell layer at the periphery of the acinus. No cases of typical BCH, by definition, contains either prominent nucleoli (their mean diameter is less than 1 μm) [46] or polymorphism; however, rare cases may show the presence of hyperchromatic nuclei, enlarged nuclei, and rare mitotic figures. BCH resembles prostate acini seen in the fetus, accounting for the synonyms "fetalization" and "embryonal hyperplasia." BCH may be composed of basal cell nests with areas of luminal differentiation resembling similar lesions of the salivary gland. This is denoted as the adenoid basal form of BCH.

Atypical adenomatous hyperplasia (AAH) is a localized proliferation of small acini within the prostate arising in intimate association with nodular hyperplasia [47, 48]. AAH varies in incidence from 19.6% (transurethral resection specimens) to 24% (autopsy series in 20- to 40-year-old men) [49]. Mean size of AAH is 0.03 cm^3, but mass-forming AAH measuring 21.1 cm^3 has been documented [50]. AAH is distinguished from well-differentiated carcinoma by the presence of inconspicuous nucleoli, partially intact but fragmented basal cell layer, and infrequent crystalloids. All measures of nucleolar size allow separation of AAH from adenocarcinoma, including mean nucleolar diameter, largest nucleolar diameter, and percentage of nucleoli greater than 1 μm in diameter. The majority of Gleason pattern 1 cancers are now thought to represent foci of AAH.

Uncommon or rare forms of hyperplasia include clear cell cribriform hyperplasia, sclerosing adenosis, stromal hyperplasia with or without atypical giant cells, verumontanum mucosal gland hyperplasia, and hyperplasia of mesonephric remnants. It is important to not misdiagnose one of these as adenocarcinoma.

Prostatic Intraepithelial Neoplasia (PIN) and Atypical Small Acinar Proliferation (ASAP)

In prostate needle biopsies, two histological findings – high-grade prostatic intraepithelial neoplasia (PIN) and atypical small acinar proliferation (ASAP) – are each predictive of subsequent prostatic adenocarcinoma, and the identification of either without concurrent cancer may warrant follow-up with repeat biopsy. ASAP is observed in about 2% of biopsies, whereas PIN is present in 9% of contemporary needle biopsies. These findings can occur together in the same biopsy set without concomitant cancer. We refer to the coexistence of the two lesions in the same high-power microscopic field as "PIN + ASAP." These histological findings are discussed in elsewhere in this book.

Adenocarcinoma

Microscopic Features of Prostatic Adenocarcinoma

Most prostatic adenocarcinomas are composed of acini arranged in one or more patterns. The diagnosis relies on a combination of architectural and cytological findings. The light microscopic features are often sufficient for diagnosis, but many cases benefit from immunohistochemical studies (Table 16.3).

Architecture

Architectural features are assessed at low to medium power magnification and include variation in acinar spacing, size, and shape. The arrangement of the acini is diagnostically useful

Table 16.3 Diagnostic immunohistochemical stains for prostatic adenocarcinoma

Prostate-specific epithelial markers
- Prostate-specific antigen (PSA): cytoplasm of all prostatic epithelial cells
- Prostatic acid phosphatase (PAP): cytoplasm of all prostatic epithelial cells
- Prostate-specific membrane antigen (PSMA): cytoplasm of all prostate epithelial cells

Cell-specific markers

Basal cells
- Cytoplasm: keratin 34 B-E12
- Cytoplasm: keratins 5, 6
- Nuclei: p63

PIN and cancer cells
- Cytoplasm: racemase (p504S)
- Nuclei: c-Myc
- Nuclei: ERG

for "prominent" nucleoli that are at least 1.25–1.50 μm in diameter or larger; however, we do not routinely measure nucleoli for diagnosis, so this determination is based on comparison with benign epithelial cells elsewhere in the specimen [51]. The identification of two or more nucleoli is virtually diagnostic of malignancy [52], particularly when the nucleoli are eccentrically located in the nucleus; we find this criterion useful, but employ it sparingly. Artifacts often obscure the nuclei and nucleoli, and overstaining of nuclei by hematoxylin creates one of the most common and difficult problems encountered in interpretation of suspicious foci. Differences in fixation and handling of biopsy specimens influence nuclear size and chromasia, so comparison with cells from the same specimen is important and serves as an internal control.

and is the basis of Gleason grade. Malignant acini usually have an irregular haphazard arrangement, randomly scattered in the stroma in clusters or single acini, usually with variation in spacing except in the lowest Gleason grades. The acini in suspicious foci are usually small or medium sized, with irregular contours that stand in contrast with the smooth round to elongated contours of benign and hyperplastic acini. Comparison with the adjacent benign prostatic acini is always of value [51]. Variation in acinar size is a particularly useful criterion, particularly when there are small irregular abortive acini with primitive lumens at the periphery of a focus of well-differentiated carcinoma.

Stroma

The stroma in cancer frequently contains young collagen that appears lightly eosinophilic, although desmoplasia may be prominent. There is sometimes splitting or distortion of muscle fibers in the stroma, but this is an inconstant and unreliable feature by itself.

Cytology

The cytological features of adenocarcinoma include nuclear and nucleolar enlargement, and these are present in the majority of malignant cells. Every cell has a nucleolus, so one searches

Luminal Mucin

Acidic sulfated and non-sulfated mucin is often seen in acini of adenocarcinoma, appearing as amorphous or delicate threadlike faintly basophilic secretions in routine sections. This mucin stains with alcian blue and is best demonstrated at pH 2.5, whereas the normal prostatic epithelium contains periodic acid Schiff-reactive neutral mucin. Acidic mucin is not specific for carcinoma [53].

Crystalloids

Crystalloids are sharp needlelike eosinophilic structures that are often present in the lumens of well-differentiated and moderately differentiated carcinoma [54]. They are not specific for carcinoma. They result from abnormal protein and mineral metabolism within benign and malignant acini and are probably related to the hard eosinophilic proteinaceous secretions commonly found in the lumens of malignant acini. Ultrastructurally, crystalloids are composed of electron-dense material that lacks the periodicity of crystals, and X-ray microanalysis reveals abundant sulfur, calcium, phosphorus, and a small amount of sodium [54]. The presence of crystalloids in metastatic adenocarcinoma of unknown site of origin is strong presumptive evidence of prostatic origin, although it is an uncommon finding and is not conclusive [55, 56].

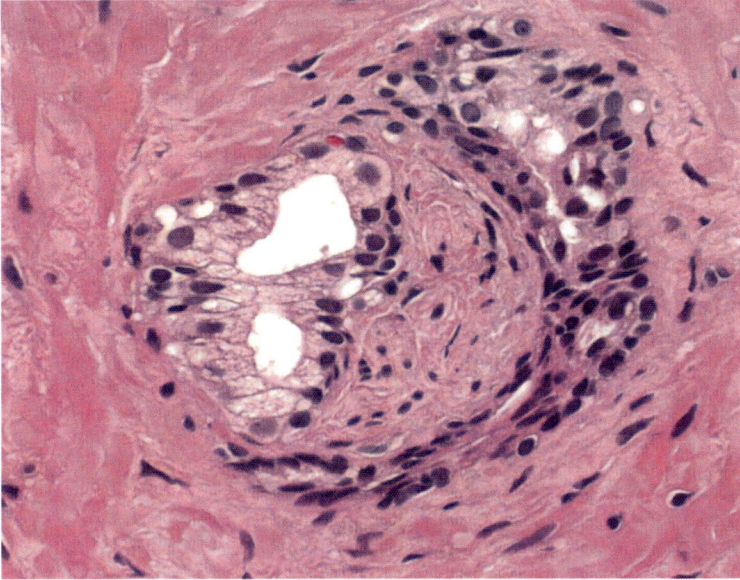

Fig. 16.6 Perineural invasion by adenocarcinoma

Collagenous Micronodules

Collagenous micronodules are a specific but infrequent and incidental finding in prostatic adenocarcinoma, consisting of microscopic nodular masses of paucicellular eosinophilic fibrillar stroma that impinge on acinar lumens [53].

Perineural Invasion

Perineural invasion is common in adenocarcinoma and may be the only evidence of malignancy in biopsy specimens. This finding is strong presumptive evidence of malignancy but may rarely occur present rarely with benign acini [53]. Complete circumferential growth and ganglionic invasion are found only with cancer (Fig. 16.6).

Vascular/Lymphatic Invasion

Microvascular invasion is a strong indicator of malignancy, and its presence correlates with histological grade, although it is sometimes difficult to distinguish from fixation-associated retraction artifact of acini [57].

Cancer Grade

Biopsy grade is one of the strongest predictors of biologic behavior in prostate cancer, including invasiveness and metastatic potential, but is not sufficiently reliable when used alone for predicting pathologic stage or patient outcome for individual patients. The Gleason score, recommended for routine use in all pre-therapy specimens, is a scalar measurement that combines discrete primary and secondary groups (patterns or grades) into a total of nine discrete groups (scores 2–10) (Fig. 16.7) [58]. The primary grade is the most common or predominant grade; the secondary grade is the next most common but should comprise at least 5% of the tumor. It is often hard to apply this rule when the amount of cancer in the specimen is small; in such cases, there may be no secondary pattern, and the primary grade is simply doubled. Score should be reported on all cases as the histological grade. Score as well as individual patterns should be reported including the most frequent pattern followed by the worst pattern. (e.g., Gleason 7 (3 + 4)). In addition to individual biopsy vial grading, global Gleason score should be given to encompass multiple biopsies containing cancer. The relative percentage or proportion of high-grade cancer (Gleason primary pattern 4 and 5) should also be included, according to the World Health Organization [58]. If a third (tertiary) pattern is present, that should also be reported. Gleason noted exact reproducibility

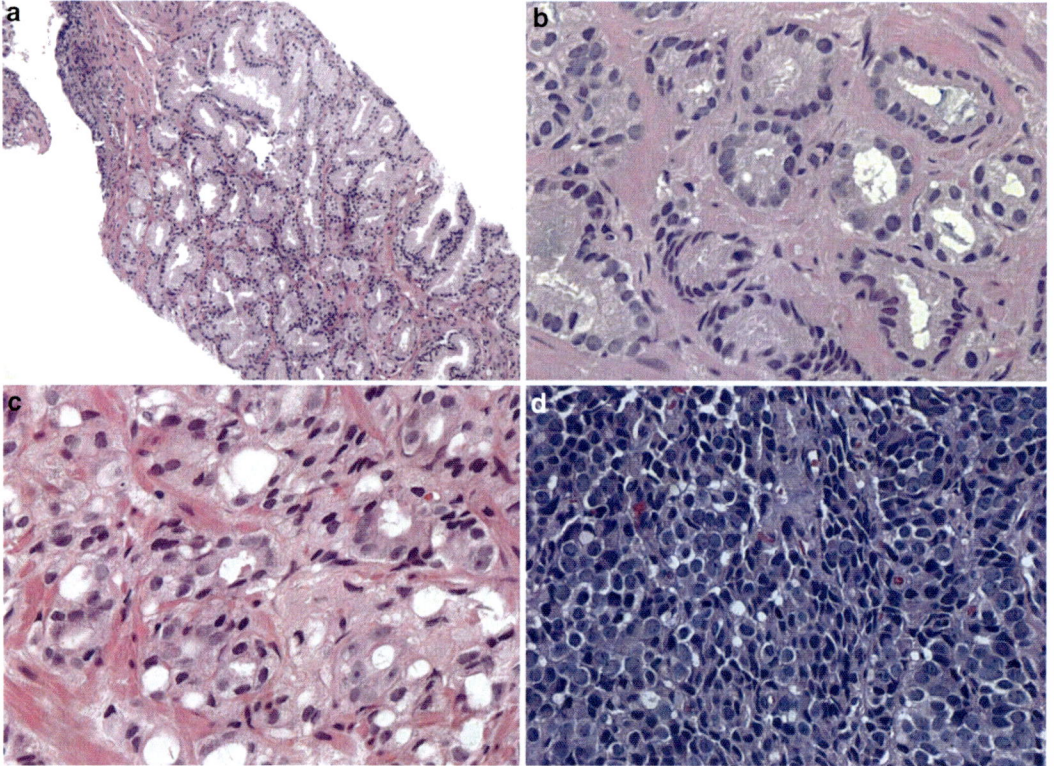

Fig. 16.7 Spectrum of Gleason scores. (**a**) 2 + 2 = 4; (**b**) 3 + 3 = 6; (**c**) 4 + 4 = 8; (**d**) 5 + 5 = 10

of score in 50% of needle biopsies and one score in 85%, similar to the findings of others [59].

Gleason pattern 1 adenocarcinoma is uncommon and difficult to diagnose and is not observed in contemporary biopsies. It consists of a circumscribed mass of simple monotonously replicated round acini that are uniform in size, shape, and spacing. Nuclear and nucleolar enlargement are moderate but allow separation from its closest mimic, atypical adenomatous hyperplasia (AAH). Crystalloids are observed in more than half of cases.

Gleason pattern 2 is very similar to pattern 1 except for the lack of circumscription of the focus, indicating the ability of the cancer to spread through the stroma. Slightly greater variation in acinar size and shape is observed, but the acinar contours are chiefly round and smoothly sculpted. Acinar packing is somewhat more variable than pattern 1, and separation is usually less than one acinar diameter. This is rarely observed in biopsies of the peripheral zone.

Gleason pattern 3 is the most common pattern of prostatic adenocarcinoma and encompasses a wide and diverse group of lesions. The hallmark of pattern 3 adenocarcinoma is prominent variation in size, shape, and spacing of acini. Despite this variation, the acini remain discrete and separate, unlike the fused acini of pattern 4 (see below). Acini are haphazardly arranged in the stroma, sometimes with prominent stromal fibrosis.

Gleason pattern 4 characteristically shows fusion of acini, with ragged infiltrating cords and nests at the edges. Unlike the simple entwined acinar tubules of pattern 3, this pattern consists of an anastomosing network or spongework of epithelium. Pattern 4 adenocarcinoma is considered poorly differentiated and is more malignant than pattern 3.

Gleason pattern 5 adenocarcinoma is characterized by fused sheets and masses of haphazardly arranged acini in the stroma, often displacing or overrunning adjacent tissues. In biopsy specimens, these cases raise the serious concern for anaplastic carcinoma or sarcoma. Cases with scattered acinar lumens indicative of glandular differentiation are included within this pattern. Comedocarcinoma is an important subtype of this pattern, consisting of luminal necrosis within an otherwise cribriform pattern. Pattern 5 also includes rare histological variants such as signet ring-cell carcinoma and small cell undifferentiated carcinoma.

Needle core biopsy underestimates tumor grade in up to 45% of cases and overestimates grade in up to 32% [60, 61]. Exact correlation is present in about one-third of biopsies and one Gleason unit in another one-third. Grading errors are common in biopsies with small amounts of tumor and low-grade tumor and are probably due to tissue sampling variation, tumor heterogeneity, and undergrading of needle biopsies. Accuracy of biopsy is highest for the primary Gleason pattern, but the secondary pattern also provides useful predictive information, particularly when combined with the primary pattern to create the Gleason score. Gleason grading should be used for all needle biopsies, even those with small amounts of tumor.

On average, there are 2.7 (range 1–5) different Gleason primary patterns (grades) in prostate cancer treated by radical prostatectomy [62]. The number of grades increases with greater cancer volume, the most common finding being high-grade cancer within the center of a larger well- or moderately differentiated cancer, occurring in some 53% of cases. Grade is an invariable component of most clinical nomograms in prostate cancer.

Reproducibility of this system is higher among urologic pathology specialists rather than general pathologists [63, 64]. Interobserver consensus among general pathologists was overall at the low end of the moderate range (Kappa=0.44). There was consistent undergrading of Gleason's score 5–6 (47%), 7 (47%) and to lesser extent (25%) among general pathologists.

Modifications to the Gleason system have been proposed by the International Society of Urologic Pathologists (ISUP) [65] to include the following: (1) Cribriform patterns are invariably Gleason pattern 4 rather than 3; (2) score is the sum of most common (primary) and highest grade (unless the primary grade is most common, rather than primary and secondary grades); and (3) the amount of high-grade cancer can be less than 1% but would still be included as secondary grade (Gleason used a 5% volume threshold for grade inclusion). If one employs this new system, it should be called the ISUP 2005 Modified Gleason Score; we report only the original (classic) Gleason score in our practice, as we believe that there are insufficient data available to warrant switching to the new system. Recent data from the dutasteride prostate cancer prevention trial revealed that the ISUP 2005 system provided no apparent advantage in predictive value when compared with the classic Gleason system [66].

Cancer Extent in Biopsies

Measurements of the extent of cancer have included the number of positive biopsies, millimeters of cancer on needle biopsy, and percentage of cancer per core. Biopsy cancer volume depends on multiple factors, including prostate volume, cancer volume, cancer distribution, number of biopsy cores obtained, the cohort of patients being evaluated, and the technical competence of the investigator. The combined results from multiple studies indicate that the biopsy extent of tumor provides some predictive value for extent in radical prostatectomy specimens and probably should be reported, although its predictive value for an individual patient is limited [67–69]. Reliance upon this measure alone may often be misleading. There is a fair [70] to good [71] correlation between amount of cancer reported in biopsies and that subsequently found in radical prostatectomy specimens. This correlation is greatest for large cancers. High cancer burden on needle biopsy is strongly suggestive of large volume high-stage cancer [67–72]. Unfortunately, low tumor burden on needle biopsy does not necessarily indicate low-volume low-stage cancer. Cupp et al. found that patients with less than 30% of needle cores replaced by cancer had a mean volume in the radical prostatectomy of 6.1 cc (range, 0.19–16.8 cc), indicating that the amount of tumor on transrectal needle biopsy was not a good predictor of tumor volume [70]. In another report, patients with less than 10% cancer in the biopsy had a 30% risk of positive surgical margins, 27% risk of extraprostatic extension, and 22% risk of PSA biochemical progression; these risks were higher in patients with more than 10% cancer [69]. Patients with less than 3-mm cancer and Gleason score 6 or less on needle biopsy had a 59% risk of cancer volume exceeding 0.5 cc [73]. Those with less than 2 mm of cancer had 26% risk of extraprostatic cancer [74], and those with less than 3 mm had 52% risk [75]. The CAP recommends that the volume of cancer in needle biopsy should be reported as the percentage of tissue involved by cancer.

Measures of cancer volume are usually [76] but not always [67, 77] predictive of cancer recurrence risk after radical prostatectomy. Accordingly, the CAP recommends that cancer volume be recorded in prostatectomy specimens, although there is no accepted universal approach [78]. Methods include computer-assisted morphometric determination [71, 76, 79], simple measurement of length X height X section thickness of the cancer (some measure the largest "index" focus, whereas others report the cumulative volumes) [80], greatest cancer dimension [1, 81], grid method [82], and visual estimate of the percentage of cancer [83, 84]. Measurements performed on fixed tissue sections may include a formalin shrinkage correction factor which varies from about 1.25 to 1.5, representing tissue shrinkage of 18–33%; conversely, Schned and colleagues demonstrated that shrinkage correction is unnecessary [85]. Cancer volume is a critical element in definitions of clinically significant and insignificant prostate cancer [80, 82]. Up to 70% of men undergoing radical prostatectomy are found to have multifocal cancer, a finding that is a major theoretical objection to focal ablation. However, about 80% of incidental tumors are less than 0.5 cc, indicating that a significant percentage of multifocal tumors, other than the largest or index cancer identified preoperatively, may not be of clinical significance. Until now, however, little attention has been paid in trying to differentiate patients with unifocal and multifocal disease since it had little clinical significance; all treatments have been aimed at total gland ablation until recently. Recently, Cheng et al. reported that small-volume prostate cancers (0.5 cc or less) are often multifocal and bilateral, with predilection for the peripheral zone. Of these small-volume prostate cases, 16% (10/62) had Gleason pattern 4 and might, therefore, be clinically significant [86].

Diagnostic Immunohistochemical Studies

Immunohistochemical studies are often used as an adjunct for the diagnosis of prostate cancer. The most important ones include PSA, PAP, basal cell-specific keratin, p63, racemase, and c-Myc. ERG has recently been described as a possible replacement for racemase and c-Myc as a marker for prostate cancer, but it is only positive in about half of cancers, so this is less likely to emerge as a purely diagnostic test.

Prostate-Specific Antigen (PSA)

Immunohistochemical staining for PSA is useful in identifying poorly differentiated prostate cancer in close proximity to the bladder and the rectum; it can also verify prostatic origin of metastatic carcinoma. The intensity of PSA immunoreactivity often varies from field to field within a tumor, and the correlation of staining intensity with tumor differentiation is inconsistent. PSA expression is generally greater in low-grade tumors than in high-grade tumors, but there is significant heterogeneity from cell to cell. Up to 1.6% of poorly differentiated cancers will be negative for both PSA and PAP. The presence of PSA-immunoreactive tumor cells in poorly differentiated carcinoma suggests that these tumors retain subpopulations of cells with properties of normal secretory prostatic epithelial cells. Extraprostatic expression of PSA has been reported in a number of tissues and tumors, including periurethral gland adenocarcinoma in women, rectal carcinoid, and extramammary Paget's disease.

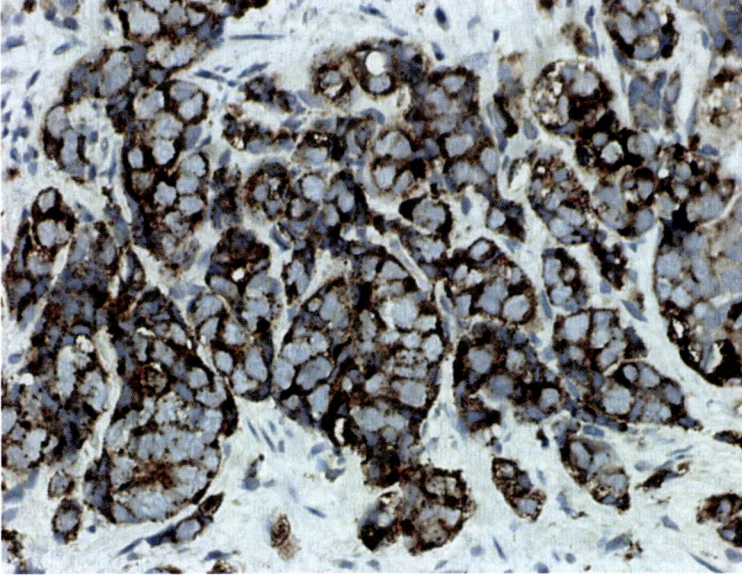

Fig. 16.8 Prostatic acid phosphatase stain. Note intense cytoplasmic immunoreactivity in virtually every cancer cell (Gleason 4 + 4 = 8) as shown by the *brown* reaction product

Prostatic Acid Phosphatase (PAP)

PAP is a valuable immunohistochemical marker for identifying prostate cancer when used in combination with stains for PSA. There is more intense and uniform staining of tumor cells and the glandular epithelium of well-differentiated adenocarcinoma, whereas less intense and more variable staining was seen in moderately and poorly differentiated adenocarcinoma (Fig. 16.8).

Basal Cell-Specific Anti-keratin 34ßE12 (Keratin 903; High Molecular Weight Keratin)

Basal cell-specific anti-keratin 34ßE12 stains virtually all of the normal basal cells of the prostate; there is no staining in the secretory and stromal cells. Basal cell layer disruption is present in 56% of cases of high-grade PIN, more commonly in glands adjacent to invasive carcinoma than in distant glands. The amount of disruption increases with increasing grades of PIN, with loss of more than one-third of the basal cell layer in 52% of foci of high-grade PIN. Early carcinoma occurs at sites of acinar outpouching and basal cell layer disruption [87]. Prostate cancer cells do not react with this antibody, although it may

stain other cancers. Basal cell layer disruption also occurs in inflamed acini, atypical adenomatous hyperplasia, and post-atrophic hyperplasia [3, 28]. In problem cases suspicious for adenocarcinoma, it may be useful to employ this immunohistochemical stain to evaluate the basal cell layer; however, this alone should not be the basis for a diagnosis of malignancy, particularly in small suspicious foci. This stain is of greatest utility in confirming the benignancy of a suspicious focus by demonstrating an immunoreactive basal cell layer. It is also valuable following treatment for separating cancer and benign mimics of cancer (see later).

p63

Recently, p63, a nuclear protein, was shown to be a diagnostically useful basal cell marker. p63 staining was reported to be at least as sensitive and specific for the identification of basal cells in diagnostic prostate specimens as is high molecular weight cytokeratin staining [88]. Shah et al. found that p63 was more sensitive than 34 βE12 in staining benign basal cells, particularly in TURP specimens, offering slight advantage over 34 βE12 in diagnostically challenging cases [89]. Zhou et al.

demonstrated basal cell cocktail (34 βE12 and p63) increased the sensitivity of the basal cell detection and reduced staining variability, thus rendering basal cell immunostaining more consistent [90]. The p63 gene is also expressed in respiratory epithelia, breast and bronchial myoepithelial cells, cytotrophoblast cells of human placenta, in scattered cells of lymph nodes and germinal centers, and in squamous cell carcinoma of the lung [91]. Triple staining with racemase, keratin 34βE12, and p63 (basal cell markers) is emerging as a standard adjunctive stain for the diagnosis of prostate cancer [92, 93].

Alpha-methylacyl-CoA Racemase/P504S (AMACR, P504S, Racemase)

Alpha-methylacyl-CoA racemase gene product, also referred to as P504S protein, is an enzyme involved in β-oxidation of branched chain fatty acids. It has recently been identified as a novel tumor marker for several human cancers and their precursor lesions, including prostate cancer [94, 95]. Initial study showed that racemase was strongly and uniformly positive in 97–100% of prostate cancers. Recent studies suggest that racemase is positive in 80–100% of small prostate cancers on needle biopsy and less intense and more heterogeneous in unusual morphologic variants of prostate cancer, including atrophic, foamy gland, and pseudohyperplastic cancers. We found that 91% of radiated prostate cancer retained racemase immunoreactivity, which was confirmed by another study [96]. In addition, positive racemase staining can also be found in the majority of cases of high-grade prostatic intraepithelial neoplasia, 10–15% of atypical adenomatous hyperplasia, occasional benign glands, and rare seminal vesicle epithelium [97, 98]. Jiang et al. found that the sensitivity and specificity of racemase immunodetection of prostatic adenocarcinoma was 97% and 92%, respectively; positive and negative predictive values were 95%. Racemase immunostaining intensity and percentage in prostatic adenocarcinoma was significantly higher than those in benign prostatic tissue [99].

Cocktail staining of racemase, keratin 34βE12, and p63 is being used increasingly in the workup of difficult prostate needle biopsies (Fig. 16.9) [100]. Negative immunohistochemical stain for basal cells is not diagnostic of carcinoma by

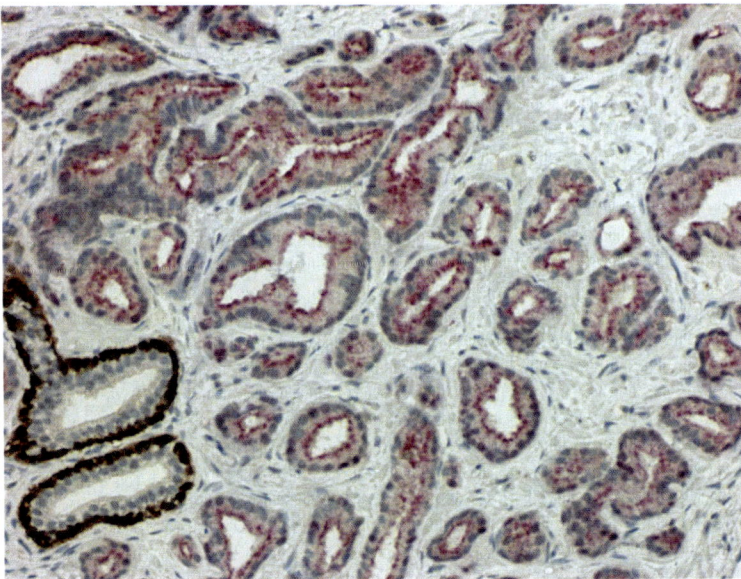

Fig. 16.9 Cocktail staining of racemase, keratin 34βE12, p63, and c-Myc. The *brown* reaction product in the *bottom left* of the image decorates the basal cells lining benign acini according to stains directed against keratin and p63. The cancer acini that populate the remainder of the image fail to contain basal cells but are decorated by the *red* reaction product that decorates cancer cells according to stains directed against racemase and c-Myc

itself as occasional benign glands may not show immunoreactivity, so a positive immunohistochemical marker specific for prostate cancer, such as racemase is of great value in confirming malignancy. A recent study showed that positive racemase staining converted an atypical diagnosis, based on suspicious histology and negative basal cell marker stains, to cancer in approximately 10% (34 of 307) of cases thought to be atypical by contributing pathologists and in approximately 50% (34 of 76) of cases thought be atypical by a specialist in genitourinary pathology. We use the cocktail staining in routine practice and find it to be very useful for the diagnosis of small prostate cancers. Polyclonal and monoclonal antibodies are available commercially [101]. Optimizing the staining conditions for cocktail antibodies is very important for staining interpretation [98]. Although it has limitations with respect to sensitivity and specificity, racemase has rapidly become a standard adjunctive stain used to reach a definitive diagnosis in prostate biopsies considered to be atypical but not diagnostic of malignancy on hematoxylin and eosin sections alone [102]. In settings where only a single section or slide is available for immunohistochemical analysis of a prostate needle biopsy specimen with a minute focus of diagnostic concern, Jiang et al. showed recently that performing immunohistochemistry with a three-antibody cocktail is a simple and easy assay that can be used as a routine test [103].

c-Myc

c-Myc appears to play an important role in the regulation of prostate growth and carcinogenesis. c-Myc is a well-known oncogene that is activated in many human cancers [104], and it has been shown to be amplified with increasing grade of prostate cancer, particularly in metastases [105, 106], and Myc expression correlates with growth of androgen-responsive prostate epithelium [107]. We routinely stain for nuclear c-Myc as a diagnostic tool to confirm the presence of PIN or adenocarcinoma.

ERG

TMPRSS2/ERG gene rearrangement was found to be highly specific for and present in about 50%

of prostate cancers and 29% of foci of PIN, according to immunohistochemical staining with a novel anti-ERG antibody that was highly correlated with TMPRSS2/ERG gene rearrangement status [108–114]. ERG rearrangements are associated with loss of the tumor suppressor gene PTEN, and this cooperation promotes progression of PIN to invasive cancer [115].

Prognostic Molecular Markers

Genetic Instability in Prostate Cancer

Prostate carcinogenesis apparently involves multiple genetic changes, including loss of specific genomic sequences that may be associated with inactivation of tumor suppressor genes and gain of some specific chromosome regions that may be associated with activation of oncogenes. The most common chromosomal aberrations in PIN and carcinoma are gain of chromosome 7, particularly 7q31; loss of 8p and gain of 8q; and loss of 10q, 16q, and 18q [116]. Fluorescence in situ hybridization (FISH) studies showed that aneusomy of chromosome 7 is frequent in prostate cancer and associated with higher cancer grade, higher pathologic stage, and early patient death from prostate cancer [117, 118]. Allelic imbalance of 7q31 was strongly correlated with cancer aggressiveness, progression, and cancer-specific death [117].

The chromosome 8 p-arm is one of the most frequently deleted regions in prostate cancer [119, 120]. The rate of 8p22 loss ranged from 29% to 50% in PIN, 32% to 69% in primary cancer, and 65% to 100% in metastatic cancer [121]. Other frequently deleted 8p regions include 8p21 and 8p12 [119, 121]. Emmert-Buck et al. found loss of 8p12–21 in 63% of PIN foci and 91% of cancer foci using microdissected frozen tissue [119]. Bostwick et al. detected loss of 8p21–12 in 37% of PIN foci and 46% of cancer foci [122]. These findings suggest that more than one tumor suppressor gene may be located on 8p, and inactivation of these tumor suppressor genes may be important for the initiation of prostate cancer. In addition to loss of the 8 p-arm, gain of the 8 q-arm has been reported in prostate cancer [105]. Bova et al. found gain of 8q in 11% of primary cancers and 40% of lymph node metastases [120]. Van Den Berg et al. found amplification of 8q DNA sequences in 75% of cancers metastatic to lymph nodes [123]. Similarly, Visakorpi et al. found gain of 8q far more frequently in locally recurrent cancer than in primary cancer [124]. Cher et al. also detected frequent gain of 8q in metastatic and androgen-independent prostate cancer [125]. Using FISH, Qian et al. observed that gain of chromosome 8 was the most frequent chromosomal anomaly in metastatic foci, and the frequency was much higher than in PIN and carcinoma [126]. Four putative target genes for 8q gain have been identified, and they are Elongin C at 8q21, as well as EIF3S3, KIAA0196, and RAD21 at 8q23–q24 regions. They seem to be overexpressed and amplified in about 20–30% of the hormone-refractory prostate carcinomas [127, 128]. Jenkins et al. identified c-Myc gene amplification, located at 8q24, in 22% of metastatic foci that was much more frequent than in primary cancer (9%), suggesting that the 8 q-arm may harbor a gene(s) whose amplification and overexpression plays a key role in the progression and evolution of prostatic carcinoma [105]. Interestingly, gain of the chromosome 8 centromere or the 8 q-arm occurs simultaneously with loss of portions of the 8 p-arm in PIN and carcinoma [105, 124, 129, 130]. One simple genetic mechanism that could explain these prior observations is the presence of multiple copies of isochromosome 8q in cancer cells.

There is also a high frequency of allelic imbalance at 10p and 10q in prostate cancer [131, 132]. The most commonly deleted region on the 10 q-arm includes bands 10q23–24, and allelic loss of this region may inactivate the MXI-1 gene. Loss of PTEN, a tumor suppressor gene on chromosome 10q23, has been reported in 25–33% of advanced prostate cancer. It has been associated with increased Gleason score and risk of clinical recurrence [133]. Chromosome 16 also had frequent allelic imbalance in prostate cancer. Allelic imbalance at 16q was present in about 30% of cases of clinically localized prostate cancer [134], and there was a high frequency of allelic imbalance at 16q23–q24 [135]. The most commonly deleted region was located at 16q24.1–q24.2, and

this deletion was significantly associated with cancer progression [135, 136]. The frequency of loss of 18q22.1 varied from 20% to 40% [131]. Other regions demonstrating frequent allelic imbalance include 3p25–26, 5q12–23, 6q, 13q, 17p31.1, and 21q22.2–22.3 [136, 137]. Loss of 10q, 16q, and 18q has also been reported in PIN [122, 138].

DNA Ploidy

DNA ploidy analysis of prostate cancer provides important predictive information that supplements histopathologic examination. Patients with diploid tumors have a more favorable outcome than those with aneuploid tumors. Among patients with lymph node metastases treated with radical prostatectomy and androgen deprivation therapy, those with diploid tumors may survive 20 years or more, whereas those with aneuploid tumors die within an average of 5 years [139]. However, the ploidy pattern of prostate cancer is often heterogeneous, creating potential problems with sampling error. Analysis of multiple biopsies is important for correct preoperative ploidy estimation [140]. A good correlation exists between DNA ploidy and histological grade, and DNA ploidy adds clinically useful predictive information for some patients [141, 142]. The incidence of aneuploidy in high-grade PIN varies from 32% to 68% and is somewhat lower than carcinoma that shows aneuploidy in 55–62% of cases [143]. There is a high level of concordance of DNA content of PIN and cancer. About 70% of aneuploid cases of PIN are associated with aneuploid carcinoma; conversely, only 29% of cases of aneuploid cancer are associated with aneuploid PIN [144]. DNA ploidy pattern by flow cytometry correlates with cancer grade [145], volume, and stage [146, 147]. Most low-stage tumors are diploid and high-stage tumors are non-diploid, but numerous exceptions occur [148]. The 5-year cancer-specific survival is about 95% for diploid tumors, 70% for tetraploid tumors, and 25% for aneuploid tumors [149]. Patients with diploid lymph node metastases treated by androgen deprivation therapy alone had longer progression-free survival and overall survival than those with aneuploid metastases [150]. Digital image analysis appears to have a high level of concordance (about 85%) with radical prostatectomy specimens evaluated by flow cytometry [151].

Apoptosis-Suppressing Oncoprotein bcl-2

Bcl-2 is widely believed to be an apoptosis-suppressor gene. Overexpression of the protein in cancer cells may block or delay onset of apoptosis, selecting and maintaining long-living cells, and arresting cells in the G0 phase of the cell cycle [152, 153]. In cancer, the prevalence and expression pattern of bcl-2 is controversial. One study found moderate heterogeneous bcl-2 overexpression in localized cancer [154] that was inversely correlated with Gleason grade. Another report described a significant elevation of bcl-2 in 45% of cases of primary cancer that was heterogeneous but did not correlate with grade. Interestingly, the area of cancer with high bcl-2 expression was devoid of apoptotic cells. One study found that over 70% of prostate carcinomas were bcl-2 negative, 18% had weak expression, and 11% exhibited strong expression [155]. Expression of bcl-2 was correlated with high stage, metastases, and high grade. Androgen deprivation therapy decreased bcl-2 expression in cancer, suggesting that these cells develop resistance to apoptotic signals [154, 156, 157].

p53

Mutant p53 expression is a late event in localized prostate cancer [158, 159], usually present in higher grade cancer [160, 161] and elevated in untreated metastatic cancer [162, 163], hormone-refractory cancer [160, 164], and recurrent cancer [162]. Inactivation of p53 (−p53) is associated with prostate cancer late progression and may be a marker of survival in stage T2-3 N1-3 M0 [165].

p21

The WAF1/CIP1 gene encodes a p21 cyclin-dependent kinase inhibitor that plays a role in the regulation of the cell cycle. Upon induction by p53, p21WAF1/CIP1 binds to cyclin-dependent kinase 2, resulting in downregulation of CDK2 activity and G1 growth arrest. Prostatic mutations in the WAF1/CIP1 gene abrogate this apparent tumor suppressor gene activity [166], thereby facilitating escape of G1/S checkpoint control with propagation into S-phase and maintenance of malignant potential. There is an increase in WAF1/CIP1 polymorphisms in prostate cancer [167], but no correlation exists between WAF1/CIP1 expression and grade, stage, or cancer progression [168].

p27Kip1

The cyclin-dependent kinase inhibitor (p27Kip1) negatively regulates cell proliferation by mediating cell cycle arrest in G1. p27Kip1 expression decreases with higher Gleason score and seminal vesicle involvement by cancer [169]. Further, p27Kip1 expression is an independent predictor of treatment failure of node-negative cancer following radical prostatectomy [169].

PCNA

Proliferating cell nuclear antigen (PCNA) is an auxiliary protein for DNA polymerase which reaches maximal expression during the S phase of the cell cycle [170]. Hence, PCNA has been widely used as an index of the proliferative activity of cancers. The PCNA labeling index is reported to be lowest in benign normal prostatic epithelium and organ-confined cancer but to increase progressively from well- to poorly differentiated invasive prostate cancer, although there is wide variance [171]. The correlation of PCNA index is strong with cancer stage [170–172]. Hence, high PCNA labeling indices may indicate progression of prostate cancer [173, 174] and may be an independent prognostic indicator [173].

Androgen Receptor (AR)

Androgen action in the target cells is mediated by androgen receptor (AR). Many studies screened prostate carcinomas for mutations of AR. AR mutations are rare in untreated prostate cancers and have been reported in 20–25% of patients treated with antiandrogens [175, 176]. No amplifications were found in untreated tumors suggesting that androgen withdrawal selected the gene amplification. The AR gene amplification leads to the overexpression of the gene, and it is now evident that almost all hormone-refractory prostate carcinomas express high levels of AR [177]. It remains still unknown what the mechanisms for the AR expression in tumors not containing the gene amplification are. It has been suggested that ERBB (HER-2/neu) could activate AR, especially when androgen levels are low.

Hypermethylation

Silencing of select genes such as GSTP1 expression by hypermethylation of the promoter region has been detected in 90% of prostate cancer and 70% of high-grade PIN. Glutathione S-transferases are detoxifying enzymes that catalyze conjugation of glutathione with harmful, electrophilic molecules either endogenously or exogenously produced, thereby protecting cells from carcinogenic factors [178]. Quantitative increase in promoter methylation levels of other genes, including APC, HOXD3, and TGFbeta2, is associated with clinical progression of prostate cancer [179].

PTEN

Loss of the tumor suppressor gene PTEN appears to promote aggressiveness in prostate cancer [180–182], as well as androgen independence [183]. Its predictive value for biochemical recurrence is enhanced by simultaneous analysis of TMPRSS2 = ERG status, according to Squire and colleagues [184, 185].

Combining Multiple Predictive Factors

The combination of predictive factors provides the greatest accuracy of predicting stage and outcome. The American Joint Committee on Cancer recommends use of neural network analysis to improve prostate cancer survival prediction [186].

Histological Variants of Prostatic Adenocarcinoma

The biologic behavior of histological variants of adenocarcinoma may differ from typical acinar adenocarcinoma, and proper clinical management depends on accurate diagnosis and separation from tumors arising in other sites (Table 16.4).

Table 16.4 Histological variants of prostate cancer

- Ductal adenocarcinoma (adenocarcinoma with endometrioid features)
- Mucinous (colloid) carcinoma
- Signet ring-cell carcinoma
- Adenocarcinoma with neuroendocrine differentiation
- Neuroendocrine carcinoma (small cell carcinoma)
- Squamous cell and adenosquamous cell carcinoma
- Sarcomatoid carcinoma
- Adenoid cystic carcinoma/basal cell carcinoma
- Lymphoepithelioma-like carcinoma
- Carcinoma with oncocytic features
- Comedocarcinoma
- Cribriform carcinoma
- Pseudohyperplastic adenocarcinoma
- Adenocarcinoma with microvacuolated cytoplasm (foamy cell carcinoma)
- Adenocarcinoma with atrophic features
- Adenocarcinoma with glomeruloid features
- Pleomorphic giant cell carcinoma
- Urothelial carcinoma (involving prostatic ducts and acini with and without stromal invasion)

Ductal carcinoma accounts for about 0.8% of prostatic adenocarcinomas [187]. It typically arises as a polypoid or papillary mass within the prostatic urethra and large periurethral prostatic ducts and may histologically resemble endometrial adenocarcinoma of the female uterus. Most refer to this tumor as *adenocarcinoma with endometrioid features* or simply *ductal carcinoma*. The term *"endometrial"* should not be used in the prostate. Bock and Bostwick reported that most cancers with papillary or cribriform pattern are located in the peripheral zone at a great distance from the urethra, indicating that these histological findings are not specific [187]. Ductal carcinoma invariably displays intense cytoplasmic immunoreactivity for PAP and PSA. Focal CEA immunoreactivity is occasionally present. The prognosis of ductal carcinoma appears to be the same as typical acinar adenocarcinoma.

Pure mucinous carcinoma of the prostate is rare [188, 189], although typical acinar adenocarcinoma often produces mucin focally, particularly following high-dose estrogen therapy. The clinical presentation of mucinous carcinoma is similar to typical acinar carcinoma, and there are no apparent differences in patient age, stage

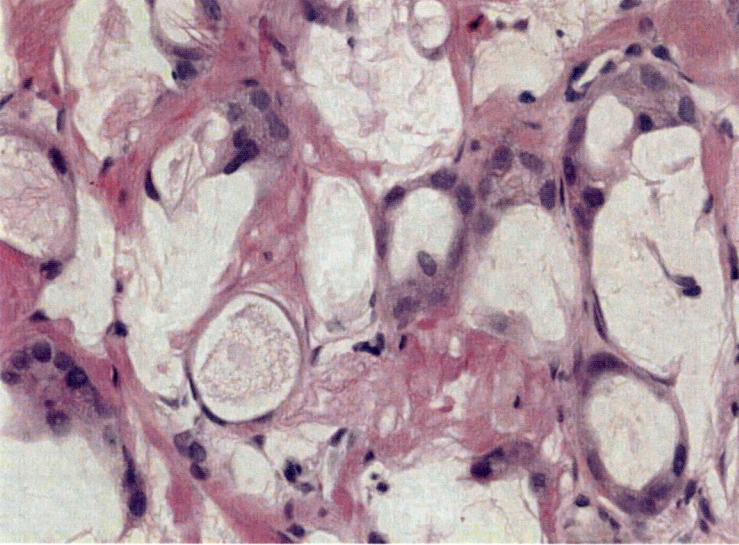

Fig. 16.10 Mucinous carcinoma

at presentation, cancer volume, serum PSA concentration, or pattern of metastases. This tumor may not respond well to endocrine therapy [190] or radiation therapy and is highly aggressive [191, 192]. Focal mucinous differentiation is observed in at least one-third of cases of prostatic carcinoma, but the accepted diagnosis of mucinous carcinoma arbitrarily requires that at least 25% of the tumor contains of pools of extracellular mucin. Mucinous carcinoma consists of tumor cell nests and clusters floating in mucin, similar to mucinous carcinoma of the breast (Fig. 16.10). Three patterns of mucinous carcinoma have been described: acinar carcinoma with luminal distension, cribriform carcinoma with luminal distension, and "colloid carcinoma" with cell nests embedded in mucinous lakes [189]. In some cases, the nuclei are low grade, with uniform finely granular chromatin and inconspicuous nucleoli, but their presence within mucin pools is diagnostic of malignancy.

Signet ring-cell carcinoma of the prostate is rare [193, 194]. The clinical presentation is similar to typical acinar adenocarcinoma except that essentially all are high stage. The prognosis is poor. The diagnosis of signet ring-cell carcinoma arbitrarily requires that 25% or more of the tumor is composed of signet ring cells, although some

authors require 50%. Most often, it is a minor component of Gleason pattern 5 carcinoma. Tumor cells show distinctive nuclear displacement by clear cytoplasm. Signet ring cells are present in 2.5% of cases of acinar adenocarcinoma but rarely in sufficient numbers to be considered signet ring-cell carcinoma [193]. Histochemical and immunohistochemical results with mucin, lipid, PSA, PAP, and CEA stains are variable, and the signet ring-cell appearance may result from cytoplasmic lumens, mucin granules, and fat vacuoles.

Small cell carcinoma (neuroendocrine carcinoma) usually has typical local signs and symptoms of prostatic adenocarcinoma, although paraneoplastic syndromes are frequent in these patients, including Cushing's syndrome, malignant hypercalcemia, syndrome of inappropriate antidiuretic hormone (SIADH) secretion, and myasthenic (Eaton-Lambert) syndrome. Small cell carcinoma is aggressive and rapidly fatal [195, 196]. Neuroendocrine carcinoma of the prostate varies histopathologically from carcinoid-like pattern (low-grade neuroendocrine carcinoma) to small cell undifferentiated (oat cell) carcinoma (high-grade neuroendocrine carcinoma) (Fig. 16.11). These tumors are morphologically identical to their counterparts in the lung

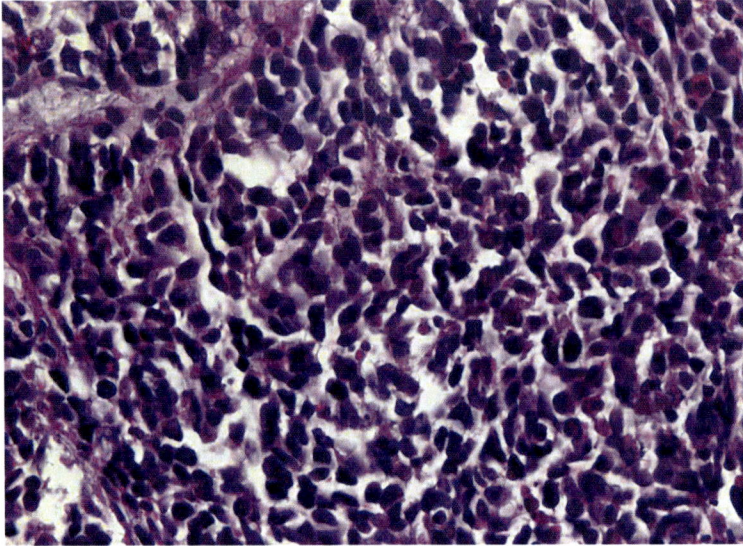

Fig. 16.11 Small cell carcinoma

and other sites. Typical acinar adenocarcinoma is present, at least focally, in about half of cases, and transition patterns may be seen. In cases with solid Gleason 5 pattern suggestive of neuroendocrine carcinoma, immunohistochemical stains are recommended. A wide variety of secretory products may be detected within the malignant cells, including serotonin, calcitonin, ACTH, human chorionic gonadotropin, thyroid stimulating hormone, bombesin, calcitonin gene-related peptide, and inhibin [195]. The same cells may express peptide hormones and PSA and PAP, but pure small cell carcinoma does not usually display immunoreactivity for PSA. Serotonin, chromogranin, and synaptophysin are the most useful markers of neuroendocrine cells in formalin-fixed sections of prostate [5, 197, 198]. Ultrastructurally, small cell carcinoma and carcinoid tumor of the prostate contain a variable number of round regular membrane-bound neurosecretory granules. Well-defined cytoplasmic processes are usually present that contain neurosecretory granules.

Other rare forms of carcinoma include squamous cell carcinoma, sarcomatoid carcinoma, adenoid cystic/basal cell carcinoma, lymphoepithelioma-like carcinoma, pseudohyperplastic carcinoma, adenocarcinoma with microvacuolated cytoplasm (xanthomatoid carcinoma; "foamy

gland" carcinoma), carcinoma with glomeruloid features, and pleomorphic giant cell carcinoma. The unusual atrophic pattern of adenocarcinoma is easily mistaken for atrophy, so caution is warranted in rendering difficult diagnoses with only a small amount of cancer. Urothelial carcinoma involving the prostate and prostatic urethra may arise primarily or from secondary spread from the bladder; it is critical that urothelial carcinoma be distinguished from adenocarcinoma owing to differences in treatment and prognosis.

Treatment Changes in Adenocarcinoma

Treatment changes in the benign and cancerous prostate create diagnostic challenges in pathologic interpretation, particularly in needle biopsies (Fig. 16.12). It is critical that the clinician provide the pertinent history of androgen deprivation or radiation therapy to assist the pathologist in rendering the correct diagnosis.

Androgen Deprivation Therapy

There are a variety of agents that are used for androgen deprivation, and the histopathologic effects of most are similar (Table 16.5). Hormonal treatment alters the benign and cancerous prostatic

Fig. 16.12 Treatment effects: (**a**) androgen deprivation, (**b**) radiation changes, (**c**) and cryosurgical ablation of epithelium with residual stromal paucicellular fibrosis

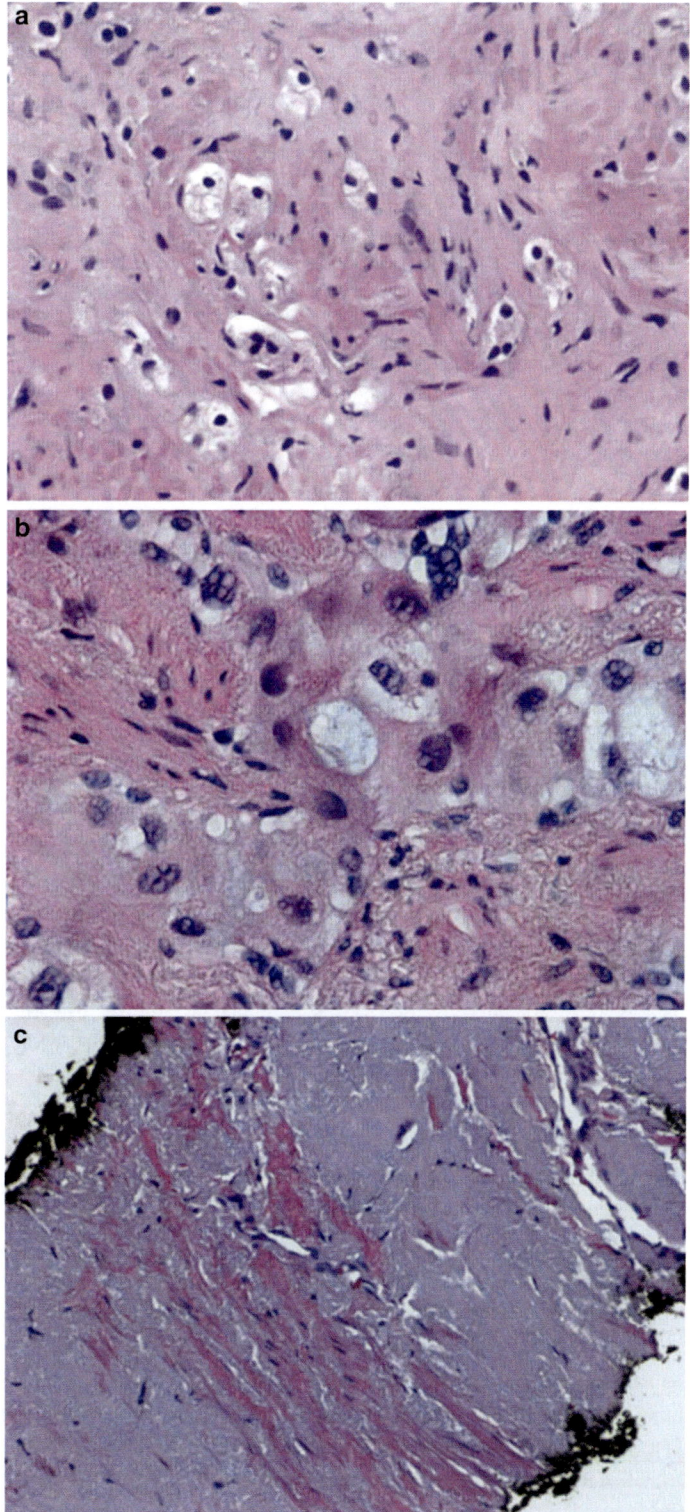

Table 16.5 Androgen deprivation therapy: histological features in the prostate

Benign epithelium
Secretory cell layer
Prominent acinar atrophy
Decreased ratio of acini to stroma
Enlargement and clearing of cytoplasm
Prominent clear cell change
Basal cell layer
Hyperplasia
Prominent component of benign acini
Squamous metaplasia
Stroma
Edema in early stages; fibrosis in late stages
Patchy condensation, resulting in focal hypercellularity
Focal chronic inflammation (lymphohistiocytic)
High-grade prostatic intraepithelial neoplasia
Decrease in prevalence and extent
Nuclear shrinkage
Nuclear hyperchromasia
Nucleolar shrinkage
Other cytological changes similar to benign secretory cell layer
Prostatic adenocarcinoma
Loss of glandular architecture
Nuclear shrinkage
Nuclear hyperchromasia and pyknosis
Nucleolar shrinkage
Mucinous degeneration
Other cytological changes similar to benign secretory cell layer

There is some variability in these changes depending on the method of therapy

epithelium, causing acinar atrophy, apoptosis (programmed cell death), cytoplasmic clearing, nuclear and nucleolar shrinkage, and chromatin condensation. Squamous metaplasia and glycogenic acanthosis are common findings after orchiectomy and diethylstilbestrol, but are uncommon after contemporary forms of treatment. Cancer usually appears as sheets and ribbons of cells with clear cytoplasm and an infiltrative pattern reminiscent of lobular carcinoma of the breast. Tumor cell nuclei are frequently small and hyperchromatic, obscuring the nucleoli and creating a "nucleolus-poor" appearance in many areas [199].

Androgen deprivation therapy causes an apparent increase in the Gleason grade of the tumor which is accompanied nuclear size reduction, loss of recognizable nucleoli, chromatin condensation, nuclear pyknosis, and clear vacuolated cytoplasm. This uncoupling of the architectural and cytological pattern is vexing due to the presence of small shrunken nuclei within malignant acini, particularly in lymph nodes submitted for frozen section evaluation [200].

Alteration in the androgen milieu by 5α-reductase inhibition may promote the growth of more aggressive tumors, but we consider this to be a likely artifact of detection. One proven effect of finasteride and dutasteride is shrinkage of the prostate, and it is likely that there is increased detection of cancer (particularly large cancers), probably accounting for the appearance of higher Gleason score (an example of sampling [detection] bias) [201]. Gleason grading after therapy is potentially misleading and is not recommended [202].

The volume of prostate cancer is reduced by more than 40% after treatment, and there is a 20–25% decline in positive margins at radical prostatectomy [203]. Pathologic stage is similar in untreated and treated prostatic adenocarcinoma, according to retrospective reports of radical prostatectomies, although there is a trend toward lower stage in treated cases. Occasional cases after therapy display the "vanishing cancer phenomenon" in which no residual cancer was found in the radical prostatectomy specimen (see below) [204].

PSA, PAP, and racemase are retained in tumor cells after 3 months of therapy, but decline with longer duration of therapy [205]; keratin 34βE12 remains negative, regardless of duration, indicating an absent basal cell layer [205]. No differences were found in expression of neuroendocrine differentiation markers such as chromogranin, neuron-specific enolase, β-HCG, and serotonin following androgen deprivation therapy. Proliferating cell nuclear antigen (PCNA) immunoreactivity declines after androgen deprivation therapy, indicating that androgens regulate cyclically expressed proteins involved in cell proliferation.

Radiation Therapy

Histological changes of radiation injury in benign and hyperplastic epithelium include acinar atrophy and distortion, marked cytological abnormalities of the epithelium, basal cell hyperplasia, stromal fibrosis, decreased ratio of acini to stroma, and vascular changes [206–208]. PIN after radiation therapy retains characteristic features of untreated PIN, but the prevalence and extent decline [206, 207]. Histological features that are helpful for the diagnosis of cancer after radiation therapy included infiltrative growth, perineural invasion, intraluminal crystalloids, blue mucin secretions, the absence of corpora amylacea, and the presence of concomitant high-grade prostatic intraepithelial neoplasia. For about 12 months after completion of external beam irradiation, needle biopsy is of limited value due to ongoing tumor cell death. After this period, however, biopsy is a good method for assessing local tumor control, with a low level of sampling variation that is minimized by obtaining multiple specimens [178, 206, 208, 209]. The changes following three-dimensional conformal therapy are similar to those after conventional external beam therapy [206]. The addition of androgen deprivation therapy has no appreciable histopathologic effect on the radiation-altered prostate [206].

PSA, PAP, keratin 34βE12, and racemase expression in the prostatic epithelium are not altered by radiation therapy and are often of value in separating treated adenocarcinoma and its mimics. Prostate cancer after radiation therapy has increased p53 nuclear accumulation and Ki-67 labeling index when compared with cancer without prior irradiation. Loss of p21^{WAF1} function has been implicated in the failure of irradiation response [210].

Persistent cancer in needle biopsies after radiation therapy has a significant impact on patient management, since positive needle biopsies portend a worse prognosis [206, 211]. Patients with positive biopsies are more likely to have local recurrence, distant metastases, and death from prostate cancer than those with negative biopsies. Postirradiation Gleason grade and DNA ploidy are independent prognostic factors in prostate cancer patients who fail radiation therapy. However, cancer grade usually shows little or no evidence of "dedifferentiation" after radiation therapy [206].

The severity and extent of radiation changes in the prostate may be of prognostic value in patients treated by external beam therapy and brachytherapy [212, 213] and appear to vary according to radiation dose [206, 214]. No definitive method exists for assessment of tumor viability after irradiation.

Ultrasound Hyperthermia, Microwave Hyperthermia, Laser Therapy, and Hot Water Balloon Thermotherapy

All forms of hyperthermia for nodular hyperplasia result in sharply circumscribed hemorrhagic coagulative necrosis that soon organizes with granulation tissue; the pattern and extent of injury is determined by the method of thermocoagulation employed, the duration of treatment, tissue perfusion factors, and the ratio of epithelium to stroma in the tissue being treated [215, 216]. Transurethral methods may be safer and more effective than transrectal methods because they appear to avoid injury to the rectal mucosa. When delivered transurethrally, laser thermocoagulation and microwave hyperthermia do not usually involve the peripheral zone or neighboring structures, presumably due to differences in tissue perfusion [216, 217]. Coagulation necrosis is greater in areas of predominantly epithelial nodular hyperplasia rather than predominantly stromal hyperplasia and the dense fibromuscular tissue of the bladder neck. Confluent coagulation necrosis occurs when multiple laser lesions are created in a single transverse plane.

Cryoablation Therapy (Cryosurgery)

Cryosurgical ablation refers to freezing of the prostate. Multiple cryoprobe needles filled with circulating liquid nitrogen transform the prostate into an ice ball, resulting in substantial tissue destruction and death of benign and malignant cells. The flow of argon gas (liquid nitrogen in prior generation technology) through the probes is adjusted to create the desired freezing pattern and extent of tissue destruction in the prostate; no freezing agent comes in contact with the tissue. Preliminary results with cryoablation for prostate cancer are encouraging, but the method is used only with select patients [218, 219].

Following cryosurgery, the prostate shows typical features of repair, including marked stromal fibrosis and hyalinization, basal cell hyperplasia with ductal and acinar regeneration, squamous metaplasia, urothelial metaplasia, and stromal hemorrhage and hemosiderin deposition [220, 221]. Coagulative necrosis is present between 6 and 30 weeks of therapy, but patchy chronic inflammation is more common. Focal granulomatous inflammation is associated with epithelial disruption due to corpora amylacea. Dystrophic calcification is infrequent and usually appears in areas with the greatest reparative response. Atypia and PIN are not seen in areas that otherwise show changes of post-cryoablation therapy. Biopsy after cryosurgery may reveal no evidence of recurrent or residual carcinoma, even in some patients with elevated PSA. In some cases, the benign prostate and tumor appear unchanged, with no change in grade or definite evidence of tissue or immune response. As the postoperative interval increases, biopsy is more likely to contain unaltered benign prostatic tissue [221]. A few radical prostatectomies have been done after cryosurgery and that was associated with an increase in morbidity, with the main problem being urinary incontinence [222].

Contemporary Questions in Biopsy Pathology of the Prostate

Can Upgrading of Biopsies Be Predicted Preoperatively?

Multiple factors have been studied to determine the cause of variance in grading between biopsy and prostatectomy (Table 16.6). Upgrading is a substantial problem owing to the strong reliance on Gleason score for treatment decisions; also, upgrading is an adverse independent predictor of patient outcome [223–226]. The upgrading problem has been somewhat mitigated in recent years with collection of increasing number of biopsies,

Table 16.6 Four contemporary questions in biopsy pathology of the prostate

- Can upgrading of biopsies be predicted preoperatively?
- Are transperineal 3-D template biopsies mapping biopsies justified for focal therapy?
- What is the vanishing cancer phenomenon (pT0 cancer)?
- What are the measures of quality control in prostate biopsies?

but upgrading persists as a potential problem for the individual patient. In 1994, we reported upgrading in 33–45% of cases based on quadrant biopsies [227]. Contemporary numbers are somewhat lower than that owing to greater sampling; for example, in men assessed with 10–12 cores, the rate of upgrading was 48% compared with 23.5% if >18 cores were taken ($P<.001$) [228].

Iremashvili compared four published nomograms developed for the purpose of predicting the likelihood of an increase in Gleason score from biopsy information [229]. They found that the combined area under the receiver operating characteristics curve (AUC-ROC) was 0.64–0.65, with upgrading in 34% of patients, and concluded that the available prognostic tools had limited ability to predict clinically significant upgrading in patients with biopsy Gleason score ≤ 6.[229].

Are Transperineal 3-D Template Biopsies Mapping Biopsies Justified for Focal Therapy?

There is a significant need for more accurate pretreatment localization, staging, and grading to ensure proper selection and appropriate management of the individual patient. Site-specific labeling and three-dimensional pathologic mapping of extended saturation biopsies (24 or more biopsies within the prostate) may avoid the sampling error biases of less-extensive biopsies, thereby potentially enabling the use of focal therapy such as cryosurgery, a controversial but potentially promising treatment modality [230]. The stated goal of minimally invasive alternative treatment (brachytherapy, cryosurgical ablation, high-intensity focused ultrasound (HIFU), and radiofrequency interstitial tumor ablation) is to eradicate localized cancers with equal efficacy, but with few or no side effects. In cases in which focal or conformal cryoablation (focal cryoablation = cryoablation on one side only; conformal cryoablation = bilateral cryoablation with sparing of at least the neurovascular bundle on the unaffected side) is carried out, the map is crucial, and therefore site-specific labeling and three-dimensional mapping of extended saturation biopsies permit selective targeted ablation of the area(s) of cancer, while sparing the uninvolved portion of the prostate. A recent consensus conference agreed that patients for focal therapy should have unilateral low- to intermediate-risk disease with clinical stage T2a or lower [231]. Prostate size, tumor volume, and tumor topography were important case selection criteria depending on the ablative technology used. All agreed that the best available method to determine these important characteristics was transperineal 3-D template mapping biopsies [231].

Comparative analysis of two prostate biopsy methods by Onik and colleagues showed that TRUS biopsy was inaccurate in assessing the extent and grade of prostate cancer, even with the extended 10-core (or more) protocol suggested by the National Comprehensive Cancer Network (NCCN) [232]. More than 60% of patients with unilateral cancer on TRUS biopsy actually had bilateral cancer by 3-D-mapping biopsy, similar to the results of others [233, 234].

All methods of biopsy sampling carry an unavoidable risk of missing prostate cancer and thus cannot be considered infallible. Onik et al. found that 36 of the 180 patients with unilateral cancer on TRUS biopsy had negative 3-D PMB, yielding a false negative rate of 20% [232]. They designed 3-D-mapping biopsies to obtain samples every 5 mm throughout the prostate to presumably avoid missing "significant" cancer 5 mm or greater in dimension. Only one such cancer was missed by this method, indicating a 3% failure rate for larger cancers [232], similar to the failure rate reported by others who studied simulations of 3-D-mapping biopsies in radical prostatectomies and autopsy prostates [233, 235, 236].

What Is the Vanishing Cancer Phenomenon (pT0 Cancer)?

In some radical prostatectomy specimens, there is minimal or no residual cancer within the specimen despite positive biopsy. This "vanishing cancer phenomenon" is increasing in incidence as more low-stage cancers are being treated by radical prostatectomy [204, 237]. However, we reported recently that the incidence of "vanishing cancer" declined between 1966 and 1995, occurring in 0.2% of radical prostatectomies and probably results of the substantial decline in the use of transurethral resection specimens. This decline may be offset by two factors: (1) an increase in patients receiving preoperative androgen deprivation therapy (or radiation therapy) and (2) an increasing vigilance in screening that shows prostate cancer is now being detected as smaller volume and lower stage than before [238]. Capitanio and colleagues recently reported an incidence of 13.9% in TURP-detected cancers [239].

The inability to identify cancer in a prostate removed for biopsy-proven carcinoma does not necessarily indicate technical failure, although it is important to exclude the possibility of improper patient identification. DNA "fingerprinting" has been used [204] as a research tool to compare the formalin-fixed paraffin-embedded biopsy and patient mouth swab, and it appears to be prudent to reassure patients in these cases [240]. Substantial resources may be needed to identify minimal residual cancer, and even exhaustive sectioning may fail. How many sections are reasonable to obtain in such cases? When can one stop sectioning if no cancer is found? We believe that it is appropriate for the pathologist to submit routine sections of the entire prostatectomy for histological evaluation in such cases; however, after submission and examination of the entire prostate, further levels and block flipping are probably not necessary, as any residual cancer at that point is likely to be extremely small and of no clinical significance.

Prognosis for pT0 cancer is excellent, with virtually no likelihood of failure [238, 240].

What Are the Measures of Quality Control in Prostate Biopsies?

Studies addressing quality control in prostate biopsy acquisition and processing are very limited. Two issues that deserve attention are (1) variance in the amount of tissue sampled by biopsy and the impact on cancer yield and (2) patient biopsy identification errors.

Urologist training and standardization of collection and processing of biopsies significantly reduced variance in prostate biopsy quality in a prospective clinical trial, thereby optimizing cancer detection and yield [241]. Biopsy quality was found to be a useful comparative measure in urologic practice that should be included in quality assurance programs.

Patient specimen switching is a common and avoidable problem, involving about 0.5% of cases [242], and may occur at any step of the workflow process in the urology clinic and pathology laboratory. The potential for patient harm is especially high in diagnostic anatomic pathology given the impact on care by each definitive diagnosis; the most significant resulting damage is to the patient who receives an erroneous diagnosis and potentially irreversible treatment (or the lack thereof) as a result. To protect patients from errors, quality control initiatives must consider every step of this process, regardless of whether the error was caused by a clinician or nurse, laboratory professional, or a non-laboratory provider. Such steps for patient identification errors include the pre-analytical phase in the clinician's office during which the biopsy is taken; the analytical phase in the laboratory during which the tissue is received, processed, and diagnosed; and the post-analytical phase in the laboratory and elsewhere during which the diagnostic report is delivered and the pathology slides and cassettes are stored. The recent Laboratory National Patient Safety Accreditation Program of the Joint Commission on Accreditation of Healthcare Organizations (JCAHO) required that each laboratory "… establishes processes to maintain specimen identity throughout the pre-analytical, analytical, and post-analytical processes" [243]. Process improvement methods include the use of two-dimensional

bar codes and radiofrequency identification (RFID) tag (DG Bostwick, manuscript in preparation). The potential for biopsy mismatches in clinical practice is an under-recognized problem that requires rigorous attention to details of chain of custody and consideration of more widespread DNA identity testing.

Editorial Comment:
No collaboration in the field of prostate cancer diagnostics is more critical than that of the urologist and pathologist. The clinician may be tempted to believe that a pathology report is immutable and all encompassing, comprising all the information that is needed to make a decision regardless of its conclusion. The author describes several issues that make clear this is not the case. For example, the pathologist can only interpret information contained in the tissue that is available to him or her. If the clinician has not supplied adequate tissue or that tissue is macerated or otherwise comprised in its ability to reflect the underlying diagnosis, the pathologist cannot overcome that. If the tissues come from parts of the prostate that do not include tumor foci, the report will be negative but the patient still has cancer.

On the pathological end, it is noted that not every single cell is included in the tissue that the pathologist examines. Furthermore, intraobserver variability can lead to some relatively small percentage of readings being equivocal, although a second pathological opinion might render a definitive diagnosis without requiring repeat biopsy. Even differences in Gleason scoring levels are important to decision-making.

Thus, we encourage a collaborative approach to this relationship. If the tissues are compromised, the pathologist should (gently) suggest critical information may be missing, and repeat biopsy can be recommended reasonably. It should also go without saying that the pathology request form should inform the pathologist of pertinent clinical information. This should not only be age and PSA value, but any treatments that might affect interpretation, such as prior radiation, LHRH use, or even use of five-ari's, plus history of any prior biopsies. If the report is in any way unclear, the clinician should likewise contact the pathologist to discuss the case, and whether anything can be done to clarify the scenario.

By working collaboratively, patient care is improved, and the risk of inaccurate decision-making can be minimized.

–J. Stephen Jones

References

1. Renshaw AA. Adequate tissue sampling of prostate core needle biopsies. Am J Clin Pathol. 1997;107(1): 26–9.
2. Brat DJ, Wills ML, Lecksell KL, Epstein JI. How often are diagnostic features missed with less extensive histologic sampling of prostate needle biopsy specimens? Am J Surg Pathol. 1999;23:257–62.
3. Brawer MK, Peehl DM, Stamey TA, Bostwick DG. Keratin immunoreactivity in the benign and neoplastic human prostate. Cancer Res. 1985;45(8): 3663–7.
4. Adlakha H, Bostwick DG. Paneth cell-like change in prostatic adenocarcinoma represents neuroendocrine differentiation: report of 30 cases. Hum Pathol. 1994;25(2):135–9.
5. Abrahamsson PA, Wadstrom LB, Alumets J, Falkmer S, Grimelius L. Peptide-hormone- and serotonin-immunoreactive tumour cells in carcinoma of the prostate. Pathol Res Pract. 1987;182(3): 298–307.
6. Aprikian AG, Cordon-Cardo C, Fair WR, Reuter VE. Characterization of neuroendocrine differentiation in human benign prostate and prostatic adenocarcinoma. Cancer. 1993;71(12):3952–65.
7. Bonkhoff H, Stein U, Remberger K. Multidirectional differentiation in the normal, hyperplastic, and neoplastic human prostate: simultaneous demonstration of cell-specific epithelial markers. Hum Pathol. 1994;25(1):42–6.
8. Shidham VB, Lindholm PF, Kajdacsy-Balla A, Basir Z, George V, Garcia FU. Prostate-specific antigen expression and lipochrome pigment granules in the differential diagnosis of prostatic adenocarcinoma versus seminal vesicle-ejaculatory duct epithelium. Arch Pathol Lab Med. 1999;123(11):1093–7.
9. Arber DA, Speights VO. Aneuploidy in benign seminal vesicle epithelium: an example of the paradox of ploidy studies. Mod Pathol. 1991;4(6):687–9.
10. Saboorian MH, Huffman H, Ashfaq R, Ayala AG, Ro JY. Distinguishing Cowper's glands from neoplastic and pseudoneoplastic lesions of prostate: immunohistochemical and ultrastructural studies. Am J Surg Pathol. 1997;21(9):1069–74.
11. Cina SJ, Silberman MA, Kahane H, Epstein JI. Diagnosis of Cowper's glands on prostate needle biopsy. Am J Surg Pathol. 1997;21(5):550–5.
12. Chughtai B, Sawas A, O'Malley RL, Naik RR, Ali Khan S, Pentyala S. A neglected gland: a review of Cowper's gland. Int J Androl. 2005;28(2):74–7.
13. Bostwick DG, de la Roza G, Dundore P, Corica FA, Iczkowski KA. Intraepithelial and stromal lymphocytes in the normal human prostate. Prostate. 2003;55(3):187–93.
14. McArdle PA, Canna K, McMillan DC, McNicol AM, Campbell R, Underwood MA. The relationship between T-lymphocyte subset infiltration and survival in patients with prostate cancer. Br J Cancer. 2004;91(3):541–3.
15. Canna K, McArdle PA, McMillan DC, McNicol AM, Smith GW, McKee RF, et al. The relationship between tumour T-lymphocyte infiltration, the systemic inflammatory response and survival in patients undergoing curative resection for colorectal cancer. Br J Cancer. 2005;92(4):651–4.
16. Blumenfeld W, Tucci S, Narayan P. Incidental lymphocytic prostatitis. Selective involvement with nonmalignant glands. Am J Surg Pathol. 1992;16(10): 975–81.
17. Zhang W, Sesterhenn IA, Connelly RR, Mostofi FK, Moul JW. Inflammatory infiltrate (prostatitis) in whole mounted radical prostatectomy specimens from black and white patients is not an etiology for racial difference in prostate specific antigen. J Urol. 2000;163(1):131–6.
18. Lopez-Plaza I, Bostwick DG. Prostatitis. In: Bostwick DG, editor. Pathology of the prostate. New York: Churchill Livingstone; 1990. p. 15–30.
19. Bostwick DG, Vonk J, Picado A. Pathologic changes in the prostate following contemporary 18-gauge needle biopsy: no apparent risk of local cancer seeding. J Urol Pathol. 1994;2:203–12.
20. Bastacky SS, Walsh PC, Epstein JI. Needle biopsy associated tumor tracking of adenocarcinoma of the prostate. J Urol. 1991;145(5):1003–7.
21. Loeb S, Gashti SN, Catalona WJ. Exclusion of inflammation in the differential diagnosis of an elevated prostate-specific antigen (PSA). Urol Oncol. 2009;27(1):64–6.
22. Terakawa T, Miyake H, Kanomata N, Kumano M, Takenaka A, Fujisawao M. Inverse association between histologic inflammation in needle biopsy specimens and prostate cancer in men with serum PSA of 10–50 ng/mL. Urology. 2008;72(6):1194–7.
23. Karakiewicz PI, Benayoun S, Begin LR, Duclos A, Valiquette L, McCormack M, et al. Chronic inflammation is negatively associated with prostate cancer and high-grade prostatic intraepithelial neoplasia on needle biopsy. Int J Clin Pract. 2007;61(3):425–30.
24. Stopiglia RM, Ferreira U, Silva Jr MM, Matheus WE, Denardi F, Reis LO. Prostate specific antigen decrease and prostate cancer diagnosis: antibiotic versus placebo prospective randomized clinical trial. J Urol. 2010;183(3):940–4.
25. Tang P, Xie KJ, Wang B, Deng XR, Ou RB. Antibacterial therapy improves the effectiveness of

prostate cancer detection using prostate-specific antigen in patients with asymptomatic prostatitis. Int Urol Nephrol. 2010;42(1):13–8.

26. Banez LL, Klink JC, Jayachandran J, Lark AL, Gerber L, Hamilton RJ, et al. Association between statins and prostate tumor inflammatory infiltrate in men undergoing radical prostatectomy. Cancer Epidemiol Biomarkers Prev. 2010;19(3):722–8.

27. Billis A, Meirelles L, Freitas LL, Magna LA, Ferreira U. Does the type of prostatic atrophy influence the association of extent of atrophy in needle biopsies and serum prostate-specific antigen levels? Urology. 2009;74(5):1111–5.

28. Cheville JC, Bostwick DG. Postatrophic hyperplasia of the prostate. A histologic mimic of prostatic adenocarcinoma. Am J Surg Pathol. 1995;19(9):1068–76.

29. Amin MB, Tamboli P, Varma M, Srigley JR. Postatrophic hyperplasia of the prostate gland: a detailed analysis of its morphology in needle biopsy specimens. Am J Surg Pathol. 1999;23(8):925–31.

30. Bardia A, Platz EA, Yegnasubramanian S, De Marzo AM, Nelson WG. Anti-inflammatory drugs, antioxidants, and prostate cancer prevention. Curr Opin Pharmacol. 2009;9(4):419–26.

31. De Marzo AM, Marchi VL, Epstein JI, Nelson WG. Proliferative inflammatory atrophy of the prostate: implications for prostatic carcinogenesis. Am J Pathol. 1999;155(6):1985–92.

32. Woenckhaus J, Fenic I. Proliferative inflammatory atrophy: a background lesion of prostate cancer? Andrologia. 2008;40(2):134–7.

33. Ulamec M, Tomas D, Ensinger C, Cupic H, Belicza M, Mikuz G, et al. Periacinar retraction clefting in proliferative prostatic atrophy and prostatic adenocarcinoma. J Clin Pathol. 2007;60(10):1098–101.

34. MacLennan GT, Eisenberg R, Fleshman RL, Taylor JM, Fu P, Resnick MI, et al. The influence of chronic inflammation in prostatic carcinogenesis: a 5-year followup study. J Urol. 2006;176(3):1012–6.

35. Borowsky AD, Dingley KH, Ubick E, Turteltaub KW, Cardiff RD, Devere-White R. Inflammation and atrophy precede prostatic neoplasia in a PhIP-induced rat model. Neoplasia. 2006;8(9):708–15.

36. Tomas D, Kruslin B, Rogatsch H, Schafer G, Belicza M, Mikuz G. Different types of atrophy in the prostate with and without adenocarcinoma. Eur Urol. 2007;51(1):98–103. Discussion –4.

37. Mikuz G, Algaba F, Beltran AL, Montironi R. Prostate carcinoma: atrophy or not atrophy that is the question. Eur Urol. 2007;52(5):1293–6.

38. Carcamo Valor PI, San Millan Arruti JP, Cozar Olmo JM, Garcia-Matres MJ, Echevarria C, Martinez-Pineiro L, Martinez-Pineiro JA. Nephrogenic adenoma of the upper and lower urinary tract. Apropos of 22 cases. Arch Esp Urol. 1992;45:423–7.

39. Malpica A, Ro JY, Troncoso P, Ordonez NG, Amin MB, Ayala AG. Nephrogenic adenoma of the prostatic urethra involving the prostate gland: a clinicopathologic and immunohistochemical study of eight cases. Hum Pathol. 1994;25(4):390–5.

40. Cheng L, Cheville JC, Sebo TJ, Eble JN, Bostwick DG. Atypical nephrogenic metaplasia of the urinary tract: a precursor lesion? Cancer. 2000;88(4):853–61.

41. Mazal PR, Schaufler R, Altenhuber-Muller R, Haitel A, Watschinger B, Kratzik C, et al. Derivation of nephrogenic adenomas from renal tubular cells in kidney-transplant recipients. N Engl J Med. 2002;347(9):653–9.

42. Shapiro E, Becich MJ, Hartanto V, Lepor H. The relative proportion of stromal and epithelial hyperplasia is related to the development of symptomatic benign prostate hyperplasia. J Urol. 1992;147(5):1293–7.

43. Bostwick DG, Cooner WH, Denis L, Jones GW, Scardino PT, Murphy GP. The association of benign prostatic hyperplasia and cancer of the prostate. Cancer. 1992;70(1 Suppl):291–301.

44. Leav I, McNeal JE, Ho SM, Jiang Z. Alpha-methylacyl-CoA racemase (P504S) expression in evolving carcinomas within benign prostatic hyperplasia and in cancers of the transition zone. Hum Pathol. 2003;34(3):228–33.

45. Untergasser G, Madersbacher S, Berger P. Benign prostatic hyperplasia: age-related tissue-remodeling. Exp Gerontol. 2005;40(3):121–8.

46. Devaraj LT, Bostwick DG. Atypical basal cell hyperplasia of the prostate. Immunophenotypic profile and proposed classification of basal cell proliferations. Am J Surg Pathol. 1993;17(7):645–59.

47. Bostwick DG, Srigley J, Grignon D, Maksem J, Humphrey P, van der Kwast TH, et al. Atypical adenomatous hyperplasia of the prostate: morphologic criteria for its distinction from well-differentiated carcinoma. Hum Pathol. 1993;24(8):819–32.

48. Bostwick DG, Qian J. Atypical adenomatous hyperplasia of the prostate. Relationship with carcinoma in 217 whole-mount radical prostatectomies. Am J Surg Pathol. 1995;19(5):506–18.

49. Brawn PN, Speights VO, Contin JU, Bayardo RJ, Kuhl DL. Atypical hyperplasia in prostates of 20 to 40 year old men. J Clin Pathol. 1989;42(4):383–6.

50. Humphrey PA, Zhu X, Crouch EC, Carbone JM, Keetch DW. Mass-forming atypical adenomatous hyperplasia. J Urol Pathol. 1998;9:73–81.

51. Bostwick DG, Cheng L.Urologic surgical pathology. Second Edition. Mosby Elsevier 2008;443–580.

52. Helpap B. Observations on the number, size and localization of nucleoli in hyperplastic and neoplastic prostatic disease. Histopathology. 1988;13(2):203–11.

53. Epstein JI. Diagnosis and reporting of limited adenocarcinoma of the prostate on needle biopsy. Mod Pathol. 2004;17(3):307–15.

54. Del Rosario AD, Bui HX, Abdulla M, Ross JS. Sulfur-rich prostatic intraluminal crystalloids: a surgical pathologic and electron probe x-ray microanalytic study. Hum Pathol. 1993;24(11):1159–67.

55. Molberg KH, Mikhail A, Vuitch F. Crystalloids in metastatic prostatic adenocarcinoma. Am J Clin Pathol. 1994;101(3):266–8.

56. Tressera F, Barastegui C. Intraluminal crystalloids in metastatic prostatic carcinoma. Am J Clin Pathol. 1995;103(5):665.

57. Salomao DR, Graham SD, Bostwick DG. Microvascular invasion in prostate cancer correlates with pathologic stage. Arch Pathol Lab Med. 1995;119(11):1050–4.

58. Bostwick DG, Foster CS. Predictive factors in prostate cancer: current concepts from the 1999 College of American Pathologists conference on solid tumor prognostic factors and the 1999 World Health Organization second international consultation on prostate cancer. Semin Urol Oncol. 1999;17(4): 222–72.

59. Gleason DF. Histologic grading of prostate cancer: a perspective. Hum Pathol. 1992;23:273–9.

60. Bostwick DG. Gleason grading of prostatic needle biopsies. Correlation with grade in 316 matched prostatectomies. Am J Surg Pathol. 1994;18(8): 796–803.

61. Steinberg DM, Sauvageot J, Piantadosi S, Epstein JI. Correlation of prostate needle biopsy and radical prostatectomy Gleason grade in academic and community settings. Am J Surg Pathol. 1997;21(5): 566–76.

62. Aihara M, Wheeler TM, Ohori M, Scardiono PT. Heterogeneity of prostate cancer in radical prostatectomy specimens. Urology. 1994;43:60–6.

63. Allsbrook WCJ, Lane RB, Lane CG, Mangold KA, Johnson M, Amin M, Bostwick D, Humphrey P, Jones E, Reuter V, Sakr W, Sesterhenn IA, Troncoso P, Wheeler T, Epstein JI. Interobserver reproducibility of Gleason's grading system: urologic pathologists. Mod Pathol. 1998;11:75A.

64. Allsbrook Jr WC, Mangold KA, Johnson MH, Lane RB, Lane CG, Epstein JI. Interobserver reproducibility of Gleason grading of prostatic carcinoma: general pathologist. Hum Pathol. 2001;32(1):81–8.

65. Lotan TL, Epstein JI. Clinical implications of changing definitions within the Gleason grading system. Nat Rev Urol. 2010;7(3):136–42.

66. Lucia MS, Somerville MC, Fowler I, Rittmaster RS, Bostwick DG. Comparison of classic and ISUP 2005 modified Gleason grading using needle biopsies from the REDUCE trial. 2011 (submitted).

67. Epstein JI, Walsh PC, Carmichael M, Brendler CB. Pathologic and clinical findings to predict tumor extent of nonpalpable (stage T1c) prostate cancer. JAMA. 1994;271(5):368–74.

68. Hammerer P, Huland H, Sparanberg S. Digital rectal examination, imaging, and systematic-sextant biopsy in identifying operable lymph node-negative prostatic carcinoma. Eur Urol. 1992;22:281–7.

69. Ravery V, Schmid HP, Toublanc M, Boccon-Gibod L. Is the percentage of cancer in biopsy cores predictive of extracapsular disease in T1-T2 prostate carcinoma? Cancer. 1996;78(5):1079–84.

70. Cupp MR, Bostwick DG, Myers RP, Oesterling JE. The volume of prostate cancer in the biopsy specimen cannot reliably predict the quantity of cancer in the radical prostatectomy specimen on an individual basis. J Urol. 1995;153(5):1543–8.

71. Stamey TA, Freiha FS, McNeal JE, Redwine EA, Whittemore AS, Schmid HP. Localized prostate cancer. Relationship of tumor volume to clinical significance for treatment of prostate cancer. Cancer. 1993;71(3 Suppl):933–8.

72. Haggman M, Nybacka O, Nordin B, Busch C. Standardized in vitro mapping with multiple core biopsies of total prostatectomy specimens: localization and prediction of tumour volume and grade. Br J Urol. 1994;74(5):617–25.

73. Terris MK, McNeal JE, Stamey TA. Detection of clinically significant prostate cancer by transrectal ultrasound-guided systematic biopsies. J Urol. 1992;148(3):829–32.

74. Bruce RG, Rankin WR, Cibull ML, Rayens MK, Banks ER, Wood Jr DP. Single focus of adenocarcinoma in the prostate biopsy specimen is not predictive of the pathologic stage of disease. Urology. 1996;48(1):75–9.

75. Weldon VE, Tavel FR, Neuwirth H, Cohen R. Failure of focal prostate cancer on biopsy to predict focal prostate cancer: the importance of prevalence. J Urol. 1995;154(3):1074–7.

76. Noguchi M, Stamey TA, McNeal JE, Yemoto CE. Assessment of morphometric measurements of prostate carcinoma volume. Cancer. 2000;89(5): 1056–64.

77. Wheeler TM, Dillioglugil O, Kattan MW, Arakawa A, Soh S, Suyama K, et al. Clinical and pathological significance of the level and extent of capsular invasion in clinical stage T1-2 prostate cancer. Hum Pathol. 1998;29(8):856–62.

78. Henson DE, Hutter RV, Farrow G. Practice protocol for the examination of specimens removed from patients with carcinoma of the prostate gland. A publication of the cancer committee, College of American Pathologists. Task force on the examination of specimens removed from patients with prostate cancer. Arch Pathol Lab Med. 1994;118(8): 779–83.

79. Stamey TA, McNeal JE, Yemoto CM, Sigal BM, Johnstone IM. Biological determinants of cancer progression in men with prostate cancer. JAMA. 1999;281(15):1395–400.

80. Babian RJ, Troncoso P, Steelhammer LC, Lloreta-Trull J, Ramirez EI. Tumor volume and prostate specific antigen: implications for early detection and defining a window of curability. J Urol. 1995;154: 1808–12.

81. Renshaw AA, Richie JP, Loughlin KR, Jiroutek M, Chung A, D'Amico AV. The greatest dimension of prostate carcinoma is a simple inexpensive predictor of prostate specific antigen failure in radical prostatectomy specimens. Cancer. 1998;83:748–52.

82. Dugan JA, Bostwick DG, Myers RP, Qian J, Bergstralh EJ, Oesterling JE. The definition and preoperative prediction of clinically insignificant prostate cancer. JAMA. 1996;275(4):288–94.

83. Humphrey PA, Vollmer RT. Percentage of carcinoma as a measure of prostatic tumor size in radical prostatectomy tissues. Mod Pathol. 1997;159:1234–7.

84. Carvalhal GF, Humphrey PA, Thorson P, Yan Y, Ramos CG, Catalona WJ. Visual estimate of the percentage of carcinoma is an independent predictor of prostate carcinoma recurrence after radical prostatectomy. Cancer. 2000;89:1308–14.

85. Schned AR, Wheeler KJ, Hodorowski CA, Heaney JA, Ernstoff MS, Amdur RJ, et al. Tissue-shrinkage correction factor in the calculation of prostate cancer volume. Am J Surg Pathol. 1996;20(12):1501–6.

86. Cheng L, Jones TD, Pan CX, Barbarin A, Eble JN, Koch MO. Anatomic distribution and pathologic characterization of small-volume prostate cancer (<0.5 ml) in whole-mount prostatectomy specimens. Mod Pathol. 2005;18(8):1022–6.

87. Bostwick DG, Brawer MK. Prostatic intra-epithelial neoplasia and early invasion in prostate cancer. Cancer. 1987;59(4):788–94.

88. Weinstein MH, Signoretti S, Loda M. Diagnostic utility of immunohistochemical staining for p63, a sensitive marker of prostatic basal cells. Mod Pathol. 2002;15(12):1302–8.

89. Shah RB, Zhou M, LeBlanc M, Snyder M, Rubin MA. Comparison of the basal cell-specific markers, 34betaE12 and p63, in the diagnosis of prostate cancer. Am J Surg Pathol. 2002;26(9):1161–8.

90. Zhou M, Shah R, Shen R, Rubin MA. Basal cell cocktail (34betaE12 + p63) improves the detection of prostate basal cells. Am J Surg Pathol. 2003;27(3):365–71.

91. Reis-Filho JS, Simpson PT, Martins A, Preto A, Gartner F, Schmitt FC. Distribution of p63, cytokeratins 5/6 and cytokeratin 14 in 51 normal and 400 neoplastic human tissue samples using TARP-4 multi-tumor tissue microarray. Virchows Arch. 2003; 443(2):122–32.

92. Signoretti S, Waltregny D, Dilks J, Isaac B, Lin D, Garraway L, et al. p63 is a prostate basal cell marker and is required for prostate development. Am J Pathol. 2000;157(6):1769–75.

93. Parsons JK, Gage WR, Nelson WG, De Marzo AM. p63 protein expression is rare in prostate adenocarcinoma: implications for cancer diagnosis and carcinogenesis. Urology. 2001;58(4):619–24.

94. Evans AJ. Alpha-methylacyl CoA racemase (P504S): overview and potential uses in diagnostic pathology as applied to prostate needle biopsies. J Clin Pathol. 2003;56(12):892–7.

95. Wu CL, Yang XJ, Tretiakova M, Patton KT, Halpern EF, Woda BA, et al. Analysis of alpha-methylacyl-CoA racemase (P504S) expression in high-grade prostatic intraepithelial neoplasia. Hum Pathol. 2004;35(8):1008–13.

96. Yang XJ, Laven B, Tretiakova M, Blute Jr RD, Woda BA, Steinberg GD, et al. Detection of alpha-methylacyl-coenzyme A racemase in postradiation prostatic adenocarcinoma. Urology. 2003;62(2):282–6.

97. Jiang Z, Fanger GR, Woda BA, Banner BF, Algate P, Dresser K, et al. Expression of alpha-methylacyl-CoA racemase (P504s) in various malignant neoplasms and normal tissues: a study of 761 cases. Hum Pathol. 2003;34(8):792–6.

98. Yang XJ, Wu CL, Woda BA, Dresser K, Tretiakova M, Fanger GR, et al. Expression of alpha-methylacyl-CoA racemase (P504S) in atypical adenomatous hyperplasia of the prostate. Am J Surg Pathol. 2002;26(7):921–5.

99. Jiang Z, Wu CL, Woda BA, Iczkowski KA, Chu PG, Tretiakova MS, Young RH, Weiss LM, Blute Jr RD, Brendler CB, Krausz T, Xu JC, Rock KL, Amin MB, Yang XJ. Alpha-methylacyl-CoA racemase: a multi-institutional study of a new prostate cancer marker. Histopathology. 2004;45(3):218–25.

100. Zhou M, Aydin H, Kanane H, Epstein JI. How often does alpha-methylacyl-CoA-racemase contribute to resolving an atypical diagnosis on prostate needle biopsy beyond that provided by basal cell markers? Am J Surg Pathol. 2004;28(2):239–43.

101. Sanderson SO, Sebo TJ, Murphy LM, Neumann R, Slezak J, Cheville JC. An analysis of the p63/alpha-methylacyl coenzyme A racemase immunohistochemical cocktail stain in prostate needle biopsy specimens and tissue microarrays. Am J Clin Pathol. 2004;121(2):220–5.

102. Tacha DE, Miller RT. Use of p63/P504S monoclonal antibody cocktail in immunohistochemical staining of prostate tissue. Appl Immunohistochem Mol Morphol. 2004;12(1):75–8.

103. Jiang Z, Li C, Fischer A, Dresser K, Woda BA. Using an AMACR (P504S)/34betaE12/p63 cocktail for the detection of small focal prostate carcinoma in needle biopsy specimens. Am J Clin Pathol. 2005;123(2):231–6.

104. Pelengaris S, Khan M, Evan G. c-MYC: more than just a matter of life and death. Nat Rev Cancer. 2002;2(10):764–76.

105. Jenkins RB, Qian J, Lieber MM, Bostwick DG. Detection of c-myc oncogene amplification and chromosomal anomalies in metastatic prostatic carcinoma by fluorescence in situ hybridization. Cancer Res. 1997;57(3):524–31.

106. Sato K, Qian J, Slezak JM, Lieber MM, Bostwick DG, Bergstralh EJ, et al. Clinical significance of alterations of chromosome 8 in high-grade, advanced, nonmetastatic prostate carcinoma. J Natl Cancer Inst. 1999;91(18):1574–80.

107. Kokontis J, Takakura K, Hay N, Liao S. Increased androgen receptor activity and altered c-myc expression in prostate cancer cells after long-term androgen deprivation. Cancer Res. 1994;54(6):1566–73.

108. Montironi R, Filho AL, Santinelli A, Mazzucchelli R, Pomante R, Colanzi P, et al. Nuclear changes in the normal-looking columnar epithelium adjacent to and distant from prostatic intraepithelial neoplasia and prostate cancer. Morphometric analysis in whole-mount sections. Virchows Arch. 2000;437(6):625–34.

109. Klezovitch O, Risk M, Coleman I, Lucas JM, Null M, True LD, et al. A causal role for ERG in neoplastic transformation of prostate epithelium. Proc Natl Acad Sci USA. 2008;105(6):2105–10.

110. Mosquera JM, Perner S, Genega EM, Sanda M, Hofer MD, Mertz KD, et al. Characterization of TMPRSS2-ERG fusion high-grade prostatic intra-epithelial neoplasia and potential clinical implications. Clin Cancer Res. 2008;14(11):3380–5.

111. Park K, Tomlins SA, Mudaliar KM, Chiu YL, Esgueva R, Mehra R, et al. Antibody-based detection of ERG rearrangement-positive prostate cancer. Neoplasia. 2010;12(7):590–8.

112. van Leenders GJ, Boormans JL, Vissers CJ, Hoogland AM, Bressers AA, Furusato B, et al. Antibody EPR3864 is specific for ERG genomic fusions in prostate cancer: implications for pathological practice. Mod Pathol. 2011;24(8):1128–38.

113. Yaskiv O, Zhang X, Simmerman K, Daly T, He H, Falzarano S, et al. The utility of ERG/P63 double immunohistochemical staining in the diagnosis of limited cancer in prostate needle biopsies. Am J Surg Pathol. 2011;35(7):1062–8.

114. Zhang S, Pavlovitz B, Tull J, Wang Y, Deng FM, Fuller C. Detection of TMPRSS2 gene deletions and translocations in carcinoma, intraepithelial neoplasia, and normal epithelium of the prostate by direct fluorescence in situ hybridization. Diagn Mol Pathol. 2010;19(3):151–6.

115. Carver BS, Tran J, Gopalan A, Chen Z, Shaikh S, Carracedo A, et al. Aberrant ERG expression cooperates with loss of PTEN to promote cancer progression in the prostate. Nat Genet. 2009;41(5):619–24.

116. Qian J, Jenkins RB, Bostwick DG. Determination of gene and chromosome dosage in prostatic intraepithelial neoplasia and carcinoma. Anal Quant Cytol Histol. 1998;20(5):373–80.

117. Takahashi S, Qian J, Brown JA, Alcaraz A, Bostwick DG, Lieber MM, et al. Potential markers of prostate cancer aggressiveness detected by fluorescence in situ hybridization in needle biopsies. Cancer Res. 1994;54(13):3574–9.

118. Takahashi S, Alcaraz A, Brown JA, Borell TJ, Herath JF, Bergstralh EJ, et al. Aneusomies of chromosomes 8 and Y detected by fluorescence in situ hybridization are prognostic markers for pathological stage C (pt3N0M0) prostate carcinoma. Clin Cancer Res. 1996;2(1):137–45.

119. Emmert-Buck MR, Vocke CD, Pozzatti RO, Duray PH, Jennings SB, Florence CD, et al. Allelic loss on chromosome 8p12-21 in microdissected prostatic intraepithelial neoplasia. Cancer Res. 1995;55(14):2959–62.

120. Bova GS, Fox WM, Epstein JI. Methods of radical prostatectomy specimen processing: a novel technique for harvesting fresh prostate cancer tissue and review of processing techniques. Mod Pathol. 1993;6(2):201–7.

121. Macoska JA, Trybus TM, Benson PD, Sakr WA, Grignon DJ, Wojno KD, et al. Evidence for three tumor suppressor gene loci on chromosome 8p in human prostate cancer. Cancer Res. 1995;55(22):5390–5.

122. Bostwick DG, Shan A, Qian J, Darson M, Maihle NJ, Jenkins RB, et al. Independent origin of multiple foci of prostatic intraepithelial neoplasia: comparison with matched foci of prostate carcinoma. Cancer. 1998;83(9):1995–2002.

123. Van Den Berg C, Guan XY, Von Hoff D, Jenkins R, Bittner, Griffin C, et al. DNA sequence amplification in human prostate cancer identified by chromosome microdissection: potential prognostic implications. Clin Cancer Res. 1995;1(1):11–8.

124. Visakorpi T, Kallioniemi AH, Syvanen AC, Hyytinen ER, Karhu R, Tammela T, Isola JJ, Kallioniemi OP. Genetic changes in primary and recurrent prostate cancer by comparative genomic hybridization. Cancer Res. 1995;55:342–7.

125. Cher ML, MacGrogan D, Bookstein R, Brown JA, Jenkins RB, Jensen RH. Comparative genomic hybridization, allelic imbalance, and fluorescence in situ hybridization on chromosome 8 in prostate cancer. Genes Chromosomes Cancer. 1994;11(3):153–62.

126. Qian J, Jenkins RB, Bostwick DG. Chromosomal anomalies in atypical adenomatous hyperplasia and carcinoma of the prostate using fluorescence in situ hybridization. Urology. 1995;46(6):837–42.

127. Nupponen NN, Porkka K, Kakkola L, Tanner M, Persson K, Borg A, et al. Amplification and overexpression of p40 subunit of eukaryotic translation initiation factor 3 in breast and prostate cancer. Am J Pathol. 1999;154(6):1777–83.

128. Porkka KP, Tammela TL, Vessella RL, Visakorpi T. RAD21 and KIAA0196 at 8q24 are amplified and overexpressed in prostate cancer. Genes Chromosomes Cancer. 2004;39(1):1–10.

129. Cher ML, Bova GS, Moore DH, Small EJ, Carroll PR, Pin SS, et al. Genetic alterations in untreated metastases and androgen-independent prostate cancer detected by comparative genomic hybridization and allelotyping. Cancer Res. 1996;56(13):3091–102.

130. Joos S, Bergerheim US, Pan Y, Matsuyama H, Bentz M, du Manoir S, et al. Mapping of chromosomal gains and losses in prostate cancer by comparative genomic hybridization. Genes Chromosomes Cancer. 1995;14(4):267–76.

131. Gray IC, Phillips SM, Lee SJ, Neoptolemos JP, Weissenbach J, Spurr NK. Loss of the chromosomal region 10q23-25 in prostate cancer. Cancer Res. 1995;55(21):4800–3.

132. Ittman M, Mansukhani A. Expression of fibroblast growth factors (FGFs) and FGF receptors in human prostate. J Urol. 1997;157(1):351–6.

133. Halvorsen OJ, Haukaas SA, Akslen LA. Combined loss of PTEN and p27 expression is associated with tumor cell proliferation by Ki-67 and increased risk of recurrent disease in localized prostate cancer. Clin Cancer Res. 2003;9(4):1474–9.

134. Carter BS, Epstein JI, Isaacs WB. ras gene mutations in human prostate cancer. Cancer Res. 1990;50(21):6830–2.

135. Latil A, Cussenot O, Fournier G, Driouch K, Lidereau R. Loss of heterozygosity at chromosome

16q in prostate adenocarcinoma: identification of three independent regions. Cancer Res. 1997; 57(6):1058–62.

136. Cunningham JM, Shan A, Wick MJ, McDonnell SK, Schaid DJ, Tester DJ, et al. Allelic imbalance and microsatellite instability in prostatic adenocarcinoma. Cancer Res. 1996;56(19):4475–82.

137. Bergheim USR, Kunimi K, Collins VP, Ekman P. Deletion of chromosome 8, 10 and 16 in human prostatic carcinoma. Genes Chromosomes Cancer. 1991;3:215–20.

138. Sakr WA, Macoska JA, Benson P, Grignon DJ, Wolman SR, Pontes JE, et al. Allelic loss in locally metastatic, multisampled prostate cancer. Cancer Res. 1994;54(12):3273–7.

139. Zincke H, Bergstralh EJ, Larson-Keller JJ, Farrow GM, Myers RP, Lieber MM, et al. Stage D1 prostate cancer treated by radical prostatectomy and adjuvant hormonal treatment. Evidence for favorable survival in patients with DNA diploid tumors. Cancer. 1992;70(1 Suppl):311–23.

140. Haggarth L, Auer G, Busch C, Norberg M, Haggman M, Egevad L. The significance of tumor heterogeneity for prediction of DNA ploidy of prostate cancer. Scand J Urol Nephrol. 2005;39(5):387–92.

141. Bantis A, Gonidi M, Athanassiades P, Tsolos C, Liossi A, Aggelonidou E, et al. Prognostic value of DNA analysis of prostate adenocarcinoma: correlation to clinicopathologic predictors. J Exp Clin Cancer Res. 2005;24(2):273–8.

142. Shankey TV, Kallioniemi OP, Koslowski JM, Lieber ML, Mayall BH, Miller G, et al. Consensus review of the clinical utility of DNA content cytometry in prostate cancer. Cytometry. 1993;14(5):497–500.

143. Amin MB, Schultz DS, Zarbo RJ, Kubus J, Shaheen C. Computerized static DNA ploidy analysis of prostatic intraepithelial neoplasia. Arch Pathol Lab Med. 1993;117(8):794–8.

144. Baretton GB, Vogt T, Blasenbreu S, Lohrs U. Comparison of DNA ploidy in prostatic intraepithelial neoplasia and invasive carcinoma of the prostate: an image cytometric study. Hum Pathol. 1994;25(5):506–13.

145. Nativ O, Winkler HZ, Raz Y, Therneau TM, Farrow GM, Myers RP, et al. Stage C prostatic adenocarcinoma: flow cytometric nuclear DNA ploidy analysis. Mayo Clin Proc. 1989;64(8):911–9.

146. Lorenzato M, Rey D, Durlach A, Bouttens D, Birembaut P, Staerman F. DNA image cytometry on biopsies can help the detection of localized Gleason 3 + 3 prostate cancers. J Urol. 2004;172(4 Pt 1):1311–3.

147. Jones EC, McNeal J, Bruchovsky N, de Jong G. DNA content in prostatic adenocarcinoma. A flow cytometry study of the predictive value of aneuploidy for tumor volume, percentage Gleason grade 4 and 5, and lymph node metastases. Cancer. 1990;66(4):752–7.

148. Tribukait B. DNA flow cytometry in carcinoma of the prostate for diagnosis, prognosis and study of tumor biology. Acta Oncol. 1991;30(2):187–92.

149. Deitch AD, deVere White RW. Flow cytometry as a predictive modality in prostate cancer. Hum Pathol. 1992;23:352–9.

150. Pollack A, Zagars GK. External beam radiotherapy dose response of prostate cancer. Int J Radiat Oncol Biol Phys. 1997;39(5):1011–8.

151. Takai K, Goellner JR, Katzmann JA, Myers RP, Lieber MM. Static image and flow DNA cytometry of prostatic adenocarcinoma: studies of needle biopsy and radical prostatectomy specimens. J Urol Pathol. 1994;2:39–48.

152. Reed JC. Bcl-2 and the regulation of programmed cell death. J Cell Biol. 1994;124:1–6.

153. Reed JC. Bcl-2: prevention of apoptosis as a mechanism of drug resistance. Hematol Oncol Clin N Am. 1995;9:451–74.

154. Hockenbery DM, Zutter M, Hickey W, Nahm M, Korsmeyer SJ. BCL2 protein is topographically restricted in tissues characterized by apoptotic cell death. Proc Natl Acad Sci USA. 1991;88(16): 6961–5.

155. Lipponen P, Vesalaninen S. Expression of the apoptosis suppressing protein bcl-2 in prostatic adenocarcinoma is related to tumour malignancy. Prostate. 1997;32:9–16.

156. Colombel M, Symmans F, Gil S, O'Toole KM, Chopin D, Benson M, et al. Detection of the apoptosis-suppressing oncoprotein bc1-2 in hormone-refractory human prostate cancers. Am J Pathol. 1993;143(2):390–400.

157. Colecchia M, Frigo B, Del Boca C, Guardamagna A, Zucchi A, Colloi D, et al. Detection of apoptosis by the TUNEL technique in clinically localised prostatic cancer before and after combined endocrine therapy. J Clin Pathol. 1997;50(5):384–8.

158. Ittman M, Wieczorek R, Heller P, Dave A, Provet J, Krolewski J. Alterations in the p53 and MDC-2 genes are infrequent in clinically localized stage B prostate adenocarcinomas. Am J Pathol. 1994; 145:287–93.

159. Mottaz AE, Markwalder R, Fey MF, Klima I, Merz VW, Thalmann GN, et al. Abnormal p53 expression is rare in clinically localized human prostate cancer: comparison between immunohistochemical and molecular detection of p53 mutations. Prostate. 1997;31(4):209–15.

160. Navone NM, Troncoso P, Pisters LL, Goodrow TL, Palmer JL, Nichols WW, et al. p53 protein accumulation and gene mutation in the progression of human prostate carcinoma. J Natl Cancer Inst. 1993;85(20): 1657–69.

161. Fan K, Dao DD, Schutz M, Fink LM. Loss of heterozygosity and overexpression of p53 gene in human primary prostatic adenocarcinoma. Diagn Mol Pathol. 1994;3(4):265–70.

162. Moul JW, Bettencourt MC, Sesterhenn IA, Mostofi FK, McLeod DG, Srivastava S, et al. Protein expression of p53, bcl-2, and KI-67 (MIB-1) as prognostic biomarkers in patients with surgically treated, clinically localized prostate cancer. Surgery. 1996;120(2): 159–66. Discussion 66–7.

163. Heidenberg HB, Sesterhenn IA, Gaddipati JP, Weghorst CM, Buzard CM, Moul JW, Srivastava S. Alternation of tumor suppressor gene p53 in a high fraction of hormone refractory prostate cancer. J Urol. 1995;154:414–21.

164. Hall MC, Navone NM, Troncoso P, Pollack A, Zagars GK, von Eschenbach AC, et al. Frequency and characterization of p53 mutations in clinically localized prostate cancer. Urology. 1995;45(3):470–5.

165. Qian J, Hirasawa K, Bostwick DG, Bergstralh EJ, Slezak JM, Anderl KL, et al. Loss of p53 and c-myc overrepresentation in stage T(2–3)N(1–3)M(0) prostate cancer are potential markers for cancer progression. Mod Pathol. 2002;15(1):35–44.

166. Gao X, Chen YQ, Wu N, Grignon DJ, Sakr W, Porter AT, Honn KV. Somatic mutations of the WAF1/CIP1 gene in primary prostate cancer. Oncogene. 1997;11:1395–8.

167. Facher EA, Becich MJ, Deka A, Law JC. Association between human cancer and two polymorphisms occurring in the p21WAF1/CIP1 cyclin-dependent kinase inhibitor gene. Cancer. 1997;79:2424–9.

168. Byrne RL, Horne CH, Robinson MC, Autzen P, Apakama I, Bishop RI, et al. The expression of waf-1, p53 and bcl-2 in prostatic adenocarcinoma. Br J Urol. 1997;79(2):190–5.

169. Tsihlias J, Kapusta LR, DeBoer G, Morava-Protzner I, Zbieranowski I, Bhattacharya N, et al. Loss of cyclin-dependent kinase inhibitor p27Kip1 is a novel prognostic factor in localized human prostate adenocarcinoma. Cancer Res. 1998;58(3):542–8.

170. Nemoto R, Kawamura H, Miyakawa I, Uchida K, Hattori K, Koiso K, et al. Immunohistochemical detection of proliferating cell nuclear antigen (PCNA)/cyclin in human prostate adenocarcinoma. J Urol. 1993;149(1):165–9.

171. Limas C, Frizelle SP. Proliferative activity in benign and neoplastic prostatic epithelium. J Pathol. 1994;174(3):201–8.

172. Carroll PR, Waldman FM, Rosenau W, Cohen MB, Vapnek JM, Fong P, et al. Cell proliferation in prostatic adenocarcinoma: in vitro measurement by 5-bromodeoxyuridine incorporation and proliferating cell nuclear antigen expression. J Urol. 1993;149(2):403–7.

173. Grignon DJ, Hammond EH. College of American Pathologists conference XXVI on clinical relevance of prognostic markers in solid tumors. Report of the prostate cancer working group. Arch Pathol Lab Med. 1995;119(12):1122–6.

174. Idikio HA. Expression of proliferating cell nuclear antigen in node-negative human prostate cancer. Anticancer Res. 1996;16(5A):2607–11.

175. Taplin ME, Bubley GJ, Shuster TD, Frantz ME, Spooner AE, Ogata GK, et al. Mutation of the androgen-receptor gene in metastatic androgen-independent prostate cancer. N Engl J Med. 1995;332(21):1393–8.

176. Haapala K, Hyytinen ER, Roiha M, Laurila M, Rantala I, Helin HJ, et al. Androgen receptor alterations in prostate cancer relapsed during a combined androgen blockade by orchiectomy and bicalutamide. Lab Invest. 2001;81(12):1647–51.

177. Linja MJ, Savinainen KJ, Saramaki OR, Tammela TL, Vessella RL, Visakorpi T. Amplification and overexpression of androgen receptor gene in hormone-refractory prostate cancer. Cancer Res. 2001;61(9):3550–5.

178. Henrique R, Jeronimo C. Molecular detection of prostate cancer: a role for GSTP1 hypermethylation. Eur Urol. 2004;46(5):660–9. Discussion 9.

179. Liu L, Kron KJ, Pethe VV, Demetrashvili N, Nesbitt ME, Trachtenberg J, et al. Association of tissue promoter methylation levels of APC, TGFbeta2, HOXD3, and RASSF1A with prostate cancer progression. Int J Cancer. 2011;129:2454–62.

180. Lewinshtein DJ, Porter CR, Nelson PS. Genomic predictors of prostate cancer therapy outcomes. Expert Rev Mol Diagn. 2010;10(5):619–36.

181. Li Y, Su J, DingZhang X, Zhang J, Yoshimoto M, Liu S, et al. PTEN deletion and heme oxygenase-1 overexpression cooperate in prostate cancer progression and are associated with adverse clinical outcome. J Pathol. 2011;224(1):90–100.

182. Lotan T, Gurel B, Sutcliffe S, Esopi D, Liu W, Xu J, et al. PTEN protein loss by immunostaining: analytic validation and prognostic indicator for a high risk surgical cohort of prostate cancer patients. Clin Cancer Res. 2011;17:6563–73.

183. Bertram J, Peacock JW, Fazli L, Mui AL, Chung SW, Cox ME, et al. Loss of PTEN is associated with progression to androgen independence. Prostate. 2006;66(9):895–902.

184. Squire JA. TMPRSS2-ERG and PTEN loss in prostate cancer. Nat Genet. 2009;41(5):509–10.

185. Yoshimoto M, Cunha IW, Coudry RA, Fonseca FP, Torres CH, Soares FA, et al. FISH analysis of 107 prostate cancers shows that PTEN genomic deletion is associated with poor clinical outcome. Br J Cancer. 2007;97(5):678–85.

186. Burke HB, Goodman PH, Rosen DB, Henson DE, Weinstein JN, Harrell Jr FE, et al. Artificial neural networks improve the accuracy of cancer survival prediction. Cancer. 1997;79(4):857–62.

187. Bock BJ, Bostwick DG. Does prostatic ductal adenocarcinoma exist? Am J Surg Pathol. 1999;23(7):781–5.

188. Ro JY, Grignon DJ, Ayala AG, Fernandez PL, Ordonez NG, Wishnow KI. Mucinous adenocarcinoma of the prostate: histochemical and immunohistochemical studies. Hum Pathol. 1990;21(6):593–600.

189. McNeal JE, Alroy J, Villers A, Redwine EA, Freiha FS, Stamey TA. Mucinous differentiation in prostatic adenocarcinoma. Hum Pathol. 1991;22(10):979–88.

190. Efros MD, Fischer J, Mallouh C, Choudhury M, Geogsson S. Unusual primary prostatic malignancies. Urology. 1992;39(5):407–10.

191. Ishizu K, Yoshihiro S, Joko K, Takihara H, Sakatoku J, Tanaka K. Mucinous adenocarcinoma of the prostate with good response to hormonal therapy: a case report. Hinyokika Kiyo. 1991;37(9):1057–60.

192. Teichman JM, Shabaik A, Demby AM. Mucinous adenocarcinoma of the prostate and hormone sensitivity. J Urol. 1994;151(3):701–2.

193. Guerin D, Hasan N, Keen CE. Signet ring cell differentiation in adenocarcinoma of the prostate: a study of five cases. Histopathology. 1993;22(4): 367–71.

194. Akagashi K, Tanda H, Kato S, Ohnishi S, Nakajima H, Nanbu A, et al. Signet-ring cell carcinoma of the prostate effectively treated with maximal androgen blockade. Int J Urol. 2003;10(8):456–8.

195. Oesterling JE, Hauzeur CG, Farrow GM. Small cell anaplastic carcinoma of the prostate: a clinical, pathological and immunohistological study of 27 patients. J Urol. 1992;147(3 Pt 2):804–7.

196. Abbas F, Civantos F, Benedetto P, Soloway MS. Small cell carcinoma of the bladder and prostate. Urology. 1995;46(5):617–30.

197. di Sant'Agnese PA. Neuroendocrine differentiation in carcinoma of the prostate. Diagnostic, prognostic, and therapeutic implications. Cancer. 1992;70(1 Suppl):254–68.

198. Bostwick DG, Dousa MK, Crawford BG, Wollan PC. Neuroendocrine differentiation in prostatic intraepithelial neoplasia and adenocarcinoma. Am J Surg Pathol. 1994;18(12):1240–6.

199. Ellison E, Chaung S-S, Zincke H, et al. Prostate adenocarcinoma after androgen deprivation therapy. A comparative study of morphology, morphometry, immunohistochemistry, and DNA ploidy. Pathol Case Rev. 1996;1:74–83.

200. Bostwick DG, Qian J, Civantos F, Roehrborn CG, Montironi R. Does finasteride alter the pathology of the prostate and cancer grading? Clin Prostate Cancer. 2004;2(4):228–35.

201. Andriole G, Bostwick D, Civantos F, Epstein J, Lucia MS, McConnell J, et al. The effects of 5alpha-reductase inhibitors on the natural history, detection and grading of prostate cancer: current state of knowledge. J Urol. 2005;174(6):2098–104.

202. Grignon DJ, Bostwick DG, Civantos F, Garnick MB, Gaudin P, Srigley JR. Pathologic handling and reporting of prostate tissue specimens in patients receiving neoadjuvant hormonal therapy: report of the Pathology Committee. Mol Urol. 1999;3:193–8.

203. Montironi R, Schulman CC. Pathological changes in prostate lesions after androgen manipulation. J Clin Pathol. 1998;51(1):5–12.

204. Goldstein NS, Begin LR, Grody WW, Novak JM, Qian J, Bostwick DG. Minimal or no cancer in radical prostatectomy specimens. Report of 13 cases of the "vanishing cancer phenomenon". Am J Surg Pathol. 1995;19(9):1002–9.

205. Patterson RF, Glave ME, Jones EC, Zubovits JT, Goldenberg SL, Sullivan LD. Immunohistochemical analysis of radical prostatectomy specimens after 8 months of neoadjuvant hormonal therapy. Mol Urol. 1999;3:277–86.

206. Gaudin PB, Zelefsky MJ, Leibel SA, Fuks Z, Reuter VE. Histopathologic effects of three-dimensional conformal external beam radiation therapy on benign and malignant prostate tissues. Am J Surg Pathol. 1999;23(9):1021–31.

207. Cheng L, Cheville JC, Pisansky TM, Sebo TJ, Slezak J, Bergstralh EJ, et al. Prevalence and distribution of prostatic intraepithelial neoplasia in salvage radical prostatectomy specimens after radiation therapy. Am J Surg Pathol. 1999;23(7):803–8.

208. Bostwick DG, Egbert BM, Fajardo LF. Radiation injury of the normal and neoplastic prostate. Am J Surg Pathol. 1982;6(6):541–51.

209. Wheeler JA, Zagars GK, Ayala AG. Dedifferentiation of locally recurrent prostate cancer after radiation therapy. Evidence for tumor progression. Cancer. 1993;71(11):3783–7.

210. Cheng L, Darson MF, Bergstralh EJ, Slezak J, Myers RP, Bostwick DG. Correlation of margin status and extraprostatic extension with progression of prostate carcinoma. Cancer. 1999;86(9):1775–82.

211. Kuban DA, el-Mahdi AM, Schellhammer PF. Prognostic significance of post-irradiation prostate biopsies. Oncology (Williston Park). 1993;7(2): 29–38. Discussion 40, 3–4, 7.

212. Crook JM, Bahadur YA, Robertson SJ, Perry GA, Esche BA. Evaluation of radiation effect, tumor differentiation, and prostate specific antigen staining in sequential prostate biopsies after external beam radiotherapy for patients with prostate carcinoma. Cancer. 1997;79(1):81–9.

213. Goldstein NS, Martinez A, Vicini F, Stromberg J. The histology of radiation therapy effect on prostate adenocarcinoma as assessed by needle biopsy after brachytherapy boost. Correlation with biochemical failure. Am J Clin Pathol. 1998;110(6):765–75.

214. Sheaff MT, Baithun SI. Effects of radiation on the normal prostate gland. Histopathology. 1997; 30(4):341–8.

215. Susani M, Madersbacher S, Kratzik C, Vingers L, Marberger M. Morphology of tissue destruction induced by focused ultrasound. Eur Urol. 1993;23 Suppl 1:34–8.

216. Orihuela E, Motamedi M, Pow-Sang M, LaHaye M, Cowan DF, Warren MM. Histopathological evaluation of laser thermocoagulation in the human prostate: optimization of laser irradiation for benign prostatic hyperplasia. J Urol. 1995;153(5):1531–6.

217. Bostwick DG, Larson TR. Transurethral microwave thermal therapy: pathologic findings in the canine prostate. Prostate. 1995;26(3):116–22.

218. Onik G. The male lumpectomy: rationale for a cancer targeted approach for prostate cryoablation. A review. Technol Cancer Res Treat. 2004;3(4): 365–70.

219. Merrick GS, Wallner KE, Butler WM. Prostate cryotherapy: more questions than answers. Urology. 2005;66(1):9–15.

220. Petersen DS, Milleman LA, Rose EF, Bonney WW, Schmidt JD, Hawtrey CE, et al. Biopsy and clinical course after cryosurgery for prostatic cancer. J Urol. 1978;120(3):308–11.

221. Shuman BA, Cohen JK, Miller Jr RJ, Rooker GM, Olson PR. Histological presence of viable prostatic glands on routine biopsy following cryosurgical ablation of the prostate. J Urol. 1997;157(2):552–5.

222. Pisters LL, Dinney CP, Pettaway CA, Scott SM, Babaian RJ, von Eschenbach AC, et al. A feasibility study of cryotherapy followed by radical prostatectomy for locally advanced prostate cancer. J Urol. 1999;161(2):509–14.

223. Corcoran NM, Hong MK, Casey RG, Hurtado-Coll A, Peters J, Harewood L, et al. Upgrade in Gleason score between prostate biopsies and pathology following radical prostatectomy significantly impacts upon the risk of biochemical recurrence. BJU Int. 2011;108:E202–10.

224. Colleselli D, Pelzer AE, Steiner E, Ongarello S, Schaefer G, Bartsch G, et al. Upgrading of Gleason score 6 prostate cancers on biopsy after prostatectomy in the low and intermediate tPSA range. Prostate Cancer Prostatic Dis. 2010;13(2):182–5.

225. Ozden C, Oztekin CV, Ugurlu O, Gokkaya S, Yaris M, Memis A. Correlation between upgrading of prostate biopsy and biochemical failure and unfavorable pathology after radical prostatectomy. Urol Int. 2009;83(2):146–50.

226. Serkin FB, Soderdahl DW, Cullen J, Chen Y, Hernandez J. Patient risk stratification using Gleason score concordance and upgrading among men with prostate biopsy Gleason score 6 or 7. Urol Oncol. 2010;28(3):302–7.

227. Bostwick DG. Grading prostate cancer. Am J Clin Pathol. 1994;102(4 Suppl 1):S38–56.

228. Capitanio U, Karakiewicz PI, Valiquette L, Perrotte P, Jeldres C, Briganti A, et al. Biopsy core number represents one of foremost predictors of clinically significant Gleason sum upgrading in patients with low-risk prostate cancer. Urology. 2009;73(5):1087–91.

229. Iremashvili V, Manoharan M, Pelaez L, Rosenberg DL, Soloway MS. Clinically significant Gleason sum upgrade: external validation and head-to-head comparison of the existing nomograms. Cancer. 2012;118:378–85.

230. Barzell WE, Melamed MR. Appropriate patient selection in the focal treatment of prostate cancer: the role of transperineal 3-dimensional pathologic mapping of the prostate–a 4-year experience. Urology. 2007;70(6 Suppl):27–35.

231. de la Rosette J, Ahmed H, Barentsz J, Johansen TB, Brausi M, Emberton M, et al. Focal therapy in prostate cancer-report from a consensus panel. J Endourol. 2010;24(5):775–80. Endourological Society.

232. Onik G, Miessau M, Bostwick DG. Three-dimensional prostate mapping biopsy has a potentially significant impact on prostate cancer management. J Clin Oncol. 2009;27(26):4321–6.

233. Barqawi AB, Rove KO, Gholizadeh S, O'Donnell CI, Koul H, Crawford ED. The role of 3-dimensional mapping biopsy in decision making for treatment of apparent early stage prostate cancer. J Urol. 2011;186(1):80–5.

234. Taira AV, Merrick GS, Galbreath RW, Andreini H, Taubenslag W, Curtis R, et al. Performance of transperineal template-guided mapping biopsy in detecting prostate cancer in the initial and repeat biopsy setting. Prostate Cancer Prostatic Dis. 2010; 13(1):71–7.

235. Ahmed HU, Hu Y, Carter T, Arumainayagam N, Lecornet E, Freeman A, et al. Characterizing clinically significant prostate cancer using template prostate mapping biopsy. J Urol. 2011;186(2):458–64.

236. Crawford ED, Barqawi A. Targeted focal therapy: a minimally invasive ablation technique for early prostate cancer. Oncology (Williston Park). 2007;21(1):27–32. Discussion 3–4, 9.

237. Gross JL, Masterson TA, Cheng L, Johnstone PA. pT0 prostate cancer after radical prostatectomy. J Surg Oncol. 2010;102(4):331–3.

238. Bostwick DG, Bostwick KC. 'Vanishing' prostate cancer in radical prostatectomy specimens: incidence and long-term follow-up in 38 cases. BJU Int. 2004;94(1):57–8.

239. Capitanio U, Briganti A, Suardi N, Gallina A, Salonia A, Freschi M, et al. When should we expect no residual tumor (pT0) once we submit incidental T1a-b prostate cancers to radical prostatectomy? Int J Urol. 2011;18(2):148–53.

240. Bessede T, Soulie M, Mottet N, Rebillard X, Peyromaure M, Ravery V, et al. Stage pT0 after radical prostatectomy with previous positive biopsy sets: a multicenter study. J Urol. 2010;183(3):958–62.

241. Bostwick DG, Qian J, Drewnowska K, Varvel S, Bostwick KC, Marberger M, et al. Prostate needle biopsy quality in reduction by dutasteride of prostate cancer events study: worldwide comparison of improvement with investigator training and centralized laboratory processing. Urology. 2010;75(6): 1406–10.

242. Marberger M, McConnell JD, Fowler I, Andriole GL, Bostwick DG, Somerville MC, et al. Biopsy misidentification identified by DNA profiling in a large multicenter trial. J Clin Oncol. 2011;29(13): 1744–9.

243. Organizations JCoAoHC. Laboratory national patient safety goals. Available from: http://www.jointcommission.org/standards_information/npsgs.aspx. Accessed 27 Dec 2011

Complications of Transrectal Ultrasound-Guided Prostate Biopsy

17

Ian M. Thompson III, Sam S. Chang,
and Michael S. Cookson

Introduction

Current estimates predict that over one million men have undergone transrectal ultrasound-guided biopsy (TRUS-Bx) of the prostate in the United States of America (USA) this year alone. Due to a variety of factors including the widespread use of PSA testing coupled with an aging population, the number of men subjected to TRUS-Bx has increased annually over the past decade and will likely continue for the foreseeable future. This trend is not limited to the USA as evidenced by a significant increase in the number of prostate biopsies performed over the past decade in other countries as well [1]. Given the volume of the procedures currently performed, coupled with the trends toward a continued increase, certainly the safety and potential morbidity of this procedure is worthy of examination.

In addition to the increasing number of procedures, recent data suggest that the morbidity from TRUS-Bx of the prostate is also increasing. In fact, a recent retrospective population-based cohort study demonstrated that complication

rates have increased fourfold during a 10-year period [2]. Although prostate biopsy is usually generally safe and usually well tolerated in the outpatient setting, it remains an invasive procedure with associated risks and potential complications. Wantanabe et al. first described transrectal ultrasound of the prostate in 1968, but its use as a guide in systematic biopsy of the prostate was first described two decades later by Hodge et al. [3, 4]. Over the past twenty-plus years, the technique and sampling strategies of TRUS-Bx have been continually refined. To improve cancer detection, there has been an increase in the number of biopsy cores obtained during a single session as well as positioning the biopsies more posteriorly and laterally to accentuate the sampling of the peripheral zone [5]. To reduce discomfort, use of local anesthesia in the form of a periprostatic block and/or use of sedation has been included in the scope of practice [1, 6].

Although these refinements represent improvements in both cancer detection and patient acceptance, they also have the potential to contribute to the overall morbidity of the procedure. Strategies designed to reduce the risks and morbidity associated with TRUS-Bx have been developed and continue to evolve as new challenges present themselves. This is especially of importance when it comes to interventions designed to reduce periprocedural infection. In this chapter, we review the morbidity associated with contemporary TRUS-Bx of the prostate, risk factors for specific complications, and present strategies to reduce these complications. The content to follow

I.M. Thompson III , M.D. • S.S. Chang, M.D.
Department of Urologic Surgery, Vanderbilt University
Medical Center, Nashville, TN, USA

M.S. Cookson, M.D., MMHC (✉)
Department of Urologic Surgery, Vanderbilt University
Medical Center, A – 1302 MCN, Nashville,
TN 37232-2765, USA
e-mail: Michael.Cookson@vanderbilt.edu

J.S. Jones (ed.), *Prostate Cancer Diagnosis: PSA, Biopsy and Beyond*, Current Clinical Urology,
DOI 10.1007/978-1-62703-188-2_17, © Springer Science+Business Media New York 2013

is designed to guide clinicians in perioperative management of patients undergoing TRUS-Bx of the prostate, as well as an aid in counseling patients utilizing the most currently available information in the context of the evidence-based medicine.

Overview of Complications

Since the inception of its use as method for cancer detection, reports on the complications associated with prostate biopsy have been widely variable. Reasons for the variability include differences in methods of data collection and reporting, biopsy technique, and patient characteristics. Additionally, the highly variable methods for pre-procedural preparation including antibiotic prophylaxis, choice and duration of antibiotic, use of anesthesia and technique, and use of a cleansing enema are some of the confounders when trying to calculate complication rates and compare series. Over the past decade, there has been a growing amount of research to further refine the risk factors for complications associated with prostate biopsy and an attempt to develop best practice guidelines to minimize the morbidity of this procedure for patients. Where available, we have incorporated this evidence and subsequent recommendations into our current chapter.

Bleeding

Bleeding is the most common complication to occur after TRUS-Bx of the prostate and can manifest as hematuria, hematospermia, and rectal bleeding [7, 8]. Hematuria is usually minor and represents the most common of these bleeding complications. It usually resolves with conservative measures within a week [9]. Up to 70% of patients undergoing prostate biopsy can be expected to experience some degree of hematuria [9, 10].

With respect to bleeding following TRUS-Bx, studies have shown conflicting data between the amount of bleeding complications and number of cores obtained. In a prospective, randomized trial of 6- versus 12-core prostate biopsy, Naughton et al. demonstrated significantly increased incidence of hematospermia and hematochezia in patients undergoing 12-core biopsy as compared to a 6-core strategy [11]. In a retrospective review of nearly 6,000 prostate biopsies, Berger et al. demonstrated and reported a significant increase in hematospermia with increasing cores taken, although no significant increase in hematuria or hematochezia was seen [12]. By comparison, Ghani et al. showed no significant increase in hematospermia or hematuria associated with increasing number of cores [13]. In addition to the number of cores, incidence of bleeding after prostate biopsy has been shown to correlate significantly with the volume of the prostate gland [8]. Of 115 sexually active men in their cohort, Peyromaure et al. found a 78% incidence of hematospermia following a 10-core biopsy strategy [14]. While the studies above show no significant difference in hematuria associated with increased number of cores taken at biopsy, Eskew et al. demonstrated a higher rate of hematuria after biopsy, 80% of patients, in their study evaluating a five-region biopsy, which included midline biopsies [15]. The increased incidence of hematuria with midline biopsy was thought to be most likely due to penetration of the urethra with the biopsy needle. Since the majority of prostate cancer arises from the peripheral zone, needle biopsies should be directed at the lateral aspects of the prostate in order to increase cancer detection and decrease morbidity that can be seen with sampling along the midline [16].

Rectal bleeding is another common complication associated with prostate biopsy with reports demonstrating an incidence of 2–37% [7]. Immediate and brisk bleeding can occur during the time of the procedure when a hemorrhoidal vessel is punctured, but this can usually be managed with manual compressions and/or temporary rectal packing. In most cases, rectal bleeding is a minor complication and usually resolves within a couple of days following the biopsy. There are rare instances when additional intervention is needed, including proctoscopy with fulguration and/or suturing.

The incidence of hematospermia after prostate biopsy is varied as well and can be seen in 10–78% of men, with it being less likely in older men and in men with history of previous transurethral resection of prostate [8]. Both hematochezia and hematospermia can be seen increasingly with extended biopsy approaches, though these are usually mild and self-limited, resolving without need for intervention [11, 12, 14]. In a prospective evaluation of bleeding-related complications in 760 men, Ghani et al. demonstrated no significant increase in hematospermia or hematuria, but did show a significant increase in rectal bleeding incidence when more than 6 cores were obtained [13]. Though the rectal bleeding was usually self-limited, duration of which was not associated with number of cores taken on biopsy; only one patient required hospitalization [13]. They also found no significant increase in rectal bleeding between patients that had received a periprostatic block and those that had not received a block [13].

Medications Associated with Bleeding Complications

When possible, it is best to reduce risk factors associated with complications in order to mitigate any morbidity of prostate biopsy. With regard to bleeding associated with biopsy, the provider should always be aware of all medications, both prescription and over-the-counter (OTC) medications, that a patient is currently taking. It is best, when safe, to have patients discontinue all medications and supplements that can alter their coagulation or platelet function prior to performing a prostate biopsy.

One of the most commonly prescribed medications in patients presenting for consultation for an elevated PSA is aspirin. In general, aspirin should be discontinued 10 days prior to procedure if possible [17]. Before discontinuing aspirin (or any antiplatelet or anticoagulant), it is a good clinic practice to consult with the prescribing physician in order to ensure that it is safe to temporarily discontinue this form of therapy. Aspirin works by irreversibly inactivating cyclooxygenase in platelets, which last for the entire circulating life of the platelet, 7–10 days [18]. Thus, if aspirin is to be temporarily withheld, it should be held 10 days prior to the procedure in order for all platelets to function properly.

Not all studies have shown that aspirin needs to be discontinued prior to TRUS-Bx. In fact, several studies have demonstrated the safety of continuing low-dose aspirin up to and after time of prostate biopsy [9, 19–21]. In a prospective evaluation of 128 men undergoing biopsy, Rodriguez et al. showed significant association of rectal bleeding with increase in number of cores, but no difference associated with use of aspirin or NSAIDs, nor the time period in which they were stopped prior to biopsy [9]. In a retrospective review of 1,438 TRUS-Bx procedures, Zaytoun et al. found an increased risk of infectious complications (OR = 2.69, 95% CI = 1.31–5.55, $P=0.007$) and clinically relevant hematospermia (OR = 3.54, 95% CI = 1.02–12.24, $P=0.046$) in those patients that had taken anticoagulant or antiplatelet therapy within 10 days of biopsy [22]. In their prospective cohort study of 200 men, Maan et al. evaluated the effect of low-dose aspirin on morbidity after sextant biopsy of the prostate [20]. Those patients that regularly took low-dose aspirin were encouraged to continue it both before and after biopsy; this included 36 patients. Twenty (56%) of those patients on aspirin had hematuria compared to 83 (59%) of those not on aspirin [20]. Overall, they found no significant difference in bleeding-related complications between those that had taken aspirin prior to biopsy and those that did not [20].

With these conflicting data, it is not surprising that there remains controversy with regard to this issue. A survey-based study conducted by Connor et al. demonstrated the variability in management of pre-procedure anticoagulation among different providers. Fifty-two percent of radiologists and 27% of urologists had patients stop aspirin prior to biopsy; 95% of radiologists and 84% of urologists stopped warfarin prior to biopsy, though urologists tended to have patients stop these medications for longer periods of time prior to biopsy [23]. A prospective study of 530 men undergoing TRUS-Bx of prostate was conducted by Kariotis et al. to determine whether the administration of periprocedural low-dose aspirin would increase the risk of bleeding complications [21]. They demonstrated no significant differences in the incidence of hematuria (64.5% vs. 60.6%, $p=0.46$), rectal bleeding (33.6% vs. 25.9%, $p=0.09$), or hematospermia (90.1% vs. 86.9%, $p=0.45$), though they did show a significantly greater duration of hematuria and rectal bleeding in the aspirin group compared to the control group [21]. Discontinuation of any medications with anticoagulation properties prior to TRUS-Bx is a good strategy for reducing the risk of bleeding complications, though the literature does support the safety of continuing low-dose aspirin and NSAIDs, and they are not an absolute contraindication to proceeding with biopsy. In fact, practices vary between the authors of this chapter regarding aspirin discontinuation.

Given the older age of most men undergoing TRUS-Bx and the likelihood of them having comorbidities, it is not uncommon for the urologist to encounter patients on other therapeutic anticoagulation modalities, such as warfarin. In our practice, it has been a policy to avoid biopsy while patients are on warfarin. In this situation, it should be discussed with the physician prescribing the warfarin as to whether it is safe for the patient to come off the anticoagulation in order to perform the prostate biopsy safely. According to the guideline put forth by the American College of Chest Physicians, warfarin should be discontinued 5 days prior to the planned procedure [24].

As previously mentioned, in a survey-based study of current practices of practitioners that perform TRUS-Bx, Connor et al. found that 16% of UK urologists they surveyed would perform TRUS-Bx on patients receiving warfarin [23]. In a prospective assessment of 1,022 patients undergoing TRUS-Bx, Ihezue et al. identified 49 patients undergoing biopsy while on warfarin, and they found that those patients on warfarin had no significant increase in bleeding complications [25]. Of the 49 patients on warfarin, 18 (36.7%) experienced hematuria, compared to 440 (60.2%) patients with no anticoagulant medication who reported hematuria, ($p=0.001$), and 7

(14.3%) patients on warfarin reported rectal bleeding compared to 95 (13%) of patients on no anticoagulant medication, ($p=0.80$) [25]. Though some reassurance might be found in these data, the numbers in this study are small, and given the risk associated with bleeding coupled with the elective nature of the procedure, it is probably best to discontinue warfarin 5 days prior to prostate biopsy to mitigate any increased risk of bleeding complications.

Additional anticoagulation medications are also commonly encountered in this patient population. One class of drugs includes clopidogrel (Plavix) and ticlopidine (Ticlid), which act by irreversibly inhibiting ADP receptors on platelets, thus inhibiting platelet aggregation and adhesiveness, though ticlopidine is no longer used because of increased risk of bleeding and severe neutropenia [26]. Newer drugs in this class that may be encountered more in the future include prasugrel, ticagrelor, cangrelor, and elinogrel [26]. As mentioned previously, discontinuation of these medications in order to perform TRUS-Bx needs to be discussed first with the prescribing physician. Patients that have had a bare-metal cardiac stent placed must continue on combination antiplatelet therapy, aspirin and clopidogrel, for at least 6 weeks after stent placement [24]. Patients that have had a drug-eluting cardiac stent placed are recommended to continue on aspirin and clopidogrel for at least 12 months before discontinuing these medications for any elective surgical procedure [24]. If surgical procedures are planned prior to reaching these 6-week and 12-month marks, it is recommended that aspirin and clopidogrel be continued up until and after the procedure [24]. Therefore, we advise delaying TRUS-Bx if at all possible until these time points are reached to reduce the risk of stent thrombosis. Since bleeding complications are the most common of those associated with TRUS-Bx, it is important that the patient be counseled regarding the incidence, severity, and the expected duration of bleeding after prostate biopsy. If these symptoms persist beyond the expected time period, the patient should contact his physician.

Infectious Complications

Infectious complications are the second most common morbidity associated with TRUS-Bx of the prostate. Even though most infections resulting from prostate biopsy are minor, the potential for serious infection certainly exists and in fact represents one of the most feared complications after prostate biopsy. The incidence of infectious complications, including sepsis and even death, after TRUS-Bx of the prostate is reported to be on the rise and poses a real challenge for patient safety as we move forward over the next several decades. As patients and physicians have now become increasingly aware of the magnitude of the problem, strategies to reduce or eliminate these infectious complications are urgently needed.

Several studies have shown that asymptomatic bacteriuria and transient bacteremia are not uncommon in patients undergoing TRUS-Bx and not receiving prophylactic antibiotics, with a reported incidence of 20–53% and 16–73%, respectively [27]. In a prospective study evaluating complications in 415 patients undergoing TRUS-Bx without prophylactic antibiotics, the incidence of infectious complications was 2.9% [10]. In the European Randomized Study of Screening for Prostate Cancer, with all men receiving prophylactic antibiotics, 3.3% developed post-procedural fever, but only ~0.4% required admission for suspected sepsis [8]. Despite these relatively low numbers, life-threatening infectious complications can occur and even result in death [28]. Unfortunately, the incidence of infectious complications has increased over the past decade due in part to the rise of organisms with various antibiotic resistances [29].

General consensus does exist among practicing urologists that the risk of infectious complications associated with TRUS-Bx are reduced, but not completely eliminated, with the use of prophylactic antibiotics [30–32]. The benefit of prophylactic antibiotics prior to TRUS-Bx has also been demonstrated in placebo-controlled studies [33, 34]. There have been numerous regimens of periprocedural antibiotics proposed to reduce the incidence of infectious complications,

though there are no clear data that support one single antibiotic or dosing regimen as superior to any other.

In fact, the results of multiple surveys of urologist's practice patterns have demonstrated quite varied approaches including at least 19 different types of antibiotics and 48 different dosages and administration schedules [31, 35, 36]. In one of these surveys inquiring as to pre-biopsy protocols, a total of 900 practicing urologists were randomly selected by the American Urological Association (AUA) to participate [36]. Of these, 568 (63%) returned the completed survey. The results demonstrated marked variability in pre-biopsy protocols among those urologists; 11 different antibiotics were used, with 20 different doses and 23 different timing-duration regimens. Nearly all of the surveyed urologists (98.6%) utilized prophylactic antibiotics, and the majority (81%) used a pre-procedural rectal enema.

Though the response of some practitioners to the risk of infectious complications has been to increase the duration of periprocedural antibiotics, several studies have demonstrated the effectiveness of even just a single dose of antibiotics prior to TRUS-Bx [34, 37, 38]. One such study prospectively randomized 537 patients from five different institutions to receive either 500-mg oral ciprofloxacin or placebo before TRUS-Bx [34]. Urinalysis and urine culture were obtained within 24 h prior to biopsy and then at 2–6 days and again at 9–15 days after TRUS-Bx. Of note, all patients in both arms received a cleansing rectal enema prior to TRUS-Bx. The primary determinant of efficacy was bacteriologic response (bacteriuria [more than 10^4 colony-forming units (CFU)/mL] vs. no bacteriuria) at the 9–15-day follow-up evaluation. Six ciprofloxacin-treated patients (3%) and 19 placebo-treated patients (8%) had post-procedure bacteriuria ($p=0.009$) [34]. Six ciprofloxacin-treated patients (3%) and 12 placebo-treated patients (5%) demonstrated signs and symptoms of urinary tract infection ($p=0.166$). One ciprofloxacin recipient (0.4%) and four placebo recipients (1.5%) were hospitalized for post-procedure febrile UTI. The ciprofloxacin recipient demonstrated pre-biopsy bacteriuria and was later disqualified from efficacy analysis.

In another study, 231 patients from a single institution were prospectively randomized to receive either placebo twice daily for 3 days, a single dose of ciprofloxacin 500 mg and tinidazole 600 mg, and then placebo twice daily for five additional doses, or ciprofloxacin 500 mg and tinidazole 600 mg in combination twice daily for a total of 3 days [33]. All patients received pre-procedural rectal enema. Urine cultures were then obtained in all patients 48 h after biopsy, and blood cultures were obtained in patients who developed fever within 7 days of biopsy. They demonstrated a significant reduction in infections among those patients treated with antibiotics versus placebo, but no significant difference was demonstrated between those patients that received the single-dose pre-biopsy versus the 3-day course. They thus concluded that a single dose of prophylactic antibiotic was sufficient [33]. Other studies have demonstrated low rates of infectious complications (2.5–3.5%) with both a pre-procedural and post-procedural dose of antibiotics [8, 9].

In the 2011 Cochrane Review, the question of antibiotic prophylaxis prior to prostate biopsy was analyzed via literature search, during which more than 3,500 references were considered and 19 original reports with a total of 3,599 patients were included [39]. Nine trials analyzing periprocedural antibiotic versus placebo or no treatment were reviewed and all outcomes have significantly favored the use of antibiotics. In short, the authors concluded that there are no definitive data to confirm that a long course of antibiotics (3 days) is superior to a short course (1 day) or that multiple dose treatment is superior to a single dose of an antibiotic [39].

Acknowledging the wide variability among urologists in administration of periprocedural antibiotics, the AUA convened a Best Practice Policy Panel to formulate recommendations for antibiotic prophylaxis during urologic surgery [40]. Based on the evidence examined (Level Ib), the panel recommended antibiotic prophylaxis for all TRUS-Bx procedures with duration of therapy of ≤ 24 h. In addition, the AUA recommendations include a fluoroquinolone as the antimicrobial of choice with alternatives to

include clindamycin or an aminoglycoside plus metronidazole [40]. Another departure from routine practice in the past is that the American Heart Association no longer recommends the use of antibiotic prophylaxis prior to urological procedures for the prevention of infective endocarditis [41].

The landscape of infectious complications resulting from TRUS-Bx is evolving and becoming more of a concern for practitioners nationally and internationally as most are seeing a rise in urosepsis and an increasing number of antibiotic-resistant organisms. The widespread use of fluoroquinolone antibiotics has undoubtedly contributed to the growing numbers of fluoroquinolone-resistant (FQR) bacteria. In their study of a 5% random sample of Medicare participants from the SEER database from 1991 to 2007, Loeb et al. sought to determine if there was evidence for increasing incidence of infectious complications after prostate biopsy [29]. They demonstrated significantly higher rates of hospitalizations for both infectious and noninfectious reasons (6.9% overall) during the 30-day post-biopsy period compared to controls (2.7%). They also demonstrated increased incidence of hospitalization for infectious diagnoses over time [29].

In their recent retrospective cohort review from 2004 to 2006, Feliciano et al. demonstrated a 2.4% post-biopsy infection rate, half of the cases (overall 1.2%) were attributable to FQR organisms [42]. When patients were stratified by year, they also demonstrated a significant increase in infectious complications and incidence of fluoroquinolone resistance year to year [42]. Recent and current research efforts have focused on identifying those patients that are at greater risk of developing post-biopsy infection with resistant organisms. Liss et al. sought to determine the incidence of FQR *E. coli* in men undergoing TRUS-Bx at three separate institutions [43]. Between January 2009 and March 2010, they enrolled 136 men who were scheduled to undergo TRUS-Bx of prostate with antibiotic prophylaxis and rectal preparation determined by the physician performing the biopsy. Immediately prior to prostate biopsy, rectal swab cultures were obtained. Overall, 30 patients (22%) had rectal cultures positive for FQR *E. coli*. 103 of the 136 men had undergone previous TRUS-Bx with 24% of those men having positive rectal cultures for FQR *E. coli* compared to 15% in those with no history of prior biopsy [43]. Batura et al. also investigated this question in their recent cohort of 592 patients undergoing TRUS-Bx, in which 75.1% underwent rectal swab culture prior to biopsy, and 10.6% of this group demonstrated FQR organisms [44]. Madden et al. observed an interesting trend when they conducted their retrospective chart review of patients undergoing TRUS-Bx, between 2008 and 2009, in a UK teaching hospital [45]. Hospitals in the UK witnessed a gradual increase in rates of Clostridium difficile infections (CDI) in the late 1990s as well as several outbreaks of a hypervirulent epidemic strain that was strongly linked to widespread use of fluoroquinolones. In 2003, mandatory reporting of CDI rates was introduced and subsequently followed with restrictions on use of broad-spectrum antibiotics, including fluoroquinolones. Prior to the implementation of these antibiotic stewardship programs, the standard antibiotic regimen for urological procedures was ciprofloxacin alone. In 2008, the standard regimen for all surgical procedures at this institution, including urological procedures, was changed to co-amoxiclav and gentamicin. During the period of study, the rate of infectious complications for all patients who received ciprofloxacin prophylaxis prior to TRUS-Bx was 2.4%, whereas the rate of infectious complications in those patients that received gentamicin and co-amoxiclav prior to TRUS-Bx was 12.9%, a significant difference ($p < 0.001$). In a retrospective review of 1,446 patients undergoing TRUS-Bx at a single institution between 2001 and 2010, Zaytoun et al. reported that 40 patients (2.77%) developed an infectious complication, 31 (2.14%) with febrile UTI and 9 (0.62%) with sepsis [46]. Of the nine patients that developed sepsis, *E. coli* was identified in the blood of seven patients, 4 (57.1%) of which were fluoroquinolone resistant; 53.8% of those patients with febrile UTI had fluoroquinolone-resistant *E. coli* identified on urine culture [46]. Based on the microbiologic characteristics of the bacteria isolates in those patients that were found to be

septic, the authors recommend empiric treatment with a broad-spectrum cephalosporin for post-biopsy infections after standard fluoroquinolone prophylaxis [46].

Given the growing concern for the rise in post-biopsy infections, Hedelin et al. recently performed a retrospective review of their patients to evaluate the incidence of febrile infections requiring hospital admission after TRUS-Bx [47]. Between January 2006 and December 2009, 1,633 patients underwent TRUS-Bx, and 57 of these (3.5%) developed febrile infections requiring admission. All patients undergoing biopsy received norfloxacin 400 mg twice daily for 3 days, beginning just prior to the procedure and no rectal enemas were used prior to biopsy. Blood and urine cultures were performed in all but 2 of the 57 men, and then IV antibiotic treatment was instituted upon admission. Urine cultures showed growth of *E. coli* in 18 patients, while *Morganella* and *Enterobacter* were cultured from another patient. Two of the *E. coli* strains were fluoroquinolone resistant. The blood cultures of 18 patients grew *E. coli* with 6 strains demonstrating FQR and 2 strains with intermediate sensitivity. Blood cultures were more often positive in patients presenting within 24–48 h after biopsy compared to patients admitted after 2–3 days post-biopsy ($p = 0.04$) [47]. Fluoroquinolone-resistant strains were more commonly isolated in blood cultures of those patients presenting within 48 h of biopsy compared to those that presented 2–3 days after biopsy ($p = 0.001$) [47]. FQR *E. coli* was often isolated on blood cultures of patients with a febrile reaction within 48 h of biopsy and never from patients after ≥2 days of biopsy ($p < 0.001$) [47].

Another less appreciated factor that could be influencing the rise of FQR organisms is the frequent use of household products containing the antiseptic triclosan, often found in "antibacterial" soaps [48]. Exposure to triclosan can induce mutations at the drug target site, chromosome-mediated drug efflux, and overexpression of the target protein [49]. Though difficult to quantify the extent to which this could be influencing the recent rise in FQR organisms in the urologic patient population, it certainly could be playing a role.

Obtaining prostate needle biopsies via the transrectal route is in part to blame for many of the infectious complications, most likely due to the seeding of the needle tract with rectal flora. There has been debate as to the value of having patients do a cleansing enema or a bowel preparation to decrease the rectal flora at time of TRUS-Bx. Some studies have recommended the use of enemas [27, 37, 50, 51]. Other studies have argued that against the need for enema prior to biopsy [52, 53]. In a survey of a randomly selected group of 900 urologists conducted in 1996, 81% reported that they utilized enema in their patient preparation for TRUS-Bx [36]. In a prospective study of 50 men undergoing TRUS-Bx, Lindert et al. randomized 25 men to receive pre-procedural enema and 25 to no enema [27]. Pre-procedural urine culture and questionnaire were obtained as well as post-procedural urine and blood cultures and post-procedural questionnaire. Bacteriuria was seen in 44% of the cases and bacteremia in 16% of the patients, 87.5% of whom did not receive pre-biopsy enema ($p=0.0003$) [27]. The patients in this study did not receive pre-procedural antibiotics, so the application of these results may be limited.

In their recent retrospective review of TRUS-Bx's at a single institution to assess for incidence of FQR infectious complications, Mosharafa et al. showed no significant reduction in infectious prostatitis with use of pre-biopsy enema [54]. Similarly, a retrospective review of prostate biopsy in 448 men was performed, 410 of whom were analyzed after exclusions [53]. A total of 225 patients received an enema prior to TRUS-Bx, while 185 did not. All patients received an identical regimen of pre-procedural ciprofloxacin. Of those that received enema, 4.4% developed significant complications compared to 3.2% of those that did not receive an enema ($p=0.614$) [53]. Of those patients that received an enema, two were hospitalized for retention and urinary tract infection, while one patient who did not receive an enema was hospitalized for hematuria and clot retention. None of the patients that did not receive an enema were admitted to the hospital for an infectious complication [53]. The conclusion from the results of this study was that a pre-biopsy enema did not significantly reduce the risk of infectious complications.

In a more recent study, a retrospective analysis of patients undergoing TRUS-Bx was done to assess difference in infectious complication before and after implementation of pre-procedural bowel cleansing regimen [55]. All patients in the cohort of 407 patients received pre-biopsy ciprofloxacin starting the day prior to the biopsy and continued for 3 days afterward. The first group, 190 patients, was instructed only to take clear liquids after midnight the day before the procedure, while the second group, consisting of 217, was instructed to consume only clear liquids 24 h prior to biopsy. In addition, this second group was also instructed to take an enema the night before and the morning of the procedure. The authors concluded no significant reduction in post-biopsy sepsis ($p=0.189$) [55].

Another recent study retrospectively assessed the influence of pre-biopsy administration of a povidone-iodine suppository prior to TRUS-Bx on infectious complications [56]. A total of 481 patients were studied, 360 of whom received the suppository immediately prior to TRUS-Bx and 121 patients who did not. All patients received a single injection of a 3rd-generation cephalosporin and oral administration of cefixime (100 mg) morning of day of biopsy and then continued for 5 days thereafter [56]. Only one infectious complication was found in the group that had received the suppository, consisting of fever without sepsis. Of the eight patients who developed an infectious complication in the group that did not receive the suppository, two developed sepsis and six developed fever without sepsis. The authors concluded that there was a significant reduction in febrile infectious complications in those patients that received the pre-biopsy povidone-iodine suppository ($p=0.001$) [56]. Rectal swabs were taken for culture before suppository placement and after TRUS-Bx for in vitro studies. They showed that the rectal preparation decreased the mean number of colony-forming units by 99.9% ($p=0.002$) [56].

Patients undergoing TRUS-Bx need to be counseled carefully regarding the risks, benefits, and alternatives of this procedure. They need to be well informed as to the signs and symptoms of post-biopsy infection and be given an action plan in case these were to occur, such as calling the clinic staff and/or reporting promptly to a local hospital for evaluation.

Infectious complications continue to be a real and growing concern. The goal of the practitioner is to undertake every effort to mitigate the risk factors for these infectious complications related to TRUS-Bx. As stated in the AUA guidelines, all patients undergoing TRUS-Bx should receive periprocedural antimicrobial prophylaxis for up to 24-h duration, with a fluoroquinolone being the drug of choice. Going forward, additional studies will need to be performed critically assessing strategies designed to the risk of infectious complications associated with TRUS-Bx while simultaneously not adding to the increasing pool of resistant organisms.

Urinary Retention

Urinary retention is a known complication of TRUS-Bx, usually occurring less than 2% of the time, though it has been reported to occur as high as 10% [8, 57, 58]. The incidence of retention tends to be higher in those patients that undergo saturation biopsy of the prostate under general anesthesia, presumably increased based on the anesthetic [57, 58]. In the series by Borboroglu et al., 57 men undergoing extensive TRUS-Bx were studied. In this cohort, where an average of 22.5 cores were taken, urinary retention was reported in six patients (10%) and resolved within 72 h [58]. Most cases of urinary retention that occur after TRUS-Bx can be managed with an indwelling catheter or self-intermittent catheterization over the short term before normal micturition ability returns. Use of an alpha-blocker, in some cases, can help to expedite the return of spontaneous voiding.

Vasovagal Episodes

Vasovagal episodes can be a common occurrence during office-based procedures, including TRUS-Bx. In their prospective series evaluating the complications associated with TRUS-Bx, Rodriguez and Terris found that 5.3% of the cohort experienced at least a moderate vasovagal episode, which was defined as a systolic blood pressure less than 90 mm Hg, diaphoresis, and bradycardia necessitating intravenous fluid resuscitation. They did have one patient that experienced a severe vasovagal episode that induced a seizure and subsequently required admission of the patient to the hospital. Anxiety itself can lead to a vasovagal episode during prostate biopsy, but it can also be caused by rectal distention with the ultrasound probe resulting in vasodilation of the gastrointestinal vasculature and subsequently lead to hypoperfusion of the brain [59]. Relative hypoglycemia is also thought to be a contributing risk factor for the development of a vasovagal episode, and as such, patients should be encouraged to eat at least a small meal prior to the procedure [59]. The clinic should be prepared to deal with such an episode including placing the patient in the Trendelenburg position as well as starting intravenous fluids.

Pain

Of the complications associated with TRUS-Bx, pain is one of the most prevalent, and practitioners have made a growing effort over the past couple of decades to mitigate this pain. Pain is a more subjectively assessed complication of the procedure compared to other assessments. In patient surveys, pain to some degree has been reported, ranging from severe in 7%, "painful" in 22%, to "acceptable discomfort" in up to 80% [60–62]. Though, Irani et al. found that 19% of 81 patients surveyed would refuse to undergo further TRUS-Bx without analgesia [63]. Predictors of a higher rate of subjective pain include increasing number of cores, repeat biopsies, and patient age with higher levels of pain associated with younger patients [64].

In an effort to reduce the pain associated with TRUS-Bx, several analgesic strategies have been employed, including intrarectal lidocaine gel, periprostatic nerve block (PNB), and general anesthesia. Pre-procedural placement of intrarectal lidocaine gel is one of the most commonly utilized techniques for the reduction of biopsy pain. Randomized studies comparing the use of intrarectal lidocaine gel compared to placebo have yielded conflicting results. Whereas some groups have reported significant benefit in pain reduction with lidocaine gel over placebo [65, 66], other groups have been unable to demonstrate any significant reduction in pain with use of lidocaine gel [67–69]. Despite lack of convincing evidence as to its efficacy, use of intrarectal lidocaine gel is still common in clinical practice.

Nash et al. first described the use of periprostatic nerve block (PNB) [6]. They conducted a randomized, double-blind study on 64 patients undergoing systematic TRUS-Bx. Patients were randomized to receive either an injection of 5 mL of 1% lidocaine or 5 mL of saline at the vascular pedicle on one side of the prostate only, and then patients were asked to score level of discomfort of both the injection and the subsequent biopsies on each side [6]. Patients reported significantly lower pain scores when the side injected with lidocaine was compared to the saline injected side ($p < 0.0001$) [6].

Subsequent studies have reported improved techniques for periprostatic nerve block with lidocaine, such as that by Soloway and Obek where they built on the original technique and recommended additional injections at the apex and between the base and apex [70]. Obek et al. later went on to assess the morbidity associated with lidocaine PNB, whereby they randomized 100 patients undergoing TRUS-Bx to receive a PNB or no anesthesia. They found significantly greater bacteriuria in post-biopsy urine cultures in those that had received a PNB as well as more frequent fever (>37.8 C) in the PNB group [71]. In fact, two patients in the PNB group required hospitalization after biopsy. They also showed similar amount of urethral bleeding between the two groups and significantly less rectal bleeding in those patients that received PNB [71].

None of the anesthetic methods, however, consistently decreased discomfort associated with rectal placement of the ultrasound probe. This is one reason why general anesthesia and sedation have become more common for TRUS-Bx in recent years, mostly dictated by patient preference. In a recent audit conducted by the Urological Society of Australia and New Zealand in 2007, a surprising 86% of urologists performed TRUS-Bx under either sedation or general anesthesia [1]. This, however, has not become a standard of care as the vast majority of these procedures are safely done in the office setting.

Conclusion

Prostate biopsy continues to be a commonly performed outpatient procedure, with relatively low rates of complications. The most common complications are related to bleeding, most of which are self-limiting and resolve with conservative measures. Measures to mitigate the risk of bleeding include periprocedural discontinuation of antiplatelet and other anticoagulant therapy, though some studies have demonstrated the safety of continuation of aspirin through time of TRUS-Bx. Pain associated with TRUS-Bx is usually minimal, especially with the use of periprostatic nerve block and/or use of sedation.

Infectious complications, including sepsis, are currently increasing and becoming more concerning. This is within the context of increasing infections due to antimicrobial-resistant organisms, often FQR *E. coli*. Despite multiple studies demonstrating considerable variance in periprocedural antibiotic administration, the AUA Best Practice Policy Statement recommends antimicrobial administration just prior to biopsy and up to a 24-h total time period. Fluoroquinolones are recommended as antibiotic of choice, but one should be aware of the patient's previous history. Despite common use, there is insufficient evidence to support the routine use of rectal enemas. Additional research is evaluating strategies to reduce risk of infection after TRUS-Bx of the prostate, including use of combinations of antimicrobials, the use of rectal swab cultures to tailor periprocedural antibiotics, and additional strategies and combinations of mechanical cleansings, suppositories, and antibiotics.

In general, the risks, benefits, alternatives, and potential harms of TRUS-Bx of the prostate should be thoroughly reviewed with patients before proceeding with biopsy. Patients should be made aware of which symptoms to be aware and when they should call the clinic or report to the emergency department, as early intervention can reduce significant morbidity and even death. Evaluation of each patient and modification of their respective risk factors is important in reducing overall risk of complications.

Editorial Commentary:

Post-biopsy infection was uncommon a decade ago, but has significantly increased in frequency based on widespread fluoroquinolone resistance. Recognizing that none of the methods described in this chapter or the earlier one on patient preparation will eliminate this risk, it is critical to assure that patients know to report fevers as soon as possible. Due to multidrug resistance, urine and blood cultures should be obtained if at all possible.

We still observe that many patients with post-biopsy infection are given fluoroquinolones by the emergency room—a completely illogical choice. The fact that the patient has developed an infection despite being on a fluoroquinolone means that he has resistant strains and that this regimen is probably destined to fail. Alternative broad-spectrum coverage is in order, with most reports suggesting a third-generation cephalosporin if the patient is hospitalized, or oral cephalexin if ambulatory management appears to be clinically reasonable.

References

1. Hossack T, Woo HH. Acceptance of repeat transrectal ultrasonography guided prostate biopsies with local anaesthesia. BJU Int. 2011;107(Suppl 3):38–42.
2. Nam RK, et al. Prospective multi-institutional study evaluating the performance of prostate cancer risk calculators. J Clin Oncol. 2011;29(22):2959–64.
3. Watanabe H, et al. Diagnostic application of ultrasonotomography to the prostate. Nippon Hinyokika Gakkai Zasshi. 1968;59(4):273–9.
4. Hodge KK, et al. Random systematic versus directed ultrasound guided transrectal core biopsies of the prostate. J Urol. 1989;142(1):71–4. Discussion 74–5.
5. Chang JJ, et al. Prospective evaluation of lateral biopsies of the peripheral zone for prostate cancer detection. J Urol. 1998;160(6 Pt 1):2111–4.
6. Nash PA, et al. Transrectal ultrasound guided prostatic nerve blockade eases systematic needle biopsy of the prostate. J Urol. 1996;155(2):607–9.
7. Djavan B, et al. Safety and morbidity of first and repeat transrectal ultrasound guided prostate needle biopsies: results of a prospective European prostate cancer detection study. J Urol. 2001;166(3):856–60.
8. Raaijmakers R, et al. Complication rates and risk factors of 5802 transrectal ultrasound-guided sextant biopsies of the prostate within a population-based screening program. Urology. 2002;60(5):826–30.
9. Rodriguez LV, Terris MK. Risks and complications of transrectal ultrasound guided prostate needle biopsy: a prospective study and review of the literature. J Urol. 1998;160(6 Pt 1):2115–20.
10. Enlund AL, Varenhorst E. Morbidity of ultrasound-guided transrectal core biopsy of the prostate without prophylactic antibiotic therapy. A prospective study in 415 cases. Br J Urol. 1997;79(5):777–80.
11. Naughton CK, et al. Pain and morbidity of transrectal ultrasound guided prostate biopsy: a prospective randomized trial of 6 versus 12 cores. J Urol. 2000;163(1):168–71.
12. Berger AP, et al. Complication rate of transrectal ultrasound guided prostate biopsy: a comparison among 3 protocols with 6, 10 and 15 cores. J Urol. 2004;171(4):1478–80. Discussion 1480–1.
13. Ghani KR, Dundas D, Patel U. Bleeding after transrectal ultrasonography-guided prostate biopsy: a study of 7-day morbidity after a six-, eight- and 12-core biopsy protocol. BJU Int. 2004;94(7):1014–20.
14. Peyromaure M, et al. Pain and morbidity of an extensive prostate 10-biopsy protocol: a prospective study in 289 patients. J Urol. 2002;167(1):218–21.
15. Eskew LA, Bare RL, McCullough DL. Systematic 5 region prostate biopsy is superior to sextant method for diagnosing carcinoma of the prostate. J Urol. 1997;157(1):199–202. Discussion 202–3.
16. Presti Jr JC, et al. The optimal systematic prostate biopsy scheme should include 8 rather than 6 biopsies: results of a prospective clinical trial. J Urol. 2000;163(1):163–6. Discussion 166–7.
17. Rietbergen JB, et al. Complications of transrectal ultrasound-guided systematic sextant biopsies of the prostate: evaluation of complication rates and risk factors within a population-based screening program. Urology. 1997;49(6):875–80.
18. Masood J, et al. Aspirin use and transrectal ultrasonography-guided prostate biopsy: a national survey. BJU Int. 2007;99(5):965–6.
19. Herget EJ, et al. Transrectal ultrasound-guided biopsy of the prostate: relation between ASA use and bleeding complications. Can Assoc Radiol J. 1999;50(3):173–6.
20. Maan Z, et al. Morbidity of transrectal ultrasonography-guided prostate biopsies in patients after the continued use of low-dose aspirin. BJU Int. 2003;91(9):798–800.

21. Kariotis I, et al. Safety of ultrasound-guided transrectal extended prostate biopsy in patients receiving low-dose aspirin. Int Braz J Urol. 2010;36(3):308–16.

22. Zaytoun OM, et al. Morbidity of prostate biopsy after simplified versus complex preparation protocols: assessment of risk factors. Urology. 2011;77(4):910–4.

23. Connor SE, Wingate JP. Management of patients treated with aspirin or warfarin and evaluation of haemostasis prior to prostatic biopsy: a survey of current practice amongst radiologists and urologists. Clin Radiol. 1999;54(9):598–603.

24. Hirsh J, et al. Executive summary: American College of Chest Physicians evidence-based clinical practice guidelines (8th edn). Chest. 2008;133(6 Suppl):71S–109.

25. Ihezue CU, et al. Biopsy of the prostate guided by transrectal ultrasound: relation between warfarin use and incidence of bleeding complications. Clin Radiol. 2005;60(4):459–63. Discussion 457–8.

26. Sikka P, Bindra VK. Newer antithrombotic drugs. Indian J Crit Care Med. 2010;14(4):188–95.

27. Lindert KA, Kabalin JN, Terris MK. Bacteremia and bacteriuria after transrectal ultrasound guided prostate biopsy. J Urol. 2000;164(1):76–80.

28. Brewster SF, et al. Fatal anaerobic infection following transrectal biopsy of a rare prostatic tumour. Br J Urol. 1993;72(6):977–8.

29. Loeb S, et al. Complications after prostate biopsy: data from SEER-Medicare. J Urol. 2011;186(5):1830–4.

30. Crawford ED, et al. Prevention of urinary tract infection and sepsis following transrectal prostatic biopsy. J Urol. 1982;127(3):449–51.

31. Taylor HM, Bingham JB. The use of prophylactic antibiotics in ultrasound-guided transrectal prostate biopsy. Clin Radiol. 1997;52(10):787–90.

32. Davison P, Malament M. Urinary contamination as a result of transrectal biopsy of the prostate. J Urol. 1971;105(4):545–6.

33. Aron M, Rajeev TP, Gupta NP. Antibiotic prophylaxis for transrectal needle biopsy of the prostate: a randomized controlled study. BJU Int. 2000;85(6):682–5.

34. Kapoor DA, et al. Single-dose oral ciprofloxacin versus placebo for prophylaxis during transrectal prostate biopsy. Urology. 1998;52(4):552–8.

35. Sieber PR, et al. Antibiotic prophylaxis in ultrasound guided transrectal prostate biopsy. J Urol. 1997;157(6):2199–200.

36. Shandera KC, Thibault GP, Deshon Jr GE. Variability in patient preparation for prostate biopsy among American urologists. Urology. 1998;52(4):644–6.

37. Shandera KC, Thibault GP, Deshon Jr GE. Efficacy of one dose fluoroquinolone before prostate biopsy. Urology. 1998;52(4):641–3.

38. Bates TS, Porter T, Gingell JC. Prophylaxis for transrectal prostatic biopsies: a randomized controlled study of intravenous co-amoxiclav given as a single dose compared with an intravenous dose followed by oral co-amoxiclav for 24h. Br J Urol. 1998;81(4):529–31.

39. Zani EL, Clark OA, Rodrigues Netto Jr N. Antibiotic prophylaxis for transrectal prostate biopsy. Cochrane Database Syst Rev. 2011;5:CD006576.

40. Wolf Jr JS, et al. Best practice policy statement on urologic surgery antimicrobial prophylaxis. J Urol. 2008;179(4):1379–90.

41. Wilson W, et al. Prevention of infective endocarditis: guidelines from the American Heart Association: a guideline from the American Heart Association Rheumatic Fever, Endocarditis, and Kawasaki Disease Committee, Council on Cardiovascular Disease in the Young, and the Council on Clinical Cardiology, Council on Cardiovascular Surgery and Anesthesia, and the Quality of Care and Outcomes Research Interdisciplinary Working Group. Circulation. 2007;116(15):1736–54.

42. Feliciano J, et al. The incidence of fluoroquinolone resistant infections after prostate biopsy–are fluoroquinolones still effective prophylaxis? J Urol. 2008;179(3):952–5. Discussion 955.

43. Liss MA, et al. Prevalence and significance of fluoroquinolone resistant *Escherichia coli* in patients undergoing transrectal ultrasound guided prostate needle biopsy. J Urol. 2011;185(4):1283–8.

44. Batura D, Rao GG, Nielsen PB. Prevalence of antimicrobial resistance in intestinal flora of patients undergoing prostatic biopsy: implications for prophylaxis and treatment of infections after biopsy. BJU Int. 2010;106(7):1017–20.

45. Madden T, et al. Infective complications after transrectal ultrasound-guided prostate biopsy following a new protocol for antibiotic prophylaxis aimed at reducing hospital-acquired infections. BJU Int. 2011;108(10):1597–602.

46. Zaytoun OM, et al. Emergence of fluoroquinolone-resistant *Escherichia coli* as cause of postprostate biopsy infection: implications for prophylaxis and treatment. Urology. 2011;77(5):1035–41.

47. Hedelin H, Claesson BE, Wilpart A. Febrile reactions after transrectal ultrasound-guided prostatic biopsy: a retrospective study. Scand J Urol Nephrol. 2011;45(6):393–6.

48. Terris MK. TRUS—is current prophylaxis appropriate and adequate? AUA News. 2011;16(8):8.

49. Aiello AE, Larson EL, Levy SB. Consumer antibacterial soaps: effective or just risky? Clin Infect Dis. 2007;45(Suppl 2):S137–47.

50. Melekos MD. Efficacy of prophylactic antimicrobial regimens in preventing infectious complications after transrectal biopsy of the prostate. Int Urol Nephrol. 1990;22(3):257–62.

51. Jeon SS, et al. Bisacodyl rectal preparation can decrease infectious complications of transrectal ultrasound-guided prostate biopsy. Urology. 2003;62(3):461–6.

52. Vallancien G, et al. Systematic prostatic biopsies in 100 men with no suspicion of cancer on digital rectal examination. J Urol. 1991;146(5):1308–12.

53. Carey JM, Korman HJ. Transrectal ultrasound guided biopsy of the prostate. Do enemas decrease clinically significant complications? J Urol. 2001;166(1):82–5.

54. Mosharafa AA, et al. Rising incidence of acute prostatitis following prostate biopsy: fluoroquinolone resistance and exposure is a significant risk factor. Urology. 2011;78(3):511–4.

55. Ruddick F, et al. Sepsis rates after ultrasound-guided prostate biopsy using a bowel preparation protocol in a community hospital. J Ultrasound Med. 2011; 30(2):213–6.

56. Park DS, Oh JJ, Lee JH, Jang WK, Hong YK, Hong SK. Simple use of the suppository type povidone-iodine can prevent infectious complications in transrectal ultrasound-guided prostate biopsy. Adv Urol. 2009:750598.

57. Stewart CS, et al. Prostate cancer diagnosis using a saturation needle biopsy technique after previous negative sextant biopsies. J Urol. 2001;166(1):86–91. Discussion 91–2.

58. Borboroglu PG, et al. Extensive repeat transrectal ultrasound guided prostate biopsy in patients with previous benign sextant biopsies. J Urol. 2000;163(1):158–62.

59. Rodriguez LV, Terris MK. Risks and complications of transrectal ultrasound. Curr Opin Urol. 2000; 10(2):111–6.

60. Aus G, et al. Transrectal ultrasound examination of the prostate: complications and acceptance by patients. Br J Urol. 1993;71(4):457–9.

61. Collins GN, et al. Multiple transrectal ultrasound-guided prostatic biopsies–true morbidity and patient acceptance. Br J Urol. 1993;71(4):460–3.

62. Bastide C, et al. Tolerance of pain during transrectal ultrasound-guided biopsy of the prostate: risk factors. Prostate Cancer Prostatic Dis. 2003;6(3):239–41.

63. Irani J, et al. Patient tolerance of transrectal ultrasound-guided biopsy of the prostate. Br J Urol. 1997;79(4):608–10.

64. Autorino R, et al. How to decrease pain during transrectal ultrasound guided prostate biopsy: a look at the literature. J Urol. 2005;174(6):2091–7.

65. Issa MM, et al. A randomized prospective trial of intrarectal lidocaine for pain control during transrectal prostate biopsy: the Emory University experience. J Urol. 2000;164(2):397–9.

66. Saad F, et al. A prospective randomized trial comparing lidocaine and lubricating gel on pain level in patients undergoing transrectal ultrasound prostate biopsy. Can J Urol. 2002;9(4):1592–4.

67. Chang SS, et al. Intrarectal lidocaine during transrectal prostate biopsy: results of a prospective double-blind randomized trial. J Urol. 2001; 166(6):2178–80.

68. Cevik I, et al. Lack of effect of intrarectal lidocaine for pain control during transrectal prostate biopsy: a randomized prospective study. Eur Urol. 2002;42(3): 217–20.

69. Desgrandchamps F, et al. The rectal administration of lidocaine gel and tolerance of transrectal ultrasonography-guided biopsy of the prostate: a prospective randomized placebo-controlled study. BJU Int. 1999;83(9):1007–9.

70. Soloway MS, Obek C. Periprostatic local anesthesia before ultrasound guided prostate biopsy. J Urol. 2000;163(1):172–3.

71. Obek C, et al. Is periprostatic local anesthesia for transrectal ultrasound guided prostate biopsy associated with increased infectious or hemorrhagic complications? A prospective randomized trial. J Urol. 2002; 168(2):558–61.

Management of High-Grade Prostatic Intraepithelial Neoplasia (HGPIN)

18

Krishna Ramaswamy, Herbert Lepor, and Samir S. Taneja

Introduction

The diagnosis of isolated high-grade prostatic intraepithelial neoplasia (HGPIN) is based on findings of atypical nuclei in cells lining architecturally benign glands. This premalignant entity is associated with increased risk of coexistent cancer or delayed progression to carcinoma. Extended biopsy schemes have improved the ability to rule out concurrent cancers, increased the detection of isolated HGPIN, and removed the routine necessity for immediate repeat biopsy. Current evidence suggests that men with isolated HGPIN have a continued risk of developing prostate cancer during long-term follow-up, regardless of the changes in the serum PSA level.

To date, no consensus has been reached with regard to interval, frequency, and technique of repeat biopsy. Our multidisciplinary group at New York University Langone Medical Center (NYULMC) suggests empiric interval biopsies every 2–3 years in the follow-up of men with isolated HGPIN found by extended core biopsy. Some authors advocate earlier biopsy for men who have high volume of HGPIN on initial biopsy, but current data are difficult to interpret.

Regardless, we believe that our approach appears to result in a diagnosis of a substantial number of clinically significant cancers that are still organ-confined at the time of pathological review.

Background

Prostatic intraepithelial neoplasia (PIN) is defined by the abnormal proliferation of the secretory epithelium within prostatic ducts and acini without the invasion of the basement membrane [1]. The diagnosis of high-grade prostatic intraepithelial neoplasia (HGPIN) is based on findings of atypical nuclei in cells lining architecturally benign glands. The nuclear atypia, specifically, the presence of prominent nucleoli, is the basic difference between low-grade PIN and HGPIN [2]. It is now widely accepted that low-grade PIN should not be reported by pathologists because of its poor interobserver reproducibility, its resemblance to benign prostate, and its lack of clinical significance [3]. The histopathologic diagnosis of HGPIN has excellent interobserver reproducibility between pathologists [4].

Incidence

Incidence in Screening Population

The incidence of HGPIN can be estimated from autopsy, cystoprostatectomy (CP), radical prostatectomy (RP), or biopsy series. It is assumed

K. Ramaswamy, M.D. • H. Lepor, M.D.
• S.S. Taneja, M.D. (✉)
Division of Urologic Oncology, Department of Urology,
New York University Langone Medical Center
(NYULMC), 150 East 32nd Street, Suite 200,
New York, NY 10016, USA
e-mail: Samir.Taneja@nyumc.org

that biopsy series greatly underestimate the incidence due to sampling error. Among autopsy series, incidence may vary with age and ethnicity. These series allow assessment of the factors that influence the prevalence of HGPIN. Additionally, the frequency of coexistent cancer can be best estimated from autopsy series as well. While biopsy series generally underestimate the true prevalence of HGPIN, they may allow selection of "clinically significant" cases through selection of higher volume HGPIN.

Autopsy and Radical (Cysto) Prostatectomy Series

The prevalence of HGPIN in autopsy series ranges from 37.8% to 84.4% [5–9]. This variability is influenced by several factors, including age, PSA, race/ethnicity, and the accurate diagnosis of HGPIN. The largest series to date was reported by Sakr et al. who showed that age and race distribution of HGPIN parallels prostate cancer. The authors retrospectively analyzed 370 prostates in a population that was comprised of African Americans (60%) and Caucasians (40%). HGPIN was observed in 18%, 3%, 69%, 78%, and 86% of African American men and in 14%, 21%, 38%, 50%, and 63% of Caucasian men in the fourth, fifth, sixth, seventh, and eighth decades, respectively. They also found more extensive HGPIN in African Americans in every decade of life

compared to a matched cohort of Caucasians. Furthermore, when compared to a matched cohort of 345 controls who underwent RP, the incidence of HGPIN was similar when stratified for age and race [7].

The incidence of concomitant HGPIN reported in RP/CP specimens provides the opportunity to examine whether there is a direct association between HGPIN and clinically relevant prostate cancer. The frequent concomitant existence of prostate cancer alongside HGPIN provides provocative evidence to the premalignant/precancerous nature of this entity. Troncoso et al. found that all 100 CP specimens that presented with incidental prostate cancer also harbored HGPIN [10]. This finding was confirmed by Kim in 2002 where all 21 CP specimens harboring incidental prostate cancer also showed HGPIN [11]. Similarly, Silvestri et al. studied 130 autopsy prostates and 70 RP and CP whole-mount specimen with prostate cancer in an Italian population and found HGPIN in 70% and 100% of the autopsy prostates and RP/CP specimens, respectively [5].

Biopsy Series

Epstein et al. reported that the incidence of HGPIN on needle biopsy varies from 0.6% to 25% (see Table 18.1 for a representative sample) with a median incidence of around 4% [2]. These investigators did not identify any trends related to the type

Table 18.1 Incidence of HGPIN in contemporary extended biopsy series and risk of prostate cancer

Author	Year	Patients	No. of cores (minimum)	Incidence of HGPIN (%)	Risk of subsequent prostate cancer (%)	Median interval to repeat biopsy (months)
Herawi [26]	2006	323	8	–	13.3	4.6
Schoenfield [35]	2007	9	24	26	33	13
Bostwick [34]	2009	594	14[a]	40.2	19	4.6
De Nunzio [38]	2009	117	12	22	18.8	6
Roscigno [24]	2010	72	12	–	21.8	12
Lee [30]	2010	328	11	18.2	36.3	Variable
Merrimen [39]	2010	120	10	53.3	20.8	9
Laurila 2010 [65][b]	2010	n/a	10	2.3/3/6.4	27.8/13.8/10.5	6
Godoy [29]	2011	112	12	–	31.2	34.4/66.2[c]

[a]Median number of cores
[b]Finland arm of the European Randomized Study of Screening for Prostate Cancer (ERSPC) only – initially used sextant biopsy schema; 10–12-core biopsies adapted after Round 2 in (2002). Figures for the three rounds of biopsies are shown in the dataset
[c]Patients underwent delayed interval biopsies at 3-year intervals

of practice setting (community hospital, commercial laboratory, or academic institution), number of cores, or era. Interestingly, Bostwick and Qian observed that the lowest likelihood of diagnosing HGPIN was in men participating in screening and early detection programs, with incidences ranging from 0.7% to 20%, whereas men seen by urologists in practice had a diagnosis of 4.4–25% [3]. The variation in incidence in some of the more contemporary series may be explained by the fact that a more extended biopsy scheme may lead to an increased sampling of the gland with a subsequent increase in the diagnosis of HGPIN.

Other factors accounting for the marked variation in the incidence of HGPIN include the absence of strict diagnostic criteria and definitions, the variable number of cores used at baseline sampling, and differences in the nonstandardized pathological techniques [2]. Additionally, differences in age, ethnicity, and familial predisposition among the study populations, and disparities in the biopsy indications, contribute to the observed prevalence of HGPIN.

As the number of prostate biopsies performed annually in the United States increases, the number of cases with isolated HGPIN similarly increases. Aggregate data on the number of prostate biopsies performed in the United States is incomplete, but some estimate the number of prostate biopsies done annually in the USA to be approximately one to one and a half million [12]. In the last decade, there has been agreement that patients with HGPIN need to be followed closely with repeat biopsies, but there exists no validated or central guidelines. The need for risk stratification in this group is becoming increasingly paramount. In this chapter we provide an evaluation of pertinent literature and an evidence-based algorithm for management.

Risk of Subsequent Prostate Cancer

Risk of Cancer on Immediate Repeat Biopsy

Following the initial descriptions of HGPIN [8], it was recognized that among men with isolated HGPIN on biopsy, immediate repeat biopsy resulted in a high likelihood of cancer detection [13, 14]. This observation was consistent with autopsy studies demonstrating a high rate of coexistent prostate cancer and HGPIN [5–9]. Therefore, after an initial sextant prostate biopsy, immediate repeat biopsy resulted in cancer detection in 13.2–100% of men [13–21]. Therefore, the standard of care generally included immediate repeat biopsy with extended core sampling (within 3 months) for all men with isolated HGPIN on sextant prostate biopsy.

In the late 1990s, the standard biopsy evaluation for men presenting with suspicion of prostate cancer evolved to a 10–12 core sampling. It was observed that when men with isolated HGPIN on 12 core biopsy underwent repeat biopsy, cancer was rarely found. In 2001, our group retrospectively evaluated 43 men from a Veterans Administration cohort who underwent repeat biopsy within one year of diagnosis of HGPIN on 12-core biopsy. Only 2.3% of men were found to have cancer [22].

Conversely, in 2004, Naya et al. biopsied 1,086 men using an extended biopsy scheme and 175 men without cancer underwent at least one repeat biopsy (range 1–3; median interval between biopsies, 3 months). Among these 175 patients, 47 had HGPIN on initial biopsy. Repeat biopsy identified cancer in 18.3% of the 175 men. Of the 47 men with HGPIN, only 5 (10.6%) were found to have cancer on repeat biopsy. The number of biopsy specimens positive for HGPIN on initial biopsy was not associated with the likelihood of prostate cancer on repeat biopsy. In follow-up, neither the presence of HGPIN nor the number of cores containing HGPIN on initial biopsy was a significant predictor for prostate cancer on repeat biopsy [23].

It is known that increasing core number on repeat biopsy increases cancer detection. In 2010 Roscigno et al. [24] reported the results of 193 men with HGPIN initial biopsy with 6–24 random cores. All patients underwent a "saturation" re-biopsy with 18–26 cores with a median time to re-biopsy of 12 months. When stratified according to number of cores sampled, prostate cancer was detected at a much higher rate in men who had less than or equal to 12 cores at initial biopsy (35.5% vs. 16.8%; HR – 3.62). They reported a much higher rate of prostate cancer diagnosis at one year, possibly explained by the much more aggressive biopsy strategy. Nonetheless, given that some patients were only biopsied with 6 cores initially, it is likely that this influenced the ultimate detection rate.

Subsequently, several investigators reported similar outcomes, concluding that immediate repeat biopsy following the diagnosis of isolated HGPIN on extended core biopsy is not necessary and that the risk of undetected cancer in these men is comparable to that of men with a benign biopsy [19, 25, 26].

Risk of Cancer in Long-Term Follow-Up

The consensus among investigators was that immediate repeat biopsy following diagnosis of isolated HGPIN on extended biopsy was not necessary [19, 22, 25, 26]; the long-term natural history of isolated HGPIN remained poorly understood. Following the observation of low likelihood of cancer on immediate repeat sampling in 2001 [22], our group followed with a second study in which empiric biopsy performed three years after the diagnosis of HGPIN on extended core prostate biopsy yielded a much higher prostate cancer detection rate of 25.8%, independent of changes in PSA [27]. In this small prospective evaluation, 31 men were invited to undergo biopsy 3 years after the diagnosis of isolated HGPIN on a minimum 12-core sampling. Neither PSA nor volume of HGPIN on baseline biopsy was predictive of the risk cancer in follow-up. All of the men with diagnosed cancers who underwent RP had pathologically organ-confined disease, suggesting that a 3-year interval for surveillance was a reasonable time interval for obligatory repeat biopsy. Based upon this study, we proposed that serial sampling on a 3-year interval was an appropriate method for surveillance of men with isolated HGPIN on biopsy. In 2008, we presented an algorithm for the management of patients with isolated HGPIN based upon further follow-up (see Fig. 18.1 for an updated version) [28].

In early 2011, Godoy et al. reported on further matured follow-up from our series previously reported by Lefkowitz et al. Using this strategy, men underwent a second mandatory surveillance biopsy regardless of changes in PSA or DRE findings, but if rising PSA was noted, earlier "for cause" biopsy was allowed. Using a surveillance strategy of empiric delayed biopsies every 2–3 years, a cancer detection rate of 22.3% was reported for 112 men undergoing biopsy at a mean of 34.4 months after baseline diagnosis of HGPIN. In follow-up, 47 men had undergone a second surveillance biopsy at 66.2 months from baseline with cancer detected in 23.4%. In total, cancer was diagnosed in 32.1% of men at a median follow-up of 46.6 months [29].

In this series, 63.6% of men had a Gleason score of ≥ 7 indicating clinically significant disease, and all men undergoing surgery had pathologically organ-confined disease. The stability of the PSA level or the absence of HGPIN on repeat biopsy did not lower the risk of subsequent cancer detection on delayed biopsies. While PSAV, defined as (>0.75 ng/ml/year) was not a significant predictor of progression in the short term, it became a significant predictor of cancer when evaluating men diagnosed with cancer in the long term [29]. We concluded that the evidence of the sustained risk of cancer on follow-up interval biopsy, the high likelihood of clinically significant cancer, and the lack of reliable indicators of cancer during follow-up suggest that active surveillance using empiric interval biopsies every 2–3 years should be the routine follow-up strategy for men with isolated HGPIN found by extended core biopsy.

Similarly, the likelihood of a delayed cancer diagnosis in men with isolated HGPIN was reported to be 19% (4 of 21) at repeat biopsy at 36 months of follow-up by Abdel-Khalek et al. in 2004 [17]. All patients in that series had undergone repeat biopsy because of either concerning changes found on DRE or an increased PSAV, unlike the data from the NYULMC series, in which men underwent repeat biopsy regardless of changes in the DRE findings or PSA level. It is important to note that the initial set of biopsies in this series was only six cores, followed by extended core sampling on repeat biopsies.

A more recent report by Lee et al. from the Cleveland Clinic Foundation (CCF) in 2010

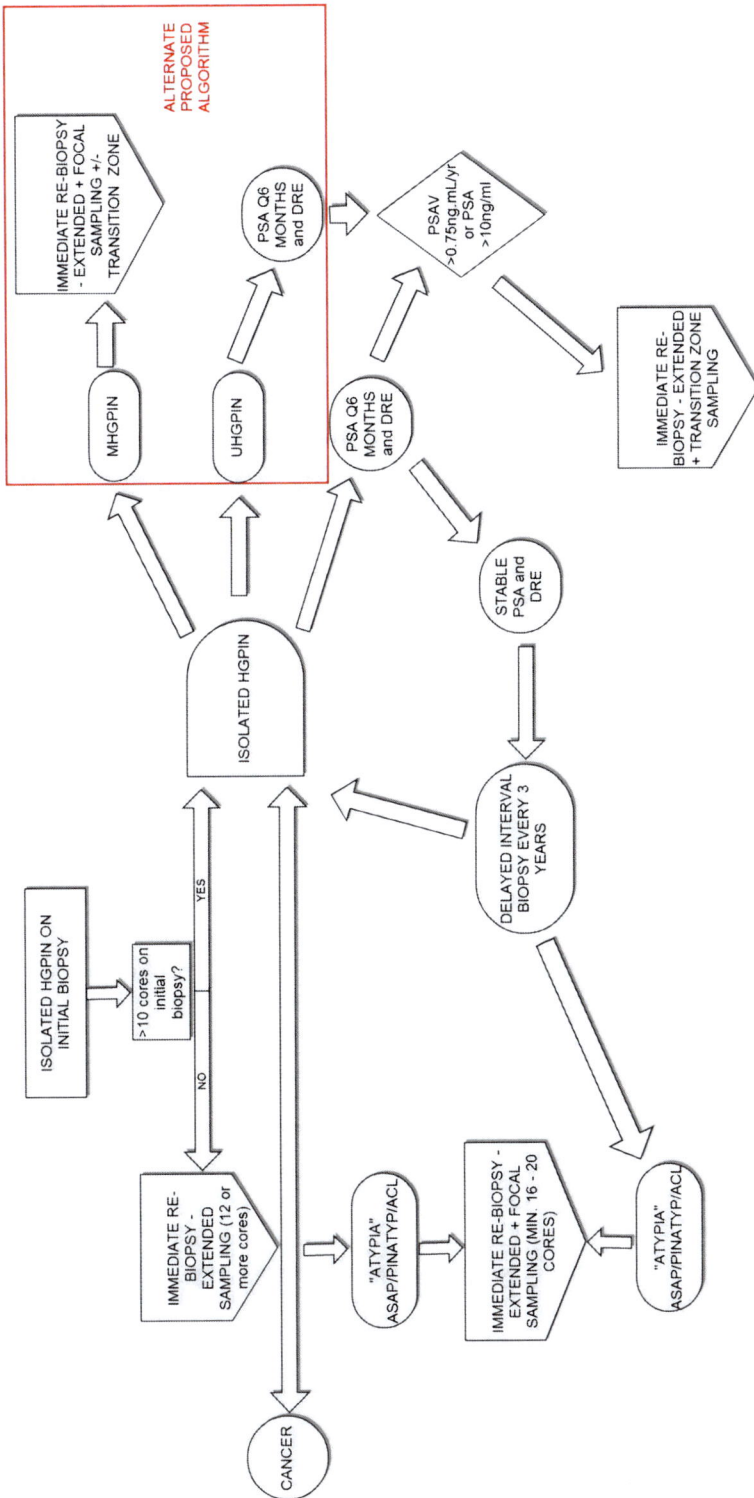

Fig. 18.1 Proposed algorithm for the management of HGPIN

compared repeat biopsy findings for 338 men initially diagnosed with HGPIN to 335 controls who underwent repeat biopsy without HGPIN based on clinical suspicion alone [30]. They found that HGPIN on initial extended core biopsy had an overall hazard ratio of 1.89 for prediction of cancer irrespective of PSA, DRE, age, or number of cores sampled [30]. It is important to note that the decision to perform repeat prostate biopsy was at the discretion of the individual surgeon and no standardized schedule was followed.

Conversely, Gallo et al. compared repeat biopsy findings for 65 patients with HGPIN who underwent repeat biopsy at 3–12, 13–24, 25–36, and 37–48 months after initial biopsy, with a mean of 16 cores, to 65 matched controls. They observed that the risk for cancer after HGPIN diagnosis (21.5%) was not higher than the risk after a benign diagnosis (23.0%) – PSA and HGPIN focality at biopsy did not enhance prostate cancer prediction. They concluded that patients with an HGPIN diagnosis do not seem to need any different follow-up re-biopsy strategy than patients with a benign diagnosis on initial biopsy [31].

Predictors of Cancer on Follow-Up

Unifocal Versus Multifocal HGPIN

HGPIN and prostate cancer are morphometrically and phenotypically similar. HGPIN occurs primarily in the peripheral zone and is typically observed adjacent to prostate cancer [3, 32–34].

While most studies have reported the associated overall risk of prostate cancer in patients with HGPIN, relatively few have evaluated the impact of focality, as a surrogate of HGPIN volume, on cancer risk [24, 30, 35–40] (see Table 18.2). For the sake of uniformity in reviewing this literature, we define unifocal HGPIN (UHGPIN) as one core with HGPIN and multifocal HGPIN (MHGPIN) as ≥2 cores positive for HGPIN.

Lee et al. stratified the patients with isolated HGPIN on biopsy by focality and found that MHGPIN significantly increased the risk of prostate cancer (HR – 2.56), resulting in estimated 3-year cancer detection rate of 29.0%. Alternatively, in UHGPIN (HR –1.19) and benign disease, the 3-year cancer rates were 14.7% and 12.5%, respectively [30]. Again it is important to note that, in this series, no standardization for repeat biopsy was followed and the decision to biopsy was at the discretion of the urologist.

Merrimen et al. examined 12,304 men who underwent initial and at least one repeat prostatic needle biopsy over an 8-year period – 564 men with HGPIN alone versus 845 matched controls with benign diagnosis. In men with HGPIN on initial biopsy, the risk of prostate cancer remained elevated (OR – 1.38) at a mean follow-up of 16 months. In men with UHGPIN, the risk of subsequent prostate cancer was almost that of benign disease (OR – 1.02). In men with MHGPIN, the risk of prostate cancer increased with the number of positive cores. Among men found to have cancer, those with MHGPIN on initial biopsy were more likely to have Gleason

Table 18.2 Risk of prostate cancer stratified by volume of HGPIN

Author	Year	% Prostate cancer in UHGPIN	Risk of prostate cancer	% Prostate cancer in MHGPIN	Risk of prostate cancer	Median interval to repeat biopsy (months)	Median follow-up (months)
Lee [30]	2010	14.7	HR 1.19	29	HR 2.56	Variable	36
Merrimen [39]	2010	–	OR 1.02	–	OR 2.66	9	16.3
Schoenfield [35]	2006	0	–	80	–	13	15
Akhavan [37]	2007	17.2	–	31	–	Immediate	28 days
Roscigno [63]	2004	10	–	70	–	Variable	11.5
Roscigno [24]	2010	21	–	35	OR 3.97	12	12
De Nunzio [38]	2009	13.7	–	36	–	6	6
Netto [40]	2006	24.3	–	39[a]	–	11	10.4

[a]Widespread as defined by four or more cores of HGPIN

4/5 component cancer, but did not have more likelihood of extracapsular disease. In the initial report of this series, the mean number of cores on initial biopsy was 7.48 and 8.09 cores in the benign group and HGPIN group, respectively. The same group reexamined their data including men who underwent an initial extended biopsy of 10 or more cores. On repeat analysis, they found that men who had two cores (OR – 2.57) and greater than two cores (OR – 3.61) involved by HGPIN carried an even greater risk of prostate cancer than men in the earlier study. Conversely, UHGPIN showed no increased risk of prostate cancer (OR – 0.68) [39].

In 2007, Shoenfield et al. reported the results of 100 consecutive men with first-time 24-core saturation biopsies for abnormal DRE or elevated PSA who underwent repeat biopsy after a median interval of 13 months. They found that in men with benign and UHGPIN on initial biopsy, none had prostate cancer on repeat biopsy, whereas men with MHGPIN had 80% incidence of prostate cancer on repeat biopsy [35]. Akhavan et al. reported the results of 577 men having extended biopsies, 48 of whom had isolated HGPIN, followed by one to four "site-directed" repeat biopsies – where three to four cores were sampled from each area of the prostate that was positive for HGPIN. The overall risk of prostate cancer after UHGPIN was 17.2% on repeat biopsy, whereas the risk of finding prostate cancer on repeat biopsy was significantly higher and related to the proportion of cores with HGPIN [37]. The median time to repeat biopsy was 28 days; thus, the cancers detected were most likely unsampled synchronous, rather than metachronous tumors. The number of cores on initial biopsy was not clearly stated.

In 2004, Bishara et al. re-biopsied 132 of 200 men with isolated HGPIN on initial biopsy and found that if multiple cores were involved by HGPIN on the repeat biopsy, 50.0% (8 of 16) had cancer on follow-up compared with 0 of 9 if there was only one core with HGPIN on repeat biopsy [19]. Of the men with HGPIN on the first repeat biopsy who had additional follow-up biopsies, 32.0% (8 of 25) eventually had prostate cancer. The time from the initial HGPIN biopsy to the first repeat biopsy ranged from 1 to 33 months

with a mean of 7 months. Again, it is important to note that 60% of men underwent only sextant biopsies and not the standard extended core biopsy raising the issue of inadequate baseline sampling.

Roscigno et al. reported the results of 47 men with an initial HGPIN diagnosis who underwent repeat biopsy (mean repeat biopsy cores 11.5) with a median follow-up of 11.4 months (range 3–24). Overall prostate cancer detection rate was 45%. The cancer detection rate was higher on repeat biopsy in those men with MHGPIN at initial biopsy than UHGPIN, 70% versus 10%, respectively (OR – 4.65) [36].

Interestingly, De Nunzio et al. reported the results of a prospective series in which 117 men with HGPIN detected on a 12-core initial biopsy underwent a repeat biopsy 6 months later independent of PSA. They observed an 18.8% prostate cancer incidence. They found that patients with widespread HGPIN (4 cores or more) had the greatest risk (39%) of subsequent diagnosis of prostate cancer on repeat biopsy. This study confirms the observation that widespread HGPIN as defined by Netto and Epstein is associated with a high risk of prostate cancer [40].

Analyzing CP specimen, Wiley et al. reported that 91% of incidental prostate cancer were found in prostates with extensive or multifocal HGPIN, whereas only 11% of cancers occurred in prostates with absent or only focal HGPIN. Extensive HGPIN was defined as involving more than 1% of the examined slide area on three or more slides totaling 2% or more of total prostate volume, and MHGPIN was defined as more than three slides but 2% or less of total prostate volume [41].

In the aforementioned study by Kim and Yang, extensive HGPIN was more likely associated with cancer compared to focal lesions (65% and 31%, respectively, $P=0.021$) [11]. This pathologic data may implicate HGPIN volume as a risk factor for occult cancer, with more extensive lesions predicting an increased likelihood of harboring histologic cancer.

Based upon this collective literature, several authors have suggested that repeat biopsy might not be necessary with a finding of UHGPIN – only requiring serial PSA and DRE for follow-up [2, 19, 20, 26, 30, 42–44].

Laterality of HGPIN

There is a paucity of literature that examines the true relationship of laterality of HGPIN and subsequent risk of prostate cancer, but there is some evidence to suggest that bilateral disease is associated with a greater risk of subsequent development of prostate cancer. The investigators from CCF found that bilateral disease had greater risk (HR – 2.20) of subsequent prostate cancer compared to unilateral disease (HR – 1.67). Three-year estimated cancer rates for unilateral and bilateral HGPIN were 29.6% and 37%, respectively [30]. Schoenfield et al. found that in cases associated with prostate cancer on repeat biopsy, bilateral HGPIN was present 38% of the time [35].

Histological Variants of HGPIN

There are four main histologic patterns of HGPIN: tufting, micropapillary, cribriform, and flat [1, 3]. Tufting pattern is the most common, present in roughly 97% of the time, but most cases harbor multiple patterns concomitantly. The risk of prostate cancer associated with the various patterns of HGPIN has yet to be resolved. There are other unusual patterns of HGPIN such as signet ring cell pattern, small cell neuroendocrine pattern, and foamy cell pattern, but their clinical and prognostic value is undetermined at this time [45, 46].

In a previously discussed series, Bishara et al. did not observe any significant differences in prostate cancer rates when comparing histologic patterns of HGPIN [19]. Their subtype analysis revealed a relative higher and statistically insignificant risk of carcinoma with the tufting/flat category (31.9%) as compared with the micropapillary/cribriform category (22.0%).This is contrary to a previous report from the same institution by Kronz et al. in 2001 who reported an increased risk of prostate cancer associated with micropapillary and cribriform HGPIN subtypes [43]. In that report, it was observed that among men with HGPIN who had more than one repeat biopsy, a predominant micropapillary or cribriform HGPIN pattern had greater than 58% chance of subsequently diagnosed with prostate cancer on third and fourth repeat biopsies. They found no significant difference in prostate cancer in patients with tufted/flat pattern. They found that a combined micropapillary/cribriform pattern and MHGPIN had the greatest risk for prostate cancer of 71%. It is important to note that the study was carried out retrospectively, and the interval to third or fourth biopsy, the number of biopsy cores, and the technique of biopsy were not standardized.

Schoenfield et al. also found no significant association of HGPIN architectural pattern with the presence of cancer on repeat biopsy in 100 men with consecutive first-time 24-core saturation biopsies [35]. Their findings were similar to what Akhavan et al. found in their small series. They reported that the histological subtype of HGPIN did not correlate with final outcome, prostate cancer or not, a finding that might also be a function of the sample size [37].

Other Lesions of the Prostate

It is important to recognize that HGPIN is distinct from the finding of HGPIN with adjacent small atypical glands, which is termed "PINATYP." Fifty-five percent of men with these lesions have cancer on follow-up biopsy [47]. Current recommendations include focal repeat saturation of the suspicious area even when coexistent with isolated HGPIN. If favorable histology is present and the original HGPIN involved only one core, then the patient may be followed without additional biopsy depending on the comfort level of the patient and urologist. The "atypical" label is particularly worrisome because of its known association with carcinoma. In a recent study by Loeb et al., 100% of men with "atypical" glands who decided to have a RP were found to have prostate cancer on final pathology [48]. In a patient with both atypia and HGPIN on biopsy, the high risk of cancer is driven by the "atypical" elements and not HGPIN [2, 48].

PSA and Other Parameters

PSA and PSA Velocity (PSAV)

It has been generally accepted that HGPIN does not raise the serum PSA [49, 50]. To date, there have been no studies showing reproducible and validated relationships between serum PSA level, PSA velocity, and PSA density as parameters of clinical importance in patients with HGPIN. Analyzing PSA kinetics, Loeb et al. showed that PSAV is greater in patients with HGPIN who were subsequently diagnosed with prostate cancer ($p < 0.03$). A PSAV threshold of >0.75 ng/ml/yr predicted which men with HGPIN would ultimately be diagnosed with prostate cancer. On multivariate analysis including PSAV, age, and initial PSA level, PSAV was the only significant predictor of subsequent prostate cancer detection (OR – 4.2). Since PSAV appeared to identify those men who are subsequently diagnosed with prostate cancer, the recommendation was made to use this parameter in the follow-up of men with HGPIN [47]. In the same study of 193 patients with HGPIN on initial biopsy (6–24 cores) who underwent repeat biopsy, Roscigno et al. observed that in patients with baseline extended sampling (>12 cores), a higher PSA was associated with an increased risk of prostate cancer detection (OR – 1.75) at re-biopsy [24].

Our group reported no relationship between cancer detection and PSAV in the 3-year follow-up period. However, PSAV became a significant predictor of cancer when evaluating men diagnosed with cancer on delayed biopsy (> 3 years) [29]. This suggests that PSAV might become more predictive of cancer over time in men with HGPIN, suggesting that a critical volume of cancer is necessary before the trends in PSA become meaningful.

Magnetic Resonance Imaging (MRI)

In 2009, Sciarra et al. compared peripheral zone MRI spectroscopy and contrast enhancement findings in a 27 peripheral zone areas of normal prostate tissue. HGPIN foci were characterized by a significantly higher ($P < 0.05$) absolute value of choline and choline + creatine/citrate ratio compared with normal tissue. On dynamic contrast-enhanced magnetic resonance (DCEMR), HGPIN foci were characterized by lower values of all parameters, but differences did not reach statistical significance ($P > 0.05$). They concluded that HGPIN lesions can be metabolically characterized by MRS through the absolute value of choline and the choline + creatine/citrate ratio. MRI has emerged as an invaluable tool in the diagnosis and treatment of prostate cancer with multiple functional sequences enhancing specificity. The role of multiparametric MRI to identify coexistence of cancer or risk of progression to cancer in cases of HGPIN has yet to be defined.

Biomarkers

The alterations in the cellular components cells have been associated with carcinogenesis in a variety of tissues, including the prostate. Biomarkers have great potential in the management of prostate cancer, but none are available that have been validated in the management of HGPIN.

Early prostate cancer antigen (EPCA) was discovered by Dhir et al. in 2004. It was found to be expressed throughout the prostate of patients with prostate cancer but not in those without the disease [51]. Recently, Zhao et al. measured an initial serum EPCA measurement in 112 men with isolated HGPIN who were followed for 5 years. All men underwent extended core follow-up biopsy within 18 months of the initial diagnosis of HGPIN. The patients with HGPIN on the first follow-up biopsy had an immediate second 12-core biopsy if they had an elevated PSA and/or suspicious DRE. Those without an elevated PSA/DRE underwent a standard biopsy at the end of the study period.

Using an enzyme-linked immunosorbent assay (ELISA) for plasma EPCA cutoff > 1.10 absorbance, the authors found that this cutoff in predicting prostate cancer in patients with HGPIN had a sensitivity and specificity of 100% and

97.5%, respectively. They found that men with isolated HGPIN who presented with an increased EPCA level in the initial serum (>1.10) were significantly more likely to develop a clinically significant cancer after the initial diagnosis than those who had an absorbance of <1.10 for serum EPCA ($P<0.001$). All men diagnosed with cancer underwent RP, and all had pathologically organ-confined disease. The predictive accuracy of parameters for the presence of subsequent cancer was quantified by using the area under the curve (AUC) of 0.839 – correlating to a significantly higher risk of developing cancer (RR – 3.32). A limitation of the study is that "clinically significant" cancer was not defined or validated [52].

Mosquera et al. recently explored the importance of *TMPRSS2-ERG* gene fusion associated with HGPIN as it relates to the development of prostate cancer. They showed that the presence of *TMPRSS2-ERG* gene fusion HGPIN is always indicative of a prostate cancer bearing the same genetic aberration [53]. Currently, the clinical importance and reproducibility of these biomarkers is unclear, but stratification of different subtypes of HGPIN at the molecular level may facilitate clinical decision making in the management of HGPIN.

Chemoprevention

Men with HGPIN are an excellent target for chemoprevention because they represent a high-risk population for developing prostate cancer. The Prostate Cancer Prevention Trial (PCPT) showed a statistically significant decrease in the incidence of HGPIN on end of study biopsy from 11.7% to 8.2% in the placebo and finasteride groups, respectively [54, 55]. The Reduction by Dutasteride of Prostate Cancer Events (REDUCE) trial demonstrated a decreased volume of HGPIN in a randomized trial of 46 patients who underwent RP that approached statistical significance ($p=0.052$) [56]. One must interpret these findings related to HGPIN with caution since these were secondary endpoints men with preexisting HGPIN were excluded from the studies. As such, the findings say little about active chemoprevention in men who are known to have HGPIN.

Supplements have also garnered attention for prostate cancer prevention in men with HGPIN. Fleshner et al. recently published a randomized phase III double-blind study of daily combination soy (40 g), vitamin E (800 U), and selenium (200 mug) versus placebo in 300 men with biopsy-confirmed HGPIN in at least one biopsy within 18 months of the study. Treatment was administered daily for 3 years. Follow-up prostate biopsies occurred at 6, 12, 24, and 36 months postrandomization. Prostate cancer developed in 26.4% of patients – the hazard ratio for the nutritional supplement to prevent prostate cancer was 1.03 (95% CI, 0.67–1.60; P=.88). They concluded that combination of vitamin E, selenium, and soy was ineffective in preventing progression from HGPIN to prostate cancer [66].

Selective estrogen receptor modulators (SERM) show much promise in preventing the progression of HGPIN to prostate cancer. Studies have shown that estrogens play a significant role in prostate carcinogenesis and prostate cancer proliferation in animal models [57]. While administration of testosterone to rodents does not induce prostate cancer, simultaneous administration of testosterone and estradiol induces prostate carcinogenesis in 100% of treated animals [58]. In a non-castrate environment, estrogen receptor alpha (ER-α) serves as mediator of growth-stimulatory signal transduction through initiation of stromal paracrine effect on prostate cancer epithelium while estrogen receptor beta (ER-β) mediates a direct antiproliferative effect on the epithelial compartment [59].

Toremifene citrate is an oral SERM approved by the Food and Drug Administration (FDA) for the treatment of advanced breast cancer. At low concentrations, toremifene selectively inhibits ER-alpha [60, 61]. Toremifene citrate reduced the progression of HGPIN to prostate cancer in a dose-finding randomized phase IIB clinical trial. In this study of 514 men with isolated HGPIN on biopsy, the incidence of prostate cancer at 1 year in the 20 mg toremifene and placebo groups was 24.4% and 31.2%, respectively [62].

The randomized phase III, double-blind, placebo-controlled clinical trial of 20 mg toremifene citrate for prevention of prostate cancer in 1,590 men with isolated HGPIN on biopsy treated for 3 years has completed, and the results are unpublished at time of this transcript.

Recommended Management of HGPIN

Two fundamental goals exist in the clinical management of isolated HGPIN: (1) to exclude malignancy at initial presentation due to tissue sampling error and (2) to monitor for development of clinically significant prostate cancer over time. In doing so, the clinician must balance the morbidity and expense of repetitive biopsy and the window of opportunity to diagnose the cancer while it is curable. Ultimately, it would be highly desirable to elucidate methods of reducing the risk of progression to prostate cancer.

National Comprehensive Cancer Network (NCCN) Guidelines

The NCCN has updated its general recommendations on the management of isolated HGPIN on initial biopsy in the Prostate Cancer Early Detection Guideline v.1.2011 (electronic access at http://www.nccn.org/professionals/physician_gls/pdf/prostate_detection.pdf). They recommend patients undergo repeat extended core biopsy if an extended scheme was not employed initially. Further, they recommend a repeat biopsy be undertaken if more than one core is positive for HGPIN (>/2 cores). Those with baseline biopsy of 10 or more cores and no prostate cancer on repeat biopsy may be considered for close follow-up with PSA and DRE. It is important to note that the aforementioned recommendations are category 2A: recommendation based on lower level evidence, but there is uniform NCCN consensus.

The NYULMC Approach and Current Recommendation

Based on the existing literature and clinical observations, the multidisciplinary prostate cancer group at NYULMC has proposed a general strategy in

the management of isolated HGPIN (see Fig. 18.1). Among men who are diagnosed with a biopsy of <10 cores, an immediate repeat extended biopsy should be performed to provide adequate baseline sampling of the gland. In men with isolated HGPIN identified on an extended core biopsy (>10 cores), if the serum PSA is markedly elevated (>10 ng/ml) or there is strong suspicion based on clinical history, then a repeat saturation biopsy with sampling of the transition zone is advised.

In those men with isolated HGPIN identified on extended core biopsy, in whom there are no high-risk features, we obtain PSA measurements every 6 months and a delayed interval biopsy at 3 years of follow-up in the absence of a rising PSA. If a rising PSA is observed, (e.g., PSAV >0.75 ng/ml/year), an earlier delayed interval biopsy (1–3 years) is often performed based on age and comorbidities. We currently do not recommended risk stratification based on number of cores positive for HGPIN (one or greater than one core), but if there is significant volume of HGPIN, an earlier interval biopsy (1–3 years) is often considered based on clinical suspicion by the physician. At the time of delayed interval biopsy in men with stable serum PSA and no other high-risk features, routine transition zone sampling is unlikely to improve prostate cancer detection.

Alternative Approaches

The NYULMC approach advocates the "active surveillance" with delayed interval biopsies in men with isolated HGPIN regardless of the number of cores positive. There are a number of other follow-up schedules that have been recommended. Lee et al. recommends that clinicians should have a low threshold for repeat biopsy of men with bilateral and/or MHGPIN. They recommend repeat biopsy within 2–3 years in these men [30]. Other recommendations include biopsy anywhere from 6 to 18 months. Each of the studies makes provocative arguments for their specific follow-up recommendations based upon small retrospective series, but the studies themselves are generally flawed because of the lack of standardization with regard to interval to follow-up biopsy and the lack of standardized repeat biopsy in all patients [2, 38, 39, 63, 64]. Nonetheless, an alternative approach including the consideration of HGPIN volume at baseline is a reasonable approach.

Conclusion

HGPIN is widely accepted as a precursor of prostate cancer and a predictor of cancer on subsequent biopsy. It does not appear that immediate repeat biopsy is necessary for men who are well sampled at baseline, but long-term follow-up with surveillance biopsy appears warranted. To date, no consensus has been reached with regard to interval, frequency, and technique of repeat biopsy. At the time of writing this chapter, the authors believe that the sustained risk of cancer on follow-up biopsy, the high likelihood of clinically significant cancer, and the lack of reliable indicators of cancer during follow-up justifies active surveillance using empiric 12-core systematic interval biopsies every 3 years would be a reasonable strategy for follow-up of men with isolated HGPIN found by extended core biopsy. Such an approach appears to result in a diagnosis of a substantial number of clinically significant cancers that are still organ-confined at the time of pathological review. As chemoprevention strategies emerge, use of nontoxic preventive agents within the periods of observation would be ideal. It is likely that multiparametric MRI will likely emerge as a useful tool to decrease the frequency of surveillance biopsies in those cases with a predictable low risk of progression to prostate cancer.

Editorial Commentary

It is pretty amazing that HGPIN has been recognized as a pathological abnormality for over a quarter century, but there remains little consensus on what it is, what it means to the individual patient's likelihood of having or developing prostate cancer, or how it should be evaluated or managed. Early practices of serial biopsy as often as every 3 months were clearly infeasible, but many of the protocols that followed had little logic or sustainability either.

The authors pose a logical, data-driven approach that minimizes excessive evaluation while limiting the risk that aggressive prostate cancer will be missed until too late to cure. Recognizing that prostate cancer prevention efforts have not achieved broad success, better markers of coexistent prostate cancer are desperately needed for this patient population.

References

1. Bostwick DG, et al. Architectural patterns of high-grade prostatic intraepithelial neoplasia. Hum Pathol. 1993;24(3):298–310.
2. Epstein JI, Herawi M. Prostate needle biopsies containing prostatic intraepithelial neoplasia or atypical foci suspicious for carcinoma: implications for patient care. J Urol. 2006;175(3 Pt 1):820–34.
3. Bostwick DG, Qian JQ. High-grade prostatic intraepithelial neoplasia. Mod Pathol. 2004;17(3):360–79.
4. Epstein JI, et al. Interobserver reproducibility in the diagnosis of prostatic intraepithelial neoplasia. Am J Surg Pathol. 1995;19(8):873–86.
5. Silvestri F, et al. Neoplastic and borderline lesions of the prostate: autopsy study and epidemiological data. Pathol Res Pract. Italy 1995;191(9):908–16.
6. Billis A. Age and race distribution of high grade prostatic intraepithelial neoplasia (HGPIN): an autopsy study in Brazil (South America). Mod Pathol. 1996; 9(1):71A.
7. Sakr WA, et al. Epidemiology of high-grade prostatic intraepithelial neoplasia. Pathol Res Pract. 1995; 191(9):838–41.
8. McNeal JE, Bostwick DG. Intraductal dysplasia: a premalignant lesion of the prostate. Hum Pathol. 1986;17(1):64–71.
9. Oyasu R, et al. Cytological atypia in the prostate gland: frequency, distribution and possible relevance to carcinoma. J Urol. 1986;135(5):959–62.
10. Troncoso P, et al. Prostatic intraepithelial neoplasia and invasive prostatic adenocarcinoma in cystoprostatectomy specimens. Urology. 1989;34(6 Suppl): 52–6.
11. Kim HL, Yang XJ. Prevalence of high-grade prostatic intraepithelial neoplasia and its relationship to serum prostate specific antigen. Int Braz J Urol. 2002;28(5):413–6. Discussion 417.
12. Jones JS. Managing patients following a negative prostate biopsy. Haymarket; Littleton, Colorado 2011.
13. Weinstein MH, Epstein JI. Significant of high-grade prostatic intraepithelial neoplasia on needle biopsy. Hum Pathol. 1993;24(6):624–9.

14. Brawer MK, et al. Significance of prostatic intraepithelial neoplasia on prostate needle biopsy. Urology. 1991;38(2):103–7.

15. Gokden N, et al. High-grade prostatic intraepithelial neoplasia in needle biopsy as risk factor for detection of adenocarcinoma: current level of risk in screening population. Urology. 2005;65(3):538–42.

16. Keetch DW, et al. Morphometric analysis and clinical followup of isolated prostatic intraepithelial neoplasia in needle biopsy of the prostate. J Urol. 1995;154(2 Pt 1):347–51.

17. Abdel-Khalek M, El-Baz M, Ibrahiem EH. Predictors of prostate cancer on extended biopsy in patients with high-grade prostatic intraepithelial neoplasia: a multivariate analysis model. BJU Int. 2004;94(4):528–33.

18. Alsikafi NF, et al. High-grade prostatic intraepithelial neoplasia with adjacent atypia is associated with a higher incidence of cancer on subsequent needle biopsy than high-grade prostatic intraepithelial neoplasia alone. Urology. 2001;57(2):296–300.

19. Bishara T, Ramnani DM, Epstein JI. High-grade prostatic intraepithelial neoplasia on needle biopsy – risk of cancer on repeat biopsy related to number of involved cores and morphologic pattern. Am J Surg Pathol. 2004;28(5):629–33.

20. Borboroglu PG, et al. Repeat biopsy strategy in patients with atypical small acinar proliferation or high grade prostatic intraepithelial neoplasia on initial prostate needle biopsy. J Urol. 2001;166(3):866–70.

21. Kamoi K, Troncoso P, Babaian RJ. Strategy for repeat biopsy in patients with high-grade prostatic intraepithelial neoplasia. J Urol. 2000;163(3):819–23.

22. Lefkowitz GK, et al. Is repeat prostate biopsy for high-grade prostatic intraepithelial neoplasia necessary after routine 12-core sampling? Urology. 2001;58(6):999–1003.

23. Naya Y, et al. Can the number of cores with high-grade prostate intraepithelial neoplasia predict cancer in men who undergo repeat biopsy? Urology. 2004;63(3):503–8.

24. Roscigno M, et al. Diagnosis of high-grade prostatic intraepithelial neoplasia: the impact of the number of biopsy cores at initial sampling on cancer detection after a saturation re-biopsy. Arch Ital Urol Androl. 2010;82(4):242–7.

25. O'Dowd GJ, et al. Analysis of repeated biopsy results within 1 year after a noncancer diagnosis. Urology. 2000;55(4):553–9.

26. Herawi M, et al. Risk of prostate cancer on first re-biopsy within 1 year following a diagnosis of high grade prostatic intraepithelial neoplasia is related to the number of cores sampled. J Urol. 2006;175(1):121–4.

27. Lefkowitz GK, et al. Followup interval prostate biopsy 3 years after diagnosis of high grade prostatic intraepithelial neoplasia is associated with high likelihood of prostate cancer, independent of change in prostate specific antigen levels. J Urol. 2002;168(4):1415–8.

28. Godoy G, Taneja SS. Contemporary clinical management of isolated high-grade prostatic intraepithelial neoplasia. Prostate Cancer Prostatic Dis. 2008;11(1):20–31.

29. Godoy G, et al. Long-term follow-up of men with isolated high-grade prostatic intra-epithelial neoplasia followed by serial delayed interval biopsy. Urology. 2011;77(3):669–74.

30. Lee MC, et al. Multifocal high grade prostatic intraepithelial neoplasia is a risk factor for subsequent prostate cancer. J Urol. 2010;184(5):1958–62.

31. Gallo F, et al. Prognostic significance of high-grade prostatic intraepithelial neoplasia (HGPIN): risk of prostate cancer on repeat biopsies. Urology. 2008;72(3):628–32.

32. Qian JQ, Wollan P, Bostwick DG. The extent and multicentricity of high-grade prostatic intraepithelial neoplasia in clinically localized prostatic adenocarcinoma. Hum Pathol. 1997;28(2):143–8.

33. Bostwick DG, Qian JQ, Frankel K. The incidence of high grade prostatic intraepithelial neoplasia in needle biopsies. J Urol. 1995;154(5):1791–4.

34. Bostwick DG, et al. High grade prostatic intraepithelial neoplasia and atypical small acinal proliferation are significant cancer risk factors: follow – up study of 1,476 cases. J Urol. 2009;181(4):2075%U.

35. Schoenfield L, et al. The incidence of high-grade prostatic intraepithelial neoplasia and atypical glands suspicious for carcinoma on first-time saturation needle biopsy, and the subsequent risk of cancer. BJU Int. 2007;99(4):770–4.

36. Roscigno M, et al. Isolated mono- and pluri-focal high grade prostatic intraepithelial neoplasia (HGPIN) on initial extended prostate needle biopsies: factors predicting cancer detection on extended re-biopsy. Eur Urol Suppl. 2004;3(2):67.

37. Akhavan A, et al. The proportion of cores with high-grade prostatic intraepithelial neoplasia on extended-pattern needle biopsy is significantly associated with prostate cancer on site-directed repeat biopsy. BJU Int. 2007;99(4):765–9.

38. De Nunzio C, et al. The number of cores positive for high grade prostatic intraepithelial neoplasia on initial biopsy is associated with prostate cancer on second biopsy. J Urol. 2009;181(3):1069–74.

39. Merrimen JL, Jones G, Srigley JR. Is high grade prostatic intraepithelial neoplasia still a risk factor for adenocarcinoma in the era of extended biopsy sampling? Pathology. 2010;42(4):325–9.

40. Netto GJ, Epstein JI. Widespread high-grade prostatic intraepithelial neoplasia on prostatic needle biopsy: a significant likelihood of subsequently diagnosed adenocarcinoma. Am J Surg Pathol. 2006;30(9):1184–8.

41. Wiley EL, et al. Risk of concurrent prostate cancer in cystoprostatectomy specimen is related to volume of high-grade prostatic intraepithelial neoplasia. Urology. 1997;49(5):692–6.

42. Hoedemaeker RF, et al. Histopathological prostate cancer characteristics at radical prostatectomy after population based screening. J Urol. 2000;164(2):411–5.

43. Kronz JD, et al. Predicting cancer following a diagnosis of high-grade prostatic intraepithelial neoplasia on needle biopsy – data on men with more than one follow-up biopsy. Am J Surg Pathol. 2001;25(8):1079–85.

44. Sakr WA. High-grade prostatic intraepithelial neoplasia: additional links to a potentially more aggressive prostate cancer? J Natl Cancer Inst. 1998;90(7):486–7.

45. Reyes AO, et al. Unusual histologic types of high-grade prostatic intraepithelial neoplasia. Am J Surg Pathol. 1997;21(10):1215–22.

46. Berman DM, Yang J, Epstein JI. Foamy gland high-grade prostatic intraepithelial neoplasia. Am J Surg Pathol. 2000;24(1):140–4.

47. Shah RB, et al. Atypical cribriform lesions of the prostate: relationship to prostatic carcinoma and implication for diagnosis in prostate biopsies. Am J Surg Pathol. 2010;34(4):470–7.

48. Loeb S, et al. Use of prostate-specific antigen velocity to follow up patients with isolated high-grade prostatic intraepithelial neoplasia on prostate biopsy. Urology. 2007;69(1):108–12.

49. Alexander EE, et al. Prostatic intraepithelial neoplasia does not appear to raise serum prostate-specific antigen concentration. Urology. 1996;47(5):693–8.

50. Yang X, Kim H, Steinberg G. High grade prostatic intraepithelial neoplasia does not cause elevation of serum prostate specific antigen. Pathol Int. 2000;50(Supplement):A108.

51. Dhir R, et al. Early identification of individuals with prostate cancer in negative biopsies. J Urol. 2004;171(4):1419–23.

52. Zhao ZG, Zeng GH. Increased serum level of early prostate cancer antigen is associated with subsequent cancer risk in men with high-grade prostatic intraepithelial neoplasia. Endocr Relat Cancer. 2010;17(2):505–12.

53. Mosquera JM, et al. Characterization of TMPRSS2-ERG fusion high-grade prostatic intraepithelial neoplasia and potential clinical implications. Clin Cancer Res. 2008;14(11):3380–5.

54. Thompson IM, et al. The influence of finasteride on the development of prostate cancer. N Engl J Med. 2003;349(3):215–24.

55. Thompson IM, et al. Finasteride decreases the risk of prostatic intraepithelial neoplasia. J Urol. 2007;178(1):107–9. Discussion 110.

56. Andriole GL, et al. Effect of dutasteride on the risk of prostate cancer. N Engl J Med. 2010;362(13):1192–202.

57. Ho SM. Estrogens and anti-estrogens: key mediators of prostate carcinogenesis and new therapeutic candidates. J Cell Biochem. 2004;91(3):491–503.

58. Risbridger GP, et al. Oestrogens and prostate cancer. Endocr Relat Cancer. 2003;10(2):187–91.

59. Leav I, et al. Comparative studies of the estrogen receptors beta and alpha and the androgen receptor in normal human prostate glands, dysplasia, and in primary and metastatic carcinoma. Am J Pathol. 2001;159(1):79–92.

60. Taneja SS. Baseline characteristics validate the inclusion criteria of a phase III comparison of toremifene and placebo for the prevention of prostate cancer in men with isolated high grade prostatic intraepithelial neoplasia (HGPIN). Eur Urol Suppl. 2008;7(3):613.

61. Taneja SS, et al. Toremifene–a promising therapy for the prevention of prostate cancer and complications of androgen deprivation therapy. Expert Opin Investig Drugs. 2006;15(3):293–305.

62. Price D, et al. Toremifene for the prevention of prostate cancer in men with high grade prostatic intraepithelial neoplasia: results of a double-blind, placebo controlled, phase IIB clinical trial. J Urol. 2006;176(3):965–70.

63. Roscigno M, et al. Monofocal and plurifocal high-grade prostatic intraepithelial neoplasia on extended prostate biopsies: factors predicting cancer detection on extended repeat biopsy. Urology. 2004;63(6):1105–10.

64. Herawi M, et al. Risk of prostate cancer on re-biopsy following a diagnosis of high-grade prostatic intraepithelial neoplasia (HGPIN) is related to the number of cores sampled. J Urol. 2005;173(4):142–3.

65. Laurila M, et al. Detection rates of cancer, high grade PIN and atypical lesions suspicious for cancer in the European randomized study of screening for prostate cancer. Eur J Cancer. 2010;46(17):3068–72.

66. Fleshner NE, et al. Progression from high-grade prostatic intraepithelial neoplasia to cancer: a randomized trial of combination vitamin-E, soy, and selenium. J Clin Oncol. 2011;29(17):2386–90.

Adriana Olar and Thomas M. Wheeler

Introduction

Atypical small acinar proliferation (ASAP) has been reported in approximately 5–6% of all of the prostate biopsies and is a clinically controversial diagnosis. Surveys have shown that many clinicians might not fully appreciate its definition finding it equivalent to high-grade prostatic intraepithelial neoplasia (HGPIN). The purpose of this chapter is to clarify the definition of ASAP, its histological findings, and clinical consequences. We propose a new follow-up approach following the diagnosis of ASAP, by increasing the number of repeat biopsies with consecutive negative results from two to three.

Definition and Incidence

Epstein and Kahane et al. [1, 2] described prostate biopsies that were "atypical but not diagnostic" and "small focus of atypical glands suspicious for, but not diagnostic of cancer." However, the acronym ASAP (atypical small acinar prolifera-

tion) was coined by Bostwick et al. that same year [3]. Since then ASAP has been the subject of numerous comments and critiques [4–6].

Isolated ASAP has been reported in approximately 5–6%* of prostate biopsy accessions (range 0.4–31%) in 30 studies (Table 19.1) [2, 3, 7–39]. (*The studies with 100% reported frequency have not been considered for average determination.)

For urologists, ASAP is a controversial diagnosis [40]. In a survey sent to 42 members of the Society of Urological Oncology, 98% would rebiopsy a patient with ASAP as a diagnosis, 52% would treat ASAP and high-grade prostatic intraepithelial neoplasia (HGPIN) the same, 29% considered ASAP to be worse than HGPIN, 12% considered HGPIN to be worse than ASAP, and 7% were unsure which was worse [41]. This survey also found that the clinicians might not fully appreciate the definition of ASAP even given the definition in a comment accompanying the diagnosis. On another survey directed to urologists, 37% of the 110 respondents considered ASAP as being equivalent to HGPIN [42].

An important fundamental difference between HGPIN and ASAP is that HGPIN is considered a dysplastic process confined to architecturally benign glands with basal cells and as such is considered to be a precursor of adenocarcinoma. ASAP, on the other hand, is a different pathological entity, representing a wide variety of histological findings that are suspicious for, but not diagnostic of, adenocarcinoma (qualitatively, quantitatively, or both). When reporting ASAP, the pathologist must convey to the urologist that the

A. Olar, M.D.
Department of Pathology and Genomic Medicine,
The Methodist Hospital, 6565 Fannin St., Houston,
TX 77030, USA

T.M. Wheeler, M.D. (✉)
Department of Pathology & Immunology,
Baylor College of Medicine, BCM 315, One Baylor
Plaza, Houston, TX 77030, USA
e-mail: twheeler@bcm.edu

Table 19.1 Literature review. The frequency of isolated ASAP, ASAP associated with HGPIN, time to repeat biopsy, and frequency of prostatic adenocarcinoma on repeat biopsy is shown

References	Year	Setting	Frequency of diagnosis of isolated ASAP per total	%	ASAP associated with HGPIN	%	Frequency of repeat biopsy in isolated ASAP	%	Time to repeat biopsy (months)	Frequency of diagnosis of cancer on subsequent biopsies (%)	%
Bostwick et al. [3]	1995	Community	3/200	1.5	2/200	1	N/A	N/A	N/A	N/A	N/A
		Academic	1/200	0.5	2/200	1	N/A	N/A	N/A	N/A	N/A
Kahane et al. [2]	1995	Laboratory	15/4,047	0.4	N/A	N/A	N/A	N/A	N/A	N/A	N/A
Roehrborn et al. [7]	1996	Academic	38/123	31	N/A	N/A	38/38	100	6	8/38	21
Cheville et al. [8]	1997	Community	48/1,009	4.8	N/A	N/A	25/54	46	N/A	15/25	60
Iczkowski et al. [9]	1997	Community	33/33	100	14/33	42	33/33	100	1–27 Median:3	15/33	45
Wills et al. [10]	1997	Academic	18/439	4.1	2/439	0.5	N/A	N/A	N/A	N/A	N/A
Allen et al. [11]	1998	Academic	124/124	100	N/A	N/A	124/124	100	N/A	56/124	45.2
Iczkowski et al. [12]	1998	Community	295/295	100	N/A	N/A	295/295	100	0.1–43.2 Mean: 5.7	125/295	42
Renshaw et al. [13]	1998	Academic	167/2,219	7.5	N/A	N/A	59/167	35	9–19	22/64	34
Reyes and Humphrey [14]	1998	Academic	128/795	16.1	10/795	1.3	N/A	N/A	N/A	N/A	N/A
Weinstein et al. [15]	1998	Community	96/1,192	8	N/A	N/A	N/A	N/A	N/A	N/A	N/A
		Community	170/2,792	6.1	N/A	N/A	N/A	N/A	N/A	N/A	N/A
		Community	62/1,306	4.7	N/A	N/A	N/A	N/A	N/A	N/A	N/A
Chan and Epstein [16]	1999	Consults	200/200	100	N/A	N/A	92/144	64	0.5–36	45/92	49
Hoedemaeker et al. [17]	1999	Screening	43/1,824	2.4	N/A	N/A	39/43	91	6	15/39	38.5
Novis et al. [18]	1999	Multiinstitutional	1,121/15,753	7.1	N/A	N/A	N/A	N/A	N/A	N/A	N/A
O'dowd et al. [19]	2000	Laboratory	3,269/132,426	2.5	440/132,426	0.3	1,321/3,269	40.4	3	529/1,321	40
Borboroglu et al. [20]	2001	Academic	53/1,391	3.8	8/1,391	0.6	48/53	91	12	23/48	48
Ouyang et al. [21]	2001	Academic	21/331	6.3	N/A	N/A	17/21	81	2–12	9/17	53
Park et al. [22]	2001	Academic	45/45	100	N/A	N/A	45/45	100	Mean: 24	23/45	51
Iczkowski et al. [23]	2002	Laboratory	184/7,081	2.6	N/A	N/A	129/227	57	12	51/129	40
Mian et al. [24]	2002	Academic	33/939	3.5	N/A	N/A	10/33	30	N/A	7/10	70
Brausi et al. [25]	2004	Academic	71/1,327	5.3	N/A	N/A	23/45	51.1	6	6/23	26

Fadare et al. [26]	2004	Academic	36/1,964	1.8	N/A	N/A	24/36	67	2–24 Mean: 8	9/24	38
Gupta et al. [27]	2004	Community	18/515	3.5	13/515	2.5	N/A	N/A	N/A	N/A	N/A
		Community	17/933	1.8	9/933	1	N/A	N/A	N/A	N/A	N/A
Kobayashi et al. [28]	2004	Academic	6/104	5.8	N/A	N/A	N/A	N/A	N/A	N/A	N/A
Naya et al. [29]	2004	Academic	12/1,086	1.1	10/1,086	1	12/12	100	3	7/12	58.3
Postma et al. [30]	2004	Screening	108/4,117	2.6	N/A	N/A	96/108	89	N/A	35/96	36.5
		Screening	50/1,840	2.7	N/A	N/A	47/50	94	N/A	8/47	17
Leite et al. [31]	2005	Laboratory	26/1,420	1.8	40/1,420	2.8	16/26	61.5	4.26	7/16	43.8
Moore et al. [32]	2005	Academic	72/1,188	6	N/A	N/A	53/72	73.6	2.5	19/53	36
Schlesinger et al. [33]	2005	Community	78/336	23	54/336	16	78/78	100	Mean: 3.8	29/78	37
Mallén et al. [34]	2006	Academic	69/3,600	1.9	N/A	N/A	64/69	92.75	1–13 Median: 2	27/64	42
Rodríguez-Patrón Rodríguez et al. [35]	2006	Academic	127/6,000	2.1	N/A	N/A	50/127	39.3	0.7–83 Mean: 13–17	20/50	40
Mearini et al. [36]	2008	Academic	76/1,274	5.9	6/1,274	0.4	65/76	85.5	5	25/65	38.4
Ploussard et al. [37]	2009	Community	23/2,006	1.2	N/A	N/A	17/23	74	5.9	7/17	41.1
Ryu et al. [38]	2010	Community	244/3,130	7.8	N/A	N/A	170/244	70	3–6	57/170	33.5
Kopp et al. [39]	2011	Academic	199/2,628	7.6	N/A	N/A	139/199	67	<4, >12.8	41/139	29

lesion is not merely *atypical* but is actually *suspicious* for adenocarcinoma. Published reports suggest that ASAP has a significantly higher likelihood of prostate cancer on a subsequent biopsy (40.2% mean) as compared with HGPIN (31.5% mean) [32, 40]. ASAP is a diagnostic category [12, 43], whereas HGPIN is a preneoplastic lesion [44]. ASAP is defined as small acini suspicious for, but not diagnostic of, malignancy. This diagnostic category arose to encompass small lesions where there was an absolute "uncertainty" regarding the definitive diagnosis of prostatic adenocarcinoma [43]. Since the diagnosis of isolated ASAP confers a substantial risk of subsequent prostatic adenocarcinoma, its identification warrants careful follow-up with repeat biopsy. Therefore, rendering a diagnosis of ASAP should indicate to the clinician that the biopsy specimen in question exhibits inconclusive histological features that are neither clearly malignant nor clearly benign [43, 45].

The mean age of patients with ASAP is in the seventh decade (60s) and does not differ significantly from patients with prostatic adenocarcinoma [46].

Difficulties in Diagnosing Small Lesions

Often, on biopsy material, the abnormal focus of interest is very small, composed of just a few acini. Deeper levels, or ancillary studies, such as immunohistochemical stains sometimes can help; however, the focus may disappear on deeper levels. The clinical consequences of a definitive diagnosis of prostatic adenocarcinoma are not trivial – radical prostatectomy or definitive radiation therapy – procedures with potentially severe morbidity for the patient. Erectile dysfunction in a middle-aged man and its resulting effects on his lifestyle is not to be ignored, especially if the radical prostatectomy specimen turns out negative for adenocarcinoma [47–50]. According to Bostwick and colleagues, there are three highly important questions needed to be answered prior to diagnosing ASAP or cancer in such small lesions [43]:

1. Would you be absolutely confident of this biopsy diagnosis if it were followed by a radical prostatectomy with negative findings?
2. Would another colleague pathologist agree with the diagnosis of cancer?

3. Can you confidently support the diagnosis of adenocarcinoma based solely on this biopsy result?

If the answer to any of the above questions is "no," Bostwick et al. recommend the use of the more conservative diagnosis of ASAP [43].

Stratification of ASAP in subcategories or levels of suspicion for malignancy (*favor benign, suspicious,* and *highly suspicious*) has been attempted; however, it has been demonstrated that it was not predictive of cancer in specimens from repeat biopsies despite multiple attempts [9, 12, 43, 51]. In clinical practice some expert pathologists occasionally subclassify an atypical diagnosis as "highly suspicious," but only if carcinoma is strongly favored. Similarly "mildly atypical" is used if there is low suspicion for adenocarcinoma [40].

Diagnosis: Lack of Distinct Criteria

A diagnosis of ASAP is not characterized by distinct morphological criteria, but rather reflects the lack of diagnostic criteria for a definitive diagnosis of adenocarcinoma [40, 43]. Urologists must understand the uncertainty the pathologist faces when confronted with such lesions. In the following discussion (and summarized in Tables 19.2 and 19.3), the "how" and "why" of this diagnostic category are discussed.

Table 19.2 Reasons for diagnosing ASAP [9, 33, 43]

Size of focus
Very small (see Table 19.3 for specifics)
Lesion present at the core edge (incomplete sampling)
Loss of focus on deeper levels
Histology
Distorted histological detail
Crush artifact
Prominent inflammation (reactive atypia)
Processing artifact (thick sections, overstaining)
Lack of convincing malignant features
Clustered growth pattern (mimicking adenosis)
Conflicting immunohistochemical findings
Focally positive for basal cell markers
Negative AMACR stain
Presence of adjacent HGPIN
Tangential cutting (budding PIN)

Table 19.3 Histological features of ASAP compared to adenocarcinoma in prostate core needle biopsies [8, 9]

	ASAP	Prostatic adenocarcinoma
Architectural		
Mean size of focus (mm)	0.4 +/− 0.3	0.8 +/− 0.5
Mean number of involved acini	11 +/− 10	17 +/− 14
Infiltrative growth	Sometimes	Always
Cytological		
Nuclear enlargement	Mild	Moderate
Nuclear hyperchromasia	More common	Less common
Prominent nucleoli	Sometimes	Always
Luminal secretions		
Blue-gray luminal mucin	Less likely	More likely
Eosinophilic proteinaceous secretions	Equally present	Equally present
Crystalloids	Equally present	Equally present
Associated pathological features		
Atrophy	More common	Less common
Inflammation	Equally present	Equally present
HGPIN	Less common	More common
Immunohistochemical features		
Racemase	Sometimes negative	Usually positive [40, 59–61]
P63	Sometimes positive	Usually negative [57, 65, 66, 74]
34betaE12	Sometimes positive	Usually negative [57, 65, 66]

Firstly one of the most important factors in consideration of the diagnosis of ASAP is the size of the focus of interest [9]. A small focus has been defined as a focus representing less than 5% of the core [3], or less than 0.4 mm, comprising less than two dozen acini [46], or being less than the size of the head of a pin [43]. In all of these instances, there is major concern for overdiagnosis of cancer based on insufficient evidence [43] (Fig. 19.1). The same applies if the focus of concern is present at the edge of the tissue core (fractured core) or disappears on deeper levels suggesting incomplete sampling [43]. Moreover, the specimen may be composed of acini of small size, that is, smaller than normal ducts and acini, but it may also include glands with a diameter similar to that of normal ducts and acini [52].

The presence of infiltrative growth, a common feature of adenocarcinoma, is not reliable as a sole criterion for malignancy in that it has been reported in up to 75% of ASAP [8, 46].

Mild nuclear enlargement (relative to the adjacent benign epithelial cells) with more prominent nuclear hyperchromasia is characteristic of ASAP as compared to more pronounced nuclear enlargement and less hyperchromasia

seen with malignancy [43]. Hyperchromasia however has to be interpreted carefully taking into account the laboratory's technical staining protocols.

The presence of mitotic figures in suspicious foci usually points to a diagnosis of adenocarcinoma; however, in small foci mitotic figures are rarely encountered (in either adenocarcinoma or its mimics) [43].

Blue-gray luminal mucin (Fig. 19.2) may be encountered in both ASAP and adenocarcinoma, and the presence of eosinophilic secretions and crystalloids is also nonspecific, found in atypical adenomatous hyperplasia and occasionally even normal glands (Fig. 19.3) (although all are encountered with a greater relative frequency in adenocarcinoma) [8, 9, 53].

Associated inflammation or mechanical distortion (crush artifact) following the biopsy procedure might also cause distorted glands with an atypical look posing further difficulty in interpretation (Fig. 19.2) [40]. The individual submission and processing of prostate biopsies in 6–12 containers decrease the rate of atypical diagnosis by preventing core entanglement and fragmentation. It is also more difficult to embed

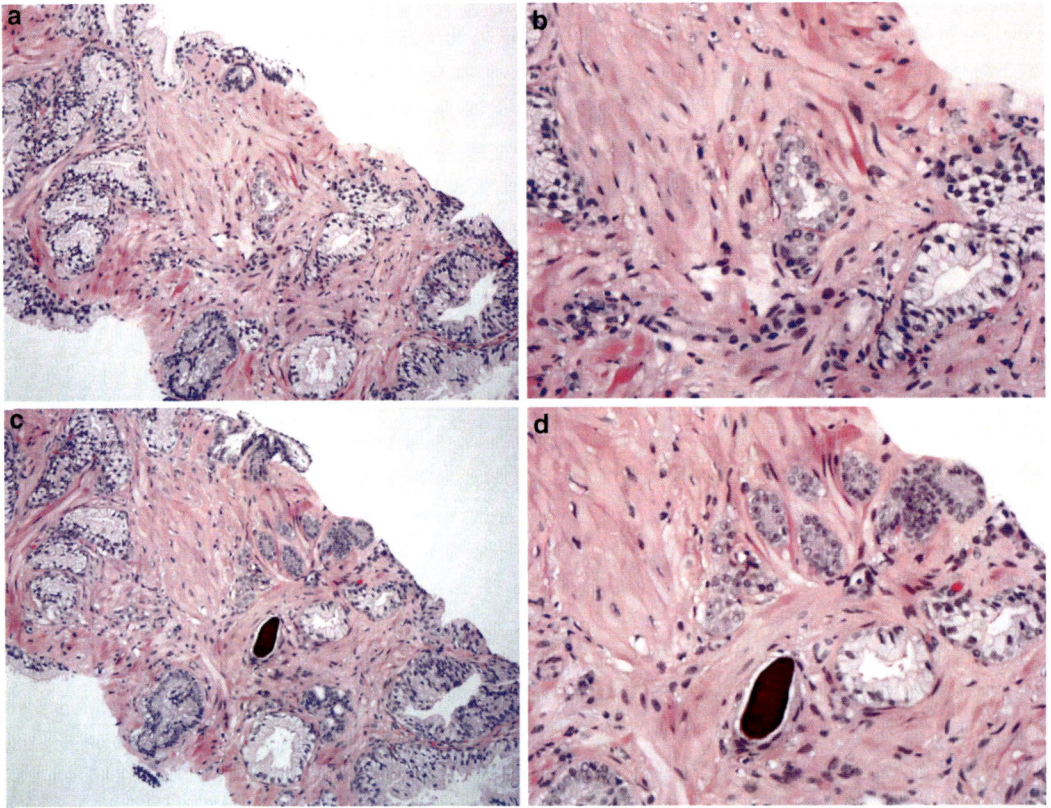

Fig. 19.1 A small focus composed of two acini shows nuclear atypia with prominent nucleoli (**a** – HE, 200×; **b** – HE, 400×). Deeper levels unveil a total of 12 acini showing the same nuclear atypical features (**c** – HE, 200×; **d** – HE, 400×). The focus is too small for a definitive diagnosis of adenocarcinoma, however is highly suspicious due to its morphology. A diagnosis of ASAP is warranted

multiple cores in a single plane following processing [27]. Epstein recommends that no more than two cores should be submitted per container to optimize sectioning and visualization [40].

Often ASAP coexists with HGPIN (see Table 19.1) [3, 9, 10, 14, 19, 20, 27, 29, 31, 33, 36]. The small foci of atypical small proliferating glands may be immediately adjacent to a focus of HGPIN (Fig. 19.4) [40]. In this instance, the concern is that the focus of ASAP actually represents budding or tangentially sectioned glands from the adjacent HGPIN gland rather than a true and independent cancer focus [8]. HGPIN with adjacent atypical (suspicious) glands shows a higher risk of cancer on subsequent biopsies compared to HGPIN alone [54, 55].

An adequate number of histological levels should be considered before a final diagnosis reflecting uncertainty is rendered. Because atypical foci sometimes may still be missed on one or two levels, Renshaw et al. recommend that a minimum of three levels should be prepared from each block for an adequate visualization of the focus [56] with additional deeper levels if warranted [14].

Ancillary studies are highly recommended and encouraged to help in differentiating these challenging situations. Appropriate controls must always be used [52]. P63, a nuclear protein, and high molecular weight cytokeratin (HMWCK) detected by antibody clone 34betaE12 are prostatic basal cell-specific immunohistochemical markers not expressed by the secretory cells [57, 58]. Alpha-methyl-CoA racemase (AMACR, P504S) is a mitochondrial and peroxisomal enzyme involved in the β (beta)-oxidation

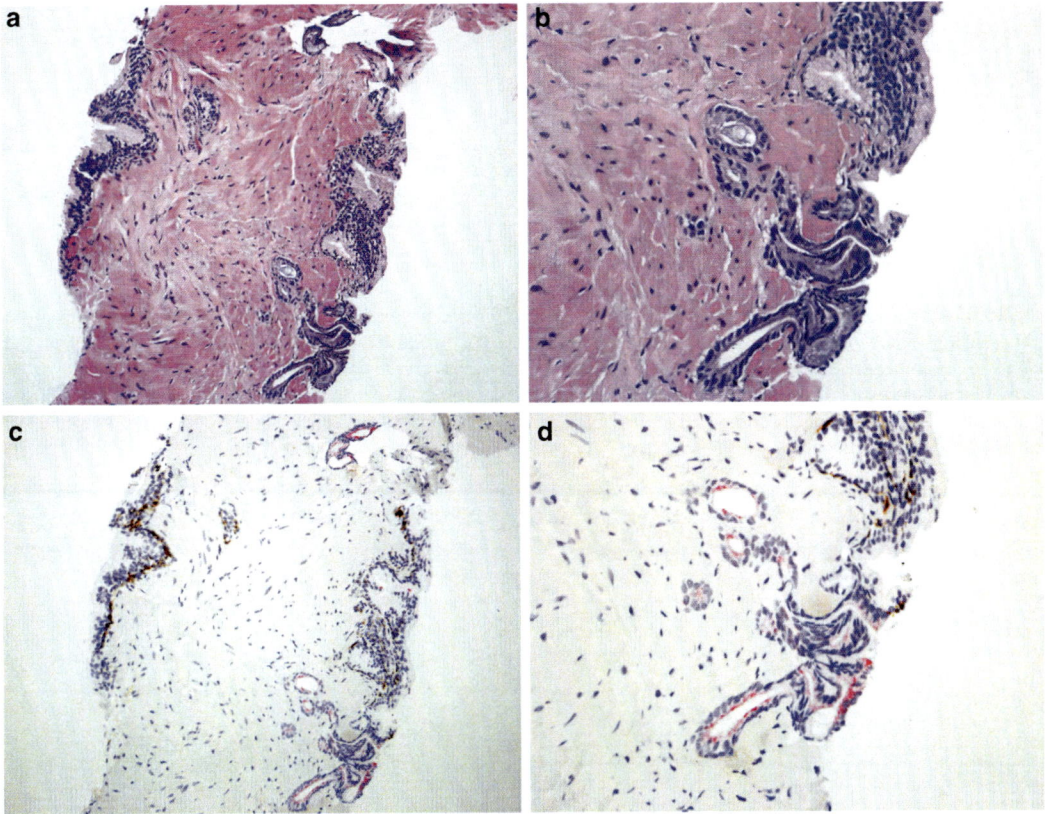

Fig. 19.2 A small distorted suspicious focus is present at the *right lower edge* of a core needle biopsy (**a** – HE, 200×). The acini show intraluminal mucin and nuclear hyperchromasia, but assessing the basal cell layer is difficult due to the distorted nature of the tissue (**b** – HE, 400×). PIN4 immunohistochemical cocktail does not identify basal cells, and the acinar cells faintly express racemase (**c** – PIN4, 200×, **d** – PIN4, 400×). An additional suspicious focus is highlighted (*right upper corner*), a focus that could have been otherwise missed on HE (**c**)

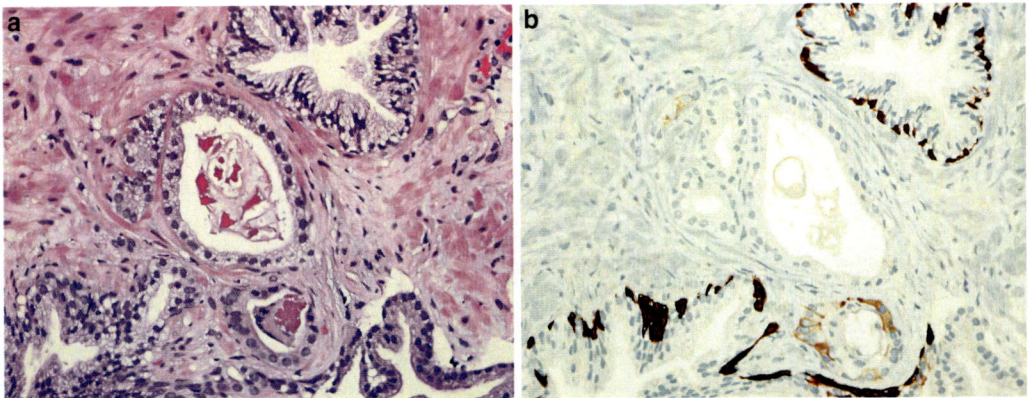

Fig. 19.3 A few small acini show prominent nucleoli and intraluminal eosinophilic secretions (**a** – HE, 400×). No basal cells are identified, but the secretory cells are not expressing racemase (**b** – PIN4, 400×). This focus is suspicious for adenocarcinoma; however, it is too small and the immunohistochemical features are atypical. A confident definite diagnosis of adenocarcinoma cannot be made.

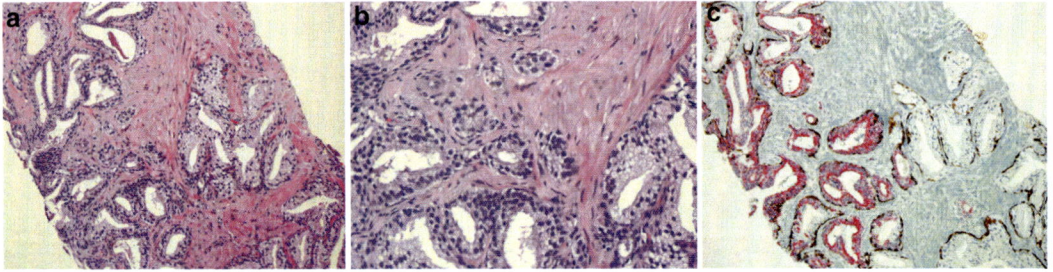

Fig. 19.4 A focus of HGPIN is identified (*left*) (**a** – HE, 200×). A higher magnification illustrates adjacent small acini with prominent nucleoli (**b** – HE, 400×). PIN4 illustrates the presence of basal cells and strong racemase staining in the focus of HGPIN compared to the negative staining of the normal glands on the *right* (**c** – PIN4, 200×). These small atypical acini present adjacent to a focus of HGPIN could be tangential sections of the dysplastic focus also known as budding PIN. However, the atypical focus is small and a confident diagnosis cannot be made. A repeat biopsy should be performed to confirm or rule out adenocarcinoma.

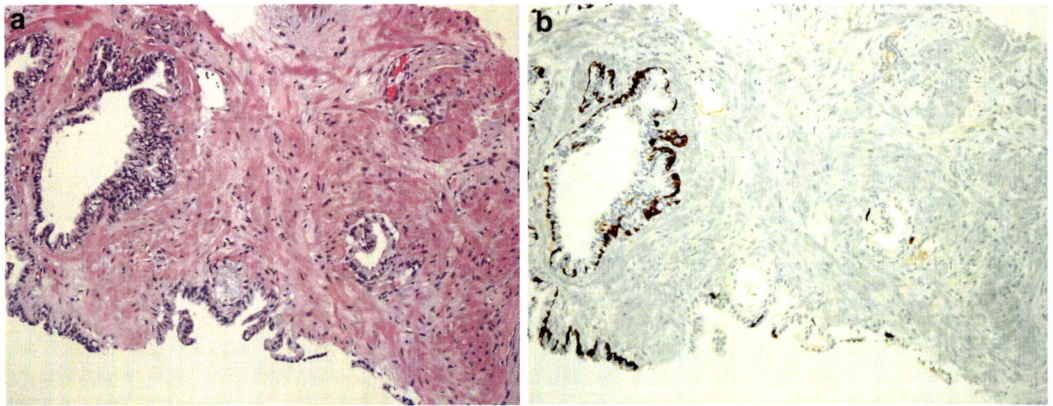

Fig. 19.5 A few scattered acini are worrisome for malignancy (*left upper* and *lower* edge) (**a** – HE, 200×). There are only a few basal cells present, and the acinar cells do not express racemase (**b** – PIN4, 200×). A diagnosis of ASAP is appropriate in this case.

branched chain fatty acids and bile acid intermediates. It is usually upregulated in malignancy and HGPIN [59]. However, numerous false-positive and false-negative results have been reported, and interpretation must be performed with caution [40].

Multiple studies have reported AMACR expression in HGPIN, atypical adenomatous hyperplasia (AAH), partial atrophy, and occasionally benign secretory cells [60, 61]. Absence of staining has been reported in approximately 18% of prostatic adenocarcinomas [62–64] and also in ASAP [61]. Due to this fact, AMACR should not be used alone for a diagnosis of adenocarcinoma [40]. Invasive adenocarcinoma invariably lacks basal cells and therefore will be negative for p63 and HMWCK [57]. However, lack of immunoreactivity should be interpreted in the context of suspicious morphology, as various mimickers of carcinoma can have an absent or partially absent basal cell layer (AAH, partial atrophy, basal cell hyperplasia) [65]. Also very rarely, small foci of adenocarcinoma can retain a few basal cells [66].

Epstein and Herawi recommend the use of basal cell immunohistochemical stains to verify suspicious foci as cancer and not to establish a diagnosis of cancer. For example, if a focus is morphologically favored benign but without confidence and the basal cell markers are negative, they diagnose the focus as suspicious (similar examples are illustrated in Figs. 19.3 and 19.5).

If benign morphology is favored with confidence and the basal markers are negative, they diagnose the focus as benign. They also recommend using a positive AMACR stain (with negative basal cell markers) to convert an atypical diagnosis to cancer in cases that are highly suspicious morphologically [40].

Maximum information should be obtained from the available tissue [33]. Careful hematoxylin-eosin interpretation, with additional deeper levels if necessary, followed by immunohistochemical and molecular studies should be integrated. The clinical parameters (PSA, age, digital rectal examination findings) should not unduly influence the morphological diagnosis of adenocarcinoma.

Last but not least, it is extremely important to note that there is interobserver reproducibility and interpretative variability depending on the experience and skill of the pathologist. Studies have shown that it is more common for an atypical case to be finalized as carcinoma as opposed to benign upon expert review [9, 12, 13, 23, 40, 67]. Cases finalized as atypical or suspicious in the community setting have a not insignificant likelihood of being changed to adenocarcinoma upon expert review. Therefore, patients and urologists should consider having such cases for expert consultation in such situations before subjecting the patient to a repeat biopsy [67]. A prudent diagnostic strategy may include review of such challenging cases by multiple general or expert pathologists to develop a consensus opinion [40].

Finally, Epstein has recommended the use of descriptive terminology (rather than a diagnostic category of ASAP), for example, "prostate tissue with small focus of atypical glands" with a comment explaining "While these findings are atypical and suspicious for adenocarcinoma, there is insufficient cytological and/or architectural atypia to establish a definitive diagnosis" [40]. In a similar view, we use "few small glands suspicious for adenocarcinoma" at our institution. Our feeling is that "suspicious" conveys a higher risk category to the urologist than "atypical."

What Is Next? Clinical Follow-Up

Repeat biopsy is warranted when faced with a diagnosis of ASAP and was performed in an average of 6–7% (Table 19.1) of the cases with a diagnosis of ASAP in 20 reviewed studies [8, 13, 16, 17, 19–21, 23–26, 30–32, 34–39].

Multiple studies have reported the presence of adenocarcinoma on subsequent follow-up biopsies initially diagnosed with ASAP ranging from 17% to 60% (see Table 19.1) with an average of 41% [7–9, 11–13, 16, 17, 19–26, 29–39].

Brausi et al. reported malignancy in 100% (25/25) radical prostatectomy specimens performed immediately following a diagnosis of ASAP without a confirmatory biopsy [25]. However, due to the aforementioned clinical implications, this radical surgical procedure is not recommended without a confirmatory repeat biopsy showing definite adenocarcinoma.

The presence of ASAP associated with HGPIN in biopsy specimens has a significant predictive value for concurrent or subsequent cancer in repeat biopsy specimens [43]. On the other hand in about 40% of cases, ASAP represents under sampled cancer that might not be detected even in multiple subsequent biopsy specimens [43].

What should the needle biopsy sampling protocol be after the diagnosis of isolated ASAP? On subsequent biopsies it is recommended to sample the entire prostate and not just the site initially diagnosed as ASAP, as multiple studies demonstrated the presence of cancer contralateral to or in a different sextant site from the initial ASAP diagnosis site in 26–39% of cases [11, 12, 20]. Based on these studies, the following recommendations emerged:

1. Increased sampling of the initial atypical site (three cores)
2. Increased sampling of the adjacent ipsilateral and contralateral sites (two cores each site)
3. Routine sampling of all sextant sites (one core)

In order for these recommendations to be carried out appropriately, it is imperative for urologists to submit biopsy specimens in a manner that the location of each core is clearly delineated [40].

The current guidelines [68] recommend extended pattern rebiopsy (12 cores) within 6 months with increased sampling of the ASAP site and adjacent areas. If no cancer is found, close follow-up with serum PSA and digital rectal examination (DRE) is recommended. According to these guidelines after two negative extended transrectal ultrasound (TRUS)-guided biopsies, cancer is not commonly found on an additional repeat biopsy.

Multiple studies analyzed the rate of cancer diagnosis following multiple repeat biopsies after a diagnosis of ASAP. Iczkowski et al. identified 99% of cancers on the second and third repeat biopsies following a diagnosis of ASAP [12]. However, in the same study, a case of cancer was diagnosed following a primary diagnosis of ASAP followed by two consecutive negative biopsies. Ryu et al. reported the cancer detection rates of the first, second, third, and fourth repeat biopsies as 24.1% (41/170), 34.1% (14/41), 18.2% (2/11), and 0% (0/2), respectively [38]. Rodríguez-Patrón Rodríguez et al. found cancer following a diagnosis of ASAP on the first, second, and third repeat biopsies of 34% (17/50), 33.3% (2/6), and 33.3% (1/3), respectively, with mean biopsy intervals approximately ranging from 13 to 17 months [35]. It appears that most of the cancers are diagnosed on the first repeat biopsy. Also Moore et al. reported cancer following ASAP in 36% (19/53) and 16% (3/19) of the first and second repeat biopsies [32].

We agree with the current guidelines, and we believe that repeat biopsy should be performed in the setting of a diagnosis of ASAP. The question is how many successive biopsies with a negative result should be performed and when should we stop? One study reported cancer following two consecutive negative biopsies and multiple studies have reported cancer on the third biopsy [12, 35, 38]; however, according to Bostwick [43], some cancers are never detected. We propose raising the number of follow-up biopsies to a total of at least three and pausing after three negative results. Additional clinical follow-up (PSA, DRE) should be continued, and a repeat biopsy protocol should be reinstated if there are strong clinical indications (rising PSA, DRE positivity).

It has been reported that there is no correlation of encountering cancer on repeat biopsy with serum PSA following an atypical diagnosis [9, 12, 16, 22, 26, 30, 32], with DRE [9, 12, 30, 32], and with transrectal ultrasound [20, 30]. Finding, however, recently PSA density (PSAD), PSA velocity (PSAV), and a decreased total prostate volume (TPV) were reported as predictive for prostate cancer in patients with an initial diagnosis of ASAP of the prostate [36, 38, 51].

Usually adenocarcinoma diagnosed following a diagnosis of ASAP is of favorable grade (likely Gleason 6), confined to the prostate, with negative margins, with a few reported exceptions [8, 13, 25].

Differential Diagnosis

Various small foci of benign pathological entities can mimic adenocarcinoma on needle biopsy and, therefore, may be occasionally diagnosed as ASAP (Table 19.4). There is a broad spectrum of entities ranging from benign glandular lesions such as atypical adenomatous hyperplasia [53, 69], atrophy, postatrophic hyperplasia [70], and sclerosing adenosis [71, 72] to treatment effect

Table 19.4 The differential diagnosis of ASAP

Adenocarcinoma
Atypical adenomatous hyperplasia [53, 69]
Sclerosing adenosis (typical and atypical) [71, 72]
Atrophy-postatrophic hyperplasia [70]
Basal cell hyperplasia [75, 76]
HGPIN
Mesonephric hyperplasia [77–79]
Nephrogenic adenoma [80, 81]
Radiation atypia [70, 73]
Androgen deprivation [70, 73]
Inflammation associated atypia
Verumontanum hyperplasia [70, 82]
Clear-cell cribriform hyperplasia [70, 76]
Xanthoma [70]
Normal anatomic structures [70, 73]
Seminal vesicles/ejaculatory ducts
Cowper's glands
Ganglia

and even normal benign prostate histology [70, 73]. Further studies such as immunohistochemistry may serve to appropriately classify these lesions as entities apart from ASAP. This has led some to suggest that ASAP is merely a "wastebasket" term for atypical proliferations that cannot be classified with certainty. For a detailed coverage of these entities, please refer to the references provided in Table 19.4 and to the corresponding chapters in this book.

Conclusions

The diagnosis of ASAP should indicate to the clinicians that the biopsy findings are "uncertain," neither clearly malignant nor clearly benign, and that follow-up biopsy is warranted [43]. It is crucial for urologists to understand the difference between HGPIN and ASAP when present on pathology reports as these two entities have different morphology and ASAP is associated with a much higher risk of cancer on repeat biopsy [40]. Extended pattern repeat biopsy is recommended every 6 months until three consecutive negative results, then clinical follow-up with serum PSA and DRE is warranted.

Editorial Commentary

ASAP seems to confuse urologists more than almost any issue in prostate cancer diagnostics. Unfortunately, the most common response that I observe – by far – is to ignore it. This is illogical, as the author describes that this pathological finding is often actually prostate cancer that has simply been under sampled.

I teach our residents that ASAP is a way for pathologists to tell urologists, "I think this is cancer, but there just isn't enough evidence on the slide to prove it." It is our job to provide that additional evidence. Regardless of your preferred biopsy technique – we use 20 core transrectal office-based saturation biopsies – it is imperative to give the pathologist more tissue. Alternatively, it is not uncommon that a subspecialty pathologist will make the call for a cancer diagnosis on the original biopsy tissue, so a second pathological opinion should be considered if there is any doubt on the part of the pathologist or if the initial

pathologist is not highly experienced with prostate biopsy interpretation.

Another issue that I see which causes problems for many people is the relatively widespread concept that repeat biopsy for ASAP should be performed within 6 months. I find that many urologists interpret this to imply that they should wait 6 months. It is not clear why this interpretation is so prevalent, but I hypothesize that it is because patients historically are not keen to proceed right back to another biopsy immediately, so the urologists probably believe they are doing the patient a favor by not recommending immediate repeat biopsy. Nevertheless, with modern periprostatic block, this is rarely a concern to the large numbers of patients that I see for second opinions for this diagnosis. Quite the opposite, many of them are unhappy that they have been told they have to wait 6 months, and they are relieved when informed that there is no reason to delay the biopsy. They usually don't want to worry another day once they know that this reading implies a high likelihood that they have unrecognized cancer, and they usually want to proceed to repeat biopsy (dare I say?), ASAP.

References

1. Epstein JI. Diagnostic criteria of limited adenocarcinoma of the prostate on needle biopsy. Hum Pathol. 1995;26(2):223–9.
2. Kahane H, Sharp JW, Shuman GB, Dasilva G, Epstein JI. Utilization of high molecular weight cytokeratin on prostate needle biopsies in an independent laboratory. Urology. 1995;45(6):981–6.
3. Bostwick DG, Qian J, Frankel K. The incidence of high grade prostatic intraepithelial neoplasia in needle biopsies. J Urol. 1995;154(5):1791–4.
4. Iczkowski KA, Cheng L, Qian J, et al. ASAP is a valid diagnosis. Atypical small acinar proliferation. Hum Pathol. 1999;30(12):1403–4.
5. Rosen S, Upton M. ASAP. Atypical small acinar proliferations. Hum Pathol. 1999;30(12):1403. author reply 1404.
6. Oxley DK. ASAP. Hum Pathol. 2000;31(6):774.
7. Roehrborn CG, Pickens GJ, Sanders JS. Diagnostic yield of repeated transrectal ultrasound-guided biopsies stratified by specific histopathologic diagnoses and prostate specific antigen levels. Urology. 1996; 47(3):347–52.
8. Cheville JC, Reznicek MJ, Bostwick DG. The focus of "atypical glands, suspicious for malignancy" in prostatic needle biopsy specimens: incidence, histo-

logic features, and clinical follow-up of cases diagnosed in a community practice. Am J Clin Pathol. 1997;108(6):633–40.

9. Iczkowski KA, MacLennan GT, Bostwick DG. Atypical small acinar proliferation suspicious for malignancy in prostate needle biopsies: clinical significance in 33 cases. Am J Surg Pathol. 1997;21(12):1489–95.

10. Wills ML, Hamper UM, Partin AW, Epstein JI. Incidence of high-grade prostatic intraepithelial neoplasia in sextant needle biopsy specimens. Urology. 1997;49(3):367–73.

11. Allen EA, Kahane H, Epstein JI. Repeat biopsy strategies for men with atypical diagnoses on initial prostate needle biopsy. Urology. 1998;52(5):803–7.

12. Iczkowski KA, Bassler TJ, Schwob VS, et al. Diagnosis of "suspicious for malignancy" in prostate biopsies: predictive value for cancer. Urology. 1998;51(5):749–57. discussion 757–8.

13. Renshaw AA, Santis WF, Richie JP. Clinicopathological characteristics of prostatic adenocarcinoma in men with atypical prostate needle biopsies. J Urol. 1998;159(6):2018–21. discussion 2022.

14. Reyes AO, Humphrey PA. Diagnostic effect of complete histologic sampling of prostate needle biopsy specimens. Am J Clin Pathol. 1998;109(4):416–22.

15. Weinstein MH, Greenspan DL, Epstein JI. Diagnoses rendered on prostate needle biopsy in community hospitals. Prostate. 1998;35(1):50–5.

16. Chan TY, Epstein JI. Follow-up of atypical prostate needle biopsies suspicious for cancer. Urology. 1999;53(2):351–5.

17. Hoedemaeker RF, Kranse R, Rietbergen JB, Kruger AE, Schröder FH, van der Kwast TH. Evaluation of prostate needle biopsies in a population-based screening study: the impact of borderline lesions. Cancer. 1999;85(1):145–52.

18. Novis DA, Zarbo RJ, Valenstein PA. Diagnostic uncertainty expressed in prostate needle biopsies. A College of American Pathologists Q-probes Study of 15,753 prostate needle biopsies in 332 institutions. Arch Pathol Lab Med. 1999;123(8):687–92.

19. O'dowd GJ, Miller MC, Orozco R, Veltri RW. Analysis of repeated biopsy results within 1 year after a noncancer diagnosis. Urology. 2000;55(4):553–9.

20. Borboroglu PG, Sur RL, Roberts JL, Amling CL. Repeat biopsy strategy in patients with atypical small acinar proliferation or high grade prostatic intraepithelial neoplasia on initial prostate needle biopsy. J Urol. 2001;166(3):866–70.

21. Ouyang RC, Kenwright DN, Nacey JN, Delahunt B. The presence of atypical small acinar proliferation in prostate needle biopsy is predictive of carcinoma on subsequent biopsy. BJU Int. 2001;87(1):70–4.

22. Park S, Shinohara K, Grossfeld GD, Carroll PR. Prostate cancer detection in men with prior high grade prostatic intraepithelial neoplasia or atypical prostate biopsy. J Urol. 2001;165(5):1409–14.

23. Iczkowski KA, Chen HM, Yang XJ, Beach RA. Prostate cancer diagnosed after initial biopsy with atypical small acinar proliferation suspicious for malignancy is similar to cancer found on initial biopsy. Urology. 2002;60(5):851–4.

24. Mian BM, Naya Y, Okihara K, Vakar-Lopez F, Troncoso P, Babaian RJ. Predictors of cancer in repeat extended multisite prostate biopsy in men with previous negative extended multisite biopsy. Urology. 2002;60(5):836–40.

25. Brausi M, Castagnetti G, Dotti A, De Luca G, Olmi R, Cesinaro AM. Immediate radical prostatectomy in patients with atypical small acinar proliferation. Over treatment? J Urol. 2004;172(3):906–8 discussion 908–9.

26. Fadare O, Wang S, Mariappan MR. Practice patterns of clinicians following isolated diagnoses of atypical small acinar proliferation on prostate biopsy specimens. Arch Pathol Lab Med. 2004;128(5):557–60.

27. Gupta C, Ren JZ, Wojno KJ. Individual submission and embedding of prostate biopsies decreases rates of equivocal pathology reports. Urology. 2004;63(1):83–6.

28. Kobayashi T, Nishizawa K, Watanabe J, Ogura K, Mitsumori K, Ide Y. Effects of sextant transrectal prostate biopsy plus additional far lateral cores in improving cancer detection rates in men with large prostate glands. Int J Urol. 2004;11(6):392–6.

29. Naya Y, Ayala AG, Tamboli P, Babaian RJ. Can the number of cores with high-grade prostate intraepithelial neoplasia predict cancer in men who undergo repeat biopsy? Urology. 2004;63(3):503–8.

30. Postma R, Roobol M, Schröder FH, van der Kwast TH. Lesions predictive for prostate cancer in a screened population: first and second screening round findings. Prostate. 2004;61(3):260–6.

31. Leite KR, Mitteldorf CA, Camara-Lopes LH. Repeat prostate biopsies following diagnoses of prostate intraepithelial neoplasia and atypical small gland proliferation. Int Braz J Urol. 2005;31(2):131–6.

32. Moore CK, Karikehalli S, Nazeer T, Fisher HA, Kaufman Jr RP, Mian BM. Prognostic significance of high grade prostatic intraepithelial neoplasia and atypical small acinar proliferation in the contemporary era. J Urol. 2005;173(1):70–2.

33. Schlesinger C, Bostwick DG, Iczkowski KA. High-grade prostatic intraepithelial neoplasia and atypical small acinar proliferation: predictive value for cancer in current practice. Am J Surg Pathol. 2005;29(9):1201–7.

34. Mallén E, Gil P, Sancho C, et al. Atypical small acinar proliferation: review of a series of 64 patients. Scand J Urol Nephrol. 2006;40(4):272–5.

35. Rodríguez-Patrón Rodríguez R, Mayayo Dehesa T, Burgos Revilla FJ, Sanz Mayayo E, García González R. Prognostic significance of PIN and atypical small acinar proliferation on transrectal ultrasound-guided prostate biopsy. Actas Urol Esp. 2006;30(4):359–66.

36. Mearini L, Costantini E, Bellezza G, et al. Is there any clinical parameter able to predict prostate cancer after initial diagnosis of atypical small acinar proliferation? Urol Int. 2008;81(1):29–35.

37. Ploussard G, Plennevaux G, Allory Y, et al. High-grade prostatic intraepithelial neoplasia and atypical small acinar proliferation on initial 21-core extended biopsy scheme: incidence and implications for patient care and surveillance. World J Urol. 2009;27(5): 587–92.

38. Ryu JH, Kim YB, Lee JK, Kim YJ, Jung TY. Predictive factors of prostate cancer at repeat biopsy in patients with an initial diagnosis of atypical small acinar proliferation of the prostate. Korean J Urol. 2010;51(11):752–6.

39. Kopp RP, Parsons JK, Shiau J, et al. Prostate atypia: clinical and pathological variables associated with cancer diagnosis on repeat biopsy. Prostate Cancer Prostatic Dis. 2011;14(2):149–54.

40. Epstein JI, Herawi M. Prostate needle biopsies containing prostatic intraepithelial neoplasia or atypical foci suspicious for carcinoma: implications for patient care. J Urol. 2006;175:820–34.

41. Rubin MA, Bismar TA, Curtis S, Montie JE. Prostate needle biopsy reporting: how are the surgical members of the Society of Urologic Oncology using pathology reports to guide treatment of prostate cancer patients? Am J Surg Pathol. 2004;28(7): 946–52.

42. Descazeaud A, Rubin MA, Allory Y, et al. What information are urologists extracting from prostate needle biopsy reports and what do they need for clinical management of prostate cancer? Eur Urol. 2005;48(6): 911–5.

43. Bostwick DG, Meiers I. Atypical small acinar proliferation in the prostate: clinical significance in 2006. Arch Pathol Lab Med. 2006;130(7):952–7.

44. Montironi R, Mazzucchelli R, Lopez-Beltran A, Cheng L, Scarpelli M. Mechanisms of disease: high-grade prostatic intraepithelial neoplasia and other proposed preoplastic lesions in the prostate. Nat Clin Pract Urol. 2007;4(6):321–32.

45. Abouassaly R, Tan N, Moussa A, Jones JS. Risk of prostate cancer after diagnosis of atypical glands suspicious for carcinoma on saturation and traditional biopsies. J Urol. 2008;180(3):911–4 discussion 914.

46. Iczkowski KA, Bostwick DG. Criteria for biopsy diagnosis of minimal volume prostatic adenocarcinoma: analytic comparison with nondiagnostic but suspicious atypical small acinar proliferation. Arch Pathol Lab Med. 2000;124(1):98–107.

47. Michaelson MD, Cotter SE, Gargollo PC, Zietman AL, Dahl DM, Smith MR. Management of complications of prostate cancer treatment. CA Cancer J Clin. 2008;58(4):196–213.

48. Wolin KY, Luly J, Sutcliffe S, Andriole GL, Kibel AS. Risk of urinary incontinence following prostatectomy: the role of physical activity and obesity. J Urol. 2010;183(2):629–33.

49. Messaoudi R, Menard J, Ripert T, Parquet H, Staerman F. Erectile dysfunction and sexual health after radical prostatectomy: impact of sexual motivation. Int J Impot Res. 2011;23(2):81–6.

50. Gallina A, Briganti A, Suardi N, et al. Surgery and erectile dysfunction. Arch Esp Urol. 2010;63(8): 640–8.

51. Scattoni V, Roscigno M, Freschi M, et al. Atypical small acinar proliferation (ASAP) on extended prostatic biopsies: predictive factors of cancer detection on repeat biopsies. Arch Ital Urol Androl. 2005;77(1):31–6.

52. Montironi R, Scattoni V, Mazzucchelli R, Lopez-Beltran A, Bostwick DG, Montorsi F. Atypical foci suspicious but not diagnostic of malignancy in prostate needle biopsies (also referred to as "atypical small acinar proliferation suspicious for but not diagnostic of malignancy"). Eur Urol. 2006;50(4):666–74.

53. Bostwick DG, Srigley J, Grignon D, et al. Atypical adenomatous hyperplasia of the prostate: morphologic criteria for its distinction from well-differentiated carcinoma. Hum Pathol. 1993;24(8):819–32.

54. Kronz JD, Shaikh AA, Epstein JI. High-grade prostatic intraepithelial neoplasia with adjacent small atypical glands on prostate biopsy. Hum Pathol. 2001;32(4):389–95.

55. Alsikafi NF, Brendler CB, Gerber GS, Yang XJ. High-grade prostatic intraepithelial neoplasia with adjacent atypia is associated with a higher incidence of cancer on subsequent needle biopsy than high-grade prostatic intraepithelial neoplasia alone. Urology. 2001;57(2): 296–300.

56. Renshaw AA. Adequate tissue sampling of prostate core needle biopsies. Am J Clin Pathol. 1997;107(1): 26–9.

57. Shah RB, Zhou M, LeBlanc M, Snyder M, Rubin MA. Comparison of the basal cell-specific markers, 34betaE12 and p63, in the diagnosis of prostate cancer. Am J Surg Pathol. 2002;26(9):1161–8.

58. Shah RB, Kunju LP, Shen R, LeBlanc M, Zhou M, Rubin MA. Usefulness of basal cell cocktail (34betaE12 + p63) in the diagnosis of atypical prostate glandular proliferations. Am J Clin Pathol. 2004;122(4):517–23.

59. Jiang Z, Woda BA, Wu CL, Yang XJ. Discovery and clinical application of a novel prostate cancer marker: alpha-methylacyl CoA racemase (P504S). Am J Clin Pathol. 2004;122(2):275–89.

60. Jiang Z, Woda BA, Rock KL, et al. P504S: a new molecular marker for the detection of prostate carcinoma. Am J Surg Pathol. 2001;25(11):1397–404.

61. Kunju LP, Rubin MA, Chinnaiyan AM, Shah RB. Diagnostic usefulness of monoclonal antibody P504S in the workup of atypical prostatic glandular proliferations. Am J Clin Pathol. 2003;120(5):737–45.

62. Browne TJ, Hirsch MS, Brodsky G, Welch WR, Loda MF, Rubin MA. Prospective evaluation of AMACR (P504S) and basal cell markers in the assessment of routine prostate needle biopsy specimens. Hum Pathol. 2004;35(12):1462–8.

63. Jiang Z, Wu CL, Woda BA, et al. P504S/alpha-methylacyl-CoA racemase: a useful marker for diagnosis of small foci of prostatic carcinoma on needle biopsy. Am J Surg Pathol. 2002;26(9):1169–74.

64. Zhou M, Aydin H, Kanane H, Epstein JI. How often does alpha-methylacyl-CoA-racemase contribute to resolving an atypical diagnosis on prostate needle biopsy beyond that provided by basal cell markers? Am J Surg Pathol. 2004;28(2):239–43.

65. Molinié V, Fromont G, Sibony M, et al. Diagnostic utility of a p63/alpha-methyl-CoA-racemase (p504s) cocktail in atypical foci in the prostate. Mod Pathol. 2004;17(10):1180–90.

66. Oliai BR, Kahane H, Epstein JI. Can basal cells be seen in adenocarcinoma of the prostate?: an immuno-histochemical study using high molecular weight cytokeratin (clone 34betaE12) antibody. Am J Surg Pathol. 2002;26(9):1151–60.

67. Chan TY, Epstein JI. Patient and urologist driven second opinion of prostate needle biopsies. J Urol. 2005;174(4 Pt 1):1390–4 discussion 1394; author reply 1394.

68. National Comprehensive Cancer Network: Practice guidelines in oncology, version 1.2011. Clinical practice guidelines in oncology, 2011. Available at: www.nccn.org. Accessed 15 July 2011

69. Midi A, Tecimer T, Bozkurt S, Ozkan N. Differences in the structural features of atypical adenomatous hyperplasia and low-grade prostatic adenocarcinoma. Indian J Urol. 2008;24(2):169–77.

70. Srigley JR. Benign mimickers of prostatic adenocarcinoma. Mod Pathol. 2004;17(3):328–48.

71. Berney DM, Fisher G, Kattan MW, et al. Pitfalls in the diagnosis of prostatic cancer: retrospective review of 1791 cases with clinical outcome. Histopathology. 2007;51(4):452–7.

72. Cheng L, Bostwick DG. Atypical sclerosing adenosis of the prostate: a rare mimic of adenocarcinoma. Histopathology. 2010;56(5):627–31.

73. Gaudin PB, Reuter VE. Benign mimics of prostatic adenocarcinoma on needle biopsy. Anat Pathol. 1997;2:111–34.

74. Parsons JK, Gage WR, Nelson WG, De Marzo AM. p63 protein expression is rare in prostate adenocarcinoma: implications for cancer diagnosis and carcinogenesis. Urology. 2001;58(4):619–24.

75. Hosler GA, Epstein JI. Basal cell hyperplasia: an unusual diagnostic dilemma on prostate needle biopsies. Hum Pathol. 2005;36(5):480–5.

76. Hameed O, Humphrey PA. Pseudoneoplastic mimics of prostate and bladder carcinomas. Arch Pathol Lab Med. 2010;134(3):427–43.

77. Chen YB, Fine SW, Epstein JI. Mesonephric remnant hyperplasia involving prostate and periprostatic tissue: findings at radical prostatectomy. Am J Surg Pathol. 2011;35(7):1054–61.

78. Tacha D, Zhou D, Cheng L. Expression of PAX8 in normal and neoplastic tissues: a comprehensive immunohistochemical study. Appl Immunohistochem Mol Morphol. 2011;19(4):293–9.

79. Laury AR, Perets R, Piao H, et al. A comprehensive analysis of PAX8 expression in human epithelial tumors. Am J Surg Pathol. 2011;35(6):816–26.

80. Ozcan A, Shen SS, Hamilton C, et al. PAX 8 expression in non-neoplastic tissues, primary tumors, and metastatic tumors: a comprehensive immunohistochemical study. Mod Pathol. 2011;24(6):751–64.

81. Tong GX, Melamed J, Mansukhani M, et al. PAX2: a reliable marker for nephrogenic adenoma. Mod Pathol. 2006;19(3):356–63.

82. Gagucas RJ, Brown RW, Wheeler TM. Verumontanum mucosal gland hyperplasia. Am J Surg Pathol. 1995;19(1):30–6.

Repeat Prostate Biopsy Strategies: How Many and Where?

20

Joseph C. Presti Jr.

Introduction

Patients with a negative prior prostate biopsy yet a persistently elevated or rising PSA level represent a challenge to the practicing urologist. Anxiety often exists in the patient, the family, and the referring primary care physician. Tremendous variation exists among physicians in the approach to these patients. Controversy exists with respect to the use of various markers to determine the need for additional biopsy, specific biopsy technique used, and significance of cancers found in this setting. Each of these will be addressed in this chapter. This chapter will not address patients who have either high-grade prostatic intraepithelial neoplasia (HGPIN) or atypical small acinar proliferation (ASAP) on their prior biopsy as this is covered elsewhere in this book.

Adequacy of Initial Biopsy

One of the first steps in the evaluation of these patients is to assess the adequacy of the initial biopsy. Adequacy of the initial biopsy depends upon 2 factors: (1) the number and location of the biopsy cores taken and (2) the size of prostate. One should ensure that the biopsy followed an

extended pattern biopsy scheme (minimum of 10–12 cores). If the prior negative biopsy was a sextant biopsy, detection rates on repeat biopsy are twofold higher than if the initial negative biopsy was an extended pattern biopsy scheme [1]. Extended pattern biopsy schemes, introduced in 1997, have undergone many refinements [2]. Although many variations of extended pattern biopsies have been described, the unifying factor common to all of these schemes is that they maximize sampling of the peripheral zone where the majority of prostate cancers arise. The most commonly used scheme today consists of a 12-core scheme where biopsies are obtained from the apex, mid, base, lateral apex, lateral mid, and lateral base from both right and left sides [3].

Prostate size also contributes to assessing the adequacy of the biopsy. Since prostate sizes vary, it seems logical to assume that larger prostates might be inadequately sampled by 12-core biopsy schemes. Indeed, investigators have noted an inverse relationship between prostate size and cancer detection rates in referral-based populations undergoing an initial sextant biopsy [4]. A similar observation is seen in patients undergoing repeat biopsies by extended pattern biopsy schemes. The chance of finding any cancer or high-grade cancer (Gleason score ≥ 7) is inversely related to prostate size [5]. While it is assumed that this is in part related to the enrichment of such populations with BPH patients (large benign prostate is associated with a higher PSA level), it is quite possible that missed cancers might also contribute to this observation.

J.C. Presti Jr., M.D. (✉)
Department of Urology, Stanford University School of Medicine, 875 Blake Wilbur Drive, Rm 2217, Stanford, CA 94305-5826, USA
e-mail: jpresti@stanford.edu

J.S. Jones (ed.), *Prostate Cancer Diagnosis: PSA, Biopsy and Beyond*, Current Clinical Urology, DOI 10.1007/978-1-62703-188-2_20, © Springer Science+Business Media New York 2013

Lastly, in some situations, a secondary review of the pathology slides from the initial biopsy may be warranted. In patients who are identified as having atypical small acinar proliferation or very small foci of cancer, a second review might shed light on any ambiguity of the initial diagnosis.

Risk Assessment in the Repeat Biopsy Population

Several markers and tools can be used to better assess the risk of a missed cancer. Refinements of PSA include corrections for prostate size, changes over time, and the different molecular forms of PSA. When looking at studies comparing the utility of different markers in predicting cancer, a commonly used statistical method involves receiver operating characteristic curves. Typically as the sensitivity of a test increases, its specificity decreases. Clinically, this means that there is always a trade-off between finding cancers and performing biopsies that come back negative. The latter is sometimes referred to as an "unnecessary biopsy," but I would argue that one should question in whose eyes were these biopsies "unnecessary." Perhaps they would be considered unnecessary from a financial perspective (cost of biopsy) or from a risk perspective (risk associated with biopsy procedure). If we want to minimize the number of negative biopsies (increase specificity), we risk missing a cancer. The impact of missing this cancer is of course related to the severity of the cancer. The latter is difficult to know *a priori*, and thus as a urologist, I feel that if the trigger has already been pulled to evaluate someone for the presence of prostate cancer (PSA is drawn), it is our job to determine whether a cancer is present and, if so, its severity. This later statement I recognize is quite controversial; however, I equate it to whether or not you want to deal with a "black box" or know what is inside. As we know, overdetection for this disease is common. It is critical to initiate the discussion early with the patient (prior to the biopsy and preferably at the time of initiating screening) that some cancers may be indolent and not require aggressive therapy. As urologists, we need to emphasize that detection must be separated from

treatment. The latter includes assessment of both the cancer (i.e., grade, stage, volume) and the host (age and comorbidities).

The inverse relationship between sensitivity of a test and its specificity is graphically depicted in a receiver operating characteristic (ROC) curve. ROC curves graphically demonstrate the performance test characteristics by plotting the sensitivity on the Y-axis and 1-specificity on the X-axis. Commonly, the area under the curves (AUCs) is then used to compare the performance of different tests. A better test typically has a larger AUC. A diagonal line drawn from the bottom left corner of the graph to the upper right corner of the graph is considered the line of no discrimination (AUC = 0.50). A test whose curve falls on this line is no better than a coin toss (50:50 chance) in its ability to predict the outcome (i.e., find cancer). In general, the more rapidly the ROC curve rises to the upper left corner of the graph, the better the test. However, when it comes to diagnostic tests, one needs to exercise some caution in just relying upon the AUC when comparing tests. As it pertains to prostate cancer detection, if we are trying to find cancer, we are most interested in the region of the curve in the upper right area of the graph (i.e., where the test has a high sensitivity). Often, although significant differences might be observed in the AUC between two tests, this region of the curves may be quite similar and thus their clinical utility might be similar. Although formal statistical analyses are possible comparing this region of the ROC curves, they are rarely reported in the literature. The downside to focusing on this area of the curve is that it will convey a lower specificity; thus, many biopsies will be negative. However, I would argue that this is not an unnecessary biopsy but rather reassurance for the patient and physician.

Markers for Detection in the Repeat Biopsy Population

One of the earliest refinements of PSA was PSA density (PSAD) that attempts to correct the PSA level for prostate size. PSAD is calculated by dividing the total serum PSA level by the entire volume of the prostate as determined by transrectal ultrasound (TRUS). It is a crude method to try to distinguish between the relative contributions of the total PSA level from BPH compared to prostate cancer [6, 7]. Typically, the prostate volume is estimated using a prolate ellipse formula, the volume equals $\Pi/6 \times$ length $\times$ width $\times$ height where length is obtained in the longitudinal plane and height and width are obtained in the axial plane. Higher PSAD levels are associated not only with higher cancer detection rates but also the presence of high-grade disease [8]. A further refinement of this index has been the realization that as a prostate enlarges with age, most of the enlargement occurs in the transition zone. Thus, one can calculate a transition zone density (PSAD-TZ) [9].

An additional refinement of PSA comes from the observation that in the serum, PSA occurs in both free and protein-bound states. The ratio of free/total PSA levels (F/T PSA) has been found to be lowered in the presence of cancer [10]. Additional assays have focused on just the component that is bound to protein (complexed PSA or cPSA) [11]. These indices have been studied by numerous investigators; however, in most series, these have relied upon sextant biopsy sampling as the gold standard for the determination of the presence or absence of prostate cancer. In one large series of 820 patients undergoing repeat biopsy, the ROC curves showed that the F/T PSA (AUC=0.745) outperformed PSA (AUC=0.603), PSAD (AUC=0.618), and PSAD-TZ (AUC=0.691) [12]. In the region of the ROC curves for high sensitivity, the differences persist; thus, F/T PSA was the best test in this study to predict cancer on repeat biopsy.

Several studies have assessed the utility of PSA kinetics in predicting the presence of cancer on repeat biopsy. In general, two parameters can be used: PSA velocity (PSAV) and/or PSA doubling time (PSADT). One series of 373 repeat biopsy patients demonstrated that a long PSADT (>5 years) was protective with respect to finding cancer on repeat biopsy [13]. Variables that were significant in multivariate analysis in predicting cancer were PSAD (>0.25), an abnormal DRE, and a positive family history for prostate cancer. One confounder in this analysis was that patients with HGPIN were included in the population.

A smaller series of 99 patients, all of whom had undergone a prior negative 12-core biopsy, showed that PSAD-TZ was an independent predictor of cancer on repeat biopsy and that PSAV was not predictive of cancer [14]. Again, HGPIN patients were included in this analysis.

A secondary analysis of the Reduction by Dutasteride of Prostate Cancer Events (REDUCE) Trial provides additional information regarding PSA velocity as well as how 5-alpha reductase inhibitors may influence cancer detection in a repeat biopsy population [15]. This trial enrolled men with PSA levels between 2.5 and 10 ng/ml who had a negative prostate biopsy within 6 months of enrollment. Biopsies were performed at 2 and 4 years following the initiation of either placebo or dutasteride. For men on placebo, PSA velocity was a poor predictor for the presence of any cancer (ROC curve AUC=0.530) but did show some improvement for detection of Gleason score 7–10 (ROC curve AUC=0.593). In patients on dutasteride, the AUC for the ROC curve for PSA velocity did show improvement compared to placebo for both the detection of any cancer (AUC=0.637) and high-grade cancer (AUC=0.699). Unfortunately, the ROC curves were not shown in this analysis to better understand where the improvement of test performance occurred. It should be noted that the authors did report positive predictive values for various cut points of PSA change to predict high-grade cancer in both the placebo and dutasteride arms. Even at changes up to 4 ng/ml, the positive predictive value in the placebo patients was less than 10% for predicting high-grade disease. In the dutasteride arm, PSA changes of 1 ng/ml conveyed a positive predictive value of 17%, while a change of 2 ng/ml conveyed a positive predictive value of 20% in predicting high-grade disease. PSA increases in patients on 5-alpha reductase inhibitors warrant further study.

One study of 343 repeat biopsy patients was used to create a nomogram specific to the population of men who had a prior negative biopsy [16]. Unique to the revised nomogram are variables such as the cumulative number of negative cores in prior biopsy sessions and the time interval from prior biopsy session [17]. Again, confounders are the presence of ASAP and HGPIN in the patient population and the lack of PSAD or F/T PSA. Additionally, although the cumulative number of negative cores was collected, the cohort may have included patients with any number of cores taken at the prior session. Thus, the likelihood of a false-negative biopsy is unknown.

Nomograms are valuable tools in medicine. By combining multiple variables in a mathematical model, a refined probability can be determined that is superior to any one given variable. Many such nomograms are available in urologic oncology. The prostate cancer risk calculator was derived from the placebo arm of the Prostate Cancer Prevention Trial [18]. By including the patient's age, race, PSA level, DRE findings, presence of a family history for prostate cancer, and whether he has had a previous biopsy, estimates were generated for finding any cancer and also high-grade (Gleason score$\geq$7) cancer. Despite studying 20 different definitions modeling various methods of PSA kinetics, this calculator showed that no measure of PSA kinetics was independently useful as identifying the presence of cancer. A more recent analysis of this data set again failed to demonstrate the utility of PSA velocity in prediction of cancer on biopsy [19]. This analysis did not provide information specific to those men who had a prior negative biopsy. The utility of the prostate cancer risk calculator for an initial biopsy patient in a referral-based population as it relates to predicting high-grade disease has recently come into question [20]. For initial biopsy patients, the risk calculator accurately predicted risk of any cancer; however, it underestimated the risk of high-grade cancer by about 50%. It is important to recognize that the study population used to generate the risk calculator represents a highly select cohort. To enter the Prostate Cancer Prevention Trial, patients had to have a PSA level <3 ng/ml and a normal DRE. They were then followed longitudinally for up to 7 years. These subjects were considered to be at low risk for developing prostate cancer. Additionally, about 80% of the patients in the Prostate Cancer Prevention Trial underwent a sextant biopsy during the trial, and details of the prior negative biopsy are unknown. Although additional work has been done on this study

cohort using other markers such as PCA3 and proPSA, the utility of this data is unknown as the patient cohort is not reflective of a referral-based population. In a urologic practice, patients are referred for either an abnormal DRE or an elevated PSA. This cohort is considered to be a much higher risk group. Additional work is needed to validate the results of the risk calculator in the repeat biopsy population.

A newer test that is approved for use in this patient population is the PCA3 test. This is a urinary test that detects the presence of prostate cancer cells in the urine using reverse transcriptase polymerase chain reaction. The PCA3 gene is expressed in a high percentage of prostate cancers, so this test is essentially a molecular cytology trying to detect small numbers of prostate cancer cells that are shed in the urine following a DRE. In 233 patients who had at least one negative prior biopsy, PCA3 demonstrated an area under the ROC curve of 0.678 [21]. A quantitative score for this assay can be obtained and its positive predictive value increases with increasing score. As with PSA, higher levels of PCA3 convey a higher risk of finding cancer on biopsy. An arbitrary cut point of 35 for PCA3 has been defined as a positive test. Investigations using this marker and other urinary markers in a multiplex fashion are ongoing [22]. The PCA3 test was more recently tested in the placebo arm of the REDUCE trial [23]. In an ancillary study, PCA3 scores were determined prior to the scheduled biopsies. In 1,072 patients, the ROC curves showed that the PCA3 (AUC=0.693) outperformed F/T PSA (AUC=0.637) and total PSA (AUC=0.612) for overall cancer detection. However, it should be noted that the difference between PCA3 and F/T PSA was not statistically significant (p=0.06). In addition, and perhaps more importantly, when looking at the regions of the ROC curves of high sensitivity, PCA3 and F/T PSA performed similarly.

More recently, a precursor of PSA has been tested in its ability for cancer detection. Proenzyme PSA is a cancer-associated form of free PSA that has an amino acid leader attached. Various forms of proPSA exist depending upon how many amino acids are attached. One form, in particular is stable, [−2]proPSA, and automated assays have been developed. Early studies suggest that the %[−2]proPSA may perform better (AUC=0.70) than F/T PSA (AUC=0.66) and PSA (AUC=0.58) in the initial biopsy population with PSA levels between 2 and 10 ng/ml [24]. However, again when looking at the regions of the ROC curves of high sensitivity, these differences seem small. Additional studies are needed with proPSA in repeat biopsy populations.

Techniques of Repeat Biopsy

The majority of prostate cancers arise from the peripheral zone [25]. It is important to understand the zonal anatomy of the prostate. As seen in the schematic drawing in Fig. 20.1, when looking in the transverse plane at the mid-gland level, the peripheral zone extends anteriorly forming anterior horns at the midlevel and base of the gland. In the sagittal plane (Fig. 20.2), the entire apex of the prostate is comprised of peripheral zone.

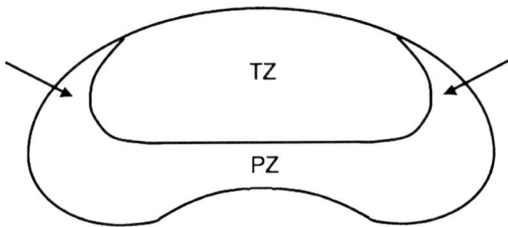

Fig. 20.1 Schematic diagram of transverse plane of prostate at the mid-gland level. Notice anterior horns of peripheral zone (*arrows*). *PZ* peripheral zone, *TZ* transition zone

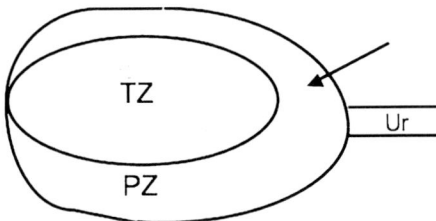

Fig. 20.2 Schematic diagram of prostate in sagittal plane. Notice anterior apical tissue (*arrow*) comprised of peripheral zone that may harbor missed cancers in a traditional 12-core biopsy scheme. *PZ* peripheral zone, *TZ* transition zone, *Ur* urethra

Extended biopsy schemes have evolved to more heavily sample the peripheral zone.

Babaian et al. evaluated an 11-core biopsy strategy in 277 patients with a prior negative biopsy [26]. Cancer was found in 81 (29%) and the regions of unique cancer detection (only region where cancer was found) were non-sextant sites for 27 cancers (33%), sextant sites for 20 cancers (25%), anterior horn sites in 15 (19%), transition zone in 9 (11%), and the midline in 2 (3%).

A larger series looked at 218 patients with a prior negative biopsy and no HGPIN or ASAP by a 10-core systematic biopsy scheme (standard sextant plus lateral mid and lateral base biopsies) [1]. A subset of 139 patients underwent six additional transition zone biopsies. A total of 77 out of 218 (35%) patients had cancer on repeat biopsy. In general, apical and laterally directed biopsies resulted in the highest overall and unique cancer detection rates. The unique cancer detection rates for the transition zone biopsies were low (<5%).

A particular region of interest in the prostate that might be undersampled with the 12-core extended pattern biopsy scheme is the anterior apex [27]. As shown in Fig. 20.2, the entire apex of the prostate is comprised of peripheral zone. In a series of 255 patients with prostates less than 50 cc in size undergoing a 12-core scheme that included a 10-core scheme plus anterior apical biopsies, cancer was found in over 30% of the anterior apical cores. In men with a normal DRE, the anterior apical core was the only site of disease in 6%. Investigations on the role of anterior apical biopsies in patients with a prior negative biopsy are ongoing.

Some investigators have advocated more aggressive biopsy schemes in patients undergoing repeat biopsy. Such biopsy schemes are referred to as "saturation schemes" and consist of obtaining 20 or more cores that emphasize sampling of the peripheral zone. One of the more common saturation schemes involves taking two cores from the lateral base, three cores from the lateral mid, three cores from the apex (including anterior apex), one core from the parasagittal mid, and one core from the parasagittal base [28].

While initial saturation schemes included two cores at both the parasagittal mid and parasagittal base, unique identification of cancer in these areas is rare, and thus it has been recommended to only obtain one core for each of these areas.

One series analyzed 224 men who underwent saturation prostate biopsies [29]. It must be noted that these biopsies were performed under anesthesia as an outpatient procedure. The mean number of cores obtained was 23 (range 14–45). Indications for repeat biopsy included elevated PSA in 108, abnormal digital rectal exam and elevated PSA in 27, abnormal digital rectal examination alone in four, high-grade prostatic intraepithelial neoplasia in 64, and atypia in 21. Cancer was detected in 77 of 224 patients (34%). Complications occurred in 27 patients (12%) and included sepsis in one, hematuria requiring hospitalization in 12, and urinary retention in 10. This study did not provide information regarding positive biopsy site identification.

More recently, investigators have demonstrated that saturation biopsies can be performed in the office using a periprostatic block [30]. The same group of investigators has assessed the utility of the saturation biopsy technique as an initial approach and in the repeat biopsy setting. They observed no improved yield by using a saturation biopsy as the initial biopsy scheme or the first repeat biopsy scheme but rather advocate it as a second repeat biopsy strategy [31]. It should be noted that no randomized trial has been performed to truly assess the utility of saturation biopsy schemes in this population.

Another approach has used a transperineal template to better sample the prostate. In this series, 88 men had a mean of 15.1 cores taken, and cancer was identified in 38 (43%) [32]. All procedures were performed in the operating room using general or regional anesthesia. The utility of such an approach seems limited.

Significance of Cancers on Repeat Biopsy

Much concern exists surrounding the overdiagnosis of prostate cancer. Clearly one needs to separate diagnosis from treatment or else overtreatment with its associated morbidity and cost will negatively impact the individual and the population. For this reason, it is important to recognize the significance of the cancers found on repeat biopsy approaches.

A large radical prostatectomy series was evaluated for the presence of clinically insignificant cancers as a function of the number of biopsy sessions performed [33]. Of 905 patients, 57% were diagnosed in the first biopsy session (group 1), 23% at the second biopsy session (group 2), and 21% at the third or greater biopsy session (group 3). The chance of bilateral disease was greatest in group 1 (43%) compared to group 2 (28%) and group 3 (25%). Using the Epstein criteria for insignificant cancer, there was no difference in the rates of insignificant disease between the three groups (7.7%, 7.0%, 8.2%), respectively [34]. The majority of the patients in this series who underwent repeat biopsies underwent either an extended pattern biopsy or a saturation biopsy. The chance of finding a significant cancer after two negative saturation biopsies was considered to be low. Of course, it should be noted that this is a retrospective surgical series. We do not understand the drivers leading to repeat biopsies in these patients who were diagnosed with cancer and then taken to surgery. We do not know how many patients may have been found to have small cancers on repeat biopsies and were then counseled to receive other therapy or be placed on active surveillance.

The REDUCE trial allows us to prospectively look at both cancer detection rates and quality of cancers in a repeat biopsy situation [35]. Recall that entry criteria for this trial mandated a prior negative biopsy (minimum of a negative sextant biopsy) within 6 months of enrollment. Men between the ages of 50 and 60 had to have a PSA level between 3 and 10 ng/ml, while men between 60 and 75 had to have a PSA level between 2.5 and 10 ng/ml. I will reserve my comments to just the placebo arm so as to avoid any controversy with respect to the action of 5-alpha reductase inhibitors on cancer prevention or influence on grade. The protocol biopsy scheme utilized was a 10-core scheme. Subjects were followed for 4 years and were asked to undergo protocol biopsies at years 2 and 4. If abnormalities were noted such as an abnormal PSA or DRE during the trial, subjects were recommended to undergo "for-cause" biopsies. In the placebo arm, 3,346 patients underwent a repeat biopsy within 1–2 years of enrollment, and 17.2% were found to have cancer of which 30% were high grade (Gleason score ≥7). At the repeat biopsy between years 3 and 4, 11.7% of 2,343 patients were found to have cancer of which 21% were high grade. If we were just to consider patients with primary Gleason pattern 4 or 5, 8.7% and 2.6% of the cancers were high grade at the 2- and 4- year biopsy, respectively. Of note, 194 underwent "for-cause" biopsy between 1 and 24 months, while 272 underwent "for-cause" biopsy between 25 and 48 months. The specific results of the "for-cause" biopsy are not known.

Algorithm for Patient with Prior Negative Biopsy

In patients with a prior negative biopsy, assessing the adequacy of the initial biopsy is important. For markers, F/T PSA is currently the most useful marker in predicting cancer on repeat biopsy although newer markers, such as PCA3 and % [−2]proPSA, are promising. Repeat biopsies should include a minimum of 14 cores, the 12 cores recommended for an initial biopsy and two additional cores obtained from the right and left anterior apex. The yield from transition zone biopsies is low. In patients whom repeat biopsies fail to identify cancer yet the clinical suspicion remains high, a saturation biopsy is warranted. After two negative saturation biopsies, the likelihood of finding cancer is extremely low and if found the clinical significance of that cancer is questionable.

Editorial Commentary

Much ado has been made regarding the concept of avoiding "unnecessary biopsies." Dr. Presti makes that point that a biopsy is not unnecessary just because it turns out to be negative. If we could have preemptively known the results, then there would be no reason to ever perform biopsy at all. Furthermore, just because the biopsy is negative does not mean that the patient

is without cancer, as evidenced by the fact that repeat biopsies are positive in approximately one fourth of cases.

The key issue is to identify cancers that have the potential to harm the patient. Dr. Presti has shown that there should be a low threshold to perform one repeat biopsy if clinical suspicion persists after a negative biopsy, but that after a second negative biopsy, it is uncommon to find clinically significant cancer so the threshold should be substantially higher. Unfortunately, this is where clinical decision making and an individualized approach come in. Using the markers for detection of prostate cancer described can improve this decision process.

–J. Stephen Jones

References

1. Hong YM, Lai FC, Chon CC, et al. Impact of prior biopsy scheme on pathologic features of cancers detected on repeat biopsies. Urol Oncol. 2004;22:7.
2. Eskew LA, Bare RL, McCullough DL. Systematic 5 region prostate biopsy is superior to sextant method for diagnosing carcinoma of the prostate. J Urol. 1997;157:199.
3. Presti Jr JC, O'Dowd G, Miller MC, et al. Extended peripheral zone biopsy schemes increase cancer detection rates and minimize variance in prostate specific antigen and age related cancer rates: results of a community multi-practice study. J Urol. 2003;169:125.
4. Karakiewicz PI, Bazinet M, Aprikian AG, et al. Outcome of sextant biopsy according to gland volume. Urology. 1997;49:55.
5. Presti JC. Repeat prostate biopsy–when, where, and how. Urol Oncol. 2009;27:312.
6. Benson MC, Whang IS, Olsson CA, et al. The use of prostate-specific antigen density to enhance the predictive value of intermediate levels of serum prostate-specific antigen. J Urol. 1992;147:817.
7. Benson MC, Whang IS, Pantuck A, et al. Prostate-specific antigen density: a means of distinguishing benign prostatic hypertrophy and prostate cancer. J Urol. 1992;147:815.
8. Elliott CS, Shinghal R, Presti JC. The performance of prostate specific antigen, prostate specific antigen density and transition zone density in the era of extended biopsy schemes. J Urol. 2008;179:1756.
9. Djavan B, Zlotta AR, Remzi M, et al. Total and transition zone prostate volume and age: how do they affect the utility of PSA-based diagnostic parameters for early prostate cancer detection? Urology. 1999;54:846.
10. Catalona WJ, Partin AW, Slawin KM, et al. Use of the percentage of free prostate-specific antigen to

enhance differentiation of prostate cancer from benign prostatic disease: a prospective multicenter clinical trial. JAMA. 1998;279:1542.

11. Stenman UH, Leinonen J, Alfthan H, et al. A complex between prostate specific antigen and alpha-1-antichymotrypsin is the major form of prostate specific antigen in serum of patients with prostate cancer: assay of the complex improves clinical sensitivity for cancer. Cancer Res. 1991;51:222.

12. Djavan B, Zlotta A, Remzi M, et al. Optimal predictors of prostate cancer on repeat prostate biopsy: a prospective study of 1051 men. J Urol. 2000;163:1144.

13. Garzotto M, Park Y, Mongoue-Tchokote S, et al. Recursive partitioning for risk stratification in men undergoing repeat prostate biopsies. Cancer. 2005; 104:1911.

14. Singh H, Canto EI, Shariat SF, et al. Predictors of prostate cancer after initial negative systematic 12 core biopsy. J Urol. 2004;171:1850.

15. Andriole GL, Bostwick D, Brawley OW, et al. The effect of dutasteride on the usefulness of prostate specific antigen for the diagnosis of high grade and clinically relevant prostate cancer in men with a previous negative biopsy- results for the REDUCE study. J Urol. 2011;185:126.

16. Lopez-Corona E, Ohori M, Scardino PT, et al. A nomogram for predicting a positive repeat prostate biopsy in patients with a previous negative biopsy session. J Urol. 2003;170:1184.

17. Errata to (Lopez-Corona E, Ohori M, Scardino PT, et al. A nomogram for predicting a positive repeat prostate biopsy in patients with a previous negative biopsy session. J Urol. 2003; 170:1184) J Urol. 2003 171:360.

18. Thompson IM, Ankerst DP, Chi C, et al. Assessing prostate cancer risk: results from the prostate cancer prevention trial. J Natl Cancer Inst. 2006;98:529.

19. Vickers AJ, Till C, Tangen CM, et al. An empirical evaluation of guidelines on prostate-specific antigen velocity on prostate cancer detection. J Natl Cancer Inst. 2011;103:1.

20. Ngo TC, Turnbull BB, Lavori PW, et al. The prostate cancer risk calculator from the prostate cancer prevention trial underestimates the risk of high grade cancer in contemporary referral patients. J Urol. 2011;185:483.

21. Marks L, Fradet Y, Deras IL, et al. PCA3 molecular urine assay for prostate cancer in men undergoing repeat biopsy. Urology. 2007;69:532.

22. Laxman B, Morris DS, Yu J, et al. A first generation multiplex biomarker analysis of urine for the early detection of prostate cancer. Cancer Res. 2008; 68:645.

23. Aubin SM, Reid J, Sarno MJ, et al. PCA3 molecular urine test for predicting repeat biopsy outcome in populations at risk: validation in the placebo arm of the dutasteride REDUCE trial. J Urol. 2010; 184:1947.

24. Sokoll LJ, Sanda MG, Feng Z, et al. A prospective, multicenter, National Cancer Institute early detection research network study of [−2]proPSA: improving prostate cancer detection and correlating with cancer aggressiveness. Cancer Epidemiol Biomarkers Prev. 2010;19:1193.

25. McNeal JE, Redwine EA, Freiha FS, et al. Zonal distribution of prostatic adenocarcinoma: correlation with histologic pattern and direction of spread. Am J Surg Pathol. 1988;12:897.

26. Babaian RJ, Toi A, Kamoi K, et al. A comparative analysis of sextant and an extended 11-core multisite directed biopsy strategy. J Urol. 2000;163:152.

27. Meng MV, Franks JH, Presti Jr JC, et al. The utility of apical anterior horn biopsies in prostate cancer detection. Urol Oncol. 2003;21:361.

28. Jones JS. Saturation biopsy for detection and characterization of prostate cancer. In: Jones JS, editor. Prostate biopsy. Totowa: Humana press; 2008. p. 217–29.

29. Stewart CS, Leibovich BC, Weaver AL, et al. Prostate cancer diagnosis using a saturation needle biopsy technique after previous negative sextant biopsies. J Urol. 2001;166:86.

30. Jones JS, Oder M, Zippe CD. Saturation biopsy with periprostatic block can be performed in the office. J Urol. 2002;168:2108.

31. Jones JS, Patel A, Schoenfield L, et al. Saturation technique does not improve cancer detection as an initial prostate biopsy strategy. J Urol. 2006;175:485.

32. Igel TC, Knight MK, Young PR, et al. Systematic transperineal ultrasound guided template biopsy of the prostate in patients at high risk. J Urol. 2001; 165:1575.

33. Tan N, Lane BR, Li J, et al. Prostate cancers diagnosed at repeat biopsy are smaller and less likely to be high grade. J Urol. 2008;180:1325.

34. Epstein JI, Walsh PC, Carmichael M, et al. Pathologic and clinical findings to predict tumor extent of nonpalpable (stage T1c) prostate cancer. JAMA. 1994; 271:368.

35. Andriole GL, Bostwick DG, Brawley OW, et al. Effect of dutasteride on the risk of prostate cancer. N Engl J Med. 2010;362:1192.

Transperineal Mapping Biopsy of the Prostate for Assessment of the Minimal Risk Patient

21

Jonathan A. Coleman

Introduction

Prostate cancer is a diverse disease requiring equally diverse strategies for diagnosis and management. Were all prostate cancers in need of treatment and only one modality available, then diagnostic strategies would require only the ability to identify prostate cancer when it exists, and to do so with a reasonable degree of accuracy. In many ways, this has been the endeavor regarding the evolution of prostate biopsy techniques: the quest to improve diagnostic yield and identify every man who has a cancer and minimize the possibility of a false-negative result. Yet, it is clear that not all prostate cancer requires detection just as it is certain that radical treatment is not always necessary if cancer is discovered. Stratification of patients in regard to their risk of disease and counseling for treatment options is a critical step in disease management and largely dependent on information obtained from biopsy. It is necessary, therefore, to develop complementary tissue sampling strategies, beyond simply identifying the presence of cancer, to more accurately quantify the extent and localization of tumors.

Toward Addressing Patient-Related Issues

Appropriate temperance in the evaluation of men for prostate cancer recognizes the requirements of screening and the impact of screening practices on patients and the realities of associated untoward outcomes. Cancer screening is not intended to find every patient with a tumor but to identify those biologically significant cancers for which treatment options may prove beneficial in improving disease-specific outcomes. Screening approaches, and indeed standard biopsy strategies for detecting prostate cancer, are far from perfect. As a result, multiple complex clinical scenarios are common. Not all men with significant cancers will meet threshold criteria for prostate biopsy at a time when their tumors are still localized and potentially curable. Conversely, of men who do ultimately undergo prostate biopsy, many are identified with tumors which have low or negligible malignant potential, while still others will have results which underrepresent the extent of their disease. Further, the screening-related stage shift which has been documented is truly a chronologic shift, intended to identify smaller volume tumors but simultaneously increasing the potential for false-negative biopsies in patients with biologically meaningful disease.

The great uncertainties from results of standard diagnostic biopsy techniques are therefore limiting in regard to interpretation. This is most relevant in clinical situations where the presumption

J.A. Coleman, M.D. (✉)
Department of Surgery/Urology, Memorial Sloan Kettering Cancer Center, 1275 York Ave.,
New York, NY 10065, USA
e-mail: colemaj1@mskcc.org

J.S. Jones (ed.), *Prostate Cancer Diagnosis: PSA, Biopsy and Beyond*, Current Clinical Urology,
DOI 10.1007/978-1-62703-188-2_21, © Springer Science+Business Media New York 2013

of disease burden is small, including patients considered for active surveillance, focal therapy, and repeat prostate biopsy following prior negative biopsy. For patients with larger disease burden on initial diagnostic biopsy or for whom organ preservation options are not being considered, the need for further tissue characterization may be less important.

Transperineal Mapping Biopsy

A number of prostate biopsy strategies have been proposed and studied, each with the intention of optimizing detection characteristics by various definitions. Transperineal stereotactic mapping biopsy (TMB) is perhaps the most thorough of these approaches. As described by Barzell [1], the technique is intended to provide detailed information regarding location and extent of tumor by use of a fixed 5×5-mm grid template for systematic biopsy.

The procedure is performed with similar equipment and setup as that of many prostate focal therapy and standard brachytherapy approaches (Fig. 21.1). Ultrasound is used to guide biopsy needles into the prostate gland with 5-mm spacing as they are placed through a brachytherapy template grid with sampling performed systematically to map the location and

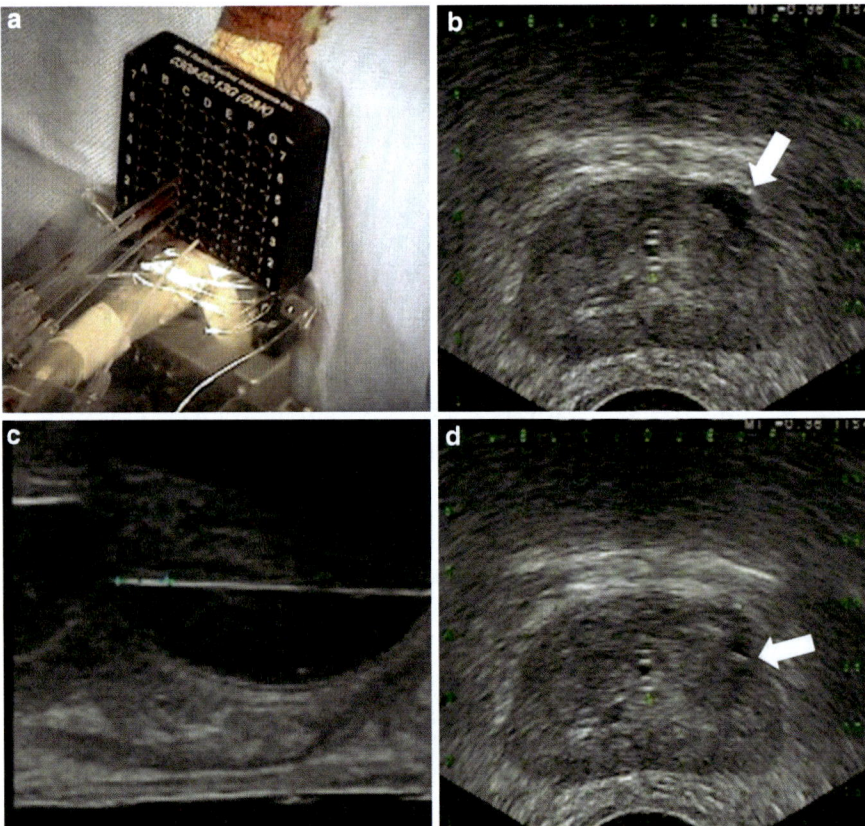

Fig. 21.1 Biopsy procedure (clockwise from *top left*). Stereotactic transrectal ultrasound guidance for transperineal prostate mapping biopsy is utilized in a manner similar to that of prostate focal therapy (**a**) including brachytherapy equipment and needle guide (grid) placed over the perineum with the patient in lithotomy position. Axial imaging planes (**b**) are useful for biometric data acquisition and may help identify hypoechoic areas of suspicion (*arrow*). Note the coordinate axes labeled in *green* across *top and sides* of the image corresponding to grid coordinates in *panel A*. Initial needle placement into the targeted area under axial imaging (**c**) will confirm needle tip placement (*arrow*) in the coordinate to be sampled. Accurate needle passage with avoidance of the urethra and symphysis pubis can be facilitated by use of a urethral catheter and parasagittal imaging during biopsy needle insertion (**d**)

extent of tumor if present. This approach is intended to control for many of the errors associated with other biopsy procedures, particularly the association between sampling density relative to prostate volume. Hypothetical advantages include reduction of random error associated with typical freehand transrectal biopsy and the greater ability to locate and quantify tumor with biometric information estimated from core data.

Mounting evidence supports the use of TMB for enhanced characterization of prostate tumors. Initial studies described by Crawford helped to establish the potential diagnostic capabilities [2]. In their retrospective analysis of ex vivo prostate specimens, TMB was simulated using two different systems to test the detection of prostate tumors based on findings from histology. Using 86 prostate glands obtained from autopsy and a subsequent 20 prostatectomy specimens, whole-mount slides were created, regions of tumor delineated, and images reconstructed into three-dimensional models to test the performance of biopsy sampling with either 5- or 10-mm needle spacing. As expected, sampling with 5-mm spacing had a higher rate of detection for all tumors, correctly identifying 86% of autopsy cases and 100% of prostatectomy cases. For localizing tumors, 5-mm biopsies identified 76% of 161 tumors, whereas 10-mm spacing identified 45%. Increased biopsy density was also better at finding the subset of defined clinically significant cancers ($>/= 5$ cc or Gleason 7), identifying these tumors among autopsy cases with both sensitivity and negative predictive values of 0.95. These results suggest TMB with 5-mm sampling can be effective at identifying and localizing a variety of tumor volumes, though discriminatory biopsy criteria for significant and more indolent cancers were not defined.

Defining Indolent Tumors

Validation studies have been performed, additionally focusing on establishing definitions to discriminate between established definitions of significant and indolent tumors based on TMB results. Pinochet and colleagues evaluated the modification of standard transrectal ultrasound biopsy (TRUS) criteria to TMB acquired data. They reported on 90 patients who met eligibility criteria for low-risk disease based on prior TRUS biopsy (Gleason ≤ 6, ≤ 3 positive cores, and $\leq 50\%$ of involvement of cancer in a single core, PSA density <0.15) and who underwent TMB within 6 months of their TRUS biopsy [3]. Results from TMB were interpreted using composite criteria modified from two prior biopsy definitions for indolent tumors, both requiring $\leq$ Gleason 6 disease and (a) maximal cancer core length ≤ 2 mm [4, 5] or (b) $\leq 25\%$ of total cores positive [6]. Biopsy density was fairly high in this series, averaging 1.8 cores per ml of prostate volume (range, 35–126 cores per case). Following repeat TMB, 14% of cases did not have cancer identified, 8% had > Gleason 6 disease, 32% had involvement of more than 50% of 1 core, and 50% had > 3 cores of cancer involvement. Regarding reclassification of the entire cohort using the modified definitions for indolent cancers, 68% did not meet indolent tumor criteria for composite definition A and 34% did not meet indolent criteria for composite definition B. It is interesting to note that the crude approximation of definition B to findings seen with standard repeat TRUS biopsy in similarly selected men resulting in approximately 70% of cases meeting criteria for indolent disease, including the subset of 26% without cancer on repeat TRUS biopsies [7].

Most recently, Ahmed and colleagues evaluated the performance characteristics of computer-simulated TMB in a series of 107 whole-mount radical prostatectomy specimens with graphically reconstructed three-dimensional images [8]. In an important modification, a uniform correction factor was utilized for tissue deformation from fixation and processing in an effort to more accurately represent the native tumor morphometry. Simulations were performed while incorporating needle error calculations to allow for 3-mm tip deflection and planar correction made for prostate orientation to the computer-generated representation of a 5×5-mm template grid. The model performed 500 simulations per case with biopsy results tabulated based on distribution and length of cancer per core within the reconstructed image. Simulation results were similar to those clinically obtained. Characteristics for prostate volume (median, 50.2 ml; range, 27–128 ml) and biopsies per gland (median, 51; range, 16–156) were comparable to clinical series. Performance of the simulated biopsies in detecting tumors was evaluated using two definitions for significant cancer: tumors ≥ 0.2 ml and tumors ≥ 0.5 ml. Variables based on biopsy result included the evaluation of maximal cancer core length (maximal measurement of cancer in any one core) and total cancer core length (sum of cancer length in all cores). Based on these variables and conditions, the authors created stratified biopsy criteria for indolent disease, tumors ≥ 0.2 ml and tumors ≥ 0.5 ml which could be discriminated with TMB. The most salient of these is the definition for indolent tumors which encompassed $\leq$ Gleason 6 disease, cumulative total cancer length ≤ 5 mm, or maximal single core cancer length ≤ 3 mm. Any Gleason 7 prostate tumor was interpreted as significant as were other definitions of cancer involvement above the indolent threshold. Further studies are needed to validate these definitions in independent data sets and clinical series.

TMB in Prior Biopsy Negative Patients

Cancer will not be identified on biopsy in the majority of patients who meet recommended criteria for prostate cancer screening. The reasons are self-evident: either tumor is not present at the time of biopsy or is missed, which may occur in an estimated 20–35% of men [9–11]. In cases of false-negative biopsy, rebiopsy of patients with prior negative biopsies will more often reveal low-risk cancer than clinically significant tumors [12]. Yet the concern for false-negative biopsy and suspicion of undiagnosed aggressive cancer often produces patient and physician anxiety during follow-up – driving the interest in repeat biopsy, particularly when abnormal screening parameters persist. Specific techniques for rebiopsy have not been defined and are typically or ideally performed in similar fashion to the initial biopsy, resampling previously negative regions of the gland. These factors raise the issue of appropriate secondary

screening practices for patients with prior negative or suspicious biopsies.

The role of TMB in this setting has been pursued as a means to obtain a more definitive form of sampling and rule out the possibility of clinically significant prostate cancer, potentially sparing some men from further screening. An early comparative study utilizing both TRUS sextant biopsy and transperineal 6-core "fan" biopsy demonstrated a rate of prostate cancer detection of 38% for transperineal biopsy compared to 32% with TRUS approach [13]. Moran et al. reported their results with TMB using more biopsies (mean, 40 cores; range 13–117) in a group of 747 men with history of prior negative TRUS biopsy [14]. The cancer detection rate was 39% with a preponderance of tumors detected in the apical and anterior segments of the gland. In a study of 102 men having undergone an average of 2.1 prior TRUS biopsy procedures with negative results, Merrick reported a 42% detection rate for prostate cancer, with an average of 50 cores obtained per procedure. Over 65% of biopsy positive patients had Gleason 7 or greater disease [15]. Dimmen and colleagues evaluated 69 men with prior negative transrectal biopsies using a more limited template than 5-mm spacing, performing an average of 18 cores using transperineal biopsy. The patients in this series had generally been well biopsied previously (mean, >2 sets of prior biopsies) though serum PSA was also quite elevated in the group of positive biopsy cases (mean, >25 ng/mL). Following transperineal biopsy just over 55% were identified with prostate cancer, the majority in the anterior prostate (85%). In a retrospective review of TMB procedures in 294 men with prior negative biopsy, Taira and colleagues found a positive cancer detection rate inversely proportional to the number of prior negative biopsies. Men with 1, 2, or 3+ prior negative biopsies had cancer detection rates of 56%, 42%, and 34%, respectively [16]. Cancers were classified as insignificant in 9–14% of these cases, though they defined indolent disease based on standard Epstein criteria which was developed from more limited sampling in TRUS biopsy data and of questionable validity for this density of prostate biopsy in which a median of 57 cores were obtained [3, 6].

These data collectively serve to demonstrate the limitations of standard TRUS biopsy techniques developed to oversample peripheral zone regions, particularly near the base of the gland [17, 18]. Rebiopsy with TMB techniques appear to yield higher than expected positive biopsy results, including higher grade cancers, in this much selected group of patients. Notable findings include the clustering of tumors seen anteriorly and centrally in this population of men, suggesting that secondary screening and rebiopsy strategies need to especially address this region with imaging and biopsy.

Adverse Outcomes and Cost

Transperineal prostate biopsy is more costly, both in terms of medical and financial resources and the risks for adverse outcomes from biopsy. One potential advantage of transperineal biopsy is their ability to be performed under clean-contaminated conditions, with standard skin preparation, in the operating room, potentially lowering the risks of infection-related events which are an increasing problem [19]. Drawbacks of TMB surround the requirements of a more invasive procedure including the need for systemic anesthetics, surgeon time, operating room access and personnel, the greater number of biopsy samples generated, their processing, and evaluation. Though several groups have investigated costs associated with saturation TRUS biopsy, little data are available on the overall cost-effectiveness of TMB which take into account these several factors [20, 21]. New CPT coding has been introduced to reflect the increase in resources needed in terms of reimbursement for procedural costs for personnel and facility, indicating an increase over twice the basis for standard transrectal biopsy. Further modeling of the impact of TMB on prostate cancer management is needed though quite complex, having to take into account the additional features of altered management pathways, potential for focal therapies, recommendations to obviate the need for further screening or treatment, and the costs associated with adverse outcomes (see Box 21.1)

Box 21.1 Terminology Confusion
The term "saturation biopsy" causes occasional confusion in the urological community. This term accurately refers to a transrectal biopsy involving 20 or greater cores and has been in the urological literature for over a decade.

Unfortunately, 8 years later, CPT created confusion by using this already-established term to code for template-guided mapping biopsy performed in the operating room under general anesthesia, as described in this and a previous chapter. It is important to recognize that any transrectal biopsy should be coded 55700.

Transperineal prostate biopsy is a more invasive procedure due to the density of biopsy samples taken using the 5-mm spacing paradigm. Mapping strategies include subdivision of the prostate typically into 24 sectors, 12 in the apex and 12 in the base, corresponding to right and left, anterior and posterior, and medial, intermediate, and lateral components [1]. According to most representations, 2–4 cores are taken from each of these sectors, theoretically yielding 48–96 biopsy cores per patient, possibly more for larger prostate glands. These numbers correlate with reported clinical data indicating average biopsy yields between 40 and 60 cores, with ranges in some series exceeding 115 cores [22]. Not surprisingly, TMB is associated with increased risk of adverse outcomes, particularly genitourinary toxicity, including urinary retention and hematuria. In full gland biopsy cases, urinary retention has been retrospectively reported most typically in the range of 11–15% of cases [22, 23]. Reporting is dependent on the definition used however, and rates of urinary retention reported in other experiences have been somewhat different, noting 39%, 7%, and 2% of cases requiring urinary catheter drainage for 0, 3, and 6 days following treatment as detailed in one series of 129 patients [24]. It is notable that several series report that patients are typically pretreated with alpha blockers prior to

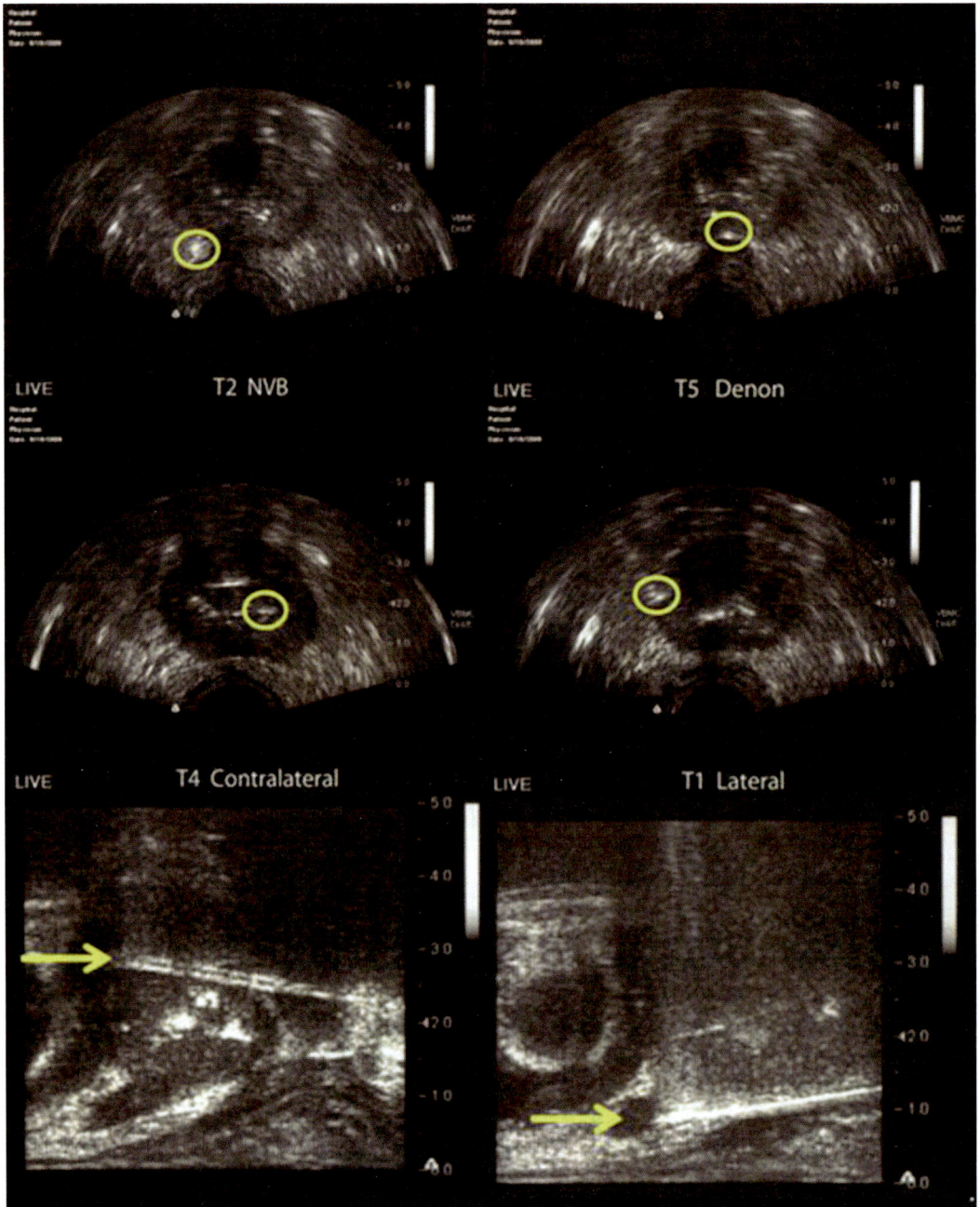

Fig. 21.2 In our example, this inaccuracy allowed us to reach almost the entire prostate through a single grid location, perhaps most graphically demonstrated by the needles shown completely missing the prostate anteriorly and posteriorly in the sagittal plane

biopsy. Although a comparative retrospective study of transperineal to transrectal biopsy failed to show a significant difference in complication rates between the two procedures, it is notable that only six cores were taken in either procedure and no events of retention occurred; sepsis events were rare and comparable between both groups [25]. Erectile dysfunction rates following TMB have also been reported with functional loss occurring in as many as 5% of cases although it is unclear whether this is a finding unique to TMB or to prostate biopsy procedures in general [24, 26].

Summary

The supporting data from retrospective studies in selected cases suggests that TMB procedures provide a higher yield of positive prostate biopsies than standard TRUS-guided prostate biopsy. Cumulatively, biopsy results from these studies have suggested a positive diagnostic rate of approximately 50% in previously biopsy negative, "at-risk" patients who have been selected, based on clinical features, for repeat biopsy using TMB. The yield from TMB appears to diminish in patients who have had multiple prior negative TRUS biopsies, though clinically significant tumors (mostly defined by Gleason Grade ≥7) are still discovered in roughly two thirds of these patients whose biopsy is positive for cancer.

Definitions of lower risk tumors based on the higher density core data of prostate biopsy mapping are under development since prior standards are likely inappropriate in this setting. These procedures appear associated with a significantly higher though manageable risk of urinary retention which may require temporary urinary catheter drainage. Larger questions yet remain as to the cost-effectiveness of these procedures in the overall role of prostate cancer management, yet it is likely that TMB will continue to be used in characterizing and localizing prostate tumors until the development of imaging studies with proven comparable accuracy.

Editorial Commentary:
The concept of transperineal mapping biopsy is dependent on the presumed fixed relationship of the brachytherapy grid to the patient's prostate. If this presumption is correct, then the findings on biopsy reflect the reality of cancer location and grade. Unfortunately, this relationship is clearly not absolute, based most obviously on the fact that 14–20% of patients with known low-volume cancer actually have negative transperineal mapping biopsies [27]. Although it is possible that this is based on cancers being so small that they exist only between the needle tracts, I believe that it is likely to be based on the needle having an unfixed trajectory once it passes through the grid. The figures below demonstrate that the needle can be placed almost anywhere in the prostate through a single brachytherapy grid hole; in fact, the sagittal view shows the needle missing the prostate entirely both anteriorly and posteriorly when passed through the same hole (Fig. 21.2, photos by Christopher Brede, MD). Thus, the surgeon must be mindful that the grid is a helpful guide, but cannot replace diligent needle placement and assuring that the needle has actually gone into the corresponding site under ultrasound guidance.

Considering the additional cost and morbidity as shown in this chapter, TMB appears to have a limited but potentially important role, which is most likely to involve patients being considered for focal therapy.

References

1. Barzell WE, Melamed MR. Appropriate patient selection in the focal treatment of prostate cancer: the role of transperineal 3-dimensional pathologic mapping of the prostate–a 4-year experience. Urology. 2007; 70(6 Suppl):27–35.
2. Crawford ED, Wilson SS, et al. Clinical staging of prostate cancer: a computer-simulated study of transperineal prostate biopsy. BJU Int. 2005;96(7):999–1004.
3. Barzell W, Pinochet R, et al. Role of 3D transperineal mapping biopsy in candidates for active surveillance. J Urol. 2010;183(4):e57–8.
4. Goto Y, Ohori M, et al. Distinguishing clinically important from unimportant prostate cancers before treatment: value of systematic biopsies. J Urol. 1996;156(3):1059–63.
5. Ochiai A, Troncoso P, et al. The relationship between tumor volume and the number of positive cores in men undergoing multisite extended biopsy: implication for expectant management. J Urol. 2005;174(6): 2164–8. discussion 2168.
6. Epstein JI, Walsh PC, et al. Pathologic and clinical findings to predict tumor extent of nonpalpable (stage T1c) prostate cancer. JAMA. 1994;271(5):368–74.
7. Berglund RK, Masterson TA, et al. Pathological upgrading and up staging with immediate repeat biopsy in patients eligible for active surveillance. J Urol. 2008;180(5):1964–7. discussion 1967–1968.

8. Ahmed HU, Hu Y, et al. Characterizing clinically significant prostate cancer using template prostate mapping biopsy. J Urol. 2011;186(2):458–64.

9. Chen ME, Troncoso P, et al. Optimization of prostate biopsy strategy using computer based analysis. J Urol. 1997;158(6):2168–75.

10. Haas GP, Delongchamps NB, et al. Needle biopsies on autopsy prostates: sensitivity of cancer detection based on true prevalence. J Natl Cancer Inst. 2007; 99(19):1484–9.

11. Rabbani F, Stroumbakis N, et al. Incidence and clinical significance of false-negative sextant prostate biopsies. J Urol. 1998;159(4):1247–50.

12. Numao N, Kawakami S, et al. Characteristics and clinical significance of prostate cancers missed by initial transrectal 12-core biopsy. BJU Int. 2011;18(10): 727–30.

13. Emiliozzi P, Corsetti A, et al. Best approach for prostate cancer detection: a prospective study on transperineal versus transrectal six-core prostate biopsy. Urology. 2003;61(5):961–6.

14. Moran BJ, Braccioforte MH. Stereotactic transperineal prostate biopsy. Urology. 2009;73(2):386–8.

15. Merrick GS, Gutman S, et al. Prostate cancer distribution in patients diagnosed by transperineal template-guided saturation biopsy. Eur Urol. 2007;52(3): 715–23.

16. Taira AV, Merrick GS, et al. Performance of transperineal template-guided mapping biopsy in detecting prostate cancer in the initial and repeat biopsy setting. Prostate Cancer Prostatic Dis. 2010;13(1):71–7.

17. Aihara M, Wheeler TM, et al. Heterogeneity of prostate cancer in radical prostatectomy specimens. Urology. 1994;43(1):60–6. discussion 66–67.

18. Chen ME, Johnston DA, et al. Detailed mapping of prostate carcinoma foci. Cancer. 2000;89(8):1800–9.

19. Loeb S, Carter HB, et al. Complications after prostate biopsy: data from SEER-Medicare. J Urol. 2011; 186(5):1830–4.

20. Heijnsdijk EA, der Kinderen A, et al. Overdetection, overtreatment and costs in prostate-specific antigen screening for prostate cancer. Br J Cancer. 2009; 101(11):1833–8.

21. Kang SG, Tae BS, et al. Efficacy and cost analysis of transrectal ultrasound-guided prostate biopsy under monitored anesthesia. Asian J Androl. 2011;13(5): 724–7.

22. Onik G, Barzell W. Transperineal 3D mapping biopsy of the prostate: an essential tool in selecting patients for focal prostate cancer therapy. Urol Oncol. 2008;26(5):506–10.

23. Buskirk SJ, Pinkstaff DM, et al. Acute urinary retention after transperineal template-guided prostate biopsy. Int J Radiat Oncol Biol Phys. 2004;59(5):1360–6.

24. Merrick GS, Taubenslag W, et al. The morbidity of transperineal template-guided prostate mapping biopsy. BJU Int. 2008;101(12):1524–9.

25. Miller J, Perumalla C, et al. Complications of transrectal versus transperineal prostate biopsy. ANZ J Surg. 2005;75(1–2):48–50.

26. Fujita K, Landis P, et al. Serial prostate biopsies are associated with an increased risk of erectile dysfunction in men with prostate cancer on active surveillance. J Urol. 2009;182(6):2664–9.

27. Onik G, Miessau M, Bostwick DG. Three-dimensional prostate mapping biopsy has a potentially significant impact on prostate cancer management. J Clin Oncol. 2009;27:4321–6.

Transrectal Saturation Biopsy

22

Vincenzo Scattoni, Carmen Maccagnano,
and Francesco Montorsi

Introduction

Prostate biopsy (PBx) is one of the most common procedures performed in the urologist's office. It has evolved from the digitally guided transrectal biopsy to the standard sextant biopsy method, described by Hodge and colleagues in 1989 [1], with a prostate cancer (PCa) detection rate (DR) between 20% and 35% [2].

Interest in defining more accurate PBx schemes has been increasing to improve PCa DR. The introduction and refinement of effective local anesthesia has allowed an increase in the number of biopsies to be taken in the outpatient setting (from 10 to 18 or 20) without significantly increasing procedure-related discomfort and pain. Consequently, the concepts of *extended biopsy* (EPBx, 10–12 cores) and *saturation biopsy* (SPBx, 20 or more cores) have rapidly evolved in the last 10 years and radically changed the general idea of PBx [3, 4]. PBx today not only is a method to diagnose PCa but also has become an informative instrument for accurate morphologic characterization of PCa, leading to new perspectives on follow-up and therapy.

Management of patients with negative biopsy often presents a dilemma. Urologists know well

that a negative biopsy does not mean the absence of cancer, and a second biopsy (with different templates and timing) is one of the options. The SPBx was initially introduced to improve PCa detection rates in the repeat setting because initial 10–12-core biopsy schemes may miss almost a third of cancers [5, 6].

Nevertheless, the most efficient scheme with the optimal number and location of cores has not been defined yet [5]. It is not clear when and how to perform a second biopsy, whether it is necessary to perform the same sampling protocol in each patient, or whether to modify the protocol for different clinical situations [7]. Moreover, it is still controversial whether the DR may increase with additional biopsies or whether it is necessary to modify the locations where the cores are taken [1, 2, 8].

Definition of and Rationale for Saturation Biopsy

The concept of increasing the number of cores led to the idea of SPBx, with 20 or more transrectal cores being taken in a systematic fashion [3, 4, 9]. In physics and chemistry, *saturation* refers to a condition or state in which a substance has reached its plateau concentration.

The term *saturation kinetics* is generally used to describe the enzyme system in which the rate of reaction tends to maximize and does not increase with additional substrate. When applied to the field of PBx, saturation should theoretically

V. Scattoni, M.D. (✉) • C. Maccagnano, M.D.
• F. Montorsi, M.D.
Department of Urology, San Raffaele Hospital,
Via Olgettina 60, Milan, 20132, Italy
e-mail: scattoni.vincenzo@hsr.it

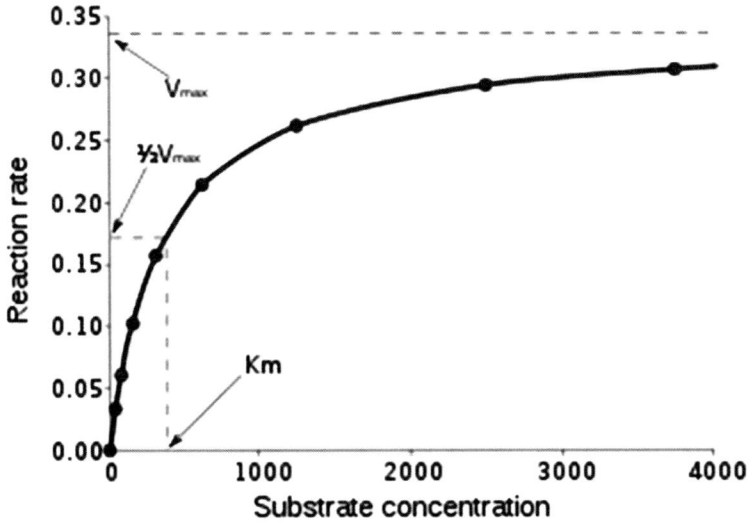

Fig. 22.1 The curve shows that the rate of reaction tends to maximum and does not increase by additional substrate

define a sampling technique whereby inclusion of additional biopsy cores, regardless of route, would not increase the cancer detection rate (Fig. 22.1).

The term *saturation biopsy* was first introduced by Stewart et al. [3] to describe the technique developed almost simultaneously with Borboroglu et al. [4] in patients with previous negative sextant PBx. These authors obtained up to 45 cores (Stewart et al. [3] mean: 23 cores; Borboroglu et al. [4] mean: 22.5 cores) and found that the additional value of taking more than 20 cores was limited in terms of PCa DR. A threshold of 22–24 cores for SPBx was set arbitrarily and is still adopted by most contemporary protocols, even in the absence of an unequivocal quantitative definition. SPBx was initially performed in the operating room using general or spinal anesthesia or intravenous sedation; however, the procedure now can be performed in an office setting using periprostatic nerve block (PNB) with minimal discomfort and pain [10–12]. The number of cores for SPBx varies widely in published studies, with a range from 20 to 24 to as many as 139 cores, as has been reported recently (Table 22.1).

The rationale for adopting an SPBx protocol in the repeat setting is due to the inability of the initial standard biopsy to detect PCa. Recognizing

that no biopsy strategy is able to detect all PCa, standard initial EPBx may miss up to 40% of cancers [13–20]. Moreover, about 10–20% of cancers not detected at initial biopsy are located in the transition zone (TZ), which is not sampled during initial biopsy [21–23]. The need to increase the cancer DR has driven the idea of increasing the number of cores taken to increase the probability of detecting more cancers.

Saturation Schemes: Clinical Data and Critical Issues

Clinical Data

Different researchers have demonstrated that SPBx techniques aimed at greatly increasing the number of samples and at varying the distribution of biopsy sites may provide a high cancer DR (Table 22.1). Studies of SPBx in the repeat-biopsy population have yielded about 30% (range: 17–41%) cancer DR, regardless of the type of previous biopsy scheme [13–19].

In 2003, de la Taille and colleagues [18] reported that SPBx detected cancer in 25% of patients undergoing their initial repeat biopsy, whereas patients who had more than one previous prostate biopsy had a cancer DR of less than 3%.

Table 22.1 Comparison of trials with saturation biopsy in the repeat setting

Reference	Setting	Route	No. of patients	Detection rate, %	No. of cores	Insignificant PCa, %
Stewart et al. [3]	Repeat	TR	224	34	Range: 14–45; mean: 23	14.3
Borboroglu et al. [4]	Repeat	TR	57	30	Mean: 22.5	7
De la Taille et al. [18]	Initial and repeat	TR	303	31.3	21	NA
Rabets et al. [24]	Repeat	TR	116	29	Range: 20–24; mean: 22.8	0
Walz et al. [26]	Repeat	TR	161	41	Range: 18–32; mean: 24.2; median: 24	15.6
Zaytoun et al. [27]	Repeat	TR	663	32.7	Range: 20–32; mean 20.7	40.1
Scattoni et al. [28]	Repeat	TR	340	27.9	24	NA
Campos-Ferdandes et al. [52]	Repeat	TR	231	25.1	21	NA
Bott et al. [48]	Repeat	TP	60	38	Mean: 24	NA
Pepe et al. [53]	Initial and Repeat	TR	189	33.8	Range: 24–37; median: 29	NA
Sajadi et al. [54]	Repeat	TR	82	19.5	Range: 24–40; median: 24	NA
Lee et al. [82]	Initial	TP	303	37.6	Range: 11–44; mean: 23.7	NA
Jones [13]	Initial	TR	139	44.6	24	15.8
Satoh et al. [125]	Repeat	TP	128	22.7	22	NA
Moran et al. [126]	Repeat	TP	180	38	Median: 41	NA
Pryor and Schellhammer [127]	Repeat	TR	35	20	Range: 14–28; median: 21	0
Fleshner et al. [128]	Repeat	TR	37	13.5	Range: 32–38	NA
Merrick et al. [129]	Repeat	TP	102	42	Mean: 51.1; median: 50	7.1
Simon et al. [130]	Repeat	TR	40	45	Range: 39–139; median: 64	NA
Novara et al. [131]	Repeat	TP	143	26	24	NA
Pinkstaff et al. [132]	Repeat	TP	210	37	Mean: 21	0

NA not assessed, *TP* transperineal, *TR* transrectal

In 2004, Patel et al. [9] reported an SPBx technique that identified five sectors of the prostate hemispheres. The overall cancer DR was 29% in 116 patients undergoing repeat biopsy. There were no reported unique medially located tumors. Consequently, sampling in the medial sectors was reduced to one core in each sector, for a total of 20 cores on repeat SPBx (Fig. 22.2). From the same series, Rabets et al. [24] noted less of a difference because patients with only one prior biopsy had a 33% cancer DR compared to 24% for patients who had more than one prior biopsy [25]. Walz et al. [26] identified cancer in 41% of patients undergoing repeat SPBx using a mean of 24 cores.

Despite the widespread assumption that SPBx increases cancer detection compared to EPBx, it is notable that few studies have actually compared cancer DR. Recently, Zaytoun et al. reported their experience at Cleveland Clinic where they compared EPBx (12–14 cores, $n = 393$) with SPBx (20–24 cores, $n = 663$) in a clearly defined, heterogeneous population of patients undergoing repeat biopsy after a single prior biopsy that failed to diagnose PCa [27]. They showed that office-based SPBx significantly increases cancer detection in repeat biopsy compared to EPBx. SPBx detected almost one-third more cancers (32.7% vs. 24.9%, $p = 0.0075$). For patients with benign initial biopsy, SPBx demonstrated significantly greater PCa detection (33.3% vs. 25.6%, $p = 0.027$). For previous atypical small acinar proliferation of prostate (ASAP) and/or high-grade prostatic intraepithelial neoplasia (HGPIN), a trend for higher PCa DR was

Fig. 22.2 Repeat saturation
biopsy scheme. The number of
parasagittal cores is reduced in
each sector since medial biopsies
have been shown to have low
yield on repeat biopsy. However,
it still is important to obtain at
least one core in these sectors
because rare cases may present
with cancer in these areas (From
Ref. [24])

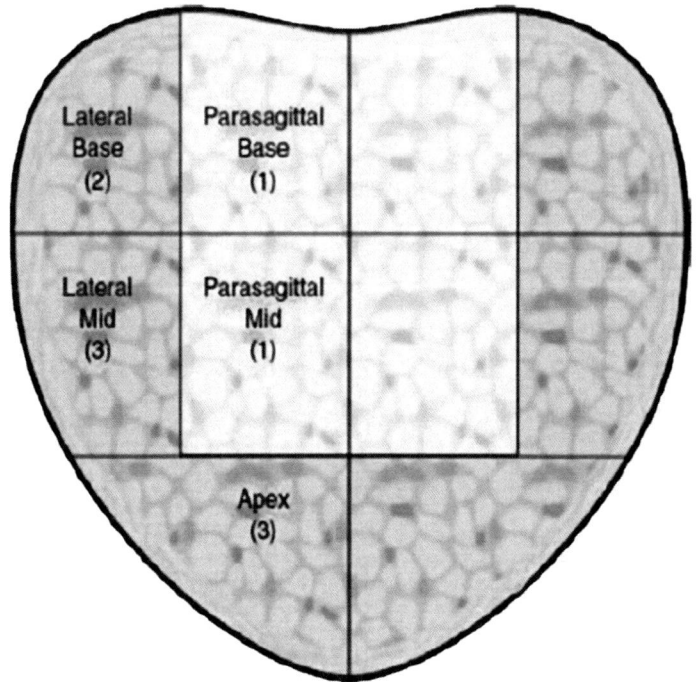

demonstrated in the saturation group but did not reach statistical significance (31.2% vs. 23.3%, $p=0.13$).

Similarly, Scattoni et al. recently tried to identify the optimal combination of sampling sites (number and location) to detect PCa in patients previously submitted to an initial negative prostatic biopsy [28]. They prospectively performed a transrectal ultrasound (TRUS)-guided systematic 24-core PBx in 340 consecutive patients after a first negative biopsy (at least 12 cores). Subsequently, they set the cancer-positive rate of the 24-core PBx at 100% and calculated PCa DR for 255 possible combinations of sampling sites. They reported that the more cores taken, the higher the cancer DR. They showed a continuum of improvement of the cancer DR when increasing the number of cores, even if the cancer DR of the 24 cores was significantly higher than only the mean cancer detection rate of 14-core schemes (Fig. 22.3). Moreover, at a given number of cores, the cancer DR varied significantly according to the different combination of sites considered.

All of these studies demonstrate that SPBx provides a higher cancer DR than the extended approach in the repeat setting and that the higher the number of cores, the higher the number of cancers detected.

Critical Issues

Saturation Biopsy in the Initial Setting

Despite the attempts of several investigators to optimize the number of cores in the single patient, Eichler and colleagues have shown that no significant benefit accrues by taking more than 12 cores as an initial biopsy strategy [20]. Jones and coworkers have suggested that further efforts at EPBx strategies beyond 10–14 cores are not appropriate in the initial setting [13, 20]. More recently, Pepe et al. reported in a retrospective study that SPBx (range: 24–37 cores) does not increase the PCa detection rate compared with an 18-core scheme in the initial setting [29]. Descazeaud and colleagues reported that the DR of their 21-core biopsy protocol was similar to their 10–12-core biopsy scheme as an initial biopsy strategy [30]. Delongchamps et al. evaluated SPBx (36 cores) on autopsied prostates for

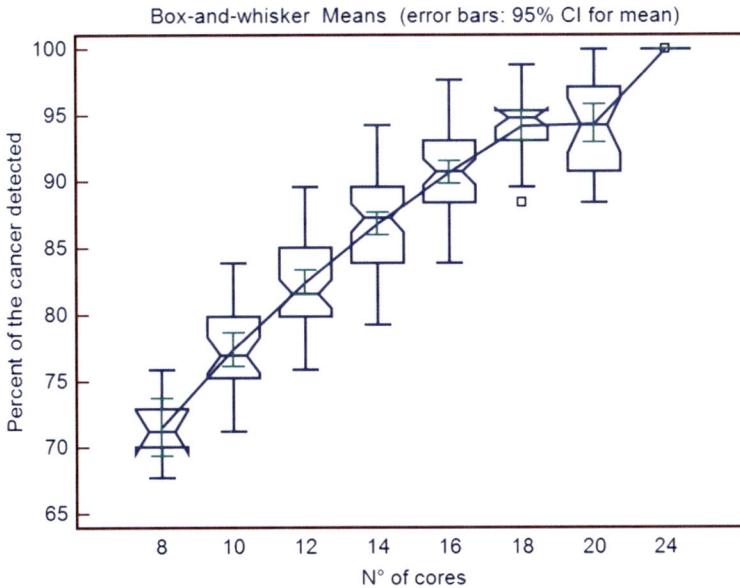

Fig. 22.3 The *bars* show the cross-validated mean percentages of cancer detected according to the number of cores at initial biopsy. Box and whisker report the range and mean values. Error bars report the 95%CI (Data from Ref. [28])

Table 22.2 Comparison of trials with saturation biopsy in the initial setting (2006–2011)

Reference	No. of patients	No. of cores	Prostate cancer detection rate, %
Lane et al. [12]	257	24	42.8
Guichard et al. [33]	1,000	21	42.5
Scattoni et al. [28]	670	24	46.8
Jones [13]	139	24	44.6
Simon et al. [130]	40	139	45

detecting PCa and concluded that the DR of the SPBx protocol did not increased with an 18-core regimen [31]. In a large retrospective study, Scattoni et al. previously showed that an initial 18-core PBx did not improve the overall PCa DR compared with a 12-core PBx (39.9% vs. 38.4%, $p=0.37$) [32]. Moreover, Lane et al. demonstrated that the false-negative rate of subsequent PBx after initial SPBx is equivalent to that following traditional PBx [12] (Table 22.2).

In contrast, Guichard et al. performed an SPBx (21 cores) as their initial PBx in 1,000 patients, including sextant biopsies, three additional posterolateral biopsies in each peripheral zone, three biopsies in each TZ, and three biopsies

in the midline peripheral zone [17]. They found an improvement, although not statistically significant, in the DR when increasing from 12 cores to 18 or 21 cores (improvement of cancer detected was about 7% with an increase of cancer DR of 2.8%) [33].

Our study group recently performed SPBx in the initial setting and has tried to identify the most advantageous PBx scheme, defined as the combination of sampling sites that detected 95% of all cancers with the minimal number of biopsy cores [34]. We reported that, despite the fact that the mean cancer DR significantly increased with an increasing number of cores, the cancer DR varied significantly according to the different combination of sites considered at a given number of cores.

We proposed a user-friendly flowchart to identify the most advantageous set of sampling sites that is able to detect 95% of the cancers with the fewest number of cores, according to patients' characteristics. The analysis revealed that the most advantageous schemes were a combination of a 16-core biopsy for patients with negative digital rectal examination (DRE), prostate volume

(PV) of 60 or less, and age 65 or younger and two different combinations of a 14-core biopsy for patients with negative DRE, PV of 60 ml or less, and age greater than 65 or with negative DRE and PV greater than 60 ml. Finally, the sampling that allows detection of 95% of cancers in patients with positive DRE was a combination of a 10-core biopsy [34]. In conclusion, sufficient evidence in the literature shows that SPBx is not necessary in the initial setting.

Saturation Biopsy in the Repeat Setting

Although SPBx has been shown to increase cancer detection and to be appropriate in men with initial negative EPBx, its regular use in clinical practice is not approved [5, 6, 35–37]. The National Comprehensive Cancer Network (NCCN) suggests performing a second extended protocol after an initial negative extended protocol and suggests considering SPBx only in patients with a high risk of cancer after multiple negative biopsies. The 2011 European Association of Urology (EAU) guidelines on PCa do not indicate the template that should be used. Consequently, the ideal strategy for a second PBX procedure has yet to be fully elucidated (Table 22.3).

Recently, interest has increased in defining more efficient biopsy schemes for PCa detection with the minimum number of cores [38–40]. Different variables, both clinical and not clinical, may have an impact on the cancer DR (as shown in Table 22.4). Apart from the clinical characteristics of the patients, some procedural character-

istics may have an even greater impact on the cancer DR. Intuitively, adding more biopsies to prostatic areas not sampled by common extended schemes should increase the DR. It should be noted, however, that increasing the number of biopsy cores is not the solution to the problem and that the relationship between the number of biopsy cores and the resulting cancer DR does not correlate linearly (Fig. 22.4). As shown in Fig. 22.4, the curve tends to plateau, and the increase of cores taken in the template is not equivalent to the increase of cancer detected.

Kawakami et al. analyzed the PCa DR by using a three-dimensional (3D) 26-core systematic super-EPBx protocol [41]. In these analyses, subset biopsy schemes were determined by recursive partitioning to achieve a maximum cancer

Table 22.4 Variables involved in cancer detection rate

Variable	Parameter
Patient characteristics	Age, race, family history
	PSA
	DRE finding
	Prostate volume
	Biopsy history
Procedure characteristics	Operator
	Route
	Number of cores
	Location of cores
Processing characteristics	Fixing
	Core length

DRE digital rectal examination, *PSA* prostate-specific antigen

Table 22.3 Recommendations according to the most important guidelines

American Urology Association (2009)	Saturation biopsy, taking tissue from >20 locations, may be considered in men with persistently elevated PSA levels and multiple previous negative prostate biopsies
European Association of Urology (2011)	Indications for repeat biopsies are rising and/or persistent PSA, suspicious digital rectal examination, and atypical small acinar proliferation of prostate. The optimal timing is still uncertain. The later the repeat biopsy is done, the higher the detection rate. High-grade prostatic intraepithelial neoplasia is only considered an indication for rebiopsy if it occurs multifocally (level of evidence: 2a). If clinical suspicion for PCa persists despite negative prostate biopsies, MRI may be used to investigate the possibility of an anteriorly located PCa, followed by transrectal ultrasound or MRI-guided biopsies of the suspicious area
National Comprehensive Cancer Network (2011)	For high-risk men with multiple negative biopsies, consideration can be given to a saturation biopsy strategy. In patients with two negative extended biopsies but a persistently rising PSA value, a saturation biopsy may be considered

MRI magnetic resonance imaging, *PCa* prostate cancer, *PSA* prostate-specific antigen

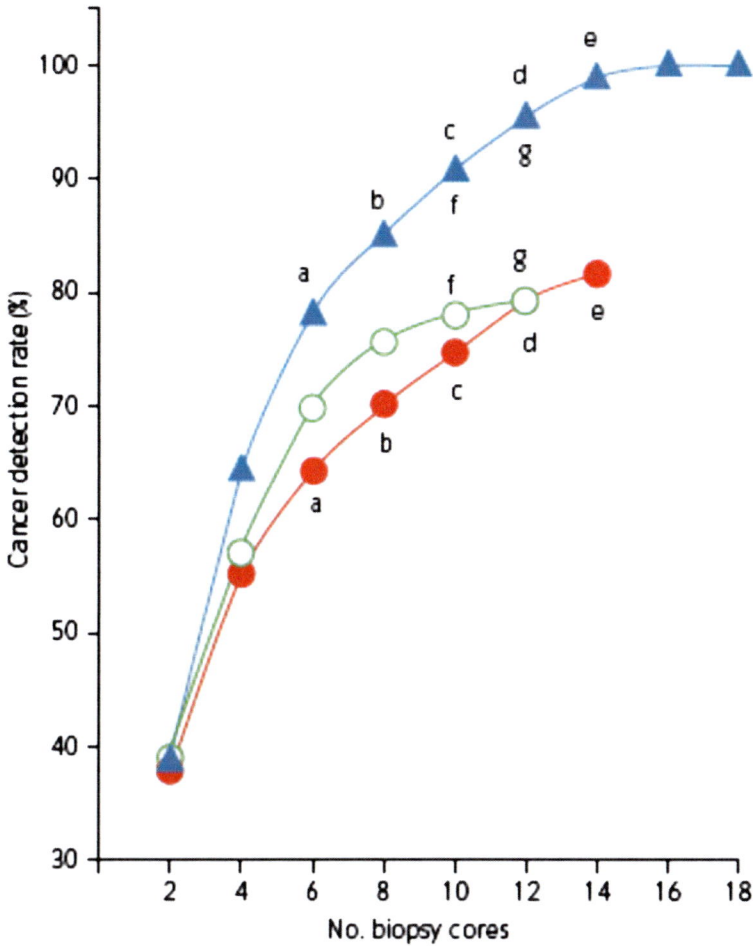

Fig. 22.4 In this analysis, it should be noted that the relationship between the number of biopsy cores and the resultant cancer detection rate does not correlate linearly. Instead, the cancer detection rate would become saturated when increasing the number of biopsy cores (From Ref. [41]). Maximum cancer detection rate achieved by the best combination of sampling sites in transrectal alone (*open circles*), transperineal alone (*closed circles*), and 3-D combination of transrectal and transperineal approaches (*closed triangles*) according to the number of biopsy cores in men who underwent repeat biopsy (Data from)

DR at a given number of biopsy cores through a single transrectal approach, a single transperineal approach, or a 3D combination of transrectal and transperineal approaches. They were able to extract a 3D 14-core biopsy protocol that could detect 95% of cancers with the fewest number of cores. Nevertheless, their approach has the disadvantage of requiring general anesthesia to perform the double approach (transrectal and transperineal). Moreover, they have not specified the most advantageous biopsy protocol according to the clinical characteristics of the patients.

All of these data demonstrate that cancer detection is influenced not only by the number of cores but also by the exact location (or route) of the cores. The optimal SPBx should be still defined.

The report by Delongchamps et al. is a reminder that the urologist needs to do a better job of biopsying the prostate. This study convincingly shows that merely increasing the number of biopsy cores will not solve the problem. A fairly extensive 36-core biopsy performed in 48 autopsied prostates (median volume: 35 ml) missed 5 of 12 (42%) cancers found on whole-mount pathologic

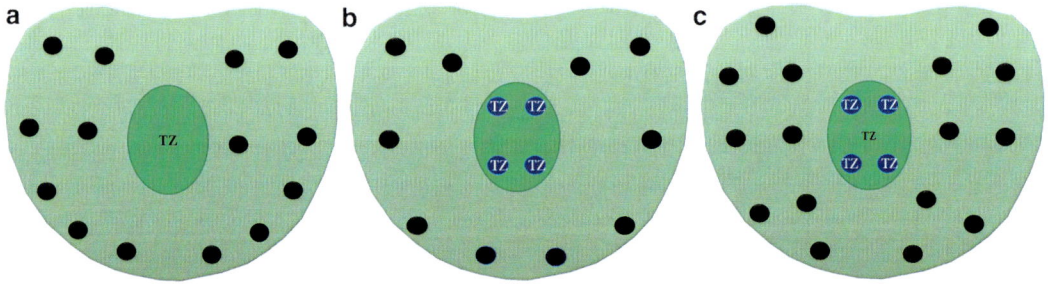

Fig. 22.5 (a–c) The figures show the location and the number of cores of the scheme that detects >95% of the cancers with the minimum number of cores, in three different risk groups. (a) Previous ASAP diagnosis (14 cores without TZ cores). (b) No previous ASAP diagnosis and fPSA/tPSA<=10% (14 cores with TZ cores). (c) No previous ASAP diagnosis and fPSA/tPSA>10% (20 cores with TZ cores)

analysis. In fact, the 36-core biopsy offered no benefit over an 18-core protocol in terms of PCa detection. Among the seven tumors that were discovered, three (43%) were incorrectly graded. Although all five of the missed tumors were small (index volume: <0.5 ml; median: 0.08 ml), two were deemed clinically significant on the basis of their relatively high Gleason score or pathologic stage [31]. These ex vivo data represent strong evidence of the limitations of conventional PBx and have been highlighted by other clinical studies.

Adopting a scheme that is able to maximize the DR with the fewest number of cores represents a possible new modality of performing PBx. This approach is clinically preferable to adopting a saturation scheme that is unable to increase the cancer DR with the same proportion of increasing numbers of cores. Scattoni et al. recently demonstrated that both the number and the location of biopsy cores taken affect cancer DR in a repeated biopsy setting [28]. They also showed that the "optimal" repeat-biopsy scheme (defined as the combination of sampling sites that detected 95% of all cancers with the minimal number of biopsy cores) varies according to the clinical characteristics of the patients.

Analysis revealed that for patients with previous ASAP diagnosis, the most advantageous scheme was a combination of a 14-core biopsy (without TZ biopsies) [28]. For patients with no previous ASAP diagnosis and percentage of free prostate-specific antigen (%fPSA) of 10% or less,

the most advantageous scheme was a 14-core biopsy (including four TZ biopsies). The most advantageous sampling scheme for patients with no previous ASAP and %fPSA greater than 10% was a combination of a 20-core biopsy (including four TZ biopsies). Even though it has to be validated with independent data, Scattoni et al. presented a flowchart that identifies the most advantageous set of sampling sites according to patient characteristics [28] (Fig. 22.5a–c).

Overdiagnosis of Clinically Insignificant Prostate Cancer

Detection of clinically insignificant PCa is an inevitable risk of repeat biopsy, and its association with the number of biopsy cores is an issue of considerable debate. To date, it must be recognized that there is no universally accepted definition of *clinically insignificant PCa* on the basis of biopsy findings. In 2004, Epstein updated the preoperative criteria, which consisted of prostate-specific antigen (PSA) density 0.15 ng/ml or less per gram, Gleason score of six or lower, fewer than three positive cores, and less than 50% of cancer involvement in any core [25]. To date, these preoperative criteria are the most widely used for predicting insignificant PCa, even though they do not take into consideration the number of cores taken.

From a theoretical point of view, the higher the number of the core taken, the higher the risk of detecting insignificant cancers. Singh et al. reported that the risk increased from 22.7% to

33.5% by increasing the number of cores from 6 to 12 [17]. In contrast, the Cancer of the Prostate Strategic Urologic Research Endeavor (CaPSURE) database shows that taking more cores improves cancer detection and does not appear to increase the risk of detecting clinically insignificant cancer [42]. Other reports suggest that SPBx may not increase the detection of clinically insignificant tumors [43, 44].

It should be considered that the Epstein criteria are not perfect and misclassify about 30% of patients who would have unfavorable pathologic features in a radical prostatectomy (RP) specimen. This risk ranges from 16% to 42% in selected series [25]. In contrast, SPBx has been evaluated as a staging tool to improve the characterization of low-volume and well-differentiated PCa, but whether SPBx improves prediction of tumor insignificance remains open to debate. It is also noteworthy that insufficient prostate sampling increases the chance of undergrading the tumor, leading to a false increase in the prevalence of insignificant PCa.

Epstein et al. have emphasized the benefit of SPBx in the measurement of tumor extent and grade and thus in the evaluation of insignificant PCa [43]. Using an SPBx scheme, the false-positive rate for the diagnosis of insignificant PCa ranged only from 8% to 11.5%, according to the algorithm chosen. This study, however, was ex vivo, and transfer to clinical practice might have limitations. Cancers originating in the TZ are more likely to behave in an indolent fashion and therefore could more easily be defined as insignificant. Consequently, EPBx schemes, including cores in the TZ, might increase the prevalence of diagnosed insignificant PCa.

Recently, Zaytoun et al. showed that SPBx detected more cases of insignificant cancer [27]. Of 315 positive biopsies, 119 (37.8%) revealed clinically insignificant cancer, as defined by the predetermined parameters. There was a trend toward increased detection of clinically insignificant cancer in the SPBx group (40.1% vs. 32.6%), but this trend did not reach statistical significance ($p=0.2$). Because the study was not powered for this finding, the authors cautioned that conclusions regarding this aspect should be tempered. Whether SPBx poses a risk of increasing detection of clinically insignificant cancer remains a matter of debate.

It should be also noted that, in general, cancer missed on initial prostate biopsy is likely to be smaller or more insignificant than those cancers identified on first attempt. Resnick et al. recently showed on pathologic analysis that increasing the number of prostate biopsies was associated with increased risk of low-volume, organ-confined disease. The risk of clinically insignificant disease was found to be 31.1%, 43.8%, and 46.8% in those undergoing one, two, and three or more PBx, respectively. Conversely, the risk of adverse pathology was found to be 64.6%, 53.0%, and 52.0% in those undergoing one, two, and three or more PBx, respectively [45]. In an editorial comment, Jones correctly noted that these data certainly demonstrate the potential to identify low-risk PCa with any biopsy strategy, even if patients undergoing repeat biopsy for any indication have real potential of harboring serious disease. The real issue with PCa detection is not overdiagnosis, since only diagnosis or misdiagnosis exists, but rather potential overtreatment. Detection and treatment of PCa should always be considered independent processes, and concern about overdetection must be weighed against the risk of missing clinically significant cancers.

Location of the Cores

The vast majority of PCa found in the contemporary series originates in the peripheral zone. Recent publications about RP specimens, however, have focused attention on the prevalence of tumors in the apex and the anterior part of the prostate (Fig. 22.6).

Takashima et al. demonstrated that tumor frequency was highest in the midgland (85.5%), followed closely by the apex (82.3%) [46]. Moussa et al. recently reported that examination of the apical cores, especially the extreme apical cores, increases PCa detection [47]. Quadrant analysis showed that tumors were significantly denser in the apex to midgland, particularly in the anterior half of the gland. Bott et al. conducted an analysis of whole-mount prostatectomy specimens with respect to the biopsy information [48].

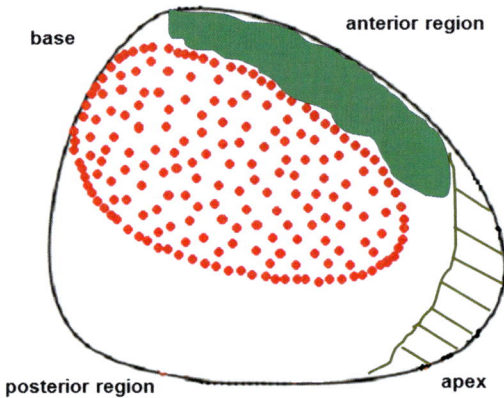

Fig. 22.6 Map of the prostate where the tumors may be located

Anterior tumors (more than 75% of tumors located anterior to the urethra) required significantly more biopsy sessions than posterior tumors (more than 75% of tumors located posterior to the urethra). They concluded that the anterior gland should be targeted in repeat biopsy in patients with clinical suspicion of PCa but persistently negative biopsies.

Bouyé et al. demonstrated that the anterior prostate harbors a significantly greater incidence of PCa than perceived, probably because biopsies more reliably target the posterior prostate [49]. The experience of Cleveland Clinic suggests increasing the cores of the apex and anterior part of the prostate when performing a second biopsy after an extended protocol. These authors also demonstrated that the end-fire probe can reach the anterior and apical aspects of the gland, regions that are likely to harbor unrecognized disease, and can identify almost 20% more cancers than the side-fire probe [50]. If the initial biopsy was performed with the more common side-fire probes, the authors will preferentially use the end-fire probe to facilitate sampling of the apex and anterior horn.

More recently, Raber et al. [51] demonstrated that PCa DR does not depend on the type of probe used in their population. They evaluated a total of 1,705 patients in the first-biopsy group and 487 patients in the repeat-biopsy group who submitted to PBx with a side-fire and an end-fire ultrasound probe [51]. The overall DR of the first-biopsy and rebiopsy groups were 37.2% and 10.1%, respectively. No significant difference was found between the two probes in the first-biopsy and rebiopsy sets (38% vs. 36.5%, $p=0.55$; 10.8% vs. 9.3%, $p=0.7$). The lack of any significant association between the type of probe used and PCa detection was confirmed by univariable and multivariable analyses in both the first-biopsy and rebiopsy sets after accounting for PSA values, %fPSA, DRE, and PV and TZ volume. The patient tolerance profile of the side-fire group was significantly better than that of the end-fire group (mean VAS: 1.78 ± 2.01 vs. 1.45 ± 2.21; $p=0.02$). The authors concluded that the side-fire transrectal probe is associated with a better patient tolerance profile than end-fire probes with a similar DR.

Recently, Walz et al. reported a high PCa DR of 41% with a 24-core protocol [24]. As with the initial biopsy protocol, it has been proven that more time and effort should be spent on lateral biopsies, which increase the cancer DR, whereas parasagittal biopsy provides a low yield on repeat biopsy [26]. Scattoni et al. selected two optimal, different schemes with different locations and numbers of cores in two groups of patients with different risks of having cancer, according to %fPSA values [34]. The parasagittal and posterior zones were omitted and two very apical biopsies were included in this scheme (Fig. 22.2).

A debate is ongoing in the literature about the role and the number of cores of the TZ biopsies in patients with an initial benign histology [21–23]. According to published reports, PCa is diagnosed on the basis of TZ biopsies in only 1.8–8% of cases [21–23]. Campos-Fernandes et al. reported that only one case (1.7%) was identified from the TZ-only cores, and they concluded that the indication of TZ biopsies alone could be discussed in their cases [52]. Nevertheless, it should be noted that the cancer DR was particularly low in their study, in which TZ biopsies were systematically performed as the initial biopsy procedure. Pepe and Aragona [29] and Pepe et al. [53] reported that sampling from the prostatic TZ by directed needle biopsies at repeated SPBx was associated with a very low incidence of PCa (2.5%),

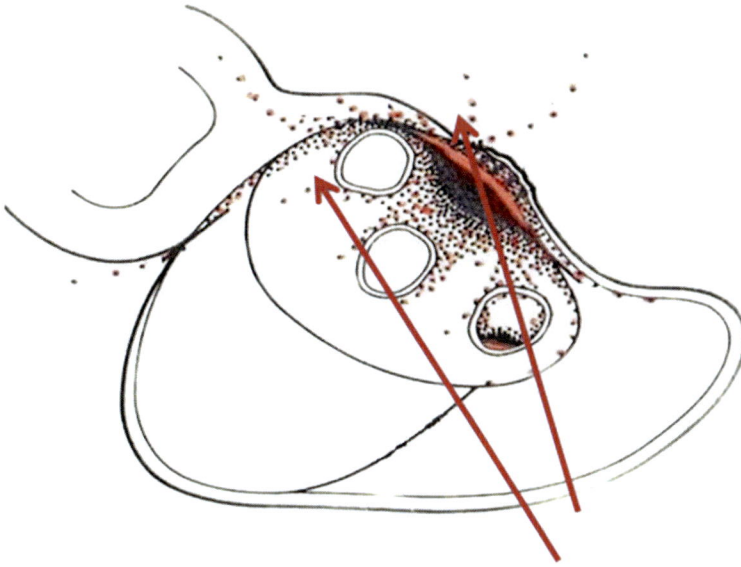

Fig. 22.7 The figure shows the right direction of the two cores for the biopsy of the TZ zone of each lobe of the prostate

especially if compared with transurethral resection of the prostate (TURP; DR: 19%). Scattoni et al. included TZ biopsies in their schemes because the majority of the patients were submitted to an extended approach without TZ biopsies [34]. They strongly suggest adding four-core TZ biopsies in the repeat setting in those patients. It should be noted that the anterior TZ cores were directed through the adenomas to the anterior capsule, whereas the other two posterior TZ cores were directed into the adenoma. The arrows in Fig. 22.7 show the direction and the position of the biopsies in each lobe.

In a study of patients undergoing repeat biopsy at Cleveland Clinic, Patel et al. were unable to identify exclusive TZ cancers and concluded that TZ biopsies may have limited utility in detecting PCa during repeat biopsy[9]. Notably, they included TZ tissue in 100% of biopsies but only as part of cores that traverse the gland and not as separately identifiable cores.

According to the 2010 EAU guidelines, TZ biopsy should be considered for men undergoing a repeat biopsy for suspicion of PCa. Recently, Ploussard et al. showed that TURP significantly increased the PCa DR by 28.5% ($p=0.035$) when used with a 21-core repeat PBx scheme [25].

Impact of Prostate Volume

The cancer DR of repeat PBx tends to decrease progressively when the prostate increases in size. Campos-Fernandes et al. reported that in multivariate analysis, PV was a significant predictive parameter of positive biopsies. The cancer DR was 21.7% in patients with PV less than 50 ml and 6.6% in patients with a PV of 50 ml or more (relative risk [RR]: 0.34; $p=0.031$) [52]. Similarly, Sajadi et al. found a much lower PCa DR with repeat SPBx in large prostates compared with smaller glands [54]. In the European Randomized Study of Screening for Prostate Cancer, Rietbergen et al. found that the most important factor related to failure to diagnose PCa at primary screening was large PV. A possible explanation is that many larger prostates have elevated PSA that is not secondary to a malignant process but rather reflects increased size and particularly TZ size [55]. Although undersampling of larger prostates (Fig. 22.8) may explain this discrepancy, it is also possible that lower prevalence of cancer exists in these large organs composed mostly of benign tissue.

In contrast, Walz et al. found a greater cancer detection rate in larger glands [26]. The Cleveland Clinic experience does not support taking more

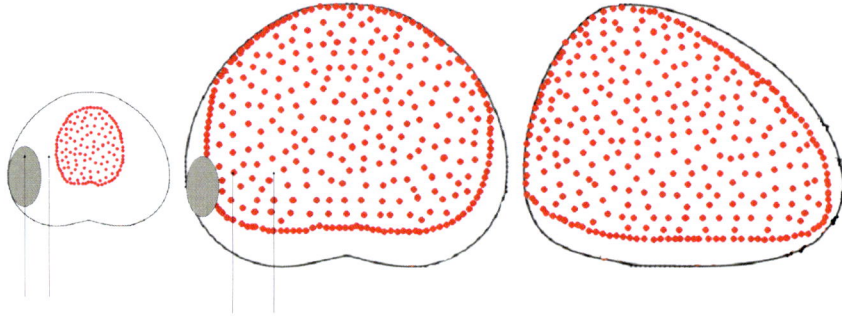

Fig. 22.8 Impact of prostate volume on prostate cancer detection

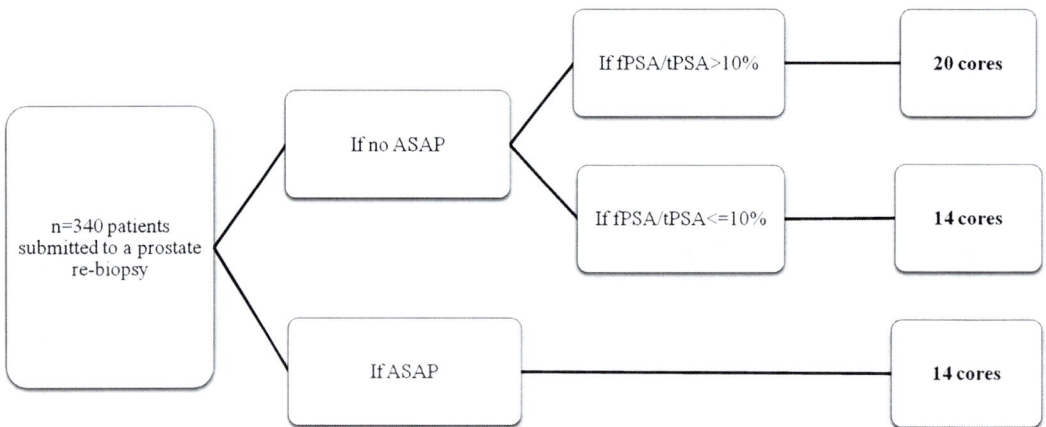

Fig. 22.9 Internally validated flowchart showing location and number of cores of the scheme that detects >95% of the cancers with the minimum number of cores, in three different risk groups (see Figs. 22.1 and 22.2 for the position of the cores). The risk groups were identified by using a classification and regression tree analysis depicting the risk to detect prostate cancer at rebiopsy

biopsies in larger prostates because no benefit has been proven. Naughton et al. have shown no correlation between the TRUS-determined PV or pathological weight and the number of biopsies needed for detecting PCa [56].

Recently, Scattoni et al. presented a flowchart to utilize the lowest core number to detect 95% of cancers that would have been detected with 24 cores [28]. PV was not included in the flowchart because PV was found to be a weak predictive factor, in contrast with results in the initial setting. Based on this experience, the number of cores should be modified according to presence of ASAP and %fPSA, which were the strongest predictive factors (Fig. 22.9).

Transrectal and Transperineal Approaches

Before the 1980s, DRE or transperineal TRUS PBx was the main method of diagnosing PCa [57, 58]. In the United States today, the transperineal approach is uncommon and is used by only 2% of urologists, although it is more common in European and Asian countries [59].

Transperineal and transrectal approaches have been shown to be equivalent for PCa detection when the same number of cores are obtained, as demonstrated by Emiliozzi et al. [60], Watanabe et al. [61], and Kawakami [41] and according to

Fig. 22.10 Double transrectal and transperineal approach (Ref. [41])

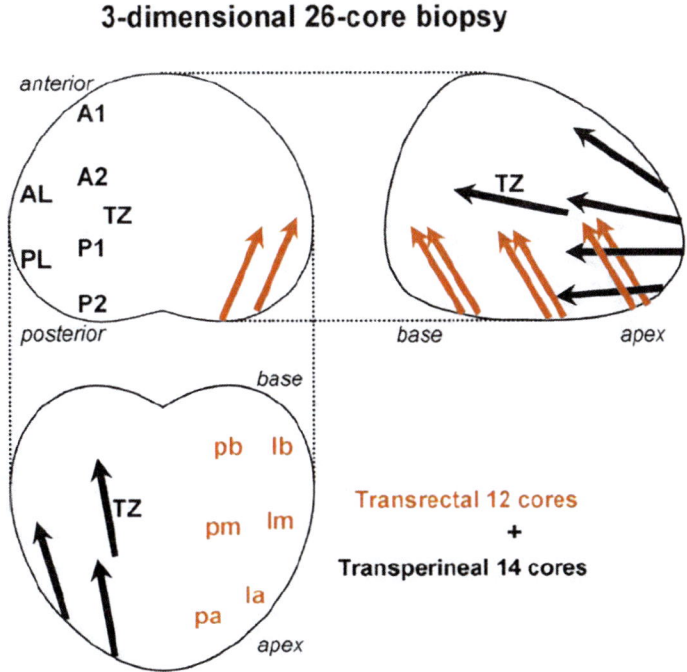

3-dimensional 26-core biopsy

anterior
A1
A2
AL
TZ
PL P1
P2
posterior

TZ

base apex

base
pb lb
TZ
pm lm
la
pa
apex

Transrectal 12 cores
+
Transperineal 14 cores

international guidelines. Over the past decade, however, several authors reported fewer complications and a greater PCa detection rate using a transperineal approach. These findings probably depend on the biopsy needle entering the prostate apex in a longitudinal direction, allowing for efficient sampling of the prostate peripheral zone. With the help of templates, the direction of the biopsy gun can be controlled and samples are uniformly distributed throughout the whole prostate. Recently, interest has been rising in taking transperineal biopsies via a brachytherapy grid to saturate the entire gland [62, 63]. Li et al. [63] recently performed an 11-region, template-guided, transperineal SPBx and obtained a mean of 23.7 cores. The authors concluded that transperineal ultrasound-guided SPBx is safe and feasible and provides an encouraging cancer DR.

Recently Abdollah et al. tested the hypothesis that there is a significant difference in the PCa DR between the transrectal and transperineal approaches in men undergoing saturation (24-core) prostate rebiopsy [64]. They evaluated 472 consecutive men submitted to 24-core prostate rebiopsy at two tertiary referral centers. Of these, 70% (332 patients) underwent a transrectal biopsy and 30% (140 patients) underwent a transperineal biopsy. Propensity score was used to match 280 patients with homogeneous characteristics, and those represented the final study cohort. No statistically significant difference in PCa DR was shown between the transrectal and transperineal approaches (31.4% vs. 25.7%, respectively; $p=0.3$). The type of approach was not an independent predictor of PCa DR at multivariable analysis (odds ratio: 0.61; $p=0.1$). The authors concluded that transrectal SPBx and transperineal SPBx have similar PCa DR in men undergoing a saturation rebiopsy and that both approaches can be offered to men undergoing a prostate rebiopsy without undermining the rate of PCa detection.

Other authors have also performed a scheme with the simultaneous combination of transrectal and transperineal PBx [61, 65]. They demonstrated that the two approaches combined were better than a single approach. Geometric considerations would dictate that the apex and the anterior region of the prostate are best sampled via the transperineal route, whereas the base is best sampled via the transrectal approach. Even if this combination provides a high DR, it is not recommended because it requires hospitalization and major anesthesia (Fig. 22.10).

Indications

The management of patients with persistently elevated PSA levels in whom a first set of PBx has been negative for cancer is a frequent problem for urologists. Although SPBx has not been shown to be beneficial in men as an initial biopsy strategy, it improves cancer detection if clinical suspicion persists after previous biopsy with negative findings and provides an accurate prediction of prostate tumor volume and grade [9, 34, 43, 66–71].

According to international guidelines, SPBx is now recommended in most clinical situations in the repeated setting:

1. Prior negative PBx but with a persistent suspicion of PCa
2. Patients with previous suspicious histological findings such as ASAP and HGPIN
3. Patients who are candidates for an active surveillance protocol
4. Patients who are candidates for focal therapy

Prior Negative Prostate Biopsy but with a Persistent Suspicion of Prostate Cancer

The persistent suspicion of PCa in patients with a prior negative PBx is based on DRE findings, repeated PSA measurements (e.g., %fPSA, complex PSA, PSA density, PSA velocity), and, rarely, the presence of a hypoechoic lesion in TRUS [3, 12, 13, 52, 53]. Different authors have reported that office-based SPBx increases the PCa DR in patients with suspicious clinical findings following previous negative standard PBx, compared with repeat standard biopsy strategies using up to 12 cores. The PCa DR of repeat SPBx has been reported to be about 30%, regardless of the type of previous biopsy scheme. Moreover, this current trend of rebiopsy schemes becoming more and more "saturated," together with acceptable side effect profiles as well as low rates of clinically insignificant disease, further supports the SPBx concept [13].

At present, only %fPSA should be considered a valid parameter for deciding to perform a second biopsy (see NCCN guidelines). Prostate cancer antigen 3 as well as PSA isoform −2proPSA and Prostate Health Index should not be considered in the decision-making process.

Patients with Previous Suspicious Histological Findings

High-Grade Prostatic Intraepithelial Neoplasia

The role of HGPIN as a precursor of PCa and, consequently, as a risk factor that improves the accuracy of repeat-biopsy outcome predictions remains controversial, even within risk-stratification analyses of repeat-biopsy outcome. Recent EAU, NCCN, and American Urological Association (AUA) guidelines reported that the presence of HGPIN diagnosis no longer represents an indication for immediate repeat biopsy [72]. Moreover, Epstein and Herawi demonstrated that the contemporary median PCa risk at repeat biopsy after HGPIN diagnosis dropped to approximately 22%. This figure almost equals the median risk of PCa detection after initial benign diagnosis (15–19%) [73]. Furthermore, prospective trials failed to demonstrate an association between the presence of HGPIN at initial biopsy and subsequent PCa at repeat biopsy [74–76].

Conversely, Benecchi et al. [77] and Rochester et al. [78] identified the presence of HGPIN as a risk factor in their analyses and included HGPIN in their novel repeat-biopsy nomograms. From a methodological viewpoint, a stepwise multivariable approach was performed in both studies and results in p values that are low, thus artificially inflating discriminative ability [77–79]. Campos-Fernandes et al. [52] performed a second extended 21-sample needle biopsy and reported a cancer DR of 17% in patients with prior benign biopsy and 16% in patients with prior HGPIN. Similarly, we reported a similar DR between patients with benign initial biopsy and patients with prior HGPIN, and we confirmed that HGPIN is not a significant predictive factor for a positive second biopsy [28].

The number of HGPIN foci appears to have a clear impact on both prognosis and suggested management protocols. Merrimen et al. showed

Fig. 22.11 Nomogram predicting the probability of a positive SPBx following diagnosis of HGPIN (Ref. [83])

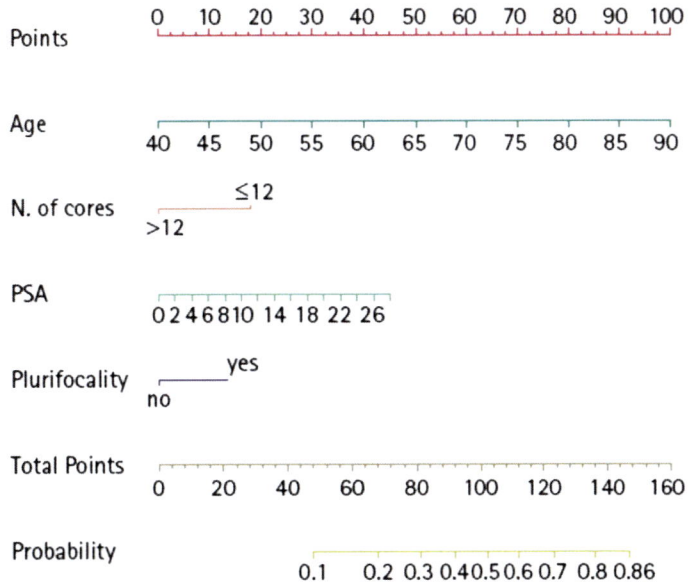

Points
0 10 20 30 40 50 60 70 80 90 100

Age
40 45 50 55 60 65 70 75 80 85 90

N. of cores
≤12
>12

PSA
0 2 4 6 8 10 14 18 22 26

Plurifocality
yes
no

Total Points
0   20   40   60   80   100   120   140   160

Probability
0.1   0.2 0.3 0.4 0.5 0.6 0.7 0.8 0.86

that unifocal HGPIN had no more likelihood of PCa detection than a benign diagnosis [80]. Similarly, Godoy et al. found that after confirming the adequacy of initial PBx (at least 10 cores), isolated HGPIN does not warrant any further PBx [81]. The original report from Cleveland Clinic showed that individuals with multifocal HPGIN versus isolated HGPIN on initial SPBx had 80% versus 0% incidence of PCa on repeat PBx, respectively. Cleveland Clinic has recently published a report on 328 men who underwent a second PBx after HGPIN diagnosis. HGPIN alone on initial PBx had a significant effect on the subsequent diagnosis of PCa (hazard ratio [HR]: 1.89; 95% confidence interval [CI], 1.39–2.55; $p < 0.0001$) [82]. Stratifying HGPIN into multifocal and bilateral disease significantly increased the HRs to 2.56 (95% CI, 1.83–3.6) and 2.2 (95% CI, 1.51–3.21), respectively.

Roscigno et al. [83] showed that PCa detection was significantly higher in patients with initial biopsy of 12 cores or less than in those with more than 12 cores (37.6% vs. 23.1%, $p = 0.01$) and in patients with plurifocal HGPIN than in those with monofocal HGPIN (40% vs. 25.1%, $p = 0.013$). At multivariable analysis, PSA value ($p = 0.041$; HR: 1.08), age ($p < 0.001$; HR: 1.09), plurifocal HGPIN ($p = 0.031$; HR: 1.97), and initial

biopsy with 12 cores or less ($p = 0.012$; HR: 1.95) were independent predictors of PCa detection. The authors presented a nomogram including these four variables that achieved 72% accuracy in predicting PCa detection after an initial HGPIN diagnosis (Fig. 22.11).

All of these data demonstrate that a single focus may be relatively meaningless, with the risk of de novo cancer development minimally increased, whereas multifocal HGPIN more than doubles the risk of de novo cancer development.

Atypical Small Acinar Proliferation of the Prostate

Isolated ASAP is a well-known risk factor for a positive second biopsy. The overall risk of harboring cancer is about 40% in recent series, slightly less than 45% observed more than a decade ago [84, 85]. In the recent study by Campos-Fernandes et al. [52], the overall risk of finding cancer is about 42%.

Repeat biopsy is mandatory at least one time, even if a pathologic second opinion may clarify the diagnosis when subspecialty pathology was not involved. In one study, 1.1% of patients with a negative biopsy were found to have cancer, and another 1.3% were found to have ASAP when cases were reviewed based on a finding of

PCa in a repeat biopsy, emphasizing the value of reinterpretation in equivocal cases [86].

For a second biopsy, Levi and colleagues found that a 20-core transrectal PBx adds no morbidity and increases cancer detection marginally compared with 12–14 cores; if a third biopsy is necessary, SPBx substantially increases cancer detection [87].

Precise labeling of initial biopsy locations is important to direct rebiopsy in a more concentrated fashion into the region of the initial atypical biopsy within 3–6 months [68, 73, 85, 88]. Allen et al. demonstrated that the chance of detecting cancer greatly increases by performing a rebiopsy not only of the atypical site but also of adjacent contralateral and adjacent ipsilateral areas [88]. Scattoni et al., however, previously reported that in a multisite study, precise spatial concordance between ASAP and cancer was present in only 33% of the cases, similar to the likelihood of finding cancer in an adjacent or a nonadjacent site [34]. They have recently reported that in this situation, the site of ASAP seems not to be so important, probably due to the multifocality of the PCa. Scattoni et al. also recently proposed a specific combination of a 14-core biopsy that is sufficient to detect 95% of the cancer. In this group of patients, the TZ biopsies were not necessary because they only slightly increased cancer detection, and the majority of cancers were situated in the peripheral gland [34] (Fig. 22.5).

Patients Who Are Candidates for an Active Surveillance Protocol

SPBx may also be performed in patients who are candidates for an active surveillance protocol. SPBx has been proven to lead to more accurate assessment of the extent and grade of disease than traditional biopsy [24, 66, 68, 89]. Even if an immediate EPBx can be performed to increase selection of patients for active surveillance up to 30%, as demonstrated by Berglund et al. [90], an SPBx protocol has been advocated to better characterize the PCa.

A minimum 12-core biopsy is now recommended, including core sampling the anterior prostate, before considering an active surveillance protocol. Some authors have advocated routine SPBx for men embarking on surveillance; however, this approach is not generally practiced in most high-volume surveillance centers [71]. In contrast, most centers recommend confirmatory biopsy if the diagnostic biopsy was not performed with an extended template or otherwise seems to be of questionable quality. Around one-third of men had more significant PCa on SPBx, and this finding probably reflects undersampling by initial EPBx rather than disease progression. The Memorial Sloan-Kettering Cancer Center criteria explicitly require confirmatory biopsy for all men before surveillance; notably, 58% of these repeat biopsies did not demonstrate cancer.

No validated criteria exist for follow-up of expectantly managed patients with low-risk PCa. Most groups advise serial biopsies at intervals varying from 1 to 4 years. The Toronto group recommends a confirmatory biopsy at 1 year to identify higher-grade disease that was missed on original biopsy; following this, biopsies are performed every 4 years to identify biological progression, a much rarer event. The Hopkins group performs biopsies annually or when a rise in PSA occurs. Unquestionably, biopsy sampling error is a significant limitation of surveillance. For this reason, some authors advocate SPBx for patients contemplating surveillance [35]. Al Otaibi et al. recommended an intensive biopsy protocol within the first 2 years for patients on active surveillance. They found that the first repeat biopsy has a strong predictive impact for disease progression. Only 25% of patients with negative first repeat biopsy had disease progression on follow-up biopsy [91]. This approach, which may identify some patients with higher-risk disease, has not been embraced by most advocates of active surveillance and does not seem necessary for the majority of patients.

Patients Who Are Candidates for Focal Therapy

The increased number of apparently small unilateral prostate tumors has led to the introduction of focal therapy as a potential alternative to radical, whole-gland therapy. In 2011 PBx, together with MRI, continues to be the most commonly used method for treatment planning [44, 92–95].

Unfortunately, the sextant and extended transrectal biopsy schemes have failed to reach a satisfactory level of accuracy with respect to identification of a unilateral tumor on the final RP pathologic specimen, minimizing the probability of achieving adequate cancer control in men treated with focal therapy based on these biopsy results. In contrast, SPBx has proved useful when focal therapy is considered but only when compared with less EPBx schemes [13, 24, 43, 59, 66, 67, 85, 89, 96]. Unfortunately, even SPBx has proved insufficiently accurate in the evaluation of tumor laterality and extension. Falzarano et al. recently reported only a minor correlation (10%) between the unilaterality of cancer on SPBx with unilateral cancer in the final pathologic specimens from RP [96]. They concluded that a negative SPBx does not confirm the absence of cancer in the corresponding side of the gland and cannot be used as single determinant when considering patients for focal treatment.

Even if SPBx may increase the certainty that a prostatic tumor is unilateral and reduce the likelihood of a lesion being present in the contralateral lobe, the most appropriate way to evaluate PCa before focal therapy is the transperineal template-guided mapping biopsy.

Pain Control

Radical improvement of anesthetic techniques in recent years has become evident and has led to diffusion of EPBx and SPBx schemes in outpatient settings and spurred rebiopsy. Different anesthetic techniques have been described in the literature, with the aim of finding the best procedure in terms of cost-benefit ratio for the patient, according to urologists' habits. Anesthesia during PBx is currently considered mandatory; performing the procedure without anesthesia is considered malpractice, according to international guidelines [71].

Various types of anesthesia have been investigated for both the transrectal and transperineal routes; however, the best method has not yet been defined for either route because many factors depend on both the patient's characteristics and the urologist's experience and habits.

Anesthetic techniques may be divided into two categories, according to route of administration and drug used: local anesthesia, with which PBx can be performed in the outpatient setting, also considering the number of cores, and systemic anesthesia, for which patients require hospitalization.

Of all anesthetic techniques, peripheral PNB (PPNB) is recommended by both conclusive expert opinion and contemporary clinical guidelines (EAU, AUA, NCCN). PPNB is generally considered the gold standard for providing comfort and no pain for patients undergoing transrectal PBx, despite the variability of location and dosage of infiltration and regardless of both patient age and number of cores. The most used drug is 1% or 2% lidocaine because of low incidence of side effects, low cost, and great efficacy. The most common injection site is the angle between the prostate base and the seminal vesicles, bilaterally [10, 97–103].

The association of PPNB and intrarectal local anesthesia (IRLA) or systemic drugs is still controversial, although an increasing number of trials demonstrate better control of discomfort caused by TRUS probe insertion, achieved with IRLA administration [104–109]. Pain control during the entire procedure seems to be superior with the aid of systemic analgesic, especially nonsteroidal anti-inflammatory drugs [110–113]. Sedoanalgesia should be preferred when extensive or repeated biopsies are needed [114].

Like the transrectal approach, transperineal PBx requires the use of local anesthesia, represented by the injection of a local anesthetic agent (analog to those used for transrectal PBx) at the prostate apex, passing through the perineal structures that may evoke significant pain during the procedure. These structures include the bulbocavernous muscle, the levator ani (both innervated by pudendal nerve), the deep transverse perineal muscle (innervated by the perineal nerves), and the prostatic capsule (innervated by the peripheral branches of the pelvic plexus) [115].

With the transperineal approach, the patient has the discomfort derived from the insertion and the movements of the probe, the injection of local anesthesia through the perineal structures, and the needle passage through the prostate capsule [116, 117]. Despite these considerations and the approach used, the choice of anesthetic technique and the drugs used actually still depend on the urologist's habits and experience.

Complications

Transrectal PBx is generally considered safe and is commonly performed in an outpatient setting. As the number of healthy men enrolled in early detection programs increases, the overall number of transrectal PBx procedures also increases [118]. In this context, reporting true morbidity and complication rates is fundamental because patients must be informed adequately. Nevertheless, comparisons among trials should be made with caution because of differences in sample size, population, biopsy protocol, definition of complications, and follow-up [119–124] (Table 22.5).

The number of samples taken is controversial as a risk factor in PBx. It was believed that increasing the number of retrieved cores, as in SPBx, was directly related to increasing the chance of complications. In fact, the act of multiple sampling may facilitate the penetration of microorganisms into the bloodstream from a prostate with latent germs, thereby favoring an infectious process. Nam et al. [119] recently reported that the hospital admission rates for complications following TRUS PBx have

increased dramatically during the last 10 years primarily due to an increasing rate of infection-related complications (Fig. 22.12).

Despite these considerations, most trials have reported a complication rate for SPBx similar to that for EPBx. Additionally, safety and efficacy of the procedure is well documented in the literature, both as a first and a repeat approach.

A review of the literature demonstrated that the most frequent early complications with increased numbers of cores are related to hemorrhagic events (i.e., hematuria and rectal bleeding). A significant number of these events are encountered in patients and often are self-limiting. Late hemorrhagic morbidity, including hematospermia and recurrent mild hematuria, shows similar recurrence rates after both first and repeat biopsy.

Different authors have reported that PV has a significant proportional correlation with the incidence of hematuria and hematospermia [27, 120–122]. The role of anticoagulant/antiplatelet medications as a cause of hemorrhagic complications in PBx is controversial. Some authors have described encountering severe hematuria often in patients on these medications. If patients were instructed to discontinue aspirin for 7 days and Coumadin for 3 days before biopsy, then the complication rate would not increase [123]. Most urologists now ask patients to discontinue anticoagulant/antiplatelet medications 5–7 days before the procedure.

Conclusions

The management of patients in whom a first set of prostate biopsies has been negative for cancer poses a problem for urologists. Although SPBx has not been shown to be beneficial in men as an initial biopsy strategy, it improves cancer detection if clinical suspicion persists after previous biopsy with negative findings and provides accurate prediction of prostate tumor volume and grade.

Despite the published trials in the literature, the issues of number and location of cores remain a matter of debate. With the development of new imaging methods that allow performance of

Table 22.5 Complications of extended and saturation biopsies

Complications	Frequency, %
Hemospermia	37.4
Urethrorrhagia	14.5
Rectorrhagia	2.2
Prostatitis	1
Fever	0.8
Epididymitis	0.7
Sepsis	0.3
Acute urinary retention	0.2

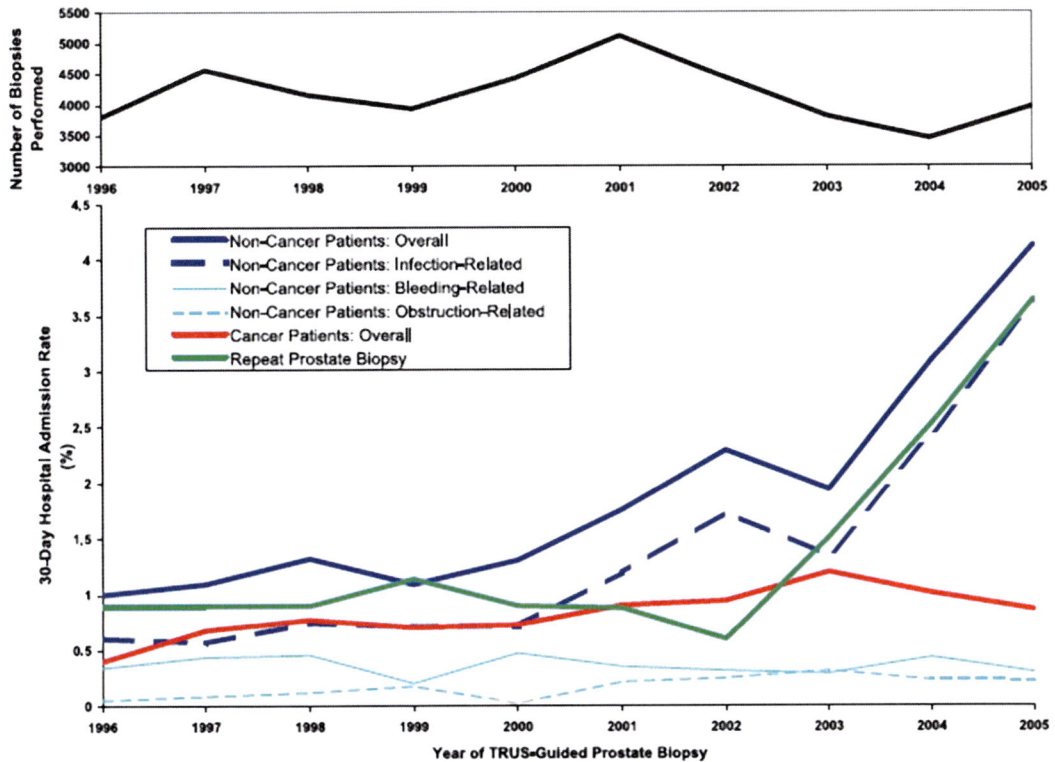

Fig. 22.12 Incidence of complications after a PBx in the last decades (Ref. [119])

targeted biopsies, the role of SPBx probably will be reconsidered. At present, SPBx seems to be necessary for men with persistent suspicion of PCa after negative initial biopsy and probably for patients with multifocal HGPIN or ASAP. In other situations, the role of transrectal SPBx is still questionable. Adopting an individualized scheme according to patients' clinical characteristics that is able to maximize the DR with the fewest number of cores seems more appealing than adopting a saturation scheme for all patients that does not increase the cancer DR in proportion to the increase in number of cores.

Editorial Commentary:

Many urologists expressed concern when Stamey originally suggested that six systematic biopsy cores should be obtained in men with high PSA. That seemed exorbitant at the time, when needle biopsy of a suspicious palpable lesion was the mainstay of PCa diagnosis. This concern was raised again when Presti and others suggested 8–10 cores and with each increasing number of cores in subsequent protocols. When Stewart and Borboroglu simultaneously reached the 22–24-core range, general anesthesia became standard, and critics were convinced that the complications would reach epic proportions.

But that did not happen.

Complication rates have still not been reported higher in the series discussed in this chapter compared to extended biopsy series. Our own publications have failed to show increased complications in direct comparative data. Furthermore, using periprostatic block, thousands of transrectal saturation biopsies have been performed in urologists' offices around the world, with detection rates almost 1/3 higher than extended repeat-biopsy strategies.

So why not go to even higher numbers of cores? The answer again lies in research and well-considered experience. Studies both in vivo and ex vivo have identified that we appear to have reached a logical "saturation point" as introduced by the authors. Nevertheless, transrectal saturation biopsy is still not universally applied for repeat biopsy despite the supporting evidence in this chapter. I believe the reasons lie in bias that more biopsy passes "surely" must have higher complication rates. Now that the literature is becoming very clear in proving this inaccurate, it is likely that the technique will become standard—and incorporated into guidelines—based on data driven logic.

–J. Stephen Jones

References

1. Hodge KK, McNeal JE, Terris MK, Stamey TA. Random systematic versus directed ultrasound guided trans-rectal core biopsies of the prostate. J Urol. 1989;142:71–4. discussion 74–5.

2. Astraldi A. Diagnosis of cancer of the prostate: biopsy by rectal route. Urol Cutan Rev. 1937;41:421.

3. Stewart CS, Leibovich BC, Weaver AL, Lieber MM. Prostate cancer diagnosis using a saturation needle biopsy technique after previous negative sextant biopsies. J Urol. 2001;166:86–91. discussion 92.

4. Borboroglu PG, Corner SW, Riffenburgh RH, Amling CL. Extensive repeat trans-rectal ultrasound guided prostate biopsy in patient with previous benign sextant biopsies. J Urol. 2000;163:158–62.

5. Schroder FH, Hugosson J, Roobol MJ, et al. Screening and prostate-cancer mortality in a randomized European study. N Engl J Med. 2009;360:1320–8.

6. Andriole GL, Crawford ED, Grubb III RL, et al. Mortality results from a randomized prostate-cancer screening trial. N Engl J Med. 2009;360:1310–9.

7. Bertaccini A, Fandella A, Prayer-Galetti T, et al. Systematic development of clinical practice guidelines for prostate biopsies: a 3-year Italian project. Anticancer Res. 2007;27:659–66.

8. Shariat SF, Roehrborn CG. Using biopsy to detect prostate cancer. Rev Urol. 2008;10:262–79.

9. Patel AR, Jones JS, Rabets J, DeOreo G, Zippe CD. Parasagittal biopsies add minimal information in repeat saturation prostate biopsy. Urology. 2004;63:87–9.

10. Nash PA, Bruce JE, Indudhara R, et al. Transrectal ultrasound guided prostatic nerve blockade eases systematic needle biopsy of the prostate. J Urol. 1996;155:607–9.

11. Crundwell MC, Cooke RW, Wallace DM. Patients' tolerance of transrectal ultrasound guided prostate biopsy: an audit of 104 cases. BJU Int. 1999;83:107.

12. Lane BR, Zippe CD, Abouassaly A, Schoenfield L, Magi-Galluzzi C, Jones SL. Saturation technique does not decrease cancer detection during follow-up after initial prostate biopsy. J Urol. 2008;179: 1749–50.

13. Jones JS. Saturation biopsy for detecting and characterizing prostate cancer. BJU Int. 2007;99: 1340–4.

14. Naughton CK, Miller DC, Mager DE, Ornsetin DK, Catalona WJ. A prospective randomized trial comparing 6 versus 12 prostate biopsy cores: impact of cancer detection. J Urol. 2000;164:388.

15. Jl G, Shariat S, Miles BJ, et al. Optimal combinations of systematic sextant and laterally directed biopsies for the detection of prostate cancer. J Urol. 2001;165:1554–9.

16. Siu W, Dunn RL, Shah RB, et al. Use of extended pattern technique for initial prostate biopsy. J Urol. 2005;174:505–9.

17. Singh H, Canto EI, Shariat SF, et al. Improved detection of clinically significant, curable prostate cancer with systematic 12-core biopsy. J Urol. 2004;171: 1089–92.

18. de la Taille A, Antiphon P, Salomon L, et al. Prospective evaluation of a 21-sample needle biopsy procedure designed to improve the prostate cancer detection rate. Urology. 2003;61:1181–6.

19. Presti Jr JC, O'Dowd GJ, Miller MC, et al. Extended peripheral zone biopsy schemes increases cancer detection rates and minimizes variance in prostate specific antigen and age related cancer rates: results of a community multi-practice study. J Urol. 2003;169:125–9.

20. Eichler K, Hempel S, Wilby J, et al. Diagnostic value of systematic biopsy methods in the investigation of prostate cancer: a systematic review. J Urol. 2006;175:1605–12.

21. Pelzer AE, Bektic J, Berger AP, et al. Are transition zone biopsies still necessary to improve prostate cancer detection? Results from the Tyrol screening project. Eur Urol. 2005;48:916–21.

22. Peyromaure M, Ravery V, Boccon-Gibod L. The role of the biopsy of the transitional zone and of the seminal vesicles in the diagnosis and staging of prostate cancer. Eur Urol Suppl. 2002;1:40–6.

23. Epstein JI, Walsh PC, Sauvageot J, Carter HB. Use of repeat sextant and transition zone biopsies for assessing extent of prostate cancer. J Urol. 1997;158:1886–90.

24. Rabets JC, Jones JS, Patel A, et al. Prostate cancer detection with office based saturation biopsy in a repeat biopsy population. J Urol. 2004;172:94–7.

25. Ploussard G, Epstein JI, Montironi R, et al. The contemporary concept of significant versus insignificant prostate cancer. Eur Urol. 2011;60:291–303.

26. Walz J, Graefen M, Chun FK, et al. High incidence of prostate cancer detected by saturation biopsy after previous negative biopsy series. Eur Urol. 2006; 50:498–505.

27. Zaytoun OM, Moussa AS, Gao T, Fareed K, Jones JS. Office based transrectal saturation biopsy improves prostate cancer detection compared to

extended biopsy in the repeat biopsy population. J Urol. 2011;186:850–4.

28. Scattoni V, Raber M, Capitanio U, et al. The optimal rebiopsy prostatic scheme depends on patient clinical characteristics: results of a recursive partitioning analysis based on a 24-core systematic scheme. Eur Urol. 2011;60:834–41.

29. Pepe P, Aragona F. Saturation prostate needle biopsy and prostate cancer detection at initial and repeat evaluation. Urology. 2007;70:1131–5.

30. Descazeaud A, Rubin M, Chemama S, et al. Saturation biopsy protocol enhances prediction of pT3 and surgical margin status on prostatectomy specimen. World J Urol. 2006;24:676–80.

31. Delongchamps NB, de la Roza G, Jones R, Jumbelic M, Haas GP. Saturation biopsies on autopsied prostates for detecting and characterizing prostate cancer. BJU Int. 2009;103:49–54.

32. Scattoni V, Roscigno M, Raber M, et al. Initial extended transrectal prostate biopsy: are more prostate cancers detected with 18 cores than with 12 cores? J Urol. 2008;179:1327–31.

33. Guichard G, Larre S, Gallina A, et al. Extended 21-sample needle biopsy protocol for diagnosis of prostate cancer in 1000 consecutive patients. Eur Urol. 2007;52:430–5.

34. Scattoni V, Raber M, Abdollah F, et al. Biopsy schemes with the fewest cores for detecting 95% of the prostate cancers detected by a 24-core biopsy. Eur Urol. 2010;57:1–8.

35. Thompson IM, Ankerst DP, Chi C, et al. Assessing prostate cancer risk: results from the Prostate Cancer Prevention Trial. J Natl Cancer Inst. 2006;98:529–34.

36. Gallina A, Chun FK, Suardi N, et al. Comparison of stage migration patterns between Europe and the USA: an analysis of 11 350 men treated with radical prostatectomy for prostate cancer. BJU Int. 2008;101:1513–8.

37. Hogarth RM, Karelaia N. Heuristic and linear models of judgment: matching rules and environments. Psychol Rev. 2007;114:733–58.

38. Chun FK, Karakiewicz PI, Briganti A, et al. Prostate cancer nomograms: an update. Eur Urol. 2006;50:914–26. discussion 926.

39. Kawakami S, Numao N, Okubo Y, et al. Development, validation, and head-to-head comparison of logistic regression-based nomograms and artificial neural network models predicting prostate cancer on initial extended biopsy. Eur Urol. 2008;54:601–11.

40. Ide H, Yasuda M, Nishio K, et al. Development of a nomogram for predicting high-grade prostate cancer on biopsy: the significance of serum testosterone levels. Anticancer Res. 2008;28:2487–92.

41. Kawakami S, Okuno T, Yonese J, et al. Optimal sampling sites for repeat prostate biopsy: a recursive portioning analysis of three-dimensional 26-core systematic biopsy. Eur Urol. 2007;51:675–83.

42. Shah JB, McKiernan JM, Elkin EP, Carroll PR, Meng MV. CaPSURE Investigators. Prostate biopsy patterns in the CaPSURE database: evolution with time and impact on outcome after prostatectomy. J Urol. 2008;179:136–40.

43. Epstein JI, Sanderson H, Carter HB, et al. Utility of saturation biopsy to predict insignificant cancer at radical prostatectomy. Urology. 2005;66:356–60.

44. Bastian PJ, Mangold LA, Epstein JI, Partin AW. Characteristics of insignificant clinical T1c prostate tumors. A contemporary analysis. Cancer. 2004;101:2001–5.

45. Resnick MJ, Lee DJ, Magerfleisch L, et al. Repeat prostate biopsy and the incremental risk of clinically insignificant prostate cancer. Urology. 2011;77:548–52.

46. Takashima R, Egawa S, Kuwao S, Baba S. Anterior distribution of stage T1c nonpalpable tumors in radical prostatectomy specimens. Urology. 2002;59:692–7.

47. Moussa AS, Meshref A, Schoenfield L, et al. Importance of additional "extreme" anterior apical needle biopsies in the initial detection of prostate cancer. Urology. 2010;75:1034–9.

48. Bott L, Langley S, Hindley L, Montgomery B. Intensifying the saturation biopsy technique for detecting prostate cancer after previous negative biopsies: a step in the wrong direction. BJU Int. 2009;103:701.

49. Bouye' S, Potiron E, Puech P, Leroy X, Lemaitre L, Villers A. Transition zone and anterior stromal prostate cancers: zones of origin and intraprostatic pattern of spread at histopathology. Prostate. 2009;69:105–13.

50. Ching CB, Moussa AS, Li J, Lane BR, Zippe C, Jones JS. Does transrectal ultrasound probe configuration really matter? End fire versus side fire probe prostate cancer detection rates. J Urol. 2009;181:2077–82. discussion 2082–3.

51. Raber M, Scattoni V, Gallina A, et al. Does the transrectal ultrasound probe influence prostate cancer detection in patients undergoing an extended prostate biopsy scheme? Results of a large retrospective study. BJU Int. 2012;109(5):672–7.

52. Campos-Fernandes JL, Bastien L, Nicolaiew N, et al. Prostate cancer detection rate in patients with repeated extended 21-sample needle biopsy. Eur Urol. 2009;55:600–6.

53. Pepe P, Galia A, Fraggetta F, et al. Prediction by quantitative histology on pathological stage in prostate cancer. Eur J Surg Oncol. 2005;31:309–13.

54. Sajadi KP, Kim T, Terris MK, Brown JA, Lewis RW. High yield of saturation prostate biopsy for patients with previous negative biopsies and small prostates. Urology. 2007;70:691–5.

55. Rietbergen JB, Hoedemaeker RF, Kruger AE, Kirkels WJ, Schröder FH. The changing pattern of prostate cancer at the time of diagnosis: characteristics of screen detected prostate cancer in a population based screening study. J Urol. 1999;161:1192–8.

56. Naughton CK, Smith DS, Humphrey PA, Catalona WJ, Keetch DW. Clinical and pathologic tumor

characteristics of prostate cancer as a function of the number of biopsy cores: a retrospective study. Urology. 1998;52:808–13.

57. Kaufman JJ, Roenthal M, Godwin WE. Methods of diagnosis of carcinoma of the prostate: a comparison of clinical impression, prostate smear, needle biopsy open perineal biopsy and transurethral biopsy. J Urol. 1954;72:450–63.

58. Ritkin MD, Kurtz AB, Goldberg BB. Sonographically guided transperineal prostate biopsy: preliminary experience with a longitudinal linear array transducer. AJR Am J Roentgenol. 1983;140:745–7.

59. Shandera KC, Thibault GP, Deshon JE, et al. Variability in patient preparation for prostate biopsy among American urologists. Urology. 1998;52:644–6.

60. Emiliozzi P, Corsetti A, Tassi B, et al. Best approach for prostate cancer detection: a prospective study on transperineal versus transrectal six core prostate biopsy. Urology. 2003;61:961–6.

61. Watanabe M, Hayashi T, Tsushima T, et al. Extensive biopsy using a combined transperineal and transrectal approach to improve prostate cancer detection. Int J Urol. 2005;12:959–63.

62. Takenaka A, Hara R, Hyodo Y, et al. Transperineal extended biopsy improves the clinically significant prostate cancer detection rate: a comparative study of 6 and 12 biopsy cores. Int J Urol. 2006;13:10–4.

63. Li H, Yan W, Zhou Y, et al. Transperineal ultrasound-guided saturation biopsies using 11-region template of prostate: report of 303 cases. Urology. 2007;70:1157–61.

64. Abdollah F, Novara G, Briganti A, et al. Trans-rectal versus trans-perineal saturation rebiopsy of the prostate: is there a difference in cancer detection rate? Urology. 2011;77:921–5.

65. Emiliozzi P, Maymone S, Paterno A, et al. Increased accuracy of biopsy Gleason score obtained by extended needle biopsy. J Urol. 2004;172:2224–6.

66. Chun FK, Epstein JR, Ficarra V, et al. Optimizing performance and interpretation of prostate biopsy: a critical analysis of the literature. Eur Urol. 2010;58:851–64.

67. Warlick C, Trock BJ, Landis B, et al. Delayed versus immediate surgical intervention and prostate cancer outcome. J Natl Cancer Inst. 2006;98:355–7.

68. Abouassaly R, Lane BR, Jones SJ. Staging saturation biopsy in patients with prostate cancer on active surveillance protocol. Urology. 2008;71:573–7.

69. Boccon-Gibod LM, de Longchamps NB, Toublanc M, et al. Prostate saturation biopsy in the reevaluation of microfocal prostate cancer. J Urol. 2006;176:971–3.

70. Patel AR, Jones JS. Optimal biopsy strategies for the diagnosis and staging of prostate cancer. Curr Opin Urol. 2009;19:232–7.

71. Scattoni V, Zlotta A, Montironi R, Schulman C, Rigatti P, Montorsi F. Extended and saturation prostatic biopsy in the diagnosis and characterisation of prostate cancer: a critical analysis of the literature. Eur Urol. 2007;52:1309–22.

72. Heidenreich A, Aus G, Bolla M, et al. EAU guidelines on prostate cancer. Eur Urol. 2008;53:68–80.

73. Epstein JI, Herawi M. Prostate needle biopsies containing prostatic intraepithelial neoplasia or atypical foci suspicious for carcinoma: implications for patient care. J Urol. 2006;175:820–34.

74. Gallo F, Chiono L, Gastaldi E, Venturino E, Giberti C. Prognostic significance of high-grade prostatic intraepithelial neoplasia (HGPIN): risk of prostatic cancer on repeat biopsies. Urology. 2008;72:628–32.

75. Gokden N, Roehl KA, Catalona WJ, Humphrey PA. High-grade prostatic intraepithelial neoplasia in needle biopsy as risk factor for detection of adenocarcinoma: current level of risk in screening population. Urology. 2005;65:538–42.

76. Bishara T, Ramnani DM, Epstein JI. High-grade prostatic intraepithelial neoplasia on needle biopsy: risk of cancer on repeat biopsy related to number of involved cores and morphologic pattern. Am J Surg Pathol. 2004;28:629–33.

77. Benecchi L, Pieri AM, Melissari M, Potenzoni M, Pastizzaro CD. A novel nomogram to predict the probability of prostate cancer on repeat biopsy. J Urol. 2008;180:146–9.

78. Rochester MA, Pashayan N, Matthews F, Doble A, McLoughlin J. Development and validation of risk score for predicting positive repeat prostate biopsy in patients with a previous negative biopsy in a UK population. BMC Urol. 2009;9:7.

79. Netto GJ, Epstein JI. Widespread high-grade prostatic intraepithelial neoplasia on prostatic needle biopsy: a significant likelihood of subsequently diagnosed adenocarcinoma. Am J Surg Pathol. 2006;30:1184–8.

80. Merrimen JL, Jones G, Srigley JR. Is high grade prostatic intraepithelial neoplasia still a risk factor for adenocarcinoma in the era of extended biopsy sampling? Pathology. 2010;42:325–9.

81. Godoy G, Huang GJ, Patel T, Taneja SS. Long-term follow-up of men with isolated high-grade prostatic intra-epithelial neoplasia followed by serial delayed interval biopsy. Urology. 2011;77:669–74.

82. Lee MC, Moussa AS, Yu C, Kattan MW, Magi-Galluzzi C, Jones JS. Multifocal high grade prostatic intraepithelial neoplasia is a risk factor for subsequent prostate cancer. J Urol. 2010;184:1958–62.

83. Roscigno M, Scattoni V, Freschi M, et al. Diagnosis of isolated high-grade prostatic intraepithelial neoplasia: proposal of a nomogram for the prediction of cancer detection at saturation re-biopsy. BJU Int. 2012;109(9):1329–34.

84. Chan TY, Epstein JI. Follow-up of atypical prostate needle biopsies suspicious for cancer. Urology. 1999;53:351–5.

85. Abouassaly R, Tan N, Moussa A, Jones JS. Risk of prostate cancer after diagnosis of atypical glands suspicious for carcinoma on saturation and traditional biopsies. J Urol. 2008;180:911–4. discussion 914.

86. Wolters T, van der Kwast TH, Vissers CJ, et al. False-negative prostate needle biopsies: frequency,

histopathologic features, and follow-up. Am J Surg Pathol. 2010;34:35–43.

87. Levy DA, Jones JS. Management of rising prostate-specific antigen after a negative biopsy. Curr Urol Rep. 2011;12:197–202.

88. Allen EA, Kahane H, Epstein JI. Repeat biopsy strategies for men with atypical diagnoses on initial prostate needle biopsy. Urology. 1998;52:803–7.

89. Chrouser KL, Lieber MM. Extended and saturation needle biopsy for the diagnosis of prostate cancer. Curr Urol Rep. 2004;5:226–30.

90. Berglund RK, Masterson TA, Vora KC, Eggener SE, Eastham JA, Guillonneau BD. Pathological upgrading and up staging with immediate repeat biopsy in patients eligible for active surveillance. J Urol. 2008;180:1964–7. discussion 1967–8.

91. Al Otaibi M, Ross P, Fahmy N, et al. Role of repeated biopsy of the prostate in predicting disease progression in patients with prostate cancer on active surveillance. Cancer. 2008;113:286–92.

92. Barqawi AB, Crawford ED. The current use and future trends of focal surgical therapy in the management of localized prostate cancer. Cancer J. 2007;13:313–7.

93. Mouraviev V, Mayes JM, Sun L, Madden JF, Moul JW, Polascik TJ. Prostate cancer laterality as a rationale of focal ablative therapy for the treatment of clinically localized prostate cancer. Cancer. 2007;110:906–10.

94. Polascik TJ, Mayes JM, Sun L, Madden JF, Moul JW, Mouraviev V. Pathologic stage T2a and T2b prostate cancer in the recent prostate-specific antigen era: implications for unilateral ablative therapy. Prostate. 2008;68:1380–6.

95. Onik G, Narayan P, Vaughan D, Dineen M, Brunelle R. Focal "nerve-sparing" cryosurgery for treatment of primary prostate cancer: a new approach to preserving potency. Urology. 2002;60:109–14.

96. Falzarano SM, Zhou M, Hernandez AV, Moussa AS, Jones JS, Magi-Galluzzi C. Can saturation biopsy predict prostate cancer localization in radical prostatectomy specimens: a correlative study and implications for focal therapy. Urology. 2010;76:682–7.

97. Aus G, Damber JE, Hugosson J. Prostate biopsy and anaesthesia: an overview. Scand J Urol Nephrol. 2005;39:124–9.

98. Soloway MS, Obek C. Periprostatic local anesthesia before ultrasound guided prostate biopsy. J Urol. 2000;163:172.

99. Leibovici D, Zisman A, Siegel YI, Sella A, Kleinmann J, Lindner A. Local anesthesia for prostate biopsy by periprostatic lidocaine injection: a double-blind placebo controlled study. J Urol. 2002;167:563–5.

100. Pareek G, Armenakas NA, Fracchia JA. Periprostatic nerve blockade for transrectal ultrasound guided biopsy of the prostate: a randomized, double blind, placebo controlled study. J Urol. 2001;166:894–7.

101. Akan H, Yildiz O, Dalva I, Yücesoy C. Comparison of two periprostatic nerve blockade techniques for transrectal ultrasound-guided prostate biopsy:

bilateral basal injection and single apical injection. Urology. 2009;73:23–6.

102. Ashley RA, Inman BA, Routh JC, et al. Preventing pain during office biopsy of the prostate: a single center, prospective, double-blind, 3-arm, parallel group, randomized clinical trial. Cancer. 2007;110: 1708–14.

103. Maccagnano C, Scattoni V, Roscigno M, et al. Anaesthesia in transrectal prostate biopsy: which is the most effective technique? Urol Int. 2011;87:1–13.

104. Cantiello F, Imperatore V, Iannuzzo M, et al. Periprostatic nerve block (PNB) alone vs. PNB combined with an anaesthetic-myorelaxant agent cream for prostate biopsy: a prospective, randomized double-arm study. BJU Int. 2009;103:1195–8.

105. Raber M, Scattoni V, Roscigno M, et al. Topical prilocaine-lidocaine cream combined with peripheral nerve block improves pain control in prostatic biopsy: results from a prospective randomized trial. Eur Urol. 2008;53:967–73.

106. Giannarini G, Autorino R, Valent F, et al. Combination of perianal-intrarectal lidocaine-prilocaine cream and periprostatic nerve block for pain control during transrectal ultrasound guided prostate biopsy: a randomized, controlled trial. J Urol. 2009;181:585–91. discussion 591–3.

107. Yurdakul T, Taspinar B, Kilic O, Kilinc M, Serarslan A. Topical and long-acting local anesthetic for prostate biopsy: a prospective randomized placebo-controlled study. Urol Int. 2009;83:151–4.

108. Bingqian L, Peihuan L, Yudong W, et al. Intraprostatic local anesthesia with periprostatic nerve block for transrectal ultrasound guided prostate biopsy. J Urol. 2009;182:479–83. discussion 483–4.

109. Skriapas K, Konstandinidis C, Samarinas M, et al. Pain level and anal discomfort during transrectal ultrasound for guided prostate biopsy. Does intrarectal administration of local anesthetic before periprostatic anesthesia makes any difference? Minerva Urol Nefrol. 2009;61:137–42.

110. Hirsh I, Kaploun A, Faris G, et al. Tramadol improves patients' tolerance of transrectal ultrasound-guided biopsy of the prostate. Urology. 2007;69:491–4.

111. Obek C, Ozkan B, Tunc B, Can G, Yalcin V, Solok V. Comparison of 3 different methods of anesthesia before transrectal prostate biopsy: a prospective randomized trial. J Urol. 2004;172:502–5.

112. Pendleton J, Costa J, Wludyka P, et al. Combination of oral tramadol, acetaminophen and 1% lidocaine induced periprostatic nerve block for pain control during transrectal ultrasound guided biopsy of the prostate: a prospective randomized, controlled trial. J Urol. 2006;176:1372–5.

113. Mireku-Boateng AO. Intravenous ketorolac significantly reduces the pain of office transrectal ultrasound and prostate biopsies. Urol Int. 2004;73: 123–4.

114. Awsare NS, Green JA, Aldwinckle B, Hanbury DC, Boustead GB, McNicholas TA. The use of propofol sedation for transrectal ultrasonography-guided prostate biopsy is associated with high patient

satisfaction and acceptability. Eur J Radiol. 2007; 63:94–5.

115. Lepor H, Gregerman M, Crosby R, Mostofi FK, Walsh PC. Precise localization of the autonomic nerves from the pelvic plexus to the corpora cavernosa: a detailed anatomical study of the adult male pelvis. J Urol. 1985;133:207–12.

116. Novella G, Ficarra V, Galfano A, et al. Pain assessment after original transperineal prostate biopsy using a coaxial needle. Urology. 2003;62:689–92.

117. Kubo Y, Kawakami S, Numao N, et al. Simple and effective local anesthesia for transperineal extended prostate biopsy: application to three-dimensional 26-core biopsy. Int J Urol. 2009;16:420–3.

118. Coplen DE, Andriole GL, Yuan JJ, Catalona WJ. The ability of systematic transrectal ultrasound guided biopsy to detect prostate cancer in men with the clinical diagnosis of benign prostatic hyperplasia. J Urol. 1991;146:75–7.

119. Nam RK, Saskin R, Lee Y, et al. Increasing hospital admission rates for urological complications after transrectal ultrasound guided prostate biopsy. J Urol. 2010;183:963–8.

120. Raaijmakers R, Kirkels WJ, Roobol MJ, Wildhagen MF, Schrder FH. Complication rates and risk factors of 5802 transrectal ultrasound-guided sextant biopsies of the prostate within a population-based screening program. Urology. 2002;60:826–30.

121. Zaytoun OM, Anil T, Moussa AS, Jianbo L, Fareed K, Jones JS. Morbidity of prostate biopsy after simplified versus complex preparation protocols: assessment of risk factors. Urology. 2011;77:910–4.

122. Utrera NM, Sánchez AT, Rodríguez-Antolín A, et al. Saturation biopsies for prostate cancer detection: effectiveness, safety and predictive factors. Arch Esp Urol. 2011;64:421–6.

123. Chiang N, Chang SJ, Pu S, et al. Major complications and associated risk factors of transrectal ultrasound guided prostate needle biopsy: a retrospective study of 1,875 cases in Taiwan. J Formos Med Assoc. 2007;106:929–34.

124. Berger AP, Gozzi C, Steiner H, et al. Complication rate of transrectal ultrasound guided prostate biopsy: a comparison among 3 protocols with 6, 10 and 15 cores. J Urol. 2004;171:1478–80.

125. Satoh T, Matsumoto K, Fujita T, et al. Cancer core distribution in patients diagnosed by extended transperineal prostate biopsy. Urology. 2005;66:114–8.

126. Moran BJ, Braccioforte MH, Conterato DJ. Re-biopsy of the prostate using a stereotactic transperineal technique. J Urol. 2006;176:1376–81. discussion 1381.

127. Pryor MB, Schellhammer PF. The pursuit of prostate cancer in patients with a rising prostate-specific antigen and multiple negative transrectal ultrasound-guided prostate biopsies. Clin Prostate Cancer. 2002;1:172–6.

128. Fleshner NE, Cookson MS, Soloway SM, Fair WR. Repeat transrectal ultrasound-guided prostate biopsy: a strategy to improve the reliability of needle biopsy grading in patients with well-differentiated prostate cancer. Urology. 1998;52:659–62.

129. Merrick GS, Gutman S, Andreini H, et al. Prostate cancer distribution in patients diagnosed by transperineal template-guided saturation biopsy. Eur Urol. 2007;52:715–23.

130. Simon J, Kuefer R, Bartsch Jr G, Volkmer BG, Hautmann RE, Gottfried HW. Intensifying the saturation biopsy technique for detecting prostate cancer after previous negative biopsies: a step in the wrong direction. BJU Int. 2008;102:459–62.

131. Novara G, Boscolo-Berto R, Lamon C, et al. Detection rate and factors predictive the presence of prostate cancer in patients undergoing ultrasonography-guided transperineal saturation biopsies of the prostate. BJU Int. 2010;105:1242–6.

132. Pinkstaff DM, Igel TC, Petrou SP, Broderick GA, Wehle MJ, Young PR. Systematic transperineal ultrasound-guided template biopsy of the prostate: three-year experience. Urology. 2005;65:735–9.

Role of Imaging as an Adjunct or Replacement for Biopsy: American Experience

23

John Kurhanewicz, Adam J. Jung, and Daniel B. Vigneron

Overview

This chapter reviews the role of magnetic resonance (MR) imaging in prostate cancer as an adjunct to ultrasound-guided biopsies for improved therapeutic selection and monitoring. Multiparametric MR imaging sequences applied for prostate cancer imaging include T2-weighted MR, proton (1H) MR spectroscopic imaging, diffusion-weighted imaging, and dynamic contrast-enhanced MR. These techniques provide information on phenotypic characteristics of normal and cancerous prostate tissue, including normal/abnormal ductal morphology, concentrations of metabolites relevant to prostate cancer, and water diffusion rates which are affected by cellularity, blood flow rates, and volumes and therefore vascularity, respectively. The information provided by this multiparametric MR imaging approach can be used to provide an improved assessment of the presence, location, and volume of prostate cancers with higher sensitivity and specificity than can be obtained for ultrasound-guided biopsy alone. Multiparametric MR data can be added to biopsy and other clinical data to better diagnose aggressive prostate cancer, predict organ-confined prostate cancer, provide improved localization of intraglandular prostate cancer, and estimation of intraglandular prostate cancer volume. It has also been applied to MR-directed transrectal ultrasound-guided biopsy, direct MR-guided biopsy, MR-ultrasound fusion-guided biopsy, and MR-guided focal therapy. This chapter also describes what is known about the potential for combining multiparametric MR data with biopsy results to improve selection, guidance, and subsequent monitoring of the effectiveness of therapy. We feel that current literature supports that multiparametric MR imaging findings can improve the correct identification of dominant tumor foci in patients with prostate cancer, add to clinical parameters and biopsy results to improve the risk assessment of individual patients, and may be useful in guiding biopsies and focal therapy directly or through fusion with TRUS imaging.

Introduction

Prostate cancer is the commonest non-cutaneous cancer and second commonest cause of cancer death in men [1]. The diagnosis, management, and prognosis of prostate cancer are largely dependent on histopathology obtained by transrectal ultrasound (TRUS)-guided biopsy. TRUS-guided biopsy uses B-mode and Doppler imaging to localize the prostate and systematically obtain anywhere from 6 to over 40 18-gauge biopsy cores. TRUS localizes the prostate; however, often it does not visualize the malignant focus

J. Kurhanewicz, Ph.D. (✉) • A.J. Jung, M.D., Ph.D. • D.B. Vigneron, Ph.D.
Department of Radiology and Biomedical Imaging, University of California, 1700 4th St. Suite 203, San Francisco, CA 94158, USA
e-mail: john.kurhanewicz@ucsf.edu

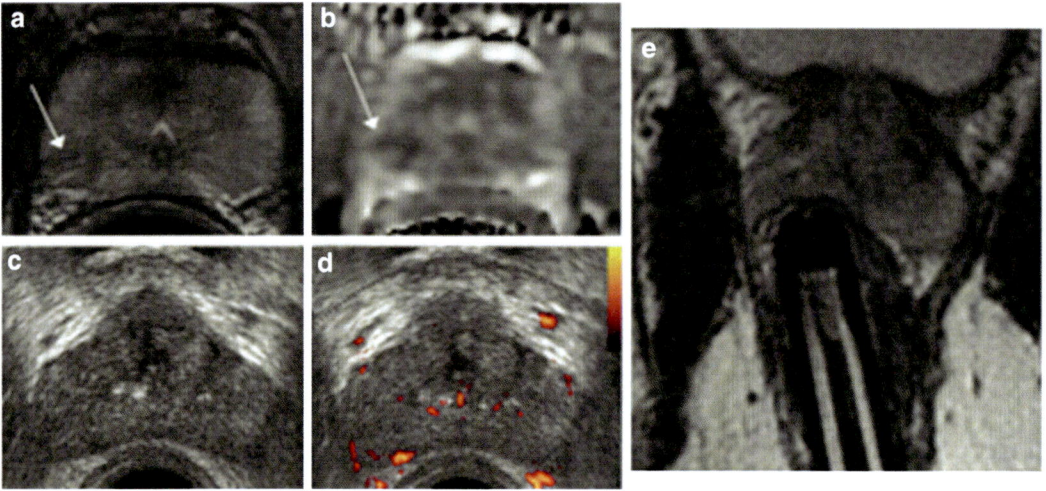

Fig. 23.1 Axial T_2-weighted (**a**) and corresponding apparent diffusion coefficient (ADC) (**b**) images demonstrating a focal area of reduced T_2 signal intensity and reduced water ADC in the right midgland in a patient who had no clear focal hypoechoic (**c**) or increased color Doppler flow (**d**) areas indicative of cancer on TRUS. The patient also had a negative systematic TRUS-guided 12-core biopsy. A subsequent MRI-guided three-core biopsy taken from the region of MRI abnormality was positive for prostate cancer (2/3 cores positive, Gleason 4 + 4, 60% of the cores positive)

because 37–50% of cancers may be isoechoic or only slightly hypoechoic [2]. Accordingly, TRUS-guided biopsy demonstrates reported false-negative rates of up to 30% [3] (Fig. 23.1). TRUS-guided biopsy Gleason scores are also often discordant with prostatectomy specimens and undergrade cancers in up to 38% of patients [4], indicating TRUS-guided biopsy results also misrepresent tumor aggressiveness. These data indicate that TRUS-guided biopsy is prone to sampling error, resulting in pathology interpretation that does not accurately depict the degree of tumor presence or volume estimated by percentage of tumor in positive cores. Multiple risk stratification schemes including the commonly used Epstein and D'Amico criteria predict prognosis and dictate the decision to undergo active surveillance versus definitive treatment [5, 6]. These criteria rely heavily on the histopathologic findings of Gleason grade and percentage of tumor seen in the core biopsy specimen [5, 6], which in turn are invariably dependent on the location of the needle tip and the region of the prostate sampled. It is clearly bad medicine and poor science for such critical decision-making algorithms to depend on flawed data regarding tumor extent and aggressiveness.

Multiparametric MRI uses a combination of anatomic T_1- and T_2-weighted imaging, diffusion-weighted imaging (DWI), proton MR spectroscopic imaging (^{1}H MRSI), and perfusion-based dynamic contrast-enhanced (DCE) imaging to better localize and characterize prostate cancers throughout the prostate, thereby addressing the sampling problem associated with TRUS-guided biopsies (Fig. 23.1). This chapter focuses on what is published about the role of multiparametric MR and multiparametric MR-guided procedures as an adjunct or replacement for more traditional ultrasound-guided biopsy and therapeutic approaches. The opinions presented reflect those of the authors and their experience with the use of transrectal ultrasound-guided biopsy and multiparametric MRI prostate data for the improved clinical management of men with prostate cancer at the University of California, San Francisco.

Multiparametric MRI Techniques: Current Clinical Status

The need for the addition of an imaging staging exam to biopsy findings is greater for prostate cancer than for many other cancers due to the pathologic and biologic complexity of the human prostate and prostate cancer. This complexity results in questions of whether and how to treat individual prostate cancer patients. Additionally, this complexity demands advanced high-spatial-resolution anatomic and metabolic/functional techniques to accurately assess disease status in individual patients. There is already a relatively large body of literature describing the clinical utility of combining the metabolic information obtained from proton magnetic resonance spectroscopic imaging (^{1}H MRSI) with the anatomic information provided by MRI [7–23]. It has been shown to be of incremental value to standard clinical parameters, weighted nomograms, to predict unfavorable pathology, such as extracapsular invasion [24] and seminal vesicle invasion [22], and favorable pathology such as organ-confined disease [25] and insignificant disease at prostatectomy [26]. A growing number of MR imaging studies have also demonstrated that the detection and characterization of prostate cancer can be significantly improved through the addition of diffusion-weighted imaging (DWI) [27–32], dynamic contrast-enhanced imaging (DCE) [33–38], quantitative T_2-mapping [39–43], and magnetization transfer imaging [44], and by performing the imaging exam on higher magnetic field strength MR scanners (3 T and 7 T) [45–47].

T_2-Weighted Magnetic Resonance Imaging

T_2-weighted MRI is the common component of all multiparametric MR approaches for imaging prostate cancer, providing the anatomy for correlation with other functional MR data, providing a majority of the information on the spread of cancer beyond the prostate, and providing the high-resolution images used for targeting subsequent biopsies and therapy. The zonal anatomy of the prostate is usually well shown on high-spatial-resolution T_2-weighted MR images acquired using an endorectal radiofrequency coil (Fig. 23.2a). The normal peripheral zone has high T_2 signal intensity similar to or greater than the signal of adjacent periprostatic fat, and the peripheral zone demonstrates higher signal intensity than prostate

cancer (red arrows) [48–52] (Fig. 23.2a). The reduction in MR image signal intensity is due to a loss of the normal glandular (ductal) morphology that typically occurs in regions of prostate cancer. Other benign pathologies (e.g., inflammation, stromal BPH) and therapy may also cause a loss of ductal morphology that is seen as low T_2 signal intensity on MRI [53]. In addition, infiltrating prostate cancer may not cause a reduction in normal glandular morphology and therefore would not be hypointense on MRI [53]. Because of these confounding factors, MRI alone has demonstrated good sensitivity (78%) but poor specificity (55%) in detecting and localizing cancer within the prostate [54]. The situation is even worse after therapy because the prostate is often significantly decreased in size, and in most cases there is a homogenous reduction in signal intensity on T_2-weighted images of the prostate resulting in a loss in distinction of normal prostatic zonal anatomy and prostate cancer (Fig. 23.3) [55, 56]. However, T_2 MRI findings remain the mainstay of assessing spread of cancer beyond the prostate [25, 57–65], a critical question for the appropriate selection of therapy.

While T_2 MRI remains a critical part of the prostate MR exam, there remains a clear need for MR data that provide a functional assessment of the prostate in order to better discriminate prostate cancer from other benign pathologies and treatment effects and to obtain assessment cancer aggressiveness within the prostate. The MR imaging detection and characterization of prostate cancer can be significantly improved through the addition of various functional sequences to the anatomic T_2-weighted imaging, such as MR spectroscopic imaging (MRSI), diffusion-weighted imaging (DWI), dynamic contrast-enhanced (DCE) imaging, and quantitative T_2 MRI, and by performing the multiparametric exam at higher magnetic field strengths (3 T)[66].

Proton Magnetic Resonance Spectroscopic Imaging (1H MRSI)

Metabolic changes that are monitored by ^{1}H MRSI have been shown to significantly improve the ability of MRI to detect and assess the location,

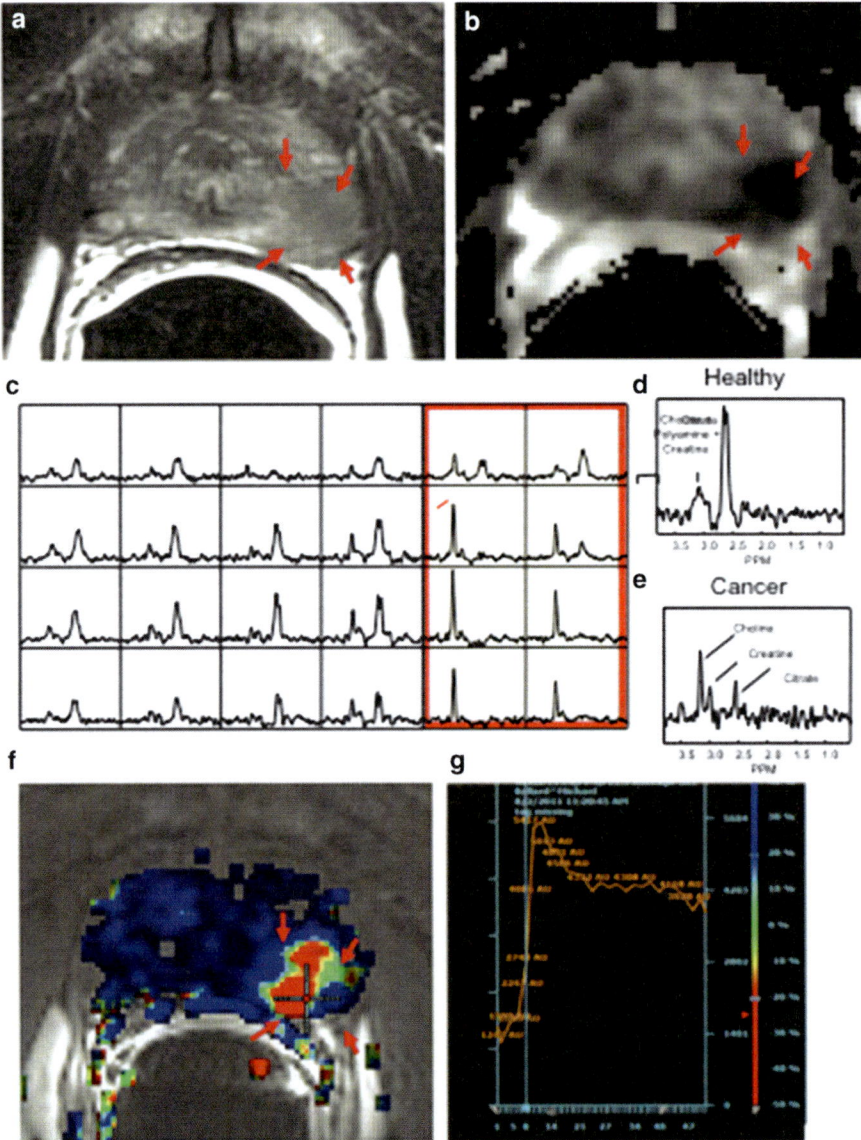

Fig. 23.2 3-T multiparametric imaging data from a 56-year-old patient with a PSA of 4.9 ng/ml with a 1.1-cc Gleason 3+4 tumor in the left apex at radical prostatectomy. (**a**) T$_2$-weighted MRI image showing a low signal intensity lesion (*red arrows*) in the left apex. (**b**) A calculated ADC map demonstrating a dramatic reduction in ADC in the region of apical cancer. (**c**) A selected 0.16-cc ^{1}H MRSI spectral array from the same apical slice shown in (**a**) demonstrating elevated choline and reduced citrate and polyamines within the left apex in the region of cancer (**c**) relative to the healthy right apex. Representative healthy (**d**) and malignant (**e**) ^{1}H spectra. (**f**) Calculated image of the slope of dynamic uptake of contrast over washout (**f**) and corresponding dynamic curve taken from the point of the cursor on the image (**g**)

volume, and aggressiveness of cancer within the prostate, as well as improve the assessment of extracapsular spread in patients [67]. It provides a noninvasive method of detecting small molecular biomarkers, specifically the metabolites choline, creatine, citrate, and polyamines, within the cytosol and extracellular spaces of the prostate and is always performed in conjunction with high-resolution anatomic imaging (Fig. 23.2c–e).

Proton (^{1}H) MRSI of the prostate is typically acquired using a combination of point-resolved spectroscopy (PRESS) volume localization and

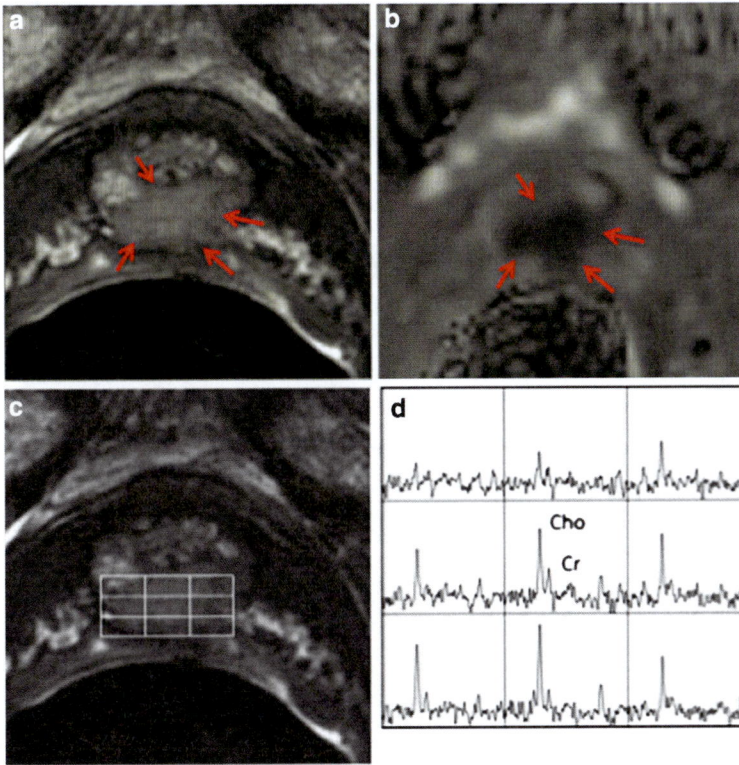

Fig. 23.3 An example of a patient with a PSA of 1.6 ng/ml 3 years after cryosurgery. On multiparametric MRI, we observed a clear-cut region of bilaterally reduced ADC and elevated choline to creatine in the apex, indicative of a high-grade recurrent disease. A subsequent MR-targeted TRUS-guided biopsy indicated the presence of Gleason 4 + 4 cancer bilaterally at the apex. There was also evidence of extracapsular extension on T_2 MRI at the left posteromedial aspect of the apex of the gland

3-dimensional (D) chemical shift imaging (CSI) to acquire arrays of ^{1}H spectra from throughout the prostate gland (Fig. 23.2C) [68]. Robust acquisition of prostate ^{1}H MRSI data has required the development of very accurate volume selection and efficient outer volume suppression techniques [69–71]. The resonances for citrate, choline, creatine, and polyamines occur at distinct frequencies or positions in the spectrum (Fig. 23.2e, f). The areas under these signals are related to the concentration of the respective metabolites, and changes in these concentrations can be used to identify cancer with high specificity [72]. In spectra taken from regions of prostate cancer (Fig. 23.2e), the citrate and polyamines are significantly reduced or absent, while choline is elevated relative to spectra taken from surrounding healthy peripheral zone tissue (Fig. 23.2d).

The specificity of ^{1}H MRSI for detecting, localizing, and characterizing the aggressiveness of prostate cancer relies on the unique metabolism of the prostate and the specific metabolic changes that occur with the evolution and progression of this disease and its response to therapy [73].

Biochemical Rationale for Metabolic Changes Prior to Therapy

Healthy prostate epithelial cells have the specialized function of synthesizing and secreting large amounts of citrate that are dramatically reduced or lost in prostate cancer [74–77]. It is believed that the transformation of prostate epithelial cells to citrate-oxidizing cells, which increases energy production capability, is essential to the process of malignancy and metastasis [75]. Additionally, both in vivo ^{1}H MRSI studies [67, 78–81] and ex

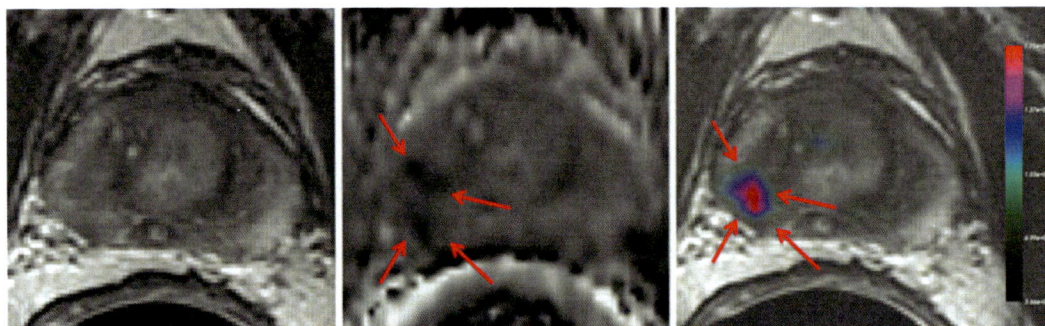

Fig. 23.4 A representative example of a patient 7 years after external beam radiation therapy with a rising PSA of 1.89 up from a nadir of <0.01 that was achieved 2 years after EBRT. The patient obtained a multiparametric 3-T exam prior to a TRUS-guided biopsy. On T_2-weighted MRI (*left*), there was no indication of residual disease within the prostate. However, there was a clear region of reduced ADC on DWI (*middle*, *red arrows*) and a corre-sponding area of elevated choline as indicated by the choline image on the *right*. The subsequent TRUS-guided biopsy demonstrated recurrent cancer in the right midgland (right midgland – 9% of 4+4, right lateral midgland – 60% – 4+4, and right apex – 17% 4+4) in the same locations as the imaging abnormality, and the patient went on to receive high-dose-rate salvage brachytherapy

vivo HR-MAS spectroscopic studies of biopsy samples and surgically removed prostate tissues [82, 83] have shown that the degree of decrease in citrate correlates with Gleason grade.

The elevation of choline-containing metabolites [phosphocholine (PC), glycerophosphocholine (GPC), and free choline (Cho)] and the over- and under-expression of key enzymes in the Kennedy cycle have been associated with the progression and therapeutic response of a variety of human cancers including prostate [67]. Specifically, HR-MAS spectroscopic studies of ex vivo surgical and biopsy prostate tissues demonstrated elevated levels of ethanolamine- and choline-containing compounds and that elevated PC and GPC were the most robust predictors of prostate cancer presence [84], and both in vivo ^{1}H MRSI studies [67, 78–81] and ex vivo HR-MAS spectroscopic studies [82, 83] have shown that the degree of elevation of choline-containing metabolites (PC and GPC) correlates with Gleason grade.

Healthy prostate epithelial cells also contain very high concentrations of polyamines, particularly spermine [67, 85, 86]. Polyamines are dramatically reduced in prostate cancer due to changes in the levels of expression of genes that regulate polyamine metabolism [67, 85]. The fact that choline and citrate change in opposite directions has led to the choline + creatine/citrate ratio (CC/C)

being one of the most widely used metabolic biomarkers for detecting prostate cancer [54] and has been used in the majority of the current ≈320 publications on prostate MRI/MRSI [87]. It has also been demonstrated that when the CC/C ratio was ≥3 standard deviations above the normal value, there was minimal overlap between spectroscopic voxels from regions of cancer and healthy peripheral zone tissues [88], and the magnitude of elevation of the CC/C ratio has shown a correlation with cancer grade [67, 78, 89]. An example of CC/C ratio indicating high-grade prostate cancer is shown in Fig. 23.4, and the elevated CC/C ratio was used to target a subsequent biopsy.

Biochemical Rationale for Metabolic Changes After Therapy

Prior published studies have indicated that the spectroscopic criteria used to identify residual/recurrent prostate cancer need to be adjusted due to a time-dependent loss of prostate metabolites following therapy. Specifically, time-dependent metabolic change after androgen deprivation therapy, a common systemic therapy for prostate cancer, has been studied using ^{1}H MRSI [90–92]. Androgen deprivation therapy (ADT) is the cornerstone of the systemic management of prostate cancer [93], and patients who succumb to prostate cancer typically do so only after ADT has ceased to be effective. ADT can take several forms – including medical castration with LHRH agonists, first-generation antiandrogens, 5-alpha-reductase inhibitors, or various combinations of these therapeutics – and can last for years. It affects both healthy and malignant prostate cells, inducing apoptosis and resulting in increasing amounts of tissue atrophy with duration of therapy [94]. Prostatic citrate production and secretion have been shown to be regulated by androgens [74], and an early dramatic reduction of citrate and polyamines after initiation of complete hormonal blockade has been observed by ^{1}H MRSI [90–92]. There was slower loss of choline and creatine with increasing duration of hormone deprivation therapy [90]. This loss of prostatic metabolites correlates with the presence of tissue atrophy and has been considered a noninvasive indicator of effective therapy [91]. Similar time-dependent reductions in prostate metabolites have also been observed after external bean radiation and brachytherapy of the entire prostate [95, 96].

Studies have also demonstrated the ability of MRI/^{1}H MRSI to discriminate residual or recurrent prostate cancer from residual benign tissue and atrophic/necrotic tissue after cryosurgery (Fig. 23.3) [97–99], hormone deprivation therapy [90, 92], and radiation therapy [95, 100] (Fig. 23.4). These studies have relied on elevated choline to creatine as a metabolic marker for prostate cancer since polyamines and citrate tend to disappear early after therapy in both residual healthy and malignant tissues. Figure 23.3 shows a patient 3 years after cryosurgery in which the goal was to ablate the entire prostate. However, on T_2-weighted imaging a small residual prostate was observed, and ^{1}H MRSI demonstrated very elevated choline to creatine ratio bilaterally at the apex of the residual gland, and this region was later biopsied and identified as Gleason 4 + 4 cancer. Figure 23.4 shows a patient with rising PSA 7 years after external beam radiation therapy, who was referred for a multiparametric MR exam to determine if the rising PSA was due to a local recurrence. We observed a clear region of elevated choline to creatine ratio in the right midgland that was identified as residual/recurrent

high-grade prostate cancer on TRUS-guided biopsy. Consistent with effective radiation therapy, the rest of the prostate demonstrated a complete loss of all prostate metabolites (metabolic atrophy). Two published MRI/^{1}H MRSI studies have demonstrated that three or more consecutive voxels having choline/creatine >1.5 resulted in the ability to predict the presence of cancer after radiation therapy with an accuracy of ≈80% [101, 102]. The detection of residual cancer at an early stage following treatment would allow earlier intervention with additional salvage therapy [103–109]. Alternatively, the lack of metabolic evidence of residual cancer after focal therapy could be used to demonstrate therapeutic success. This is a clinically important determination since residual benign tissue in the prostate will result in a nonzero serum PSA value, thereby diminishing its utility for predicting cancer presence relative to complete prostate ablation approaches such as radical prostatectomy.

Recent studies in early stage prostate cancer patients have indicated that combined 1.5 MRI/MRSI does poorly at detecting and localizing small low-grade tumors [78, 110–112]. One study demonstrated that overall sensitivity of MR spectroscopic imaging was 56% for tumor detection, increasing from 44% in lesions with Gleason score of 3 + 3–89% in lesions with Gleason score greater than or equal to 4 + 4 [78]. The inability to detect small low-grade tumors by 1.5 T 1H MRSI is primarily due to the partial voluming of surrounding benign tissue in spectroscopic volumes containing cancer due to the relatively coarse spatial resolution of 1.5 T MRSI (0.34 cc, ≈7 mm on a side). At 3 T, spatial resolution of ^{1}H MRSI can be increased ≈twofold (0.16 cc, ≈5 mm on a side) and the spectral data acquired in 8 min with better spectral signal to noise as compared to 0.34 cc ^{1}H MRSI spectra acquired at 1.5 T in 17 min (Fig. 23.1c, d, e) [47]. This should improve the ability of ^{1}H MRSI to detect small low-grade tumors and increase its clinical utility. However, the robust acquisition of ^{1}H MRSI has been technically challenging and beyond the expertise of many sites. Through the use of an inflatable endorectal coil with a compound that matches the susceptibility of tissue and a pulse sequences

(MLEV-PRESS) specifically designed for prostate spectroscopy at 3 T [47], high-spatial-resolution and high-temporal-resolution 3-D MRI/^{1}H MRSI data can be more robustly obtained. However, due to the pathologic and biologic complexity of prostate cancer, the addition of other high-spatial-resolution functional information to the MRI/^{1}H MRSI staging exam has proven key to the characterizing of prostate cancer in individual patients.

Diffusion-Weighted Imaging (DWI)

With the advent of hardware and software capable of acquiring single-shot images, and ways to reduce the magnetic susceptability at the air tissue interface of the rectum, diffusion-weighted MR imaging has become not only feasible but widely used and potentially one of the most powerful clinical imaging techniques for imaging prostate cancer [113]. Prostate DWI is most often performed using a single-shot echo planar imaging sequence [114–116] but have also been performed using a single-shot fast spin echo sequence [117] and line scan diffusion imaging techniques [39, 118]. Diffusion-weighted imaging (DWI) is sensitive to the motion of water molecules at microscopic spatial scales within biological tissues and can provide unique information about microscopic tissue compartments, structural anisotropy, and the pathology of tissues [119–122]. The rate of diffusion in tissues is lower than in free solution and is described by an apparent diffusion coefficient (ADC), which largely depends on the number, permeabilities, and separation of barriers that a diffusing water molecule encounters, and variations in ADC have been shown to roughly correlate inversely with tissue cellularity [113, 123]. The MR apparent diffusion coefficient (ADC) has been shown to be lower in prostate cancer than in surrounding benign prostate tissues (Fig. 23.2b). The loss of normal ductal architecture and increased cellularity that occurs with prostate cancer results in a smaller extracellular space and corresponding reduction in ADC [124]. However, overlap exists between individual benign and malignant peripheral zone prostate tissues, with typical ADC values ranging from 2.0 to 1.4 and 1.6 to 0.9×10^{-3} mm^2/s, respectively [41, 113]. ADC values in the central gland (central and transition zones) are reduced relatively to the periphral zone, typcially ranging from 1.7 to 1.3×10^{-3} mm^2/s, and central gland tumor ADCs on average are also slightly lower than those in the peripheral zone, $1.4–0.8 \times 10^{-3}$ and $1.6–0.9 \times 10^{-3}$ mm^2/s, respectively [41, 113]. In particular, there is significant overlap between the low ADC values observed for predominately stromal BPH and tumors within the central gland. However, DWI imaging has still proven clinically useful in detecting central gland tumors, which are often missed on TRUS-guided biopsies (Fig. 23.5) [125]. MR diffusion has also recently shown promise for reflecting the pathologic grade of prostate cancer, with lower ADC values found in higher Gleason grade cancers [125–128]. For example, in one study, ADC values decreased from 1.2×10^{-3} mm^2/s in Gleason score 6 tumors to 0.8×10^{-3} mm^2/s in Gleason score 8 prostate cancers [127], and in another study ADC decreased from $1.08 \pm 0.02 \times 10^{-3}$ mm^2/s in cancers with Gleason score ≤ 6 to $0.94 \pm 0.03 \times 10^{-3}$ mm^2/s for Gleason $4+3$ cancer [128]. In another recent study, the mean and standard deviation of the ADC values for patients with GS $3+3$, GS $3+4$, and GS $4+3$ were 1.135 ± 0.119, 0.976 ± 0.103, and 0.831 ± 0.087 mm^2/s [129].

It has been shown that the addition of DWI to T$_2$-weighted imaging increased the accuarcy of cancer diagnosis over T$_2$-weighted imaging alone. Kim et al., investigating 3-T diffusion-weighted MR imaging in 36 patients, but without an endorectal coil, found that the combination of diffusion-weighted MR imaging and T$_2$-weighted MR imaging led to an improvement in the area under the ROC curve from 0.61 to 0.88 [130]. A pilot study of 50 patients with up to 2-year follow-up by Morgan etal. demonstrated that DW-MRI has potential for monitoring patients with early prostate cancer who opt for active surveillance [131]. Specifically, a 10% reduction in tumor ADC indicated progression with a 93% sensitivity and 40% specificity (area under the receiver operating characteristic

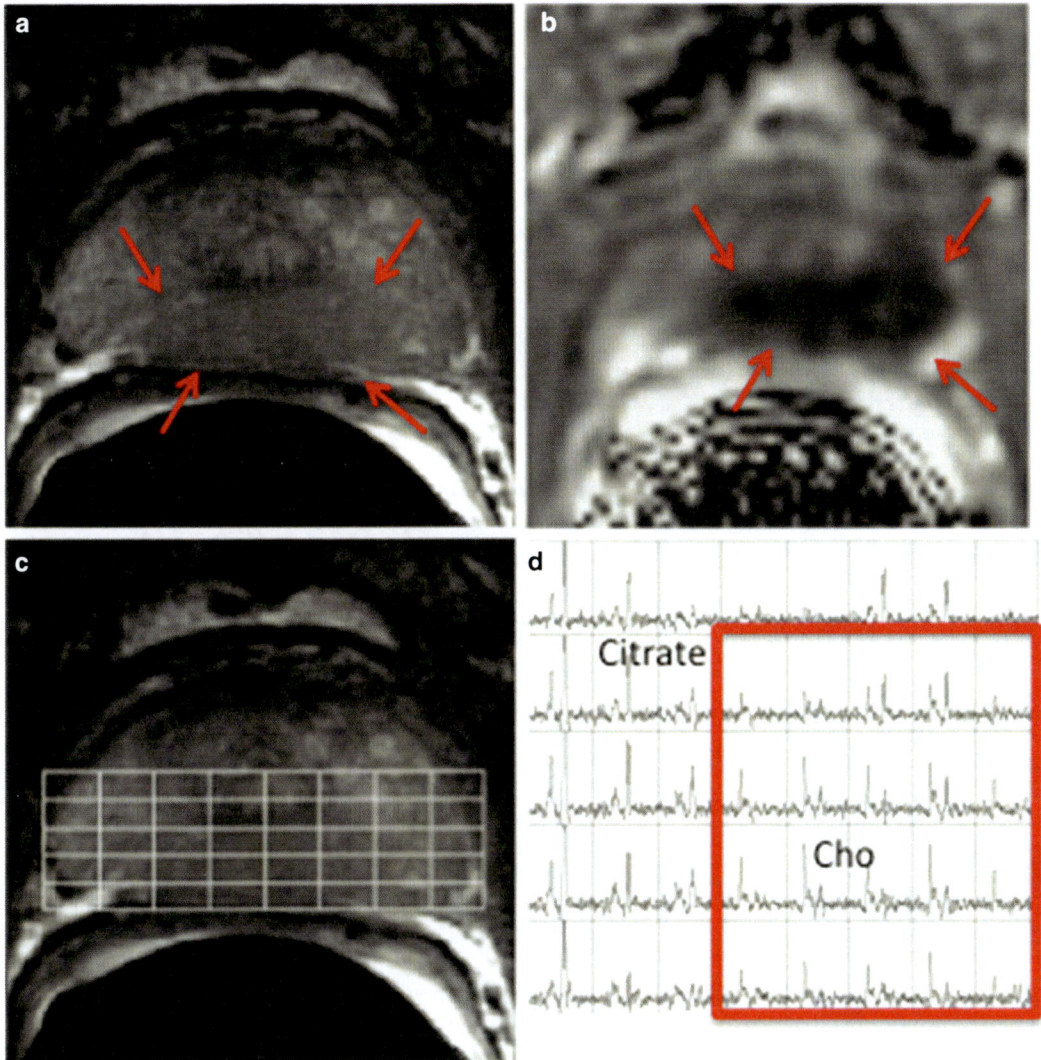

Fig. 23.5 Example of a patient with a (3.9 ng/ml) small amount of biopsy-proven cancer in the right midgland (12-core TRUS-guided biopsy, 1/12 cores positive, Gleason 3+3, 20% of the core) that was interested in "active surveillance." A subsequent multiparametric MR exam demonstrated a large volume of clear-cut, aggressive appearing, metabolic abnormality within the apex, predominately on the left but crossing the midline into the right gland. There was a region of suspicious T_2 reduction (**a**), dramatically reduced ADC on DWI (**b**), and a corresponding regions of very elevated choline to creatine on ^{1}H MRSI (**d**). A follow-up 12-core systematic TRUS-guided biopsy with an additional four cores targeted to the regions of the imaging abnormality demonstrated a large volume of high-grade prostate cancer (three positive cores in the right apex of Gleason 4+3 cancer, one core in the left apex of Gleason 3+4 cancer and one core in the left midgland of Gleason 3+4 cancer). The MRI staging exam indicated that the cancer was localized to the prostate, and the patient went on for a robotic prostatectomy

(ROC) curve = 0.68) [131]. The ability to detect and localize aggressive cancers at diagnosis is key for the accurate selection of patients for active surveillance, focal therapy, or more aggressive therapeutic approaches (Figs. 23.1, 23.2, 23.5, and 23.6).

It has also been shown that exposure of tumors to both chemotherapy and radiotherapy consistently leads to measurable increases in water diffusion in cases of favorable treatment response; however, regions of cancer still remained lower than surrounding benign and atrophic tissues

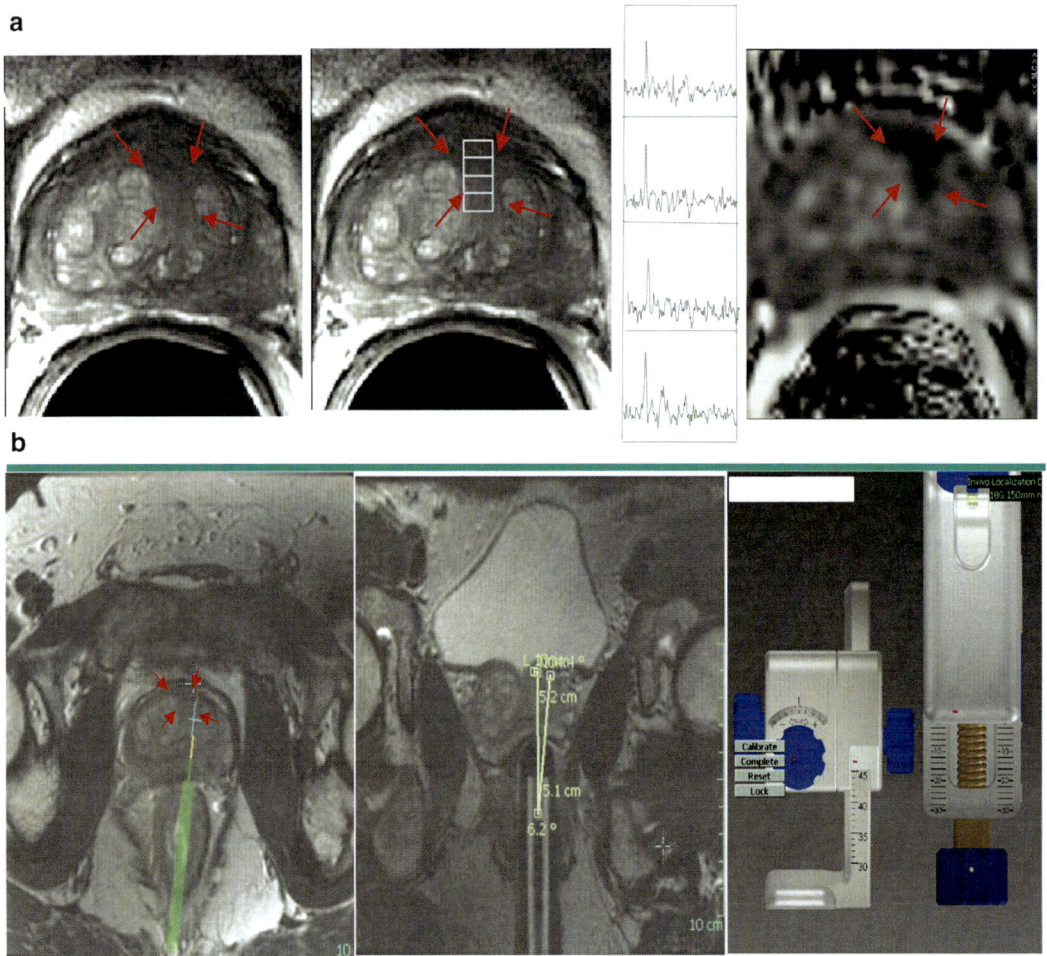

Fig. 23.6 This is a patient with a current PSA of 6.02 and a prior negative TRUS-guided biopsy. On multiparametric MR a clear-cut metabolic abnormality and reduced ADC at the anterior aspect of the LCG at the midgland to apex was observed (**a**). Given relative inaccessibility of this lesion on TRUS and history of negative biopsy, this patient was placed on a list for possible MR-guided biopsy. For initial positioning of the probe, localizer and multiplanar T_2-weighted FSE imaging was used to measure the coordinates of the biopsy guide (*green*, **b**) relative to the target determined in the staging exam (**a**). The software then provided a projection of the biopsy needle onto the T2-weighted image (**b**, *center*). The coordinates of the target on the biopsy guy were then dialed into the biopsy device (**b**, *right*); the biopsy probe adjusted accordingly, and the prostate reimaged using oblique axial images in the plane of the biopsy guide. Due to distortion of the prostate by the biopsy guide, additional needle adjustments were required prior to the biopsy. The patient was found to have Gleason 3+4 cancer (45% and 35% of two cores from that location)

[132, 133]. After radiation therapy, the mean ADC values of the biopsy-proven cancer areas $(0.98 \pm 0.23 \times 10^{-3}$ mm^2/s) were shown to be significantly lower than those of benign tissue (1.60 Å) 0.21 Å $\sim 10^{-3}$ mm^2/s [132] (Fig. 23.4). A significantly greater area under the receiver operating characteristics curve (Az) was determined for combined T_2 MRI and DWI (Az=0.879, $p < 0.01$) as compared to T_2 MRI alone (Az=0.612). Preliminary study also showed that DWI has potential for detecting residual cancer after systemic androgen deprivation therapy [133] and focal-focused ultrasound therapy [134].

High-spatial-resolution DWI images can be easily and robustly acquired within a matter of minutes and therefore easily added to an MR staging exam, and the production of ADC maps quickly and easily performed [66]. The ease of acquisition and analysis combined with initial findings demonstrating clinical utility have led to great excitement over DWIs role in prostate cancer focal therapy. However, in spite of significant differences between malignant and benign tissues in the peripheral zone before and after therapy, there is variability between patients as well as overlap of ADC values between malignant and benign prostatic tissues. This is not suprising since benign pathologies such as prostatis and predominately stromal benign prostatic hyperplasia are often associated with pathologic changes that would lead to decreases in the extracellular space and corresponding reduction in ADC. The qunatitative nature of DWI is also appealing; however, there remains a need for the test-retest validation of the quantitation of ADC values. There is also initial data suggesting that while ADC is increased in regions of prostate cancer after therapy, it remains lower than surrounding regions of treated benign and atrophic tissues [132, 133], but more studies after therapy are necessary to establish DWI utility for identifying residual disease and predict clinical outcomes.

Dynamic Contrast-Enhanced MRI

DCE MRI is currently performed by injecting a small-molecular-weight MR contrast agent (gadolinium-DTPA) into the patient, typically via the antecubital vein, and measuring the increase in signal intensity on fast T_1-weighted images of the prostate [135]. The MR contrast agent, gadolinium-DTPA (Gd-DTPA), does not penetrate prostate cells but can collect in the extracellular space [136]. The rate of enhancement reflects the volume and permeability of the blood vessels bringing the contrast agent to the tissue. Once the contrast agent is mixed in the vasculature, the peak enhancement in the tissue is due to the size of the extracellular space in which the Gd-DTPA can accumulate (both the interstitium and vasculature) [137, 138]. An additional factor that needs to be considered in interpreting DCE MRI of prostate cancer is the inability of Gd-DTPA to enter the ductal morphology of healthy glandular tissues and its subsequent ability to access residual ductal morphology in regions of prostate cancer [139].

Numerous qualitative and quantitative methods to summarize the large amounts of DCE MRI data have been suggested. Qualitatively, the characteristics of the dynamic uptake and washout curves (Fig. 23.2g) can be used to generate images that can be overlaid over the corresponding high-spatial-resolution anatomic images (Fig. 23.2f). Quantitatively, the MR data is fit to mathematical (pharmacokinetic) models of the tissue behavior. To determine underlying physiologic parameters with these models, other tissue parameters must be measured or assumed such as the concentration of the contrast agent in the vasculature, referred to as the arterial input function (AIF), and the original T_1 of the tissue. Modeling offers great benefits in terms of understanding physiology and in allowing comparisons across patients, scanners, and days. Pharmacokinetic modeling of DCE MRI data is based upon the work of Tofts and Kermode [136–138]. In this, the contrast agent is assumed to diffuse out of blood vessels into the extracellular, extravascular space (EES) based upon the concentration gradient and simple diffusion. Concentrations within compartments are assumed to be constant and parameters time-invariant. Water throughout the voxel studied is presumed to interact with the Gd causing a decrease in T_1 relaxation time, with there being a fast exchange of protons. The concentration of Gd in the tissue is modeled as in the extended Tofts-Kermode model [137]. SPGR signals are fit to the modeled equations and the parameters determined: (1) K_{trans} (the transfer of the contrast agent from the vasculature into the EES), (2) k_{ep} (the transfer back to the blood), (3) v_p (the blood plasma volume fraction), and (4) v_e (the EES volume fraction, = Ktrans/kep). The $1/T_1$ is assumed to linearly increase with the tissue concentration of gadolinium.

A number of groups have used DCE MRI to characterize differences between cancer and noncancerous prostate tissues [12, 42, 124, 135, 139–162. These typically find cancer to have a faster uptake and higher enhancement than healthy tissues. For example, in one study, regions of cancer had a higher peak enhancement ($p<0.006$), faster enhancement rate ($p<0.0008$), and faster washout slope ($p<0.05$) than normal PZ tissues. However, stromal BPH had the fastest enhancement rate ($p<0.003$) of all prostate tissues and tended to have the greatest enhancement [155]. In another study, K_{trans} and v_e were positively correlated with cell density for all prostate tissues [154].

In comparisons of DCE MRI to histopathology post-prostatectomy, a rapidly increasing then decreasing uptake curve or high v_e, peak enhancement, slope, and K_{trans} have been used as criteria for cancer [12, 35, 141, 146]. Reported sensitivities for cancer detection were typically in the 50s and 60s percent, while specificities were high, in the high 80s to low 90s in percent. In one study, dynamic contrast-enhanced MRI improved the performance of T_2 MRI for cancer localization, and volume estimation was significantly improved by the addition of DCE MRI, with area under the ROC curve of 0.83 for the PZ and 0.81 for the TZ cancers (0.7 and 0.75, respectively, for the T_2 MRI) [142]. The accuracy of detecting prostate cancer was more accurate for larger (foci >0.5 mL) and higher-grade prostate cancers ($>10\%$ of Gleason grade 4/5) [157]. DCE MRI has also been found useful for the detection, localization, and volume assessment of anterior prostate cancers [153]. Moreover, in several preliminary DCE MRI studies, poorly differentiated tumors demonstrated the earliest and greatest rate of enhancement [144, 163, 164].

While there are very few studies of DCE MRI after prostate cancer therapy, there is a recent study demonstrating that peak enhancement was useful in detecting residual disease after external beam radiation therapy [143]. Specifically, on a sextant basis, DCE MRI had significantly better sensitivity (72% [21of 29] vs. 38% [11 of 29]), positive predictive value (46% [21 of 46] vs. 24% [11 of 45]), and negative predictive value (95% [144 of 152] vs. 88% [135 of 153]) than T_2 MRI. Specificities were high for both DCE MRI and T_2w imaging (85% [144 of 169] vs. 80% [135 of 169]) [143]. There are also several preclinical studies indicating that antiangiogenic therapies

can be monitored by DCE MRI [165, 166] and one preliminary patient study. For prediction of local tumor progression of prostate cancer after high-intensity-focused ultrasonic ablation, DCE MRI was more sensitive than T_2-weighted MRI with DWI, but T_2-weighted MRI with DWI was more specific than DCE MRI. The areas under the receiver operating characteristic curve for DCE MRI and T_2-weighted MRI with DWI were 0.77 and 0.77 for reader 1 and 0.85 and 0.81 for reader 2 [134].

The superior sensitivity of DCE MRI compared with T_2 MRI, together with its high specificity, is arguably sufficient for its use for localizing cancerous lesions within the prostate for focal treatment [146]. Additionally, there is data suggesting that DCE MRI can provide information on cancer aggressiveness, although there remains conflicting views as to how well DCE MRI parameters correlate with histological grade [167]. Similar to ^{1}H MRSI, the acquisition and analysis of DCE MRI data of the prostate is more challenging and takes longer than T_2-weighted MRI and DWI. There also remains a need to determine whether qualitative versus quantitative DCE MRI parameters present the most robust predictive value and for the test-retest validation of DCE MRI results. There is also initial evidence that DCE MRI may be to detect residual cancer after therapy based on a more dramatic contrast uptake and washout compared to surrounding regions of atrophy and residual benign tissues, but this needs to be proven in a larger number of studies.

Multiparametric MR and Biopsy: Selection of Active Surveillance and Focal Therapy Patients

Given the often indolent course of many screen-detected prostate cancers [168], active surveillance – or careful monitoring of prostate-specific antigen (PSA) kinetics alongside serial biopsy sampling – is an increasingly accepted initial management approach [169]. However, concerns regarding under-sampling of prostate cancer, even with extended-core prostate biopsies [170, 171], continue to impede greater acceptance of active surveillance or focal therapy. Under-staging and/or under-grading is found in a substantial number of apparent surveillance candidates who proceed to prostatectomy [172–175]. These concerns contribute to patient anxiety, which in turn leads to dropout from surveillance protocols and treatment in the absence of any objective evidence of disease progression [176]. The same under-sampling concerns plague the use of systematic transrectal ultrasound-guided biopsy approaches alone to select patients for focal therapy and for targeting the lesions being treated. Repeat prostate biopsies, or 3-D transperineal prostate mapping (TPM) biopsies [177] without imaging could theoretically be used to determine the target of MR-guided focal therapy [178]. However, these approaches are painful and carry their own short and long-term risks.

Additionally, focal therapy seems best suited to patients with a visible dominant tumor at MR imaging, so that treatment is delivered to a tumor depicted by the same modality being used to guide therapy. This avoids the potential inaccuracies in "blindly" treating a designated portion of the prostate based purely on positive biopsies. This could be accomplished through testing of quantifiable properties such as tumor volume, grade, and other biological markers of disease progression. However, to date, it has not been possible to obtain this information noninvasively at the time of diagnosis. Multiparametric prostate cancer magnetic resonance imaging (MRI) has potential for providing this information and thereby improving the selection of low-risk patients appropriate for active surveillance, for following disease progression on active surveillance, and for more accurately localizing cancer within the prostate for focal therapy. Those patients with clinically low-risk tumors that can be confirmed with MR imaging as low risk with greater accuracy could be spared the cost and quality-of-life impact of multiple invasive diagnostic and therapeutic maneuvers. Conversely, those men with apparent low-risk disease who in fact harbor higher-risk tumors could likewise be better identified with MRI, thus avoiding under-treatment of high-risk prostate cancer – whether

with active surveillance or insufficiently aggressive focal therapy [179].

To date, there are few studies that have attempted to combine all MR biomarkers from a multiparametric MR staging exam at diagnosis to achieve the best selection of active surveillance and focal therapy patients, nor to best target intraprostatic cancer for treatment. However, there have been a number of clinical studies that have combined multiple MR parameters for the improved staging and intraglandular localization of prostate cancer. The published clinical applications of multiparametric MR imaging that could provide a significant impact on focal therapy patient selection and tumor targeting for focal therapy are reviewed in the following sections.

Predicting Organ-Confined Prostate Cancer

A more accurate prediction of organ-confined prostate cancer at the time of diagnosis would allow the determination of whether "active surveillance" or "focal therapy" is appropriate for a given patient. At 1.5 T MRI, it has been demonstrated that anatomical features on MRI such as bulging of the prostate, obliteration of the recto-prostatic angle, and asymmetry of the neurovascular bundle can predict extracapsular extension (ECE), with a specificity (up to 95%) but with low sensitivity (38%) [180]. Two studies have suggested that the addition of ^{1}H MRSI to MRI data can improve prostate cancer staging. In one study, it was found that tumor volume per lobe, estimated by ^{1}H MRSI, was significantly ($p < 0.01$) higher in patients with ECE than in patients without ECE. Moreover, the addition of an ^{1}H MRSI estimate of tumor volume to high specificity MRI findings for ECE [180] improved the diagnostic accuracy and decreased the interobserver variability of MRI in the diagnosis of extracapsular extension of prostate cancer [63].

An important advance in the staging of prostate cancer has been the development of multivariable risk prediction instruments such as the Partin tables [181], the CAPRA score [182], and various nomograms, which combine clinical stage, serum

PSA levels, and grade of biopsy results to predict at the time of diagnosis the pathologic stage of the cancer and insignificant disease, respectively [183, 184]. Two recent studies demonstrated that addition of MRI/¹H MRSI findings could significantly improve the predictive ability of biopsy-based staging nomograms for predicting seminal vesicle invasion and organ-confined cancer. It was found that the nomogram plus endorectal MR imaging (0.87) had a significantly larger ($p<0.05$) area under the curve than either endorectal MR imaging alone (0.76) or the nomogram alone (0.80) [22]. In another study of prostate cancer patients prior to radical prostatectomy, 1.5 T MRI/¹H MRSI data were added to a nomogram for predicting (no ECE or SVI) in order to assess its incremental value. The contribution of MR/¹H MRSI findings to predicting organ-confined prostate cancer was also significant [25].

Due to increased screening using serum prostate-specific antigen (PSA) and extended-template transrectal ultrasound (TRUS)-guided biopsies, thousands of patients with prostate cancer are being identified at an earlier and potentially more treatable stage [185]. However, the risk of over-detection, detecting a cancer that would not become clinically significant during that patient's lifetime if left untreated, has been estimated to vary between 15% and 84% [186–188]. Therefore, there is an increased interest in "active surveillance," but clinical parameters alone are not sufficient to predict a benign disease course. The addition of MRI/¹H MRSI data to clinical parameters has been shown to improve this prediction. In a study of 220 patients prior to surgery, the addition of MRI (AUC – 0.803) and MRI/MRSI (AUC 0.854) to biopsy-based nomograms was found to significantly improve the prediction of indolent prostate cancer using a surgical definition of indolent disease (no ECE or SVI and <0.5 cm³ of cancer with no pattern 4 or 5 cancer) as the standard of reference [26]. In another study of 114 active surveillance patients who received a MRI/¹H MRSI at baseline, with a median follow-up time of 59 months, it was demonstrated that patients with a lesion suspicious for cancer noted on a MRI/¹H MRSI staging exam had a greater risk of Gleason upgrade at subsequent biopsy (HR 4.0; 95%CI 1.1–14.9) than patients without such a lesion (Fig. 23.5) [189]. This study suggests that an abnormal MRI/¹H MRSI prostate exam at diagnosis that is suspicious for cancer may confer an increased risk of Gleason upgrade at subsequent biopsy and may help counseling potential candidates about active surveillance and whether they are more appropriate candidates for focal therapy. Specifically, MR imaging could play a role in selecting the subset of patients with indolent or subclinical disease that would be more appropriately managed with active surveillance versus patients with more aggressive localized disease that would benefit from focal therapy. Clearly, the higher spatial resolution functional MR data provided by DWI and DCE MRI could further improve this assessment. More recently, the D'Amico risk stratification was found to correlate with the degree of suspicion of prostate cancer on multiparametric magnetic resonance imaging [190].

Multiparametric MR: Targeting Clinically Significant Cancer Within the Prostate

Localizing Cancer Within the Prostate

T_2-weighted MRI alone has demonstrated good sensitivity but poor specificity in detecting cancer in the prostate [38, 54, 191]. Recent estimates using T_2-weighted sequences and endorectal coils vary from 60% to 96% [36]. The poor specificity is due to other benign pathologies (inflammation, stromal BPH) and therapy also causing a loss of ductal morphology and low T_2 on MRI [192]. Additionally, infiltrating prostate cancer may not cause a reduction in normal glandular morphology and therefore will not be hypointense on MRI [192]. Similar to imaging at 1.5 T, T_2-weighted image quality, prostate cancer localization and staging is significantly improved at 3 T with the use of an endorectal coil as compared with an external phased array coil [193]. Identifying prostate cancer within the central gland is particularly difficult for MRI due to the overlap of T_2-weighted signal intensity in predominately stromal BPH. In a recent study of 148 prostate cancer patients prior to radical prostatectomy, MR imaging alone detected zone prostate cancers with modest accuracy with areas under the reader operator curve (AUC) ranging from 0.73 to 0.75 [194].

The higher specificity of ^{1}H MRSI to metabolically identify cancer can be used to improve the ability of MRI to identify the location and volume of cancer within the prostate [110, 111, 195–198]. A study of 53 biopsy-proven prostate cancer patients prior to radical prostatectomy and step-section pathologic examination demonstrated a significant improvement in cancer localization to a prostatic sextant (left and right – base, midgland, and apex) using combined MRI/^{1}H MRSI versus MRI alone [198]. A combined positive result from both MRI and MRSI indicated the presence of tumor with high specificity (91%), while high sensitivity (95%) was attained when either test alone indicated the presence of cancer [198]. The addition of positive sextant biopsy findings to concordant MRI/MRSI findings further increased the specificity (98%) of cancer localization [197]. However, as previously discussed, ^{1}H MRSI suffers from the inability to detect small low-grade tumors, and there is a clear need for the addition of other higher spatial resolution functional imaging data.

DWI and DCE images can be acquired within a matter of minutes at very high-spatial-resolution ($0.9 \times 1.8 \times 4$ mm^3), allowing their addition to a clinically reasonable MRI/^{1}H MRSI exam and potentially improving MR detection of small low-grade tumors [66]. DCE imaging at 1.5 and 3.0 T demonstrated similar sensitivities (73% and 73%, respectively) and specificities (81% and 77%, respectively) for identifying cancer within the prostate [38, 199]. In another study of prostate cancer patients who received an MRI/^{1}H MRSI/DCE exam prior to radical prostatectomy, it was demonstrated that reader accuracy in tumor detection was significantly ($p<0.01$) better for 3-D MRSI (AUC=0.80) and DCE (AUC=0.91) than T_2-weighted imaging (AUC 0.68) [35]. However, no attempt was made to determine the accuracy when all three techniques were combined. In a recent study, combination of T_2-weighted imaging, DWI, DCE, and MRSI were used to identify the regions suspicious for prostate cancer that were biopsied under MR guidance. They showed that all areas that were determined to be suspicious or indeterminate on T_2-weighted MRI were suspicious on at least one advanced imaging technique and that the combination of the three advanced techniques depicted more prostate cancer areas than the combination of any two of them [200]. Three tesla DWI studies also demonstrated good sensitivity (84%) and specificity (80%) for identifying cancer within the prostate [32], and the overall accuracy (AUC=0.89) was found to be better than that of T_2 imaging (AUC=0.82) [27]. A positive correlation was also found between ^{1}H MRSI and DWI findings for prostate cancer [201]. Another study that utilized combined DWI and MRSI of 61 prostate cancer patients demonstrated that the combination (AUC=0.85) performed significantly better than MRSI alone (AUC=0.74; $p=0.005$) and was also better than <D> alone (AUC=0.81, $p=0.09$) for differentiating between benign and malignant ROIs in the PZ [202]. Multiparametric MR holds great potential for predicting presence or absence of high-grade tumors in men with elevated PSA. This can be important in the selection of patients for active surveillance versus more aggressive therapy, or in the decision to rebiopsy patients with prior negative biopsies [203]. Two single institutional studies reported independently in 2011 that negative MP MRI can reliably exclude clinically significant Gleason pattern (grade)≥ 4, with negative predictive value (NPV) as high as 97% [204] and 98% [205].

Estimation of Intraglandular Prostate Cancer Volume

The reliable assessment of the extent or volume of prostate cancer is also critical for MR-guided biopsy and therapy and in the risk assessment of individual patients. Two recent studies suggest that MRI/^{1}H MRSI and DCE imaging may noninvasively provide estimates of cancer volume at diagnosis. One study demonstrated that for nodules greater than 0.5 cm^3, tumor volume measurements by MRI, ^{1}H MRSI, and combined MRI and MRSI were all positively correlated with histopathologic volume (Pearson's correlation coefficients of 0.49, 0.59, and 0.55, respectively), but only measurements by ^{1}H MRSI and combined MRI/^{1}H MRSI reached statistical significance ($p < 0.05$) [110]. The addition of ^{1}H MRSI to MRI also increased the overall accuracy of prostate cancer tumor volume measurement, although measurement variability still limited consistent quantitative tumor volume estimation, particularly for small tumors (<0.5 cm^3) [110]. Another study demonstrated that DCE imaging determined the volume of smaller foci of prostate cancer with greater overall accuracy than MRI/^{1}H MRSI. Sensitivity, specificity, and positive and negative predictive values for cancer detection by DCE imaging were 77%, 91%, 86%, and 85% for foci greater than 0.2 cc, and 90%, 88%, 77%, and 95% for foci greater than 0.5 cc, respectively [33]. In another study, the sensitivity and specificity of detecting intraprostatic prostate cancer by DCE MRI was determined to be 86% and 94%, respectively, with a ROC of 0.874 [157]. Mean volume of DCE MRI detected and missed cancers were 2.44 mL (0.02–14.5) and 0.16 mL (0.005–2.4), respectively [157]. In a study of 42 patients, the addition of DWI to T$_2$ MRI can significantly improved the accuracy of prostate peripheral zone tumor volume measurement [206]. Specifically, using an ADC cutoff of 0.0016 mm^2/s for cancer, the concordance correlation coefficient of combined T$_2$ MRI and DWI MR imaging was significantly higher ($p = 0.006$) than that of T$_2$ MRI imaging alone.

Multiparametric MR-Guided Biopsy and Therapy

The ability of multiparametric MR to provide more accurate localization of clinically significant cancer within the prostate can be used to directly target biopsies and therapy (Fig. 23.3). The development of the field of direct prostate MR-guided interventions (biopsy and therapy)

began with the introduction of a low-field (0.5 T) open MRI device at the Brigham and Women's Hospital (Boston, MA) [207], in 1993. They utilized this low-field open magnet and real-time image guidance to perform transperineal biopsies of 50 patients, with a 30% cancer positive sampling rate [5, 208–210]. The joint team from Johns Hopkins University and the National Institutes of Health moved the MR-guided biopsy procedure to a closed-bore 1.5 T MRI scanner in order to acquire superior quality MR data for biopsy targeting. They initially used a transperineal biopsy approach similar to the open MRI low-field approach, but which required moving the patient in and out of magnet. They used this approach to biopsy and place HDR brachytherapy catheters in four patients with intermediate to high-risk prostate cancer [211]. The same group also developed a transrectal biopsy approach using a remotely operated needle guide, in combination with an endorectal coil for image reception and an associated biopsy planning and imaging control method [212]. They utilized this approach for MR-guided intraprostatic placement of gold fiducial markers (four procedures) and/or prostate biopsy (three procedures) to patients scheduled to receive a standard course of conformal external beam radiation therapy [213].

In the setting of focal therapy, an MRI-targeted biopsy could be used prior to treatment to confirm the region for treatment, as well as the effectiveness of the focal therapy. Moreover, to successfully perform focal therapy, there must be real-time imaging guidance of the treatment. The approaches that have been clinically used for multiparametric MR-guided prostate biopsy and therapy are described in more detail below.

MR-Directed TRUS Biopsy

Numerous studies reported in the literature have used the results from multiparametric MR staging exams, performed prior to the transrectal ultrasound (TRUS) biopsy, to identify regions of MRI suspicious cancer for subsequent real-time TRUS-guided biopsy [179, 214–217]. This MRI-targeted biopsy approach has been utilized in several studies of patients with negative prior biopsies and rising PSA. These patients typically have cancers in locations such as the anterior aspect of the prostate that are difficult to biopsy or in patients with large prostates where the sampling error of TRUS-guided systematic biopsy approaches are reduced. Specifically, in two studies, the accuracy of cancer detection of MRI/^{1}H MRSI-targeted biopsy in men with a prior negative biopsy was reported to be ≈80% [214, 215]. Combining DCE MRI with ^{1}H MRSI demonstrated a further improvement to guide biopsy needles to cancer foci in patients with previously negative TRUS biopsy [218, 219]. The combination of ^{1}H MRSI and DCE MRI yielded 93.7% sensitivity, 90.7% specificity, 88.2% PPV, 95.1% NPV, and 90.9% accuracy in detecting prostate carcinoma in a prior negative biopsy population [219]. In addition to improving cancer detection, MRI-targeted, TRUS-guided biopsies also improved estimates of cancer volume and pathologic grade as compared to a TRUS-guided systematic biopsy approach [220]. Additionally, combined T_2-weighted and DCE MRI was shown to be useful for guiding TRUS biopsies toward areas containing recurrent cancer after HIFU [221] and radiation therapy [143]. It is clear that the MR-directed TRUS biopsy approach is limited by inaccuracy in targeting small tumors as there is guesswork involved in triangulating lesions seen on multiparametric MRI to ultrasound. To date studies have added MR-targeted biopsies to a systematic TRUS biopsy protocol and whether a targeted approach alone is clinically sufficient requires further study [217]. The guesswork involved with transferring the multiparametric MR identified foci of cancer onto ultrasound data may be overcome by performing MRI-guided biopsy within the bore of the magnet.

Direct MRI-Guided Biopsy

The recent development and implementation of MR-guided biopsy devices allows for a direct means of taking a biopsy of prostate cancer identified using multiparametric data. As shown in Fig. 23.6, the current commercially available MR-guided biopsy device (DynaTRIM, In vivo Corporation, Orlando, FL) uses a transrectal biopsy approach. The patient is placed in the prone position inside the magnet. A body phased array coil is placed on the patient's lower back and abdomen, and an MR visible needle guide that is attached to the MR biopsy device is inserted into the rectum (Fig. 23.6). Based on imaging findings the MR-compatible biopsy device is adjusted using software that interfaces with the scanner and manual adjusts in all three spatial dimensions to obtain a biopsy core from the region of interest within the prostate. The needle guide is tracked by fast anatomic MR imaging during the adjustment of the biopsy device. Several studies have demonstrated the clinical potential of MRI-guided biopsies for detecting clinically significant prostate cancer prior to therapy [222–227] and residual disease after therapy [161]. Prior to therapy, the detection rate of multiparametric 3-T magnetic resonance imaging-guided biopsy was 59% (40 of 68 cases), which was significantly greater than transrectal ultrasound (15%), and 37 of the 40 patients (93%) with positive biopsies were considered highly likely to harbor clinically significant disease [226]. In a study of 24 patients with rising PSA after external beam radiation therapy, multiparametric MR identified areas of residual/recurrent prostate cancer a positive predictive value of 75% based on MR-targeted biopsies of the MR suspicious area [161]. We have recently demonstrated that MRI-guided biopsies significantly upgraded percentage of cancer within each positive core and total number of positive cores when compared to TRUS-guided biopsies in patients with highly suspicious cancer foci seen on MRI. Most of the men we have utilized MRI-guided biopsy approach on have been on active surveillance, and the MRI-guided biopsy histopathology led to a change in management recommendation to active treatment for men with an increase in pathologic grade or significant increase in the amount of cancer present [228].

Several other direct MR-guided biopsy approaches have been performed. One approach used a custom endorectal MR probe that incorporated an imaging coil, a biopsy needle, and tracking coils. The tracking coils provided the real-time location of the endorectal probe in three-dimensional space, and the imaging coil was used to acquire the anatomic images that were used to target the biopsy [211–213]. Others have used more sophisticated robotic-driven biopsy devices [229, 230].

Direct MR-targeted biopsy approaches have the potential to reduce the number of invasive biopsies required for the diagnosis and characterization of prostate cancer in individual patients and for more confidently providing a target for focal therapy. However, the approach is currently plagued by relatively long time required for the acquiring individual biopsies which limits the number of biopsies that can be performed in a clinically reasonable amount of time and increases the cost of the procedure.

MRI-TRUS Fusion

The fusion of MRI and TRUS technology offers a promising alternative to performing targeted prostate biopsies. Recent advances have made co-registration between pre-acquired MRI images and real-time TRUS feasible, thereby allowing the merging of the superior ability of multiparametric MR for cancer detection and characterization with the real-time imaging and low cost of TRUS. MRI-TRUS fusion biopsy techniques were initially developed for brachytherapy [231, 232]. These systems used fiducial markers for image registration but were limited by prostate motion, which resulted in loss of accuracy. Improved 3-D ultrasound and TRUS/MRI fusion techniques combined with ultrasound transducers with spatial tracking sensors have since been developed that address these early issues and making MRI-TRUS fusion a clinically viable approach [233–240].

MR-Guided Therapy

A number of published studies have integrated MRI/^{1}H MRSI data into the radiation treatment plan in order to optimize radiation dose selectively to regions of prostate cancer using either intensity-modulated radiotherapy (IMRT) [21, 241, 242] or brachytherapy [243–246] while treating the whole gland. A combination of MRI/^{1}H MRSI and MR-targeted biopsy has also been used to identify and treat recurrent residual cancer in the transition zone after radiation therapy using MR-guided brachytherapy [247]. In another small study of patients interested in focal salvage high-dose-rate brachytherapy, it was found that T_2-weighted and dynamic contrast-enhanced magnetic resonance imaging could provide an improved means to localize residual disease leading to an improved radiation treatment plan for salvage therapy [104].

The recent emergence of endorectal MR-guided focused ultrasound surgery as a method of prostate cancer ablation provides a novel and exciting approach to focal therapy that promises precisely targeted tissue necrosis with real-time monitoring by MR thermometry [248]. Some human subjects have already undergone technically successful endorectal MR-guided focused ultrasound surgery outside the United States. In this country, FDA approval will be required before interested institutions can provide this investigational technology to American men. While saturation biopsy without imaging could theoretically be used to determine the target of MR-guided focal therapy [178], MR-guided focused ultrasound surgery seems best suited to patients with a visible dominant tumor at multiparametric MR imaging and potentially an MR-guided biopsy, so that treatment is delivered to a tumor depicted by the same modality being used to guide therapy. This avoids the potential inaccuracies in "blindly" treating a designated portion of the prostate based purely on positive biopsies.

MRI-guided focal laser therapy has been recently performed in patients with low-risk prostate cancer [249]. Early clinical, histological, and MRI responses in 12 patients receiving MRI-guided focal laser therapy suggest that the targeted region can be ablated with minimal adverse effects [250, 251].

Summary

In summary, the available literature supports that multiparametric MR imaging findings can improve the correct identification of dominant tumor foci in patients with prostate cancer, add to clinical parameters and biopsy results to improve the risk assessment of individual patients, and may be useful in guiding biopsies and focal therapy directly or through fusion with TRUS imaging. Larger multicenter studies are clearly needed to confirm the initial promising results and to establish guidelines for the use of multiparametric MRI as a surrogate for biopsy results and for guiding biopsies and therapy. However, it is our opinion that multiparametric MRI will not be a replacement for biopsy results, due to the tremendous value of the pathologic and tissue level molecular biomarker information that can be obtained from biopsy samples.

Editorial Commentary:
These authors continue to blaze the North American trail for prostatic MRI. The challenge remains of scaling this technology across multiple centers based on the highly complex and rapidly evolving nature of this field. For most urologists, the ability to identify cancers or extraprostatic extension to this level will remain elusive for the foreseeable future, but that should not dissuade enthusiastic research and development to that end.

MRI-guided or MRI-facilitated biopsy is technically very difficult, mostly due to the physical nature of MRI machines and the inability to utilize certain metals inside the unit. The ability to couple MRI findings post hoc to a real-time ultrasound-guided approach would significantly advance the ability to biopsy specific lesions.

–J. Stephen Jones, MD

References

1. Siegel R, Naishadham D, Jemal A. Cancer statistics, 2012. (Translated from eng) CA Cancer J Clin. 2012;62(1):10–29 (in eng).
2. Vo T, Rifkin MD, Peters TL. Should ultrasound criteria of the prostate be redefined to better evaluate when and where to biopsy. (Translated from eng) Ultrasound Q. 2001;17(3):171–6 (in eng).
3. Rabbani F, Stroumbakis N, Kava BR, Cookson MS, Fair WR. Incidence and clinical significance of false-negative sextant prostate biopsies. (Translated from eng) J Urol. 1998;159(4):1247–50 (in eng).
4. Kvale R, et al. Concordance between Gleason scores of needle biopsies and radical prostatectomy specimens: a population-based study. (Translated from eng) BJU Int. 2009;103(12):1647–54 (in eng).
5. D'Amico AV, et al. Transperineal magnetic resonance image guided prostate biopsy. (Translated from eng) J Urol. 2000;164(2):385–7 (in eng).
6. Epstein JI, Walsh PC, Carmichael M, Brendler CB. Pathologic and clinical findings to predict tumor extent of nonpalpable (stage T1c) prostate cancer (see comments). JAMA. 1994;271(5):368–74.
7. Carroll PR, Coakley FV, Kurhanewicz J. Magnetic resonance imaging and spectroscopy of prostate cancer. Rev Urol. 2006;8(Suppl 1):S4–10.
8. Casciani E, Gualdi GF. Prostate cancer: value of magnetic resonance spectroscopy 3D chemical shift imaging. Abdom Imaging. 2006;31(4):490–9.
9. Coakley FV, et al. Validity of prostate-specific antigen as a tumour marker in men with prostate cancer managed by watchful-waiting: correlation with findings at serial endorectal magnetic resonance imaging and spectroscopic imaging. BJU Int. 2007;99(1):41–5.
10. Costouros NG, et al. Diagnosis of prostate cancer in patients with an elevated prostate-specific antigen level: role of endorectal MRI and MR spectroscopic imaging. AJR Am J Roentgenol. 2007;188(3):812–6.
11. Futterer JJ, et al. Prostate cancer: comparison of local staging accuracy of pelvic phased-array coil alone versus integrated endorectal-pelvic phased-array coils. Local staging accuracy of prostate cancer using endorectal coil MR imaging. Eur Radiol. 2007;17(4):1055–65.
12. Girouin N, et al. Prostate dynamic contrast-enhanced MRI with simple visual diagnostic criteria: is it reasonable? Eur Radiol. 2007;17(6):1498–509.
13. Hom JJ, et al. High-grade prostatic intraepithelial neoplasia in patients with prostate cancer: MR and MR spectroscopic imaging features–initial experience. Radiology. 2007;242(2):483–9.
14. Kwock L, et al. Clinical role of proton magnetic resonance spectroscopy in oncology: brain, breast, and prostate cancer. Lancet Oncol. 2006;7(10):859–68.
15. Manenti G, et al. Magnetic resonance imaging of the prostate with spectroscopic imaging using a surface coil. Initial clinical experience. Radiol Med (Torino). 2006;111(1):22–32.
16. Mueller-Lisse UG, Scherr MK. Proton MR spectroscopy of the prostate. (Translated from eng) Eur J Radiol. 2007;63(3):351–60 (in eng).
17. Pels P, et al. Quantification of prostate MRSI data by model-based time domain fitting and frequency domain analysis. NMR Biomed. 2006;19(2):188–97.
18. Shukla-Dave A, et al. The utility of magnetic resonance imaging and spectroscopy for predicting insignificant prostate cancer: an initial analysis. BJU Int. 2007;99(4):786–93.

19. Taouli B. MR spectroscopic imaging for evaluation of prostate cancer. J Radiol. 2006;87(2 Pt 2):222–7.

20. Testa C, et al. Prostate cancer: sextant localization with MR imaging, MR spectroscopy, and 11C-choline PET/CT. Radiology. 2007;244(3):797–806.

21. van Lin EN, et al. IMRT boost dose planning on dominant intraprostatic lesions: gold marker-based three-dimensional fusion of CT with dynamic contrast-enhanced and 1H-spectroscopic MRI. Int J Radiat Oncol Biol Phys. 2006;65(1):291–303.

22. Wang L, et al. Prediction of seminal vesicle invasion in prostate cancer: incremental value of adding endorectal MR imaging to the Kattan nomogram. Radiology. 2007;242(1):182–8.

23. Wang L, et al. Incremental value of multiplanar cross-referencing for prostate cancer staging with endorectal MRI. AJR Am J Roentgenol. 2007; 188(1):99–104.

24. Wang L, et al. Prostate cancer: incremental value of endorectal MR imaging findings for prediction of extracapsular extension. (Translated from eng) Radiology. 2004;232(1):133–9 (in eng).

25. Wang L, et al. Prediction of organ-confined prostate cancer: incremental value of MR imaging and MR spectroscopic imaging to staging nomograms. Radiology. 2006;238(2):597–603.

26. Shukla-Dave A, et al. The utility of magnetic resonance imaging and spectroscopy for predicting insignificant prostate cancer: an initial analysis. (Translated from eng) BJU Int. 2007;99(4):786–93 (in eng).

27. Miao H, Fukatsu H, Ishigaki T. Prostate cancer detection with 3-T MRI: comparison of diffusion-weighted and T2-weighted imaging. Eur J Radiol. 2007;61(2):297–302.

28. Pickles MD, Gibbs P, Sreenivas M, Turnbull LW. Diffusion-weighted imaging of normal and malignant prostate tissue at 3.0T. (Translated from eng). J Magn Reson Imaging. 2006;23(2):130–4 (in eng).

29. Mulkern RV, et al. Biexponential characterization of prostate tissue water diffusion decay curves over an extended b-factor range. Magn Reson Imaging. 2006;24(5):563–8.

30. Manenti G, et al. In vivo measurement of the apparent diffusion coefficient in normal and malignant prostatic tissue using thin-slice echo-planar imaging. Radiol Med (Torino). 2006;111(8):1124–33.

31. Hacklander T, Scharwachter C, Golz R, Mertens H. Value of diffusion-weighted imaging for diagnosing vertebral metastases due to prostate cancer in comparison to other primary tumors. Rofo. 2006;178(4):416–24.

32. Gibbs P, Pickles MD, Turnbull LW. Diffusion imaging of the prostate at 3.0 tesla. Invest Radiol. 2006; 41(2):185–8.

33. Villers A, et al. Dynamic contrast enhanced, pelvic phased array magnetic resonance imaging of localized prostate cancer for predicting tumor volume: correlation with radical prostatectomy findings. (Translated from eng). J Urol. 2006;176(6 Pt 1): 2432–7 (in eng).

34. Dafni H, Kim SJ, Panda K, Bankson JA, Ronen SM. Signal loss in DCE-MRI associated with tumor progression in prostate cancer bone metastasis. In: Proceedings of the 14th ISMRM, Seattle; 2006. p. 118.

35. Futterer JJ, et al. Prostate cancer localization with dynamic contrast-enhanced MR imaging and proton MR spectroscopic imaging. Radiology. 2006; 241(2):449–58.

36. Kirkham AP, Emberton M, Allen C. How good is MRI at detecting and characterising cancer within the prostate? Eur Urol. 2006;50(6):1163–74. discussion 1175.

37. Prando A. Dynamic contrast enhanced, pelvic phased array magnetic resonance imaging of localized prostate cancer for predicting tumor volume: correlation with radical prostatectomy findings. Int Braz J Urol. 2006;32(6):727–8.

38. Kim CK, Park BK, Kim B. Localization of prostate cancer using 3T MRI: comparison of T2-weighted and dynamic contrast-enhanced imaging. J Comput Assist Tomogr. 2006;30(1):7–11.

39. Chan I, et al. Detection of prostate cancer by integration of line-scan diffusion, T2-mapping and T2-weighted magnetic resonance imaging; a multichannel statistical classifier. Med Phys. 2003;30(9): 2390–8.

40. Gibbs P, Tozer DJ, Liney GP, Turnbull LW. Comparison of quantitative T2 mapping and diffusion-weighted imaging in the normal and pathologic prostate. (Translated from eng). Magn Reson Med. 2001;46(6):1054–8 (in eng).

41. Jacobs MA, Ouwerkerk R, Petrowski K, Macura KJ. Diffusion-weighted imaging with apparent diffusion coefficient mapping and spectroscopy in prostate cancer. (Translated from eng) Top Magn Reson Imaging. 2008;19(6):261–72 (in eng).

42. Langer DL, et al. Prostate cancer detection with multi-parametric MRI: logistic regression analysis of quantitative T2, diffusion-weighted imaging, and dynamic contrast-enhanced MRI. (Translated from eng) J Magn Reson Imaging. 2009;30(2):327–34 (in eng).

43. Liney GP, et al. Comparison of conventional single echo and multi-echo sequences with a fast spin-echo sequence for quantitative T2 mapping: application to the prostate. (Translated from eng) J Magn Reson Imaging. 1996;6(4):603–7 (in eng).

44. Kumar V, et al. Evaluation of the role of magnetization transfer imaging in prostate: a preliminary study. (Translated from eng) Magn Reson Imaging. 2008;26(5):644–9 (in eng).

45. Cunningham C, et al. Design of flyback echo-planar readout gradients for MR spectroscopic imaging. In: Proceedings of the 13th international society for magnetic resonance in medicine, South beach, Miami; 7–13 May 2005.

46. Scheenen TW, et al. Optimal timing for in vivo 1H-MR spectroscopic imaging of the human prostate at 3T. Magn Reson Med. 2005;53(6): 1268–74.

47. Chen AP, et al. High-speed 3T MR spectroscopic imaging of prostate with flyback echo-planar encoding. J Magn Reson Imaging. 2007;25(6):1288–92.
48. Phillips ME, et al. Prostatic disorders: MR imaging at 1.5 T. Radiology. 1987;164(2):386–92.
49. Hricak H, Dooms GC, McNeal JE, et al. MR imaging of the prostate gland. Normal anatomy. AJR. 1987;148:51–5.
50. Hricak H, et al. Prostatic carcinoma: staging by clinical assessment, CT, and MR imaging. Radiology. 1987;162(2):331–6.
51. Carrol CL, Sommer FG, McNeal JE, Stamey TA. The abnormal prostate: MR imaging at 1.5 T with histopathologic correlation. Radiology. 1987;163(2):521–5.
52. Bezzi M, et al. Prostatic carcinoma: staging with MR imaging at 1.5 T. Radiology. 1988;169(2):339–46.
53. Hom JJ, et al. Endorectal MR and MR spectroscopic imaging of prostate cancer: histopathological determinants of tumor visibility. Am J Roentgenol. 2005;184(4):62–62.
54. Hricak H, Kurhanewicz J, Proctor E, Bruce N, Vigneron DB. Phased-array endorectal coil MRI of prostate cancer. GE Clin Symp. 1994;7(4):1–12.
55. Chen M, et al. Hormonal ablation of prostatic cancer: effects on prostate morphology, tumor detection, and staging by endorectal coil MR imaging. (Translated from eng) AJR Am J Roentgenol. 1996;166(5):1157–63 (in eng).
56. Coakley FV, Hricak H. Radiologic anatomy of the prostate gland: a clinical approach. Radiol Clin North Am. 2000;38(1):15–30.
57. Wang L, et al. Are histopathological features of prostate cancer lesions associated with identification of extracapsular extension on magnetic resonance imaging? (Translated from eng) BJU Int. 2010;106(9):1303–8 (in eng).
58. Nogueira L, et al. Focal treatment or observation of prostate cancer: pretreatment accuracy of transrectal ultrasound biopsy and T2-weighted MRI. (Translated from eng) Urology. 2010;75(2):472–7 (in eng).
59. Westphalen AC, McKenna DA, Kurhanewicz J, Coakley FV. Role of magnetic resonance imaging and magnetic resonance spectroscopic imaging before and after radiotherapy for prostate cancer. (Translated from eng) J Endourol. 2008;22(4):789–94 (in eng).
60. McKenna DA, et al. Prostate cancer: role of pretreatment MR in predicting outcome after external-beam radiation therapy – initial experience. (Translated from eng) Radiology. 2008;247(1):141–6 (in eng).
61. Sala E, et al. Endorectal MR imaging before salvage prostatectomy: tumor localization and staging. Radiology. 2006;238(1):176–83.
62. Hricak H, et al. The role of preoperative endorectal magnetic resonance imaging in the decision regarding whether to preserve or resect neurovascular bundles during radical retropubic prostatectomy. Cancer. 2004;100(12):2655–63.
63. Yu KK, et al. Prostate cancer: prediction of extracapsular extension with endorectal MR imaging and three-dimensional proton MR spectroscopic imaging. (Translated from eng) Radiology. 1999;213(2):481–8 (in eng).
64. Hricak H, et al. Carcinoma of the prostate gland: MR imaging with pelvic phased-array coils versus integrated endorectal – pelvic phased-array coils. (Translated from eng) Radiology. 1994;193(3):703–9 (in eng).
65. Rosen MA, Goldstone L, Lapin S, Wheeler T, Scardino PT. Frequency and location of extracapsular extension and positive surgical margins in radical prostatectomy specimens. (Translated from eng) J Urol. 1992;148(2 Pt 1):331–7 (in eng).
66. Kurhanewicz J, Vigneron D, Carroll P, Coakley F. Multiparametric magnetic resonance imaging in prostate cancer: present and future. (Translated from eng) Curr Opin Urol. 2008;18(1):71–7 (in eng).
67. Kurhanewicz J, Swanson MG, Nelson SJ, Vigneron DB. Combined magnetic resonance imaging and spectroscopic imaging approach to molecular imaging of prostate cancer. J Magn Reson Imaging. 2002;16(4):451–63.
68. Kurhanewicz J, Vigneron DB, Nelson SJ. Three-dimensional magnetic resonance spectroscopic imaging of brain and prostate cancer. (Translated from eng) Neoplasia. 2000;2(1–2):166–89 (in eng).
69. Tran TK, Vigneron DB, Sailasuta N, Tropp J, Le Roux P, Kurhanewicz J, Nelson S, Hurd R. Very selective suppression pulses for clinical MRSI studies of brain and prostate cancer. Magn Reson Med. 2000;43(1):23–33.
70. Schricker AA, Pauly JM, Kurhanewicz J, Swanson MG, Vigneron DB. Dualband spectral-spatial RF pulses for prostate MR spectroscopic imaging. Magn Reson Med. 2001;46(6):1079–87.
71. Cunningham CH, et al. Design of symmetric-sweep spectral-spatial RF pulses for spectral editing. Magn Reson Med. 2004;52(1):147–53.
72. Kurhanewicz J, Vigneron DB, Hricak H, Narayan P, Carroll P, Nelson SJ. Three-dimensional H-1 MR spectroscopic imaging of the in situ human prostate with high (0.24-0.7-cm3) spatial resolution. Radiology. 1996;198(3):795–805.
73. Kurhanewicz J, Vigneron DB. Advances in MR spectroscopy of the prostate. Magn Reson Imaging Clin N Am. 2008;16(4):697–710.
74. Costello LC, Franklin RB. Concepts of citrate production and secretion by prostate: 2. Hormonal relationships in normal and neoplastic prostate. Prostate. 1991;19(3):181–205.
75. Costello LC, Franklin RB. Bioenergetic theory of prostate malignancy. Prostate. 1994;25(3):162–6.
76. Costello LC, Franklin RB. Novel role of zinc in the regulation of prostate citrate metabolism and its implications in prostate cancer. Prostate. 1998;35(4):285–96.
77. Franklin RB, et al. Human ZIP1 is a major zinc uptake transporter for the accumulation of zinc in prostate cells. J Inorg Biochem. 2003;96(2–3):435–42.
78. Zakian KL, et al. Correlation of proton MR spectroscopic imaging with gleason score based on

step-section pathologic analysis after radical prostatectomy. Radiology. 2005;234(3):804–14.

79. Garcia-Martin ML, et al. Quantitative (1) H MR spectroscopic imaging of the prostate gland using LCModel and a dedicated basis-set: correlation with histologic findings. (Translated from eng) Magn Reson Med. 2011;65(2):329–39 (in eng).

80. Casciani E, et al. Prostate cancer: evaluation with endorectal MR imaging and three-dimensional proton MR spectroscopic imaging. (Translated from eng ita) Radiol Med. 2004;108(5–6):530–41 (in eng ita).

81. Kumar R, Kumar M, Jagannathan NR, Gupta NP, Hemal AK. Proton magnetic resonance spectroscopy with a body coil in the diagnosis of carcinoma prostate. (Translated from eng) Urol Res. 2004;32(1):36–40 (in eng).

82. Keshari KR, et al. Correlation of phospholipid metabolites with prostate cancer pathologic grade, proliferative status and surgical stage: impact of tissue environment. (Translated from eng) NMR Biomed. 2011;24(6):691–9 (in eng).

83. Stenman K, et al. H HRMAS NMR derived biomarkers related to tumor grade, tumor cell fraction, and cell proliferation in prostate tissue samples. (Translated from eng) Biomark Insights. 2011;6:39–47 (in eng).

84. Keshari K, et al. Quantification of choline and ethanolamine containing phospholipids in healthy and malignant prostate tissue. In: Proceedings of the international society of magnetic resonance in medicine, Berlin; 2007.

85. Saverio B, et al. Tumor progression is accompanied by significant changes in the levels of expression of polyamine metabolism regulatory genes and clusterin (sulfated glycoprotein 2) in human prostate cancer specimens. Cancer Res. 2000;60(1): 28–34.

86. Swanson MG, et al. Single-voxel oversampled J-resolved spectroscopy of in vivo human prostate tissue. Magn Reson Med. 2001;45(6):973–80.

87. Umbehr M, et al. Combined magnetic resonance imaging and magnetic resonance spectroscopy imaging in the diagnosis of prostate cancer: a systematic review and meta-analysis. (Translated from eng) Eur Urol. 2009;55(3):575–90 (in eng).

88. Kurhanewicz J, et al. Three-dimensional H-1 MR spectroscopic imaging of the in situ human prostate with high (0.24-0.7-cm3) spatial resolution. Radiology. 1996;198(3):795–805.

89. Westphalen AC, et al. Peripheral zone prostate cancer: accuracy of different interpretative approaches with MR and MR spectroscopic imaging. Radiology. 2008;246(1):177–84.

90. Mueller-Lisse UG, et al. Time-dependent effects of hormone-deprivation therapy on prostate metabolism as detected by combined magnetic resonance imaging and 3D magnetic resonance spectroscopic imaging. (Translated from eng) Magn Reson Med. 2001;46(1):49–57 (in eng).

91. Mueller-Lisse UG, Swanson MG, Vigneron DB, Kurhanewicz J. Magnetic resonance spectroscopy in patients with locally confined prostate cancer: association of prostatic citrate and metabolic atrophy with time on hormone deprivation therapy, PSA level, and biopsy Gleason score. (Translated from eng) Eur Radiol. 2007;17(2):371–8 (in eng).

92. Mueller-Lisse UG, et al. Localized prostate cancer: effect of hormone deprivation therapy measured by using combined three-dimensional 1H MR spectroscopy and MR imaging: clinicopathologic case-controlled study. Radiology. 2001;221(2):380–90.

93. Ryan CJ, Small EJ. Role of secondary hormonal therapy in the management of recurrent prostate cancer. (Translated from eng) Urology. 2003;62(Suppl 1):87–94 (in eng).

94. Montironi R, Pomante R, Diamanti L, Magi-Galluzzi C. Apoptosis in prostatic adenocarcinoma following complete androgen ablation. Urol Int. 1998;60(Suppl 1):25–9. discussion 30.

95. Roach 3rd M, Kurhanewicz J, Carroll P. Spectroscopy in prostate cancer: hope or hype? Oncology (Williston Park). 2001;15(11):1399–410. discussion 1415–1396, 1418.

96. Pickett B, et al. Time to metabolic atrophy after permanent prostate seed implantation based on magnetic resonance spectroscopic imaging. Int J Radiat Oncol Biol Phys. 2004;59(3):665–73.

97. Kalbhen CL, et al. Prostate carcinoma: MR imaging findings after cryosurgery. Radiology. 1996;198: 807–11.

98. Parivar F, et al. Detection of locally recurrent prostate cancer after cryosurgery: evaluation by transrectal ultrasound, magnetic resonance imaging, and three-dimensional proton magnetic resonance spectroscopy. Urology. 1996;48(4):594–9.

99. Parivar F, Kurhanewicz J. Detection of recurrent prostate cancer after cryosurgery. Curr Opin Urol. 1998;8:83–6.

100. Pickett B, et al. Use of MRI and spectroscopy in evaluation of external beam radiotherapy for prostate cancer. Int J Radiat Oncol Biol Phys. 2004;60(4):1047–55.

101. Coakley FV, et al. Endorectal MR imaging and MR spectroscopic imaging for locally recurrent prostate cancer after external beam radiation therapy: preliminary experience. Radiology. 2004;233(2):441–8.

102. Westphalen AC, Coakley FV, Roach M, 3rd, McCulloch CE, Kurhanewicz J. Locally recurrent prostate cancer after external beam radiation therapy: diagnostic performance of 1.5-T endorectal MR imaging and MR spectroscopic imaging for detection. (Translated from eng) Radiology. 2010;256(2):485–492 (in eng).

103. Rouviere O, Vitry T, Lyonnet D. Imaging of prostate cancer local recurrences: why and how? (Translated from eng) Eur Radiol. 2010;20(5):1254–66 (in eng).

104. Moman MR, et al. Focal salvage guided by T2-weighted and dynamic contrast-enhanced magnetic resonance imaging for prostate cancer

recurrences. (Translated from eng) Int J Radiat Oncol Biol Phys. 2010;76(3):741–6 (in eng).

105. Jabbari S, et al. High-dose-rate brachytherapy for localized prostate adenocarcinoma post abdomino-perineal resection of the rectum and pelvic irradiation: technique and experience. (Translated from eng) Brachytherapy. 2009;8(4):339–44 (in eng).

106. Blana A, et al. High-intensity focused ultrasound for prostate cancer: comparative definitions of biochemical failure. (Translated from eng) BJU Int. 2009;104(8):1058–62 (in eng).

107. Stephenson AJ, et al. Predicting the outcome of salvage radiation therapy for recurrent prostate cancer after radical prostatectomy. J Clin Oncol. 2007;25(15):2035–41.

108. Lee B, et al. Feasibility of high-dose-rate brachytherapy salvage for local prostate cancer recurrence after radiotherapy: the University of California-San Francisco experience. (Translated from eng) Int J Radiat Oncol Biol Phys. 2007;67(4):1106–12 (in eng).

109. Bong GW, Keane TE. Salvage options for biochemical recurrence after primary therapy for prostate cancer. Can J Urol. 2007;14(Suppl 1):2–9.

110. Coakley FV, et al. Prostate cancer tumor volume: measurement with endorectal MR and MR spectroscopic imaging. Radiology. 2002;223(1):91–7.

111. Dhingsa R, et al. Prostate cancer localization with endorectal MR imaging and MR spectroscopic imaging: effect of clinical data on reader accuracy. Radiology. 2004;230(1):215–20.

112. Weinreb JC, et al. Prostate cancer: sextant localization at MR imaging and MR spectroscopic imaging before prostatectomy – results of ACRIN prospective multi-institutional clinicopathologic study. (Translated from eng) Radiology. 2009;251(1):122–33 (in eng).

113. Jagannathan NR, Kumar V, Kumar R, Thulkar S. Role of magnetic resonance methods in the evaluation of prostate cancer: an Indian perspective. MAGMA. 2008;21(6):393–407.

114. Manenti G, Squillaci E, Di Roma M, Carlani M, Mancino S, Simonetti G. In vivo measurement of the apparent diffusion coefficient in normal and malignant prostatic tissue using thin-slice echo-planar imaging. Radiol Med (Torino). 2006;111(8):1124–33.

115. Pickles MD, Gibbs P, Sreenivas M, Turnbull LW. Diffusion-weighted imaging of normal and malignant prostate tissue at 3.0T. Journal of magnetic resonance imaging : JMRI. 2006;23(2):130–4.

116. Nasu K, Kuroki Y, Kuroki S, Murakami K, Nawano S, Moriyama N. Diffusion-weighted single shot echo planar imaging of colorectal cancer using a sensitivity-encoding technique. Japanese journal of clinical oncology. 2004;34(10):620–26.

117. Kozlowski P, Chang SD, Goldenberg SL. Diffusion-weighted MRI in prostate cancer: comparison between single-shot fast spin echo and echo planar imaging sequences. Magn Reson Imaging. 2008;26(1):72–6.

118. Yoshizako T, et al. Apparent diffusion coefficient of line scan diffusion image in normal prostate and prostate cancer – comparison with single-shot echo planner image. (Translated from eng) Magn Reson Imaging. 2011;29(1):106–10 (in eng).

119. Horsfield MA, Jones DK. Applications of diffusion-weighted and diffusion tensor MRI to white matter diseases: a review. NMR Biomed. 2002;15(7–8):570–7.

120. Kubicki M, et al. Diffusion tensor imaging and its application to neuropsychiatric disorders. Harv Rev Psychiatry. 2002;10(6):324–36.

121. Moseley M. Diffusion tensor imaging and aging: a review. NMR Biomed. 2002;15(7–8):553–60.

122. Sotak CH. The role of diffusion tensor imaging in the evaluation of ischemic brain injury: a review. NMR Biomed. 2002;15(7–8):561–9.

123. Tan CH, Wang J, Kundra V. Diffusion weighted imaging in prostate cancer. (Translated from eng) Eur Radiol. 2011;21(3):593–603 (in eng).

124. Zelhof B, Lowry M, Rodrigues G, Kraus S, Turnbull L. Description of magnetic resonance imaging-derived enhancement variables in pathologically confirmed prostate cancer and normal peripheral zone regions. (Translated from eng) BJU Int. 2009;104(5):621–7 (in eng).

125. Yoshimitsu K, et al. Usefulness of apparent diffusion coefficient map in diagnosing prostate carcinoma: correlation with stepwise histopathology. J Magn Reson Imaging. 2008;27(1):132–9.

126. De Souza NM, et al. Diffusion-weighted magnetic resonance imaging: a potential non-invasive marker of tumour aggressiveness in localized prostate cancer. (Translated from eng) Clin Radiol. 2008;63(7):774–82 (in eng).

127. Turkbey B, et al. Is apparent diffusion coefficient associated with clinical risk scores for prostate cancers that are visible on 3-T MR images? (Translated from eng) Radiology. 2011;258(2):488–95 (in eng).

128. Verma S, et al. Assessment of aggressiveness of prostate cancer: correlation of apparent diffusion coefficient with histologic grade after radical prostatectomy. (Translated from eng) AJR Am J Roentgenol. 2011;196(2):374–81 (in eng).

129. Nagarajan R, et al. Correlation of Gleason scores with diffusion-weighted imaging findings of prostate cancer. (Translated from eng) Adv Urol. 2012;374805 (in eng).

130. Kim CK, Park BK, Lee HM, Kwon GY. Value of diffusion-weighted imaging for the prediction of prostate cancer location at 3T using a phased-array coil: preliminary results. (Translated from eng) Invest Radiol. 2007;42(12):842–47 (in eng).

131. Morgan VA, et al. Diffusion-weighted magnetic resonance imaging for monitoring prostate cancer progression in patients managed by active surveillance. (Translated from eng) Br J Radiol. 2011;84(997):31–7 (in eng).

132. Kim CK, Park BK, Lee HM. Prediction of locally recurrent prostate cancer after radiation therapy: incremental value of 3T diffusion-weighted MRI.

(Translated from eng) J Magn Reson Imaging. 2009;29(2):391–7 (in eng).

133. Nemoto K, Tateishi T, Ishidate T. Changes in diffusion-weighted images for visualizing prostate cancer during antiandrogen therapy: preliminary results. (Translated from Eng) Urol Int. 2010;85(4):421–6 (in Eng).

134. Kim CK, Park BK, Lee HM, Kim SS, Kim E. MRI techniques for prediction of local tumor progression after high-intensity focused ultrasonic ablation of prostate cancer. AJR Am J Roentgenol. 2008; 190(5):1180–6.

135. Alonzi R, Padhani AR, Allen C. Dynamic contrast enhanced MRI in prostate cancer. Eur J Radiol. 2007;63(3):335–50.

136. Tofts PS, Wicks DA, Barker GJ. The MRI measurement of NMR and physiological parameters in tissue to study disease process. (Translated from eng) Prog Clin Biol Res. 1991;363:313–25 (in eng).

137. Tofts PS. Modeling tracer kinetics in dynamic Gd-DTPA MR imaging. J Magn Reson Imaging. 1997;7(1):91–101.

138. Tofts PS, et al. Estimating kinetic parameters from dynamic contrast-enhanced T(1)-weighted MRI of a diffusable tracer: standardized quantities and symbols. J Magn Reson Imaging. 1999;10(3):223–32.

139. Noworolski SM, Vigneron DB, Chen AP, Kurhanewicz J. Dynamic contrast-enhanced MRI and MR diffusion imaging to distinguish between glandular and stromal prostatic tissues. Magn Reson Imaging. 2008;26(8):1071–80.

140. Bonekamp D, Macura KJ. Dynamic contrast-enhanced magnetic resonance imaging in the evaluation of the prostate. (Translated from eng) Top Magn Reson Imaging. 2008;19(6):273–84 (in eng).

141. Carlani M, Mancino S, Bonanno E, Finazzi Agro E, Simonetti G. Combined morphological, [1H]-MR spectroscopic and contrast-enhanced imaging of human prostate cancer with a 3-Tesla scanner: preliminary experience. Radiol Med (Torino). 2008;113(5):670–88.

142. Cornud F, et al. Quantitative dynamic MRI and localisation of non-palpable prostate cancer. (Translated from fre) Prog Urol. 2009;19(6):401–13 (in fre).

143. Haider MA, et al. Dynamic contrast-enhanced magnetic resonance imaging for localization of recurrent prostate cancer after external beam radiotherapy. Int J Radiat Oncol Biol Phys. 2008;70(2):425–30.

144. Hara N, Okuizumi M, Koike H, Kawaguchi M, Bilim V. Dynamic contrast-enhanced magnetic resonance imaging (DCE-MRI) is a useful modality for the precise detection and staging of early prostate cancer. Prostate. 2005;62(2):140–7.

145. Ito H, Kamoi K, Yokoyama K, Yamada K, Nishimura T. Visualization of prostate cancer using dynamic contrast-enhanced MRI: comparison with transrectal power Doppler ultrasound. Br J Radiol. 2003; 76(909):617–24.

146. Jackson AS, et al. Dynamic contrast-enhanced MRI for prostate cancer localization. (Translated from eng) Br J Radiol. 2009;82(974):148–56 (in eng).

148. Jacobs MA, et al. Combined dynamic contrast enhanced breast MR and proton spectroscopic imaging: a feasibility study. J Magn Reson Imaging. 2005;21(1):23–8.

149. Jordan BF, et al. Dynamic contrast-enhanced and diffusion MRI show rapid and dramatic changes in tumor microenvironment in response to inhibition of HIF-1alpha using PX-478. (Translated from eng) Neoplasia. 2005;7(5):475–85 (in eng).

149. Kiessling F, et al. Dynamic magnetic resonance tomography and proton magnetic resonance spectroscopy of prostate cancers in rats treated by radiotherapy. Invest Radiol. 2004;39(1):34–44.

150. Kim CK, Park BK, Park W, Kim SS. Prostate MR imaging at 3T using a phased-arrayed coil in predicting locally recurrent prostate cancer after radiation therapy: preliminary experience. (Translated from eng) Abdom Imaging. 2010;35(2):246–52 (in eng).

151. Kim JK, et al. Wash-in rate on the basis of dynamic contrast-enhanced MRI: usefulness for prostate cancer detection and localization. J Magn Reson Imaging. 2005;22(5):639–46.

152. Kozlowski P, et al. Combined diffusion-weighted and dynamic contrast-enhanced MRI for prostate cancer diagnosis–correlation with biopsy and histopathology. J Magn Reson Imaging. 2006;24(1):108–13.

153. Lemaitre L, et al. Dynamic contrast-enhanced MRI of anterior prostate cancer: morphometric assessment and correlation with radical prostatectomy findings. (Translated from eng) Eur Radiol. 2009;19(2):470–80 (in eng).

154. Lowry M, et al. Analysis of prostate DCE-MRI: comparison of fast exchange limit and fast exchange regimen pharmacokinetic models in the discrimination of malignant from normal tissue. (Translated from eng) Invest Radiol. 2009;44(9):577–84 (in eng).

155. Noworolski SM, Henry RG, Vigneron DB, Kurhanewicz J. Dynamic contrast-enhanced MRI in normal and abnormal prostate tissues as defined by biopsy, MRI, and 3D MRSI. (Translated from eng) Magn Reson Med. 2005;53(2):249–55 (in eng).

156. Padhani AR, Hayes C, Landau S, Leach MO. Reproducibility of quantitative dynamic MRI of normal human tissues. NMR Biomed. 2002;15(2): 143–53.

157. Puech P, et al. Dynamic contrast-enhanced-magnetic resonance imaging evaluation of intraprostatic prostate cancer: correlation with radical prostatectomy specimens. (Translated from eng) Urology. 2009;74(5):1094–9 (in eng).

158. Ren J, et al. Dynamic contrast-enhanced MRI of benign prostatic hyperplasia and prostatic carcinoma: correlation with angiogenesis. Clin Radiol. 2008;63(2):153–9.

159. Schlemmer HP, et al. Can pre-operative contrast-enhanced dynamic MR imaging for prostate cancer

predict microvessel density in prostatectomy specimens? Eur Radiol. 2003;14(2):309–17.

160. Storaas T, Gjesdal KI, Svindland A, Viktil E, Geitung JT. Dynamic first pass 3D EPI of the prostate: accuracy in tumor location. Acta Radiol. 2004;45(5):584–90.

161. Yakar D, et al. Feasibility of 3T dynamic contrast-enhanced magnetic resonance-guided biopsy in localizing local recurrence of prostate cancer after external beam radiation therapy. (Translated from eng) Invest Radiol. 2010;45(3):121–5 (in eng).

162. van Dorsten FA, et al. Combined quantitative dynamic contrast-enhanced MR imaging and (1)H MR spectroscopic imaging of human prostate cancer. J Magn Reson Imaging. 2004;20(2):279–87.

163. Jager GJ, et al. Local staging of prostate cancer with endorectal MR imaging: correlation with histopathology. AJR. 1996;166(4):845–52.

164. Schlemmer HP, et al. Can pre-operative contrast-enhanced dynamic MR imaging for prostate cancer predict microvessel density in prostatectomy specimens? Eur Radiol. 2004;14(2):309–17.

165. Checkley D, Tessier JJ, Kendrew J, Waterton JC, Wedge SR. Use of dynamic contrast-enhanced MRI to evaluate acute treatment with ZD6474, a VEGF signalling inhibitor, in PC-3 prostate tumours. Br J Cancer. 2003;89(10):1889–95.

166. Nakamura K, et al. KRN951, a highly potent inhibitor of vascular endothelial growth factor receptor tyrosine kinases, has antitumor activities and affects functional vascular properties. Cancer Res. 2006;66(18):9134–42.

167. Padhani AR, et al. Dynamic contrast enhanced MRI of prostate cancer: correlation with morphology and tumour stage, histological grade and PSA. (Translated from eng) Clin Radiol. 2000;55(2):99–109 (in eng).

168. Lu-Yao GL, et al. Outcomes of localized prostate cancer following conservative management. (Translated from eng) JAMA. 2009;302(11):1202–9 (in eng).

169. Dall'Era MA, et al. Active surveillance for early-stage prostate cancer: review of the current literature. (Translated from eng) Cancer. 2008;112(8):1650–9 (in eng).

170. Presti JC Jr, O'Dowd GJ, Miller MC, Mattu R, Veltri RW. Extended peripheral zone biopsy schemes increase cancer detection rates and minimize variance in prostate specific antigen and age related cancer rates: results of a community multi-practice study. (Translated from eng) J Urol. 2003;169(1):125–9 (in eng).

171. Scattoni V, et al. Extended and saturation prostatic biopsy in the diagnosis and characterisation of prostate cancer: a critical analysis of the literature. (Translated from eng) Eur Urol. 2007;52(5):1309–22 (in eng).

172. Suardi N, et al. Currently used criteria for active surveillance in men with low-risk prostate cancer: an analysis of pathologic features. (Translated from eng) Cancer. 2008;113(8):2068–72 (in eng).

173. Conti SL, et al. Pathological outcomes of candidates for active surveillance of prostate cancer. (Translated from eng) J Urol. 2009;181(4):1628–33; discussion 1633–1624 (in eng).

174. Duffield AS, Lee TK, Miyamoto H, Carter HB, Epstein JI. Radical prostatectomy findings in patients in whom active surveillance of prostate cancer fails. (Translated from eng) J Urol. 2009;182(5):2274–8 (in eng).

175. Smaldone MC, Cowan JE, Carroll PR, Davies BJ. Eligibility for active surveillance and pathological outcomes for men undergoing radical prostatectomy in a large, community based cohort. (Translated from eng) J Urol. 2010;183(1):138–143 (in eng).

176. Latini DM, et al. The relationship between anxiety and time to treatment for patients with prostate cancer on surveillance. (Translated from eng) J Urol. 2007;178(3 Pt 1):826–31; discussion 831–822 (in eng).

177. Taira AV, et al. Performance of transperineal template-guided mapping biopsy in detecting prostate cancer in the initial and repeat biopsy setting. (Translated from eng) Prostate Cancer Prostatic Dis. 2010;13(1):71–7 (in eng).

178. Falzarano SM, et al. Can saturation biopsy predict prostate cancer localization in radical prostatectomy specimens: a correlative study and implications for focal therapy. (Translated from eng) Urology. 2010;76(3):682–7 (in eng).

179. Lawrentschuk N, Fleshner N. The role of magnetic resonance imaging in targeting prostate cancer in patients with previous negative biopsies and elevated prostate-specific antigen levels. (Translated from eng) BJU Int. 2009;103(6):730–3 (in eng).

180. Yu KK, et al. Detection of extracapsular extension of prostate carcinoma with endorectal and phased-array coil MR imaging: multivariate feature analysis. Radiology. 1997;202(3):697–702.

181. Partin AW, et al. The use of prostate specific antigen, clinical stage and Gleason score to predict pathological stage in men with localized prostate cancer. J Urol. 1993;150(1):110–4.

182. Cooperberg MR, et al. Multiinstitutional validation of the UCSF cancer of the prostate risk assessment for prediction of recurrence after radical prostatectomy. Cancer. 2006;107(10):2384–91.

183. Graefen M, et al. Can predictive models for prostate cancer patients derived in the United States of America be utilized in European patients? A validation study of the Partin tables. Eur Urol. 2003;43(1):6–10. discussion 11.

184. Steyerberg EW, et al. Prediction of indolent prostate cancer: validation and updating of a prognostic nomogram. J Urol. 2007;177(1):107–12. discussion 112.

185. Han M, Partin AW, Piantadosi S, Epstein JI, Walsh PC. Era specific biochemical recurrence-free survival following radical prostatectomy for clinically localized prostate cancer. J Urol. 2001;166(2):416–9.

186. Draisma G, et al. Lead times and overdetection due to prostate-specific antigen screening: estimates from the European randomized study of screening for prostate cancer. J Natl Cancer Inst. 2003; 95(12):868–78.

187. Etzioni R, et al. Overdiagnosis due to prostate-specific antigen screening: lessons from U.S. prostate cancer incidence trends. J Natl Cancer Inst. 2002;94(13):981–90.

188. Carroll PR. Early stage prostate cancer–do we have a problem with over-detection, overtreatment or both? J Urol. 2005;173(4):1061–2.

189. Fradet V, et al. Prostate cancer managed with active surveillance: role of anatomic MR imaging and MR spectroscopic imaging. (Translated from eng) Radiology. 2010;256(1):176–83 (in eng).

190. Rastinehad AR, et al. D'Amico risk stratification correlates with degree of suspicion of prostate cancer on multiparametric magnetic resonance imaging. (Translated from eng) J Urol. 2011;185(3):815–20 (in eng).

191. Okamura T, et al. Pitfalls with MRI evaluation of prostate cancer detection: comparison of findings with histopathological assessment of retropubic radical prostatectomy specimens. Urol Int. 2006; 77(4):301–6.

192. Hom JJ, et al. Prostate cancer: endorectal MR imaging and MR spectroscopic imaging–distinction of true-positive results from chance-detected lesions. Radiology. 2006;238(1):192–9.

193. Heijmink SW, et al. Prostate cancer: body-array versus endorectal coil MR imaging at 3T–comparison of image quality, localization, and staging performance. Radiology. 2007;244(1):184–95.

194. Akin O, et al. Transition zone prostate cancers: features, detection, localization, and staging at endorectal MR imaging. Radiology. 2006;239(3): 784–92.

195. Hasumi M, et al. The combination of multi-voxel MR spectroscopy with MR imaging improve the diagnostic accuracy for localization of prostate cancer. Anticancer Res. 2003;23(5b):4223–7.

196. Hasumi M, et al. MR spectroscopy as a reliable diagnostic tool for localization of prostate cancer. Anticancer Res. 2002;22(2B):1205–8.

197. Wefer AE, et al. Sextant localization of prostate cancer: comparison of sextant biopsy, magnetic resonance imaging and magnetic resonance spectroscopic imaging with step section histology. J Urol. 2000; 164(2):400–4.

198. Scheidler J, et al. Prostate cancer: localization with three-dimensional proton MR spectroscopic imaging–clinicopathologic study. Radiology. 1999; 213(2):473–80.

199. Jager GJ, et al. Dynamic TurboFLASH subtraction technique for contrast-enhanced MR imaging of the prostate: correlation with histopathologic results. Radiology. 1997;203(3):645–52.

200. Franiel T, et al. Areas suspicious for prostate cancer: MR-guided biopsy in patients with at least one transrectal US-guided biopsy with a negative finding – multiparametric MR imaging for detection and biopsy planning. (Translated from eng) Radiology. 2011;259(1):162–72 (in eng).

201. Kumar V, et al. Correlation between metabolite ratios and ADC values of prostate in men with increased PSA level. Magn Reson Imaging. 2006; 24(5):541–8.

202. Mazaheri Y, et al. Prostate cancer: identification with combined diffusion-weighted MR imaging and 3D 1H MR spectroscopic imaging – correlation with pathologic findings. (Translated from eng) Radiology. 2008;246(2):480–8 (in eng).

203. Villeirs GM, et al. Combined magnetic resonance imaging and spectroscopy in the assessment of high grade prostate carcinoma in patients with elevated PSA: a single-institution experience of 356 patients. (Translated from eng) Eur J Radiol. 2011;77(2):340–5 (in eng).

204. Turkbey B, et al. Multiparametric 3T prostate magnetic resonance imaging to detect cancer: histopathological correlation using prostatectomy specimens processed in customized magnetic resonance imaging based molds. (Translated from eng) J Urol. 2011;186(5):1818–24 (in eng).

205. Sciarra A, et al. Advances in magnetic resonance imaging: how they are changing the management of prostate cancer. (Translated from eng) Eur Urol. 2011;59(6):962–77 (in eng).

206. Mazaheri Y, et al. Prostate tumor volume measurement with combined T2-weighted imaging and diffusion-weighted MR: correlation with pathologic tumor volume. (Translated from eng) Radiology. 252(2):449–57 (in eng).

207. Schenck JF, et al. Superconducting open-configuration MR imaging system for image-guided therapy. (Translated from eng) Radiology. 1995; 195(3):805–14 (in eng).

208. Cormack RA, et al. Feasibility of transperineal prostate biopsy under interventional magnetic resonance guidance. (Translated from eng) Urology. 2000;56(4):663–4 (in eng).

209. Hata N, et al. MR imaging-guided prostate biopsy with surgical navigation software: device validation and feasibility. (Translated from eng) Radiology. 2001;220(1):263–8 (in eng).

210. Tempany C, Straus S, Hata N, Haker S. MR-guided prostate interventions. (Translated from eng) J Magn Reson Imaging. 2008;27(2):356–67 (in eng).

211. Susil RC, et al. System for prostate brachytherapy and biopsy in a standard 1.5 T MRI scanner. Magn Reson Med. 2004;52(3):683–7.

212. Krieger A, et al. Design of a novel MRI compatible manipulator for image guided prostate interventions. (Translated from eng) IEEE Trans Biomed Eng. 2005;52(2):306–13 (in eng).

213. Susil RC, et al. Transrectal prostate biopsy and fiducial marker placement in a standard 1.5 T magnetic resonance imaging scanner. J Urol. 2006;175(1):113–20.

214. Yuen JS, et al. Endorectal magnetic resonance imaging and spectroscopy for the detection of tumor foci in men with prior negative transrectal ultrasound prostate biopsy. (Translated from eng) J Urol. 2004;171(4):1482–6 (in eng).

215. Prando A, Kurhanewicz J, Borges AP, Oliveira EM Jr, Figueiredo E. Prostatic biopsy directed with endorectal MR spectroscopic imaging findings in patients with elevated prostate specific antigen levels and prior negative biopsy findings: early experience. (Translated from eng) Radiology. 2005; 236(3):903–10 (in eng).

216. Labanaris AP, Engelhard K, Zugor V, Nutzel R, Kuhn R. Prostate cancer detection using an extended prostate biopsy schema in combination with additional targeted cores from suspicious images in conventional and functional endorectal magnetic resonance imaging of the prostate. (Translated from eng) Prostate Cancer Prostatic Dis. 2010;13(1):65–70 (in eng).

217. Haffner J, et al. Role of magnetic resonance imaging before initial biopsy: comparison of magnetic resonance imaging-targeted and systematic biopsy for significant prostate cancer detection. (Translated from Eng) BJU Int. 2011;108(8 Pt 2):E171–8 (in Eng).

218. Sciarra A, et al. Value of magnetic resonance spectroscopy imaging and dynamic contrast-enhanced imaging for detecting prostate cancer foci in men with prior negative biopsy. (Translated from eng) Clin Cancer Res. 2010;16(6):1875–83 (in eng).

219. Panebianco V, et al. Role of magnetic resonance spectroscopic imaging ([(1)H]MRSI) and dynamic contrast-enhanced MRI (DCE-MRI) in identifying prostate cancer foci in patients with negative biopsy and high levels of prostate-specific antigen (PSA). (Translated from eng ita) Radiol Med (Torino). 2010;115(8):1314–29 (in eng ita).

220. Ouzzane A, et al. Combined multiparametric MRI and targeted biopsies improve anterior prostate cancer detection, staging, and grading. (Translated from Eng) Urology. 2011;78(6):1356–62 (in eng).

221. Rouviere O, et al. Prostate cancer transrectal HIFU ablation: detection of local recurrences using T2-weighted and dynamic contrast-enhanced MRI. (Translated from eng) Eur Radiol. 2010;20(1):48–55 (in eng).

222. Anastasiadis AG, et al. MRI-guided biopsy of the prostate increases diagnostic performance in men with elevated or increasing PSA levels after previous negative TRUS biopsies. Eur Urol. 2006;50(4):738–48. discussion 748–739.

223. Beyersdorff D, et al. MRI of prostate cancer at 1.5 and 3.0 T: comparison of image quality in tumor detection and staging. (Translated from eng) AJR Am J Roentgenol. 2005;185(5):1214–20 (in eng).

224. Engelhard K, et al. Prostate biopsy in the supine position in a standard 1.5-T scanner under real time MR-imaging control using a MR-compatible endorectal biopsy device. Eur Radiol. 2006;16(6): 1237–43.

225. Hambrock T, et al. Thirty-two-channel coil 3T magnetic resonance-guided biopsies of prostate tumor suspicious regions identified on multimodality 3T magnetic resonance imaging: technique and feasibility. (Translated from eng) Invest Radiol. 2008;43(10):686–94 (in eng).

226. Hambrock T, et al. Magnetic resonance imaging guided prostate biopsy in men with repeat negative biopsies and increased prostate specific antigen. (Translated from eng) J Urol. 2010;183(2):520–7 (in eng).

227. Hambrock T, et al. Relationship between apparent diffusion coefficients at 3.0-T MR imaging and Gleason grade in peripheral zone prostate cancer. (Translated from eng) Radiology. 2011;259(2):453–61 (in eng).

228. Jung A, Coakley F, Westphalen A, Vigneron D, Kurhanewicz J. Comparison of TRUS vs. MRI guided biopsy in MRI apparent prostate cancers: preliminary results. International Society for Magnetic Resonance in Medicine 20th scientific meeting; 2012, Melbourne, Australia.

229. Muntener M, et al. Transperineal prostate intervention: robot for fully automated MR imaging – system description and proof of principle in a canine model. (Translated from eng) Radiology. 2008;247(2):543–9 (in eng).

230. Stoianovici D, et al. "MRI stealth" robot for prostate interventions. (Translated from eng) Mini Invasive Ther Allied Technol. 2007;16(4):241–8 (in eng).

231. Reynier C, et al. MRI/TRUS data fusion for prostate brachytherapy. Preliminary results. (Translated from eng) Med Phys. 2004;31(6):1568–75 (in eng).

232. Daanen V, et al. MRI/TRUS data fusion for brachytherapy. (Translated from eng) Int J Med Robot. 2006;2(3):256–61 (in eng).

233. Xu S, et al. Closed-loop control in fused MR-TRUS image-guided prostate biopsy. (Translated from eng) Med Image Comput Comput Assist Interv. 2007;10(Pt 1):128–35 (in eng).

234. Singh AK, et al. Initial clinical experience with real-time transrectal ultrasonography-magnetic resonance imaging fusion-guided prostate biopsy. (Translated from eng) BJU Int. 2008;101(7):841–5 (in eng).

235. Xu S, et al. Real-time MRI-TRUS fusion for guidance of targeted prostate biopsies. (Translated from eng) Comput Aided Sur. 2008;13(5):255–64 (in eng).

236. Ukimura O, et al. Technique for a hybrid system of real-time transrectal ultrasound with preoperative magnetic resonance imaging in the guidance of targeted prostate biopsy. (Translated from eng) Int J Urol. 2010;17(10):890–3 (in eng).

237. Kuru TH, et al. MRI navigated stereotactic prostate biopsy: fusion of MRI and real-time transrectal ultrasound images for perineal prostate biopsies. (Translated from Ger) Urologe A. 2011;51(1):50–6 (in Ger).

238. Natarajan S, et al. Clinical application of a 3D ultrasound-guided prostate biopsy system. (Translated from eng) Urol Oncol. 2011;29(3):334–42 (in eng).

239. Turkbey B, et al. Documenting the location of prostate biopsies with image fusion. (Translated from eng) BJU Int. 2011;107(1):53–7 (in eng).

240. Turkbey B, et al. Documenting the location of systematic transrectal ultrasound-guided prostate biopsies: correlation with multi-parametric MRI. (Translated from eng) Cancer Imaging. 2011;11:31–6 (in eng).

241. Pickett B, Vigneault E, Kurhanewicz J, Verhey L, Roach M. Static field intensity modulation to treat a dominant intra-prostatic lesion to 90 Gy compared to seven field 3-dimensional radiotherapy. Int J Radiat Oncol Biol Phys. 1999;44(4):921–9.

242. Xia P, Pickett B, Vigneault E, Verhey LJ, Roach 3rd M. Forward or inversely planned segmental multileaf collimator IMRT and sequential tomotherapy to treat multiple dominant intraprostatic lesions of prostate cancer to 90 Gy. Int J Radiat Oncol Biol Phys. 2001;51(1):244–54.

243. DiBiase SJ, et al. Magnetic resonance spectroscopic imaging-guided brachytherapy for localized prostate cancer. Int J Radiat Oncol Biol Phys. 2002;52(2):429–38.

244. Pouliot J, et al. Inverse planning for HDR prostate brachytherapy used to boost dominant intraprostatic lesions defined by magnetic resonance spectroscopy imaging. Int J Radiat Oncol Biol Phys. 2004;59(4):1196–207.

245. Zaider M, et al. Treatment planning for prostate implants using magnetic-resonance spectroscopy imaging. Int J Radiat Oncol Biol Phys. 2000;47(4):1085–96.

246. Kim Y, et al. Class solution in inverse planned HDR prostate brachytherapy for dose escalation of DIL defined by combined MRI/MRSI. (Translated from eng) Radiother Oncol. 2008;88(1):148–55 (in eng).

247. Barnes AS, et al. Magnetic resonance spectroscopy-guided transperineal prostate biopsy and brachytherapy for recurrent prostate cancer. (Translated from eng) Urology. 2005;66(6):1319 (in eng).

248. Pauly KB, et al. Magnetic resonance-guided high-intensity ultrasound ablation of the prostate. (Translated from eng) Top Magn Reson Imaging. 2006;17(3):195–207 (in eng).

249. Raz O, et al. Real-time magnetic resonance imaging-guided focal laser therapy in patients with low-risk prostate cancer. (Translated from eng) Eur Urol. 2010;58(1):173–7 (in eng).

250. Lindner U, et al. Focal laser ablation for prostate cancer followed by radical prostatectomy: validation of focal therapy and imaging accuracy. (Translated from eng) Eur Urol. 2010;57(6):1111–4 (in eng).

251. Lindner U, et al. Image guided photothermal focal therapy for localized prostate cancer: phase I trial. (Translated from eng) J Urol. 2009;182(4):1371–7 (in eng).

Role of Imaging as an Adjunct or Replacement for Biopsy: European Experience

24

Arnauld Villers, Philippe Puech,
Hashim Uddin Ahmed, and Mark Emberton

Introduction

The use of MRI in prostate cancer management remains controversial, but its use is growing fast. As a result, current clinical-practice guidelines fail to keep up with developments that are both technological and clinical. In this chapter we, rather controversially, propose that an increase in the use of mp-MRI within the diagnostic pathway would result in an enhanced detection of clinically significant disease, fewer men diagnosed with clinically insignificant disease, fewer men biopsied overall, and fewer needle deployments in those that are.

The optimal prostate cancer diagnostic strategy would reliably identify all cancers that could harm the patient at a time when cure is possible as well as causing very little harm in a cost-effective

A. Villers, M.D. (✉)
Department of Urology, Hospital Huriez, University
Lille Nord de France, Lille, France
e-mail: arnauld.villers@wanadoo.fr

P. Puech, M.D.
Department of Radiology, CHRU, Hospital Huriez,
University Lille Nord de France, Lille 59037, France

H.U. Ahmed, MRCS, BM, B.Ch. (Oxon), B.A. (Hon)
M. Emberton, FRCS (Urol), FRCS, M.D., MBBS, B.Sc.
Department of Urology, University College London
Hospitals, NHS Foundation Trust, London, UK

Division of Surgery and Interventional Science,
University College London, London, UK

manner. Implicit in the above strategy is that men with clinically insignificant disease—the majority of men over the age of 60 years—could safely avoid a biopsy.

Traditional biopsy indication based on PSA threshold and the traditional biopsy technique such as TRUS-guided 12–14-core systematic (posterior prostate) biopsies can lead to a misdiagnosis, i.e., overdiagnosis of clinically insignificant cancer or underdetection of clinically significant cancer. There are also parts of the prostate where, in even with an extended systematic biopsy scheme, the needle cannot easily reach, so biopsy results can be misleading.

The evolution of prostate biopsy over the last few decades can be represented by 4 ages of prostate biopsy. The old pathway before the PSA era was based on rectal examination and finger-guided biopsies followed closely by our current diagnostic pathway can be seen as the *Stone and Dark Ages*, respectively, since both procedures were carried out blind to the location of the cancer. The *Modern Age* can be seen as that based on prebiopsy anatomical and functional imaging to target the needle to significant cancer that is "seen" so that detection and personalized risk stratification are improved. Indeed, this era is with us now and a number of expert centers internationally are using it and have demonstrated excellent results. The future lies in diffusion and dissemination to demonstrate that the techniques and expertise can be replicated and reproduced.

We believe that the agent to deliver this optimal pathway—multiparametric MRI (mp-MRI)—is widely available, but its application requires a degree of discipline in its conduct, reporting, and evaluation [1].

One proof of concept relating to the criterion validity of mp-MRI against histopathology relates to the concept of image-targeted biopsies. Targeted biopsies to the clinical phenotype are the norm in all other solid organ cancers—whether by direct visualization or by use of imaging. The strategy of targeted biopsies to an mp-MRI suspicious area has the potential to improve biopsy results by improving detection of clinically significant cancers, reduced detection of clinically insignificant cancer, and more representative sampling of cancer (length and grade on biopsy) which allows improved risk stratification. It could do all this and use fewer number of biopsy cores required to obtain this information. For instance, in men with previous negative biopsies, a number of centers have independently obtained detection rates ranging from 30% to 59% (mostly anterior cancers), performing targeted biopsies to an MRI suspicious lesion [2–7]. Indeed, as an additional benefit, cancer upstaging and upgrading were also improved by 44% using targeted biopsies [8]. Overall, the targeted biopsies-only strategy without systematic biopsies was proven to be superior to standard TRUS-guided biopsies [9].

In addition to the role of mp-MRI as a target-generation test prior to a first or a subsequent biopsy, mp-MRI may have an even more important role in deferring prostate biopsy in men who have a low probability of harboring clinically significant disease. A normal mp-MRI, due to its very high negative predictive value for clinically significant disease, can be used as a triage test, much in the way that a normal mammogram will be used to reassure a woman that she is at low risk of breast cancer. Recent work by Haffner and colleagues from Lille University-France and Cleveland Clinic Foundation-USA illustrates just what benefits might result [9]. Just under half of subjects (42%) might be able to avoid a biopsy by virtue of a normal mp-MRI. This translates to a 13% reduction in the proportion of men that are diagnosed as having clinically insignificant prostate cancer.

This idea has been around for some time but has not yet been embraced by the wider urological community [10]. The reason why this is the case remains both important and interesting. Ahmed and colleagues advocate increased use of mp-MRI prior to biopsy but acknowledge that the will and competencies required to deliver this may be nested in just a few centers at present. The authors highlight reasons why mp-MRI may underperform when used informally. The problems of postbiopsy artifact have almost certainly been underestimated as a confounder affecting the performance of mp-MRI as have issues of optimal sequences and machine setups.

The economic implications for carrying out mp-MRI in every man who requires a prostate biopsy need careful consideration. Our proposed prebiopsy mp-MRI strategy involves a resource adjustment and may require initial investment. In pure cost terms the prospect does not look too daunting as within the European Union an mp-MRI costs about 300 € (USD 424). However, in the USA, charges for a three-part mp-MRI begin at 1,400 € (USD 2,000), a discrepancy in charge that we do not fully understand. In both jurisdictions the charges associated with TRUS-guided biopsy, including pathology costs and biopsy-related complications, exceed the charges associated with TRUS-guided biopsy. Moreover, it should be acknowledged that men who test positive on biopsy increasingly do subsequently get an MRI, albeit one compromised by artifact and as a result subject to an increased rate of both false positives and false negatives. True reductions in the cost of care will result from fewer men biopsied and better risk stratification in those that are. This should translate to fewer prostate cancer labels (clinically insignificant cancer) that serve no benefit to the patient and as such can only confer harm and cost.

Ultrasound Techniques

Prior to discussing the role of MRI in prostate cancer detection and characterization, it would be prudent to summarize the role that ultrasound and modern ultrasound techniques have in this field.

Transrectal ultrasonography imaging has reasonable accuracy for lesions located in the peripheral zone (PZ), but the observed heterogeneity of the transition zone (TZ) during TRUS prevents consistent visualization of TZ cancers. In a study by Toi et al., suspicious lesions detected during TRUS significantly increased the likelihood of cancer detection by a factor of 1.8 (57.8% vs. 30.8%). Likewise, subsequent biopsies from these lesions had an increased median percent of cancer involvement in each biopsy core versus randomly acquired biopsies (50% vs. 10%, $p<0.001$) and were more likely to have Gleason score 7 or higher (69.3% vs. 28.3%, $p<0.001$) [11]. However, no specific information was provided by the authors in regard to biopsy location (anterior vs. posterior gland). In a different study, consisting of 544 patients with abnormal PSA and a 35% prostate cancer prevalence, TRUS was found to have sensitivity and specificity of 41% and 85%, respectively [12].

Real-time elastography is a promising modality for identification of posterior cancers although it remains to be robustly validated. In one study by Walz [13], real-time elastography alone did not allow the operator to identify the prostate cancer index lesion with satisfactory reliability. In another study [14], 84 patients with suspected prostate cancer and scheduled for prostate biopsies underwent real-time elastography, TRUS, and MRI. The findings of real-time elastography were compared with those of other examinations and pathological findings. Of these 84 patients, 36 had benign lesions and 48 had prostate cancer, from peripheral zone. The diagnostic sensitivity, specificity, accuracy, positive predictive value, and negative predictive value were 91.7%, 72.2%, 83.3%, 81.5%, and 86.7% for real-time elastography and 85.4%, 63.9%, 76.2%, 75.9%, and 76.7% for TRUS ($p>0.05$). The real-time elastography findings were not significantly correlated with the pathological findings and PSA ($p>0.05$), and the diagnostic sensitivity of real-time elastography decreased along with the enlargement of prostate. If real-time elastography can be used as a diagnostic test to supplement clinical diagnosis of cancer, it has to be validated against a detailed accurate reference standard such as radical prostatectomy.

Contrast-enhanced color Doppler ultrasound (CECD-US) necessitates intravenous injection of microbubble US contrast agent. In one study, a significant benefit of CECD-US targeted biopsy relative to systematic biopsies was demonstrated [14]. Targeted biopsies were performed in hypervascular areas in the peripheral zone and compared to systematic biopsy. Of 1,776 patients, cancer was detected in 559 patients (31%), including 476 of the 1,776 patients (27%) with CECD-US and 410 (23%) with systematic biopsy ($p<0.001$). The detection rate for CECD-US targeted biopsy cores (10.8% or 961 of 8,880 cores) was significantly better than for systematic biopsy cores (5.1% or 910 of 17,760 cores, $p<0.001$). Among patients with a positive biopsy for prostate cancer, cancer was detected by CECD-US alone in 149 patients (27%) and by systematic biopsy alone in 83 (15%) ($p<0.001$). Again, the diagnosis of anterior tumors was not studied, with radical prostatectomy specimens as reference standard.

Multiparametric MRI (mp-MRI)

Multiparametric MRI (mp-MRI) of the prostate obtained prior to biopsy is effective for prostate cancer identification and characterization.

Multiparametric MRI (mp-MRI) of the prostate of patients with suspicious lesions for malignancy is shown to be effective in both anterior and posterior areas of the gland [1, 15, 16] (Fig. 24.1). A recent European MRI consensus panel [1] recommended that this modern imaging modality needs to be delivered in a quality-controlled manner with uniformly high standards and incorporated as a test prior to biopsy. The panel reached agreement on 67% of 260 items related to imaging sequence parameters. For instance, T2-weighted, dynamic contrast-enhanced, and diffusion-weighted MRI were the key sequences incorporated into the minimum requirements, but spectroscopy was not recommended. Consensus was also reached on 54% of

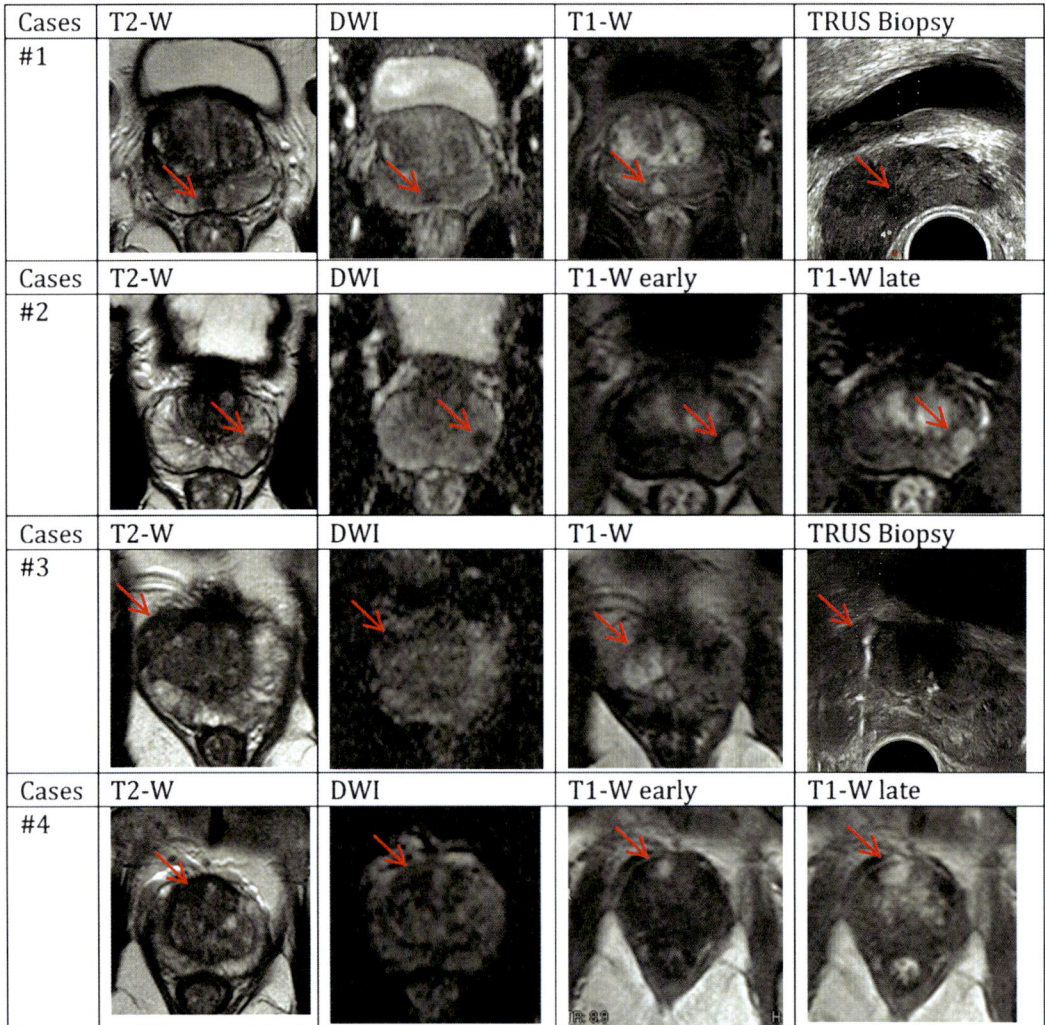

Fig. 24.1 Four cases of prostate cancers identified at multiparametric 1.5 T MRI and diagnosed by targeted biopsies. Axial T2-W, DW, T1-W DCE, and axial TRUS images. Visual reading of all sequences allows suspicious score and location determination. Suspicious areas at MRI are shown with *red arrows*. Case #1: cancer located in PZ at midline with 7-mm hyposignal area (T2-W), low ADC (DW), and intense early enhancement (T1-W DCE) with a suspicious score of 5. TRUS showed hypoechoic corresponding area. PSA = 7.9 ng/ml. Maximal cancer length was 6 mm at targeted biopsies Gleason score 4 + 4. Systematic biopsies were negative. Case #2: cancer located in the left lobe of PZ with 10-mm hyposignal area (T2-W), low ADC (DW), and intense early enhancement (T1-W DCE) with a suspicious score of 5. TRUS showed hypoechoic corresponding area. PSA = 6.9 ng/ml. Maximal cancer length was 6 mm at targeted biopsies Gleason score 4 + 4. Systematic biopsies were negative. Case #3: cancer located in right anterolateral horn of PZ with 19-mm hyposignal area (T2-W), low ADC (DW), and weak enhancement (T1-W DCE) with a suspicious score of 4. TRUS showed equivocal hypoechoic corresponding area. PSA = 7.8 ng/ml. Maximal cancer length was 4 mm at targeted biopsies Gleason score 3 + 4. Systematic biopsies were negative. Case #4: APC located in AFMS anterior to right TZ at apex with 13-mm hyposignal area (T2-W), low ADC (DW), and intense early enhancement (T1-W DCE) with a suspicious score of 5. TRUS showed equivocal hypoechoic corresponding area. Maximal cancer length was 7 mm at targeted biopsies and systematic biopsies were negative

Fig. 24.2 Twenty-seven-sector standardized MRI report prostate scheme. Average axial sections at prostate base, midgland, and apex are subdivided into four posterior regions (*p*) (midlobar and lateral), four anterior regions (*a*) (midlobar and lateral), and three anterior stroma regions (*as*), at the *center*, anterior to glandular zones. Twelve-core biopsy scheme samples the 12 posterior sectors [16] (Adapted from Dickinson et al. [1])

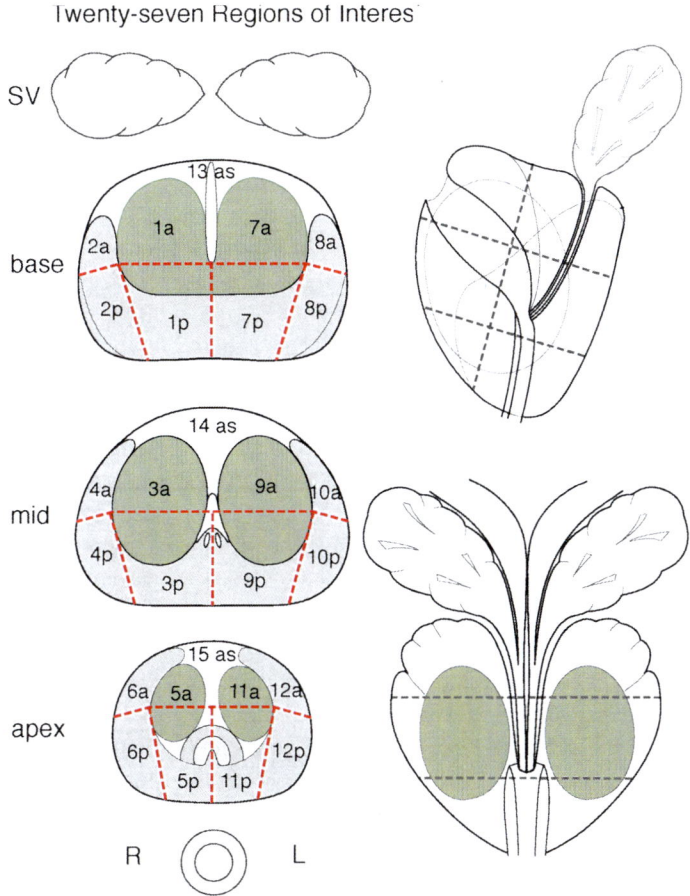

Twenty-seven Regions of Interest

260 items related to image interpretation and reporting, including features of malignancy on individual sequences. A five-point scale was agreed on for communicating the probability of malignancy, with a minimum of 16–27 prostatic sectors of analysis to include a pictorial representation of suspicious foci (Fig. 24.2). Due to the increase in signal-to-noise ratio, 3 T MRI clearly improves spatiotemporal and spectral resolutions of prostate imaging on all sequences. However, imaging criteria for malignancy seem to be comparable at 3 and 1.5 T with pelvic coil. A pelvic-phased array coil for 1.5 T MRI was deemed sufficient for standard clinical practice, and endorectal coil is not mandatory anymore for prostate cancer detection.

Mp-MRI is very sensitive and specific for anterior and posterior cancers [15, 17, 18]. At volume >0.5 cm^3, sensitivity and specificity were 86% and 94% (area under receiver operating characteristic curve [AUC] 0.874). Negative predictive value was 95%. Mean cancer volume detected at MRI was 2.44 ml (0.02–14.5), and those lesions not detected at MRI were mean 0.16 ml (0.01–2.4) in size. Correlation between cancer volumes using T1-W MRI sequences with dynamic gadolinium contrast sequences and histopathology for large tumors (>0.2 cm^3) detected by MRI (n=30) is good (r^2 value of 0.530741) [19].

Magnetic resonance spectroscopy imaging (MRSI) allows assessment of tissue metabolism in a single or in a grid of multiple voxels. Technically, an endorectal coil is required because of its high signal-to-noise ratio (SNR), but new HR-PPA at 3 T may challenge the need for endorectal coils [20, 21] in the near future. The added value of MRSI for identification of confined PZ or TZ cancers and treatment planning is still controversial with large multicentre series questioning its value [22].

Historically, imaging tests have been used to contribute little other than anatomical information about the location and extent of the cancer to aid loco-regional staging. Increasingly, functional imaging techniques provide information not just about tumor location but also about cancer behavior. For example, degree of enhancement on *T1-W sequences with gadolinium* may be related to Gleason grade [23]. In a series of 93 patients, AUC for detection of cancers with Gleason grade 4 or 5 at T1-W sequences with gadolinium was 0.819. Also, numerous early studies have documented correlations between apparent diffusion coefficient (ADC) values obtained with diffusion-weighted MR imaging and Gleason scores [24–28]. Less differentiated and dense cancers are associated with lower *ADC values at DWI* and higher detection rates [27, 29, 30]. In a study with cases performed at 3.0 T, ADC values showed an inverse relationship to Gleason grades in peripheral zone prostate cancer. A high discriminatory performance was achieved in the differentiation of low-, intermediate-, and high-grade cancer [31]. Significant differences between the ADC values of low- and intermediate-risk prostate cancer have been found, and in a cohort of patients on active surveillance, the baseline ADC value was an independent predictor of both adverse repeat biopsy findings and time to radical treatment [29, 32].

The Role of Prebiopsy MRI with Targeted Biopsies

The current diagnostic process, which has inherent random and systematic errors related to the biopsy technique, underestimates the true cancer grade in up to one third and the cancer burden in up to one half of men diagnosed with low-risk disease [33]. As a result of these errors, localization of individual tumors within the prostate is poor, whereas mp-MRI is very sensitive for both anterior and posterior cancer detection; recent published data support the concept of MRI-targeted biopsy [18, 34].

TRUS Guidance-Only Biopsies Without Prebiopsy MRI. Standard practice is to use TRUS guidance to take 10–14 transrectal needle biopsies in a systematic fashion. TRUS is used to locate the prostate gland itself but otherwise plays little part in guiding the biopsy procedure. Consequently, random error occurs, as the operator has no knowledge of where the cancerous areas may be. In addition, systematic error occurs because primarily the peripheral zone is sampled during an initial biopsy, and sampling of the anterior peripheral and transition zones is inadequate [35], whereas extreme anterior apical biopsies were shown to improve detection [36]. One way to overcome these errors is to sample the gland using more and more biopsies. Saturation TRUS biopsies have shown minimal utility in this regard [37].

3-D transperineal template prostate mapping biopsies provide several benefits compared to the conventional TRUS-guided biopsy. First, it is able to detect disease with greater accuracy by overcoming random and systematic errors of TRUS-guided biopsy since it fixes the sampling frame to 5 mm and samples the whole gland [38, 39]. Although 3-D TPM biopsy is a reliable and detailed method of mapping individual prostate tumors, it may remain a temporary step in our quest for image-guided diagnosis and treatment, as it has several disadvantages that may limit its long-term use.

Targeted biopsies-only strategy without systematic biopsies was retrospectively studied, in a series of 555 men referred for elevated PSA [9]. MRI was positive in 351 (63%) patients and overall 302 (54%) had cancer at systematic biopsies and/or targeted biopsies. This 54% detection rate is consistent with the average 50% detection rate observed in a European population of unselected newly screened patients with no history of biopsy and a median PSA of 6.75 [0.18–100]. Detection accuracy of significant prostate cancer by targeted biopsies was higher than systematic biopsies ($p < 0.001$). Furthermore, targeted biopsies detected 16% more Gleason grade 4 or 5 cancers and better quantified the burden of cancer than systematic biopsies, with a cancer core length involvement of 5.56 mm versus 4.70 mm ($p = 0.0018$). These results demonstrate the role of prebiopsy MRI with targeted biopsies.

Targeting biopsies guidance to an MRI suspicious area can be carried out in several ways. Targeting biopsies to an MRI suspicious area was proven to be very effective in improving detection of anterior-located cancers, beyond the area sampled by posterior biopsies, which represent 20% of the largest cancers in unselected patients suspected to have prostate cancer [18]. This was true when tissue biopsy was performed under TRUS guidance with MRI "cognitive" coregistration [8].

Free-hand cognitive targeted biopsies under TRUS guidance is easy to perform as office-based procedure by the urologist. There is indeed a fundamental methodological limitation of the biopsy technique to use virtual MR data for TRUS-guided biopsy, in which the biopsy is not truly MR guided. The accuracy of TRUS-guided biopsy with cognitive virtual use of MR-detected suspicious findings has not been formally studied. However, there are convincing results that additional two cores from operator use of MR data for TRUS-guided free-hand cognitive biopsy accurately hit the lesion. Hence, the correlation coefficient between the cancer length on targeted biopsies (median 8 mm, IQR: 7–12) and the anteroposterior diameter of the largest area suspicious for malignancy on MRI (median 10 mm, IQR: 8–14) was $r^2 = 0.6$ ($p < 0.001$) [8]. In this study, MRI was performed immediately before each biopsy. For each area of suspicion (anterior or posterior gland), 2–4 additional targeted biopsy cores were obtained (Fig. 24.1), resulting in a total mean of 15 (range 14–18) biopsy cores per patient. Each MRI scheme was evaluated simultaneously by both a radiologist and an urologist, which allowed the urologist performing the biopsies to localize the suspicious areas during TRUS. Targeted biopsies were performed by free hand, sampling each one of the suspicious areas based on the 27-section MRI scheme (Fig. 24.2).

Suspicious posterior areas at MRI are mostly associated with corresponding hypoechoic areas at TRUS, which help needle guidance. Suspicious anterior areas on TRUS are not identified in all cases due to the heterogeneity of the transition zone at TRUS and the normal hypoechogenicity of the AFMS. However, in some cases, the anterior area corresponding to the MRI abnormality shows equivocal hypoechoic areas with contours roughly similar to the contours seen at MRI. These TRUS anterior abnormalities are used as well as anatomic landmarks to target the biopsies despite their (very) low suspicious pattern in all cases and the fact that they would not have even been identified without prebiopsy MRI.

MRI-directed real-time biopsy (MRI guidance) was also proven to be very effective in improving detection [2–7]. In these studies of patients with negative first biopsy, the detection rate with MRI guidance were 59%, 30%, and 52% and 41%, 45.5%, and 31.5%, respectively. However, in-bore MRI guidance requires specialist expertise and additional equipment and is lengthy and expensive. No comparative study of various targeting modalities is available.

The concept of fusion of the MR images to the ultrasound images used at the time of biopsy, using virtual navigation systems with rigid registration or 3-D acquisition with elastic registration, is under evaluation. In one study, this fusion of real-time TRUS and prior MR images of the prostate proved its feasibility and enables MRI-guided biopsies outside of the MRI suite [40].

Quality of sampling is higher than with systematic biopsies. There is clear evidence of TRUS-guided targeted biopsy to image suspicious areas for malignancy that can reveal greater volume of cancers and higher grade than systematic 12-core posterior biopsies. In a study of 46 anterior cancer cases, median cancer length of the most involved core in targeted compared to systematic biopsies was 8 mm versus 1 mm ($p < 0.001$), respectively, for the 25 cases sampled by both targeted and systematic biopsies [8]. Sensitivity of biopsy for high-grade disease was also improved with biopsies targeted to MRI lesion. Significant Gleason score upgrading was observed in 11 of 25 (44%) cases.

Prebiopsy MRI to Rule Out Cancer and Avoid Biopsies: mp-MRI as a Triage Test

The Negative Predictive Value of mp-MRI to Rule Out Significant Cancer Foci (>0.5 cm³) in Clinically Localized Disease. Prostatic biopsy strategies aim to improve cancer detection and sample the cancer for volume estimation and grade. The standardization of extended biopsy protocols (10–12 cores) over the past decade improved cancer diagnosis, but is associated with detection of micro-focal cancer lesions (≤0.5 cc) [41] that may be clinically insignificant and are unlikely to require treatment. Targeted biopsies-only strategy without systematic biopsies would have the potential to avoid the unnecessary diagnosis of these micro-focal cancer lesions. This was observed in the simulation study in which 13% (53/302) of nonsignificant prostate cancer diagnosis was avoided while necessitating an average of 3.8 cores performed in only 63% of patients with positive MRI [9]. It was also demonstrated in a study by Rouse et al. that mp-MRI has a role in ruling in and ruling out clinically significant prostate cancer in men at risk prior to biopsy [42]. Negative predictive value (NPV) of 94% is high enough for ruling out clinically significant disease and may act as triage test for biopsy (rebiopsy) indication and may result in fewer men needing to undergo further biopsy. Therefore, prebiopsy MR imaging could be added to men before diagnosis of prostate cancer or to men referred to active surveillance protocols.

MR imaging could be added to active surveillance protocols as a replacement for biopsies. If the test-retest reliability of imaging is shown to be good, it may even be possible to replace serial biopsy during active surveillance with serial imaging, supplemented by biopsy only as needed. Nomograms have been shown to be useful for the prediction of a number of outcomes in men with

prostate cancer [43–45]. In a meta-analysis, it was concluded that a limited number of small studies suggest that MRI combined with MRSI could be a rule-in test for low-risk patients. This finding needs further confirmation in larger studies and cost-effectiveness needs to be established [46]. When considering the use of imaging as a predictive tool for men considering or undergoing active surveillance, one option is to compare different imaging approaches for their ability to predict pathological outcomes at radical prostatectomy. However, pathological outcomes do not directly reflect long-term clinical outcomes. It would, therefore, be valuable to compare imaging at diagnosis with the longer-term outcomes of treated or untreated disease. For example, some early work suggests that ADC values on diffusion-weighted MRI may be a better predictor of clinical outcome than Gleason score [32].

Ongoing or Future Protocols

Evaluating Imaging in the Selection of Patients for Prostate Biopsy

Three aspects of any novel imaging approach must be evaluated if we are to integrate it into the diagnostic pathway. First, can imaging confidently rule out clinically insignificant cancer to negative predictive values approaching 90–95% (need for biopsy surrogate to monitor the prostate)? Second, can imaging reliably detect cancer which could be located in the various prostatic zones (posterior, transition, central, and anterior fibromuscular stroma) [47, 48] (Fig. 24.3)? Third, can imaging provide detailed characterization of a lesion based on grade and burden?

One way of improving identification in individuals referred for screening is prebiopsy mp-MRI which would provide guidance for targeting biopsies and for selecting and monitoring patients who will undergo tissue-preserving therapies such as active surveillance or focal therapy. A recent transatlantic consensus group met to consider the potential role of emerging diagnostic tools such as precision imaging and transperineal prostate mapping biopsy in improving

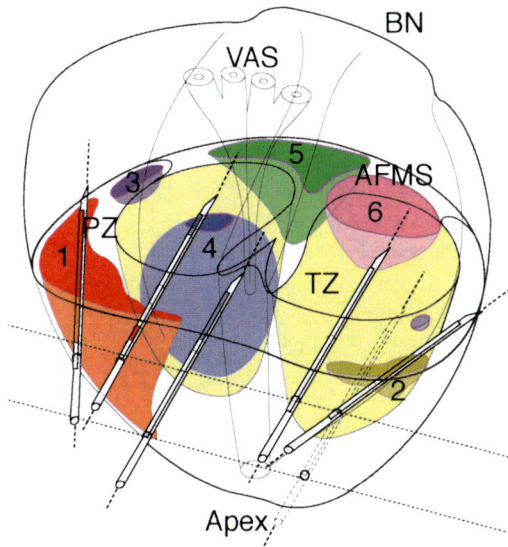

Fig. 24.3 D posterolateral view of a schematic prostate gland showing zonal anatomy. Peripheral zone (*PZ*), transition zone (*TZ*), anterior fibromuscular stroma (*AFMS*), average cancer size, and location are displayed. Posterior systematic biopsy needles and tracks are displayed (lateral and medio-lobar at midgland and medio-lobar at apex). (*1*) PZ posterolateral cancer 4 cc sampled by both lateral and midlobar biopsies. (*2*) PZ posterolateral cancer 0.9 cc sampled by lateral biopsy. (*3*) PZ anterolateral cancer 0.6 cc not sampled by posterior systematic biopsies. (*4*) TZ anterior cancer 2 cc sampled by midlobar biopsies. (*5*) AFMS anterior cancer 1 cc not sampled by posterior systematic biopsies. (*6*) TZ/AFMS anterior cancer 1 cc not sampled by posterior systematic biopsies (Adapted from Bouye et al. and Haffner et al. [47, 48])

prostate cancer care (Ahmed et al., BJUI 2011, accepted in print). It is proposed that integrating these tools into prostate cancer research and management could lead to better risk stratification and more effective treatment allocation than we have at present. Also, besides the role of imaging as an adjunct for biopsy in case of suspicious PSA for cancer identification and biopsy targeting, it has a role after the diagnosis of cancer for monitoring in case of active surveillance or ablative treatment.

Rationale for MRI Study as a Triage Test

Most overdiagnosis occurs as a result of random interrogation of the prostate. Poor risk stratification results from poor representation of maximum Gleason grade and tumor volume by virtue of maximal cancer core length. Most important underdiagnosis occurs as a result of underrepresentation of anterior, midline, and apex during sampling. Negative TRUS biopsy status has limited clinical utility, given its low negative predictive value for clinically important disease. Image-guided biopsies may result in fewer biopsies (high negative predictive value), better biopsies (high positive predictive value), and better risk stratification (high sensitivity and specificity).

PROMIS Study

The validation of MRI as a triage test for biopsy indication has to be conducted in a randomized controlled study against standard systematic TRUS biopsies or within a large paired validating cohort study in which all men are subjected to the novel strategy (mp-MRI), the standard test (TRUS systematic posterior biopsies), and the reference standard for all men at risk of prostate (template prostate mapping). The latter is currently under way in the UK. Called the PROstate MR Imaging Study, or PROMIS, this will provide level 1 evidence on this issue (http://clinicaltrials.gov/ct2/show/NCT01292291). PROMIS will involve recruitment of more than 500 men with suspected prostate cancer to take part in a trial to show whether noninvasive MRI scanning can be safely used to reduce the number of men having invasive biopsies across several major cancer centers in the UK.

Canada-UK-France-USA Consortium

It consists of a pivotal study project that would be of sufficient quality to change practice if a positive result is obtained.

A population of men referred for a biopsy, with PSA <20ug/L and no contraindications to mp-MRI, is randomized 1:1. Intervention arm referred for mp-MRI. For scores 1–2 (nonsuspicious), no biopsies performed for scores 3 (equivocal), 4, and 5 (suspicious), only two targeted biopsies per lesion are performed. Control arm patients were referred for standard of care with 12-core +/− 2-core TRUS-guided biopsy.

Outcomes consist of:

- Primary end points (based on biopsy results). Proportion of men diagnosed with clinically important prostate cancer (equivalence or superiority in intervention arm)
- Proportion of men diagnosed with clinically unimportant prostate cancer (inferiority in intervention arm)
- Secondary end points. Cancer cores length on most involved core. Maximum Gleason score on most involved core. Proportion of positive cores with any cancer
- Image-guided biopsies (principally MRI and TRUS) appear to confer sensitivities in excess of 80% for a variety of target thresholds: in a study, it was shown that TRUS-MRI fusion after biopsy can be used to document the location of each biopsy site, which can then be correlated with MRI findings (Turkbey 2011 #4274).

Key Points 1:

- *Multiparametric MRI (mp-MRI) of the prostate obtained prior to biopsy is accurate in identifying and characterizing prostate cancer.* Its sensitivity and specificity at identifying cancer foci of clinically significant volume (>0.5 cm³) is over 80% for anterior disease and over 90% for posterior disease. Mp-MRI predicts tumor volume accurately. It shows promise in grade prediction.
- *Ultrasound-based imaging is currently not as accurate as mp-MRI* with concerns over performance in the anterior gland. Correlation with radical prostatectomy specimens as a reference standard is required.
- *Prebiopsy MRI with targeted biopsies can be effective* in detecting a greater proportion of cancers that are clinically significant compared to standard TRUS-guided biopsies. The improved detection of mp-MRI-targeted biopsies has been seen with both MRI-directed real-time biopsy and TRUS guidance with MRI "cognitive" coregistration. Mp-MRI-targeted biopsies result in more representative sampling of the tumor and will aid in better risk stratification of disease. In a retrospective simulation study of 555 patients who had both systematic and targeted biopsies to MRI

suspicious abnormality, detection accuracy of 249 significant prostate cancer by targeted biopsy was higher than systematic biopsies ($p < 0.001$) [9].

- *Prebiopsy mp-MRI is able to rule out clinically significant cancer and may allow some men to avoid biopsies*
- The negative predictive value of mp-MRI to rule out clinically significant cancer foci (>0.5 cm³) in clinically localized disease is over 90%.
- *Strategy of targeted-only biopsies without* systematic sampling can reduce the detection of indolent cancer by over 10% of men sampled using fewer cores.
- *Ongoing or future protocols involve* role of mp-MRI as an adjunct for guiding TRUS biopsy, role of prebiopsy imaging as a triage test to determine those who need a biopsy, and role of MRI after the diagnosis of cancer for monitoring of progression or recurrence as part of tissue-preserving therapies such as active surveillance and minimally invasive focal ablative treatments.

Key Points 2:

MRI as an Adjunct for Biopsies

The standard of care for men with suspected prostate cancer is to have TRUS-guided biopsies. This might be considered as a reference standard to evaluate diagnostic tests for prostate cancer detection, but it is subject to a large verification bias [49]. There are several important reasons why this occurs and why TRUS-guided biopsy would serve as a poor reference test:

1. TRUS-guided biopsies have a false negative rate of up to 30% [50].
2. They systematically undersample the anterior, the midline, and the apical parts of the prostate.
3. The deployment of the biopsy needle is tangential (neither sagittal nor transverse), so it is difficult to attribute any sample to any particular location (i.e., base, midgland, or apex) within the prostate.
4. TRUS biopsies are unrepresentative of the true disease burden or grade of the cancer in more than one third of cases and therefore a poor indicator of prognostic factors such as Gleason grade and cancer burden [51–53].

5. This method may be leading to overdiagnosis and unnecessary surgery, as well as missing some important cancers.

Key Points 3:
MRI as a Triage Test Prior to Biopsy in Men at Risk
• At present, MRI is the only clinically available imaging modality that depicts the zonal anatomy of the prostate in detail.
• Anatomic MR imaging can be combined with functional and metabolic MR techniques such as dynamic contrast enhancement, diffusion weighting, and MR spectroscopy to facilitate better tumor detection and characterization and to obtain quantitative predictive and prognostic biomarkers [10].
• The optimal prostate cancer diagnostic strategy would involve low morbidity and cost to reliably identify cancers that present potential harm to the patient. It would also minimize unnecessary biopsy or other invasive procedures in patients that do not have harmful cancers, decreasing invasiveness—particularly in the number of biopsy cores.
• Furthermore, if a cancer exists that poses no potential to harm that patient, diagnosing cancer would cause potential psychological harm and unnecessary treatments with their attendant additional costs and morbidity. To date, no diagnostic strategy approaches this ideal [9].

Editorial Commentary:
Two issues have limited widespread use of MRI for prostate cancer detection. The first—cost—really reflects charges instead of the true cost of providing the examination. Thus, the "costs" vary greatly from country to country.
The second barrier is more significant, in that MRI requires a highly skilled team to obtain information adequate to drive clinical decisions. The authors have demonstrated this expertise for many years and have taught many of us—this editor included—much about the nuances of prostate imaging. Nevertheless, many centers just cannot achieve the results of the centers of excellence using current technology, so the challenge

remains to bring all centers up to standards approaching those of the teams in London, Lille, and similar institutions. As these and other authors continue to refine techniques, it will inevitably become possible for this technology to become adaptable throughout the urological community both for diagnosis and management of prostate cancer.

–J. Stephen Jones

References

1. Dickinson L, Ahmed HU, Allen C, Barentsz JO, Carey B, Futterer JJ, et al. Magnetic resonance imaging for the detection, localisation, and characterisation of prostate cancer: recommendations from a European consensus meeting. Eur Urol. 2011;59(4):477–94.
2. Hambrock T, Somford DM, Hoeks C, Bouwense SA, Huisman H, Yakar D, et al. Magnetic resonance imaging guided prostate biopsy in men with repeat negative biopsies and increased prostate-specific antigen. J Urol. 2010;183:520–8.
3. Franiel T, Stephan C, Erbersdobler A, Dietz E, Maxeiner A, Hell N, et al. Areas suspicious for prostate cancer: MR-guided biopsy in patients with at least one transrectal US-guided biopsy with a negative finding–multiparametric MR imaging for detection and biopsy planning. Radiology. 2011;259(1):162–72.
4. Roethke M, Anastasiadis AG, Lichy M, Werner M, Wagner P, Kruck S, et al. MRI-guided prostate biopsy detects clinically significant cancer: analysis of a cohort of 100 patients after previous negative TRUS biopsy. World J Urol. 2012;30:213–8.
5. Testa C, Schiavina R, Lodi R, Salizzoni E, Tonon C, D'Errico A, et al. Accuracy of MRI/MRSI-based transrectal ultrasound biopsy in peripheral and transition zones of the prostate gland in patients with prior negative biopsy. NMR Biomed. 2010;23(9):1017–26. Evaluation studies.
6. Sciarra A, Panebianco V, Ciccariello M, Salciccia S, Cattarino S, Lisi D, et al. Value of magnetic resonance spectroscopy imaging and dynamic contrast-enhanced imaging for detecting prostate cancer foci in men with prior negative biopsy. Clin Cancer Res. 2010;16(6):1875–83. Clinical trial randomized controlled trial.
7. Cirillo S, Petracchini M, Della Monica P, Gallo T, Tartaglia V, Vestita E, et al. Value of endorectal MRI and MRS in patients with elevated prostate-specific antigen levels and previous negative biopsies to localize peripheral zone tumors. Clin Radiol. 2008;63(8):871–9.
8. Ouzzane A, Puech P, Lemaitre L, Leroy X, Nevoux P, Betrouni N, et al. Combined multiparametric MRI and targeted biopsies improve anterior prostate cancer detection, staging and grading. Urology. 2011;78:1356–62.
9. Haffner J, Lemaitre L, Puech P, Haber GP, Leroy X, Jones JS, et al. Role of magnetic resonance imaging

before initial biopsy: comparison of magnetic resonance imaging-targeted and systematic biopsy for
significant prostate cancer detection. BJU Int. 2011;
108:E171–8.

10. Ahmed HU, Kirkham A, Arya M, Illing R, Freeman
A, Allen C, et al. Is it time to consider a role for MRI
before prostate biopsy? Nat Rev Clin Oncol.
2009;6(4):197–206. Review.

11. Toi A, Neill MG, Lockwood GA, Sweet JM, Tammsalu
LA, Fleshner NE. The continuing importance of tran-
srectal ultrasound identification of prostatic lesions.
J Urol. 2007;177(2):516–20.

12. Kuligowska E, Barish MA, Fenlon HM, Blake M.
Predictors of prostate carcinoma: accuracy of gray-
scale and color Doppler US and serum markers.
Radiology. 2001;220(3):757–64. Comparative study.

13. Walz J, Marcy M, Pianna JT, Brunelle S, Gravis G,
Salem N, et al. Identification of the prostate cancer
index lesion by real-time elastography: considerations
for focal therapy of prostate cancer. World J Urol.
2011;29:589–94.

14. Mitterberger MJ, Aigner F, Horninger W, Ulmer H,
Cavuto S, Halpern EJ, et al. Comparative efficiency of
contrast-enhanced colour Doppler ultrasound targeted
versus systematic biopsy for prostate cancer detection. Eur Radiol. 2010;20(12):2791–6. Comparative
study evaluation studies.

15. Puech P, Potiron E, Lemaitre L, Leroy X, Haber GP,
Crouzet S, et al. Dynamic contrast-enhanced-magnetic
resonance imaging evaluation of intraprostatic prostate cancer: correlation with radical prostatectomy
specimens. Urology. 2009;74(5):1094–9. Epub 24
Sep 2009.

16. Delongchamps NB, Rouanne M, Flam T, Beuvon F,
Liberatore M, Zerbib M, et al. Multiparametric magnetic resonance imaging for the detection and localization of prostate cancer: combination of T2-weighted,
dynamic contrast-enhanced and diffusion-weighted
imaging. BJU Int. 2011;107(9):1411–8.

17. Villers A, Puech P, Mouton D, Leroy X, Ballereau C,
Lemaitre L. Dynamic contrast-enhanced, pelvic
phased array magnetic resonance imaging of localized prostate cancer for predicting tumor volume: correlation with radical prostatectomy findings. J Urol.
2006;176(6 Pt 1):2432–7.

18. Lemaitre L, Puech P, Poncelet E, Bouye S, Leroy X,
Biserte J, et al. Dynamic contrast-enhanced MRI of
anterior prostate cancer: morphometric assessment
and correlation with radical prostatectomy findings.
Eur Radiol. 2009;19(2):470–80.

19. Villeirs GM, De Meerleer GO. Magnetic resonance
imaging (MRI) anatomy of the prostate and application of MRI in radiotherapy planning. Eur J Radiol.
2007;63(3):361–8.

20. Morakkabati-Spitz N, Bastian PJ, Gieseke J, Traber F,
Kuhl CK, Wattjes MP, et al. MR imaging of the prostate at 3.0T with external phased array coil—preliminary results. Eur J Med Res. 2008;13(6):287–91.

21. Carlani M, Mancino S, Bonanno E, Finazzi Agro E,
Simonetti G. Combined morphological, [1H]-MR

spectroscopic and contrast-enhanced imaging of human
prostate cancer with a 3-Tesla scanner: preliminary
experience. Radiol Med. 2008;113(5):670–88.

22. Weinreb JC, Blume JD, Coakley FV, Wheeler TM,
Cormack JB, Sotto CK, et al. Prostate cancer:
sextant localization at MR imaging and MR spectroscopic imaging before prostatectomy–results of
ACRIN prospective multi-institutional clinicopathologic study. Radiology. 2009;251(1):122–33.
Controlled clinical trial multicenter study research support, N.I.H., Extramural.

23. Girouin N, Mege-Lechevallier F, Tonina Senes A,
Bissery A, Rabilloud M, Marechal JM, et al. Prostate
dynamic contrast-enhanced MRI with simple visual
diagnostic criteria: is it reasonable? Eur Radiol.
2007;17(6):1498–509.

24. Gibbs P, Liney GP, Pickles MD, Zelhof B, Rodrigues
G, Turnbull LW. Correlation of ADC and T2 measurements with cell density in prostate cancer at 3.0 Tesla.
Invest Radiol. 2009;44(9):572–6. Evaluation studies
research support, non-U.S. Gov't.

25. Itou Y, Nakanishi K, Narumi Y, Nishizawa Y, Tsukuma
H. Clinical utility of apparent diffusion coefficient
(ADC) values in patients with prostate cancer: can
ADC values contribute to assess the aggressiveness of
prostate cancer? J Magn Reson Imaging. 2011;33(1):
167–72.

26. Woodfield CA, Tung GA, Grand DJ, Pezzullo JA,
Machan JT, Renzulli 2nd JF. Diffusion-weighted MRI
of peripheral zone prostate cancer: comparison of
tumor apparent diffusion coefficient with Gleason
score and percentage of tumor on core biopsy. AJR
Am J Roentgenol. 2010;194(4):W316–22.

27. Yoshimitsu K, Kiyoshima K, Irie H, Tajima T,
Asayama Y, Hirakawa M, et al. Usefulness of apparent diffusion coefficient map in diagnosing prostate
carcinoma: correlation with stepwise histopathology.
J Magn Reson Imaging. 2008;27(1):132–9.

28. Zelhof B, Pickles M, Liney G, Gibbs P, Rodrigues G,
Kraus S, et al. Correlation of diffusion-weighted magnetic resonance data with cellularity in prostate cancer. BJU Int. 2009;103(7):883–8. Evaluation studies
research support, non-U.S. Gov't.

29. deSouza NM, Riches SF, Vanas NJ, Morgan VA,
Ashley SA, Fisher C, et al. Diffusion-weighted
magnetic resonance imaging: a potential noninvasive
marker of tumor aggressiveness in localized prostate
cancer. Clin Radiol. 2008;63(7):774–82.

30. Langer DL, van der Kwast TH, Evans AJ, Sun L, Yaffe
MJ, Trachtenberg J, et al. Intermixed normal tissue
within prostate cancer: effect on MR imaging measurements of apparent diffusion coefficient and T2–sparse
versus dense cancers. Radiology. 2008;249(3):900–8.

31. Hambrock T, Somford DM, Huisman HJ, van Oort
IM, Witjes JA, Hulsbergen-van de Kaa CA, et al.
Relationship between apparent diffusion coefficients
at 3.0-T MR imaging and Gleason grade in peripheral
zone prostate cancer. Radiology. 2011;259:453–61.

32. van As NJ, de Souza NM, Riches SF, Morgan VA,
Sohaib SA, Dearnaley DP, et al. A study of diffusion-

weighted magnetic resonance imaging in men with untreated localised prostate cancer on active surveillance. Eur Urol. 2009;56(6):981–7. Research support, non-U.S. Gov't.

33. Crawford ED, Wilson SS, Torkko KC, Hirano D, Stewart JS, Brammell C, et al. Clinical staging of prostate cancer: a computer-simulated study of transperineal prostate biopsy. BJU Int. 2005;96(7): 999–1004. Comparative study research support, N.I.H., Extramural research support, U.S. Gov't, P.H.S.

34. Puech P, Huglo D, Petyt G, Lemaitre L, Villers A. Imaging of organ-confined prostate cancer: functional ultrasound, MRI and PET/computed tomography. Curr Opin Urol. 2009;19(2):168–76. Epub 04 Feb 2009.

35. Presti JC. Prostate biopsy: current status and limitations. Rev Urol. 2007;9(3):93–8.

36. Moussa AS, Meshref A, Schoenfield L, Masoud A, Abdel-Rahman S, Li J, et al. Importance of additional "extreme" anterior apical needle biopsies in the initial detection of prostate cancer. Urology. 2010;75: 1034–9. Epub 19 Jan 2010.

37. Delongchamps NB, Haas GP. Saturation biopsies for prostate cancer: current uses and future prospects. Nat Rev Urol. 2009;6(12):645–52. Review.

38. Taira AV, Merrick GS, Galbreath RW, Andreini H, Taubenslag W, Curtis R, et al. Performance of transperineal template-guided mapping biopsy in detecting prostate cancer in the initial and repeat biopsy setting. Prostate Cancer Prostatic Dis. 2010;13(1):71–7.

39. Ahmed HU, Hu Y, Carter T, Arumainayagam N, Lecornet E, Freeman A, et al. Characterizing clinically significant prostate cancer using template prostate mapping biopsy. J Urol. 2011;186(2):458–64.

40. Singh AK, Kruecker J, Xu S, Glossop N, Guion P, Ullman K, et al. Initial clinical experience with real-time transrectal ultrasonography-magnetic resonance imaging fusion-guided prostate biopsy. BJU Int. 2008;101(7):841–5. Evaluation studies multicenter study.

41. Stenman UH, Abrahamsson PA, Aus G, Lilja H, Bangma C, Hamdy FC, et al. Prognostic value of serum markers for prostate cancer. Scand J Urol Nephrol Suppl. 2005;216:64–81.

42. Rouse P, Shaw G, Ahmed HU, Freeman A, Allen C, Emberton M. Multi-parametric magnetic resonance imaging to rule-in and rule-out clinically important prostate cancer in men at risk: a cohort study. Urol Int. 2011;87:49–53.

43. Shariat SF, Kattan MW, Vickers AJ, Karakiewicz PI, Scardino PT. Critical review of prostate cancer predictive tools. Future Oncol. 2009;5(10):1555–84.

Research support, N.I.H., Extramural research support, non-U.S. Gov't review.

44. Pauly KB, Diederich CJ, Rieke V, Bouley D, Chen J, Nau WH, et al. Magnetic resonance-guided high-intensity ultrasound ablation of the prostate. Top Magn Reson Imaging. 2006;17(3):195–207. Research support, N.I.H., Extramural research support, non-U.S. Gov't review.

45. Shukla-Dave A, Hricak H, Kattan MW, Pucar D, Kuroiwa K, Chen HN, et al. The utility of magnetic resonance imaging and spectroscopy for predicting insignificant prostate cancer: an initial analysis. BJU Int. 2007;99(4):786–93. Evaluation studies research support, N.I.H., Extramural.

46. Umbehr M, Bachmann LM, Held U, Kessler TM, Sulser T, Weishaupt D, et al. Combined magnetic resonance imaging and magnetic resonance spectroscopy imaging in the diagnosis of prostate cancer: a systematic review and meta-analysis. Eur Urol. 2009;55(3):575–90. Epub 28 Oct 2008.

47. Bouye S, Potiron E, Puech P, Leroy X, Lemaitre L, Villers A. Transition zone and anterior stromal prostate cancers: zone of origin and intraprostatic patterns of spread at histopathology. Prostate. 2009;69(1): 105–13.

48. Haffner J, Potiron E, Bouye S, Puech P, Leroy X, Lemaitre L, et al. Peripheral zone prostate cancers: location and intraprostatic patterns of spread at histopathology. Prostate. 2009;69(3):276–82.

49. Punglia RS, D'Amico AV, Catalona WJ, Roehl KA, Kuntz KM. Effect of verification bias on screening for prostate cancer by measurement of prostate-specific antigen. N Engl J Med. 2003;349(4):335–42. Research support, non-U.S. Gov't research support, U.S. Gov't, P.H.S.

50. Merrick GS, Gutman S, Andreini H, Taubenslag W, Lindert DL, Curtis R, et al. Prostate cancer distribution in patients diagnosed by transperineal template-guided saturation biopsy. Eur Urol. 2007;52(3): 715–23.

51. Bott SR, Henderson A, Halls JE, Montgomery BS, Laing R, Langley SE. Extensive transperineal template biopsies of prostate: modified technique and results. Urology. 2006;68(5):1037–41.

52. Scattoni V, Zlotta A, Montironi R, Schulman C, Rigatti P, Montorsi F. Extended and saturation prostatic biopsy in the diagnosis and characterisation of prostate cancer: a critical analysis of the literature. Eur Urol. 2007;52(5):1309–22.

53. Djavan B, Milani S, Remzi M. Prostate biopsy: who, how and when an update. Can J Urol. 2005;12 (Suppl 1):44–8. Comparative study review; discussion 99–100.

Prostate Cancer Detection: Lessons Learned in the Cleveland Clinic Experience with Focus on the Negative Biopsy

25

Ayman S. Moussa, Ahmed El-Shafei,
Osama Zaytoun, and J. Stephen Jones

Twelve biopsy cores using an 18-gauge needle allow histological examination of only 0.04% of an average-size prostate [1]. Recognizing that repeat biopsy is positive in 20–35% of cases, especially if saturation biopsy is performed, it is clear that any biopsy technique involves significant sampling error. As a referral center that often ends up being the final common pathway for large numbers of patients with suspicion of prostate cancer following one, two, or often many more prior negative biopsies, we have had the opportunity to explore the issues in depth.

We have focused not on increasing cancer detection but on improving it, both from the standpoint of accuracy and patient experience. This has involved a large number of our staff urologists, fellows, residents, and medical students, as well as multidisciplinary work with pathologists, medical and radiation oncologists, and radiologists, all of whom we are grateful to. We have also benefited from collaboration with colorectal surgeons, neurologists, and anesthesiologists regarding work on pain management.

Furthermore, we have leashed the power of high-quality databases comprising over 18,645 prostate biopsies (as of the date of this writing) plus the searchable electronic medical record to answer questions that we previously could not using traditional research approaches.

This chapter summarizes over a decade of innovation and discovery in prostate cancer diagnostics at Cleveland Clinic and embodies the value and critical nature of teamwork in healthcare.

Impact of Technique on Likelihood that Initial Biopsy Simply Missed a Tumor

The first step in the evaluation of patients suspected of having unrecognized prostate cancer following a negative biopsy is to assess the adequacy of initial procedure. Seventy percent of PCa cases are detected on initial PBx; optimization of the initial PBx intuitively reduces the likelihood of facing the "repeat biopsy dilemma" and can help the patient avoid unnecessary second biopsy to find a cancer that should have been detected on initial biopsy [2]. PCa detection on repeat biopsies varies primarily as a function of how many cores were obtained on initial PBx. In the Stanford series, PCa detection was 39% in men with a prior sextant biopsy compared to 28% in men with a previous ePBx [3]. Eskicorapci et al. demonstrated that 14-core repeat biopsy detected PCa in 36.1% and 18.7% of the patients who had a previous sextant biopsy and 10-core

A.S. Moussa, M.D., Ph.D. • A. El-Shafei, M.D., Ph.D.
Glickman Urological and Kidney Institute,
Cleveland Clinic, Cleveland, OH, USA

O. Zaytoun, M.D., Ph.D.
Department of Urology, Cleveland Clinic,
Cleveland, OH, USA

J.S. Jones, M.D., FACS, MBA(✉)
Cleveland Clinic, Cleveland Clinic Lerner College
of Medicine at Case Western Reserve,
Cleveland 9500, OH, USA
e-mail: joness7@ccf.org

J.S. Jones (ed.), *Prostate Cancer Diagnosis: PSA, Biopsy and Beyond*, Current Clinical Urology,
DOI 10.1007/978-1-62703-188-2_25, © Springer Science+Business Media New York 2013

biopsy protocol, respectively ($P=0.005$) [4]. Thus, a patient who underwent initial sextant biopsy has a chance of repeat biopsy being positive which is functionally as high as had he not truly ever undergone biopsy at all.

As defined by the National Comprehensive Cancer Network, ePBx is essentially a sextant template with at least four additional cores from the lateral peripheral zone [5]. Sampling of the prostate lateral horn, obtained with laterally directed biopsies, increases the detection rate by about 25% [6, 7]. Importantly, Presti observes that apical cores are associated with the highest cancer detection on repeated biopsies [8] and that this is based largely on the apex being comprised entirely of the peripheral zone tissue known to be the source of almost all prostate cancer cases. He, along with Wright and Ellis, showed that the most common unique site of cancer was the anterior apex, where 17% of cancers would have been missed by standard peripheral zone biopsies [9].

Cancers that arise in this apico-anterior peripheral zone may be difficult to palpate by DRE [10]. In addition, apical biopsy is widely recognized as being more painful than biopsy of the remainder of the gland, so urologists are likely to avoid this area to minimize pain [11].

Recently, we published our experience regarding the yield of apical biopsies using the standard 12-core biopsy scheme plus two additional cores taken from the extreme anterior apex. The apical cores (three on each side) achieved the highest cancer detection rate (73.6% of all cancers), and the additional extreme anterior apical cores (one additional core on each side of the apex at its most extreme caudal position) achieved the highest rate of unique cancer detection [12].

In contrast, routine biopsy explicitly from the transitional zone (TZ) has not been found to be valuable by most authors [13–17]. Furthermore, in a study on patients undergoing repeat transrectal saturation PBx (sPBx, ≥20 cores), we found no exclusive TZ cancers [18]. So we introduce our model for the initial population based on 14-core biopsy as an optimal biopsy strategy for this population, with additional cores obtained from apex instead of from the transition zone as suggested by previous authors.

Intuition Overridden by Discovery in Prostate Cancer Diagnostics

It is intuitive that adding ever more cores may enhance PCa detection in any setting. However, in the field of prostate cancer diagnostics, we have repeatedly found intuition to be a poor predictor of outcomes in scientific inquiry. Because we had demonstrated that 24 cores could be routinely obtained in the office setting under periprostatic block with no increase in complications, cost, or pain compared even to sextant biopsy (below), we enthusiastically investigated the role of transrectal saturation biopsy as a method we hoped would identify the overwhelming majority of cancers during initial biopsy, which we believed would also obviate the need for repeat biopsy if the initial biopsy was benign. Counterintuitively, this yielded no higher detection rate than comparative patients who underwent 10-core biopsies (44.6% vs. 51.7% respectively, $p>0.9$) [19]. Even more disappointing, we subsequently reported follow-up of these patients and showed that when repeat biopsy was performed, 24% still had cancer despite an initially negative transrectal saturation biopsy [20], which is notably the same that Presti found in patients who had undergone initial standard extended biopsy. This has subsequently been confirmed in the literature, so going beyond the 12–14-core level for patients undergoing initial biopsy is unfounded [21–23]. This is in contrast to patients undergoing repeat biopsy, as discussed below.

PSA Issues for Repeat PBx

The traditional PSA threshold for biopsy of 4 ng/mL has now been clearly debunked and shown to be artificial; large numbers of men with prostate cancer actually have a PSA level below that threshold [24], and using that hard cut point would have missed half of all high-grade cancers found in the PCPT trial. Thus, it becomes clear that PSA is a continuous, not categorical, variable, and biopsy may be positive at any PSA level. It now becomes imperative to make the decision for biopsy based not only on the risk of finding cancer but also the potential that treatment will affect its outcome while incurring acceptable risk of morbidity related not only to the treatment but also to the diagnosis. As a result, we convinced the Cleveland Clinic Laboratory to discontinue reporting PSA values as normal or abnormal depending on whether they are above or below 4.0. Instead, the risk ranges from PCPT are included in PSA result reporting to allow the patient to understand the likelihood that he has prostate cancer based on his PSA level.

An inverse relationship exists between PCa detection and %fPSA value. Nevertheless, this important marker is used by a minority of urologists. We believe this is due to misinterpretation of the data. This is unfortunate and misses out on great opportunity to improve prostate cancer diagnosis.

Catalona et al. demonstrated that %fPSA cutoff of <25% corresponded with the highest PCa detection rate and the least number of what is often termed "unnecessary" biopsies among men seeking an initial PBx [25]. We actually do not believe that it is an accurate term, because using that logic would mean that every negative biopsy was unnecessary. This is unreasonable because if we could have known the result of any biopsy in either direction – positive or negative – then it would have been unnecessary. Quite contrary, biopsy is necessary to elucidate the cause of suspicious findings for any potential malignancy in which there is believed to be potential to have an impact on its outcome. Therefore, we do not believe the value of %free PSA is to avoid biopsy because it has not been shown to be effective at that goal. By contrast, we believe that the real value of %free PSA is its prediction strength in men who have very high likelihood of having unrecognized prostate cancer.

A multicenter study revealed that %fPSA cutoff of 26% detected 95% with PCa and eliminated 29% of negative biopsies [26]. Subsequently, the predictive role of %fPSA was similarly suggested for repeat PBx population [27]. Morgan et al. demonstrated that a %fPSA <10% was a strong predictor for PCa even after two negative

prior biopsies with a sensitivity of 91% and a specificity of 86% [28].

As mentioned, we observe that many urologists do not use %free PSA based on it being in a "gray zone" in large numbers of men. This is ironic, in that total PSA gives equivocal results in far larger numbers of men. In all studies comparing %free PSA to total PSA, the performance of %free PSA was clearly superior, but counterintuitively few urologists avoid total PSA based on its imprecision.

The second limitation to %free PSA has traditionally been that it had not been validated outside the total PSA "reflex zone" of 4–10 mg/dL, and had not been evaluated thoroughly in the setting of contemporary extended biopsy. Therefore, we recently evaluated the performance of %fPSA on 1,077 patients who underwent initial extended prostate biopsy [29] and 683 repeat extended or saturation biopsies [30]. The area under the ROC curve (AUC) for %fPSA was maintained at 0.65 for men who underwent both initial and repeat biopsy and 0.72 for men who underwent >one repeat biopsy. A %fPSA cutoff of 11% achieved 85% and 86% specificity in both categories, respectively ([29, 30] as above). The important lesson from this is that it is acceptable for most men to be in a gray zone, in which case the %free PSA does not alter management. However, for the patient with a very low %free PSA (approximately 11–12% or below), there is a very high probability of underlying malignancy regardless of total PSA level at least as far down as 2.5, so biopsy should certainly be entertained in such patients in order to avoid missing high-grade prostate cancer.

While PSA velocity (PSAV) has been a useful marker for identifying men at risk of aggressive PCa, its utility to predict PCa on repeat biopsies remains under debate [31, 32]. Keetch et al. reported that PSAV>0.75 would reduce the number who required repeat biopsies, but that velocity alone would have missed 40% of cancers without the use of other parameters (i.e., PSAD) [33]. However, Borboroglu et al. found that a PSAV>0.75 was the only statistically significant risk factor for PCa detection on repeat biopsy [34].

Loeb et al. depicted that the median PSAV was significantly greater in men with HGPIN who were subsequently diagnosed with PCa. Moreover, a PSAV threshold of 0.75 predicted which men with HGPIN would ultimately be diagnosed with PCa [35]. Okada et al. found that PSAV>0.48 was statistically significant predictor of PCa in 140 repeat PBx men ($p=0.0011$) [36]. We recently evaluated the predictive ability of PSAV on 449 patients undergoing a first repeat PBx. PSAV had the highest predictive value alone with AUC of 0.54 for all PCa and 0.68 for high-grade PCa. We found that in men pursuing a second biopsy after an initial negative biopsy, PSA slope has higher predictive value than total PSA for both PCa and high-grade PCa with the best cutoff of PSAV to 0.75 with sensitivity of 0.88 and specificity of 0.45 [37]. By contrast, we have found PSA density (PSAD) to have limited predictability in our analyses of all its permutations, including PSAD-transition zone, PSAD-peripheral zone, and several ratios that have simply not supported our hypotheses in this area.

The Impact of Suspicious Pathological Findings on Prior Biopsy

High-Grade Prostatic Intraepithelial Neoplasia

The reported incidence of HGPIN on needle biopsies varies considerably at 0.6–24% (mean 7.7%) [38, 39]. In the early 1990s, the risk of finding PCa after diagnosis of HGPIN was thought to be very high, with most studies citing a probability of ≈50% [38]. Initially it was believed that HGPIN was simply a marker of coexistent cancer missed on sextant biopsy, so repeat biopsy was mandatory. However, in the era of extended biopsy, the need for automatic repeat biopsy has been questioned, and the premalignant potential of HGPIN has been unclear in the literature.

Merrimen and Godoy showed that unifocal HGPIN had no more likelihood of PCa detection than a benign diagnosis [40, 41]. The initial report from our institution demonstrated that individuals

with multifocal HPGIN versus isolated HGPIN on initial sPBx had 80% versus 0% incidence of PCa on repeat PBx, respectively [42]. Taneja and Lepor showed that men who had undergone extended biopsy had minimal likelihood of cancer on immediate repeat biopsy but had approximately 25% chance of cancer on delayed interval biopsies at both 3 and 6 years later, suggesting that HGPIN was premalignant as described in their chapter in this book. Nevertheless, there had been no comparison to the cancer detection rate in men without HGPIN, so we recently published 328 men who underwent a second PBx after HGPIN diagnosis. HGPIN alone on initial PBx had a significant effect on the subsequent diagnosis of PCa (Hazard ratio 1.89; 95% CI 1.39, 2.55; $p<0.0001$). The most important finding was that stratifying HGPIN into multifocal and bilateral disease significantly increased the hazard ratios to 2.56 (95% CI 1.83, 3.6) and 2.2 (95% CI 1.51, 3.21), respectively, resulting in estimated 3-year cancer rates of 29.0% and 37.0% compared to 12.5% and 18.9%, respectively, following benign biopsy [43]. By contrast, men with unifocal HGPIN actually had the same risk of a positive biopsy as men who had completely benign initial biopsy. Thus, we identified that unifocal HGPIN is essentially a benign or normal condition, whereas multifocal HGPIN is a premalignant condition. Thus, we follow the lead of Taneja and Lepor and recommend delayed interval biopsy approximately every 3 years for healthy men with a history of multifocal HGPIN and recommend routine surveillance for men with unifocal HGPIN. The only exception to this is for men with an inadequate initial biopsy, in whom immediate repeat biopsy is recommended for unifocal HGPIN as well as focal HGPIN.

Moreover, this category might be an excellent target for chemoprevention. The Prostate Cancer Prevention Trial (PCPT) showed a statistically significant decrease in the diagnosis of HGPIN from 11.7% to 8.2% when administered placebo or finasteride, respectively [44]. The REDUCE trial demonstrated a decreased volume of HGPIN in a randomized trial of 46 patients who underwent radical prostatectomy that approached statistical significance at $p=0.052$ [45]

Selective estrogen receptor modulators also show promise in preventing the progression of HGPIN to PCa. In a large phase IIB clinical trial men with HGPIN who were given 20 mg toremifene had a decreased incidence of PCa at 24.4% versus 31.2% with placebo at 1 year [46]. Because they are the only FDA-approved medications with data to support their role in risk reduction, we recommend men with multifocal HGPIN consider management with 5ari's but inform them of the controversy regarding high-grade prostate cancer and that this is an off-label recommendation.

Atypical Small Acinar Proliferation

Unlike HGPIN, ASAP indicates the presence of suspicious glands with insufficient cytological or architectural atypia for a definitive diagnosis of PCa [47]. Most studies show a PCa detection rate of 34–60% on repeat biopsies in such men [38]. We interpret this finding as a message from the pathologist that he or she believes the diagnosis is prostate cancer, but simply has inadequate evidence on the slide to confirm this.

Although we hypothesized that saturation biopsy would have provided more adequate sampling, our research actually showed that that the risk of cancer on repeat biopsy is in that same range even if ASAP was identified on sPBx. Additionally, we found that the presence of inflammation increased the likelihood of ASAP, potentially because the background changes of inflammation make interpretation more difficult [48]. Most of PCa detected after initially diagnosed ASAP are proved to be clinically significant (69.8%), so repeat biopsy is always in order [49]. Most recommendations are to do so within 6 months, but we have found that many urologists interpret this to mean they have to wait 6 months. As a result, we see many patients that are inordinately worried that they must wait that long to find out whether they have cancer. We proceed to immediate repeat transrectal saturation biopsy in order to clarify the situation, and patients are grateful that we will do so without delay.

One scenario that remains unclear is how to manage a patient who has ASAP on the repeat biopsy. Even with what may be the largest experience in this unique situation, we have found it in fewer than 100 cases. Our initial evaluation of the data suggest that biopsy for the indication of ASAP even found on repeat biopsy still is likely o identify cancer in at approximately half of patients [50].

What Is the Optimal Repeat PBx Procedure?

Since 2002, we have used 20-core office-based transrectal saturation for all repeat biopsies, and others now support this practice [7]. After being described almost simultaneously by Borboroglu and Stewart performing the procedure in the operating room under general anesthesia [35, 51], we demonstrated that sPBx can be effectively performed in the office routinely using periprostatic block [52] and have performed the procedure more than 2,000 times with morbidity and tolerability identical to extended biopsy. Moreover, others confirmed its safety when compared to ePBx [7, 21].

We originally used a 24-core transrectal template with cores concentrated laterally and apically based on the preponderance of cancer in these locations (Fig. 25.1). Based on our experience with site-specific labeling, it soon became clear that the lateral sectors (dark shading) were the site of all unique tumors in the repeat biopsy setting. As a result, we reduced sampling from two cores to one core per medial sector (midgland and base), resulting in a 20-core template for patients undergoing repeat biopsy [18] (Fig. 25.2).

It is important to adequately biopsy areas likely to harbor cancer undiagnosed during previous biopsy sessions. As previously mentioned, the apex is the most likely site for this to occur, so focus of at least three cores is made at that level, especially during repeat biopsy [3]. We demonstrated that the pain of apical biopsy can be avoided by using the rectal sensation test to bypass anal pain fibers [11].

Although we demonstrated that sPBx did not increase cancer detection as an initial biopsy

Fig. 25.1 Initial sPBx template showing sectors and number of cores obtained from each during our developmental studies

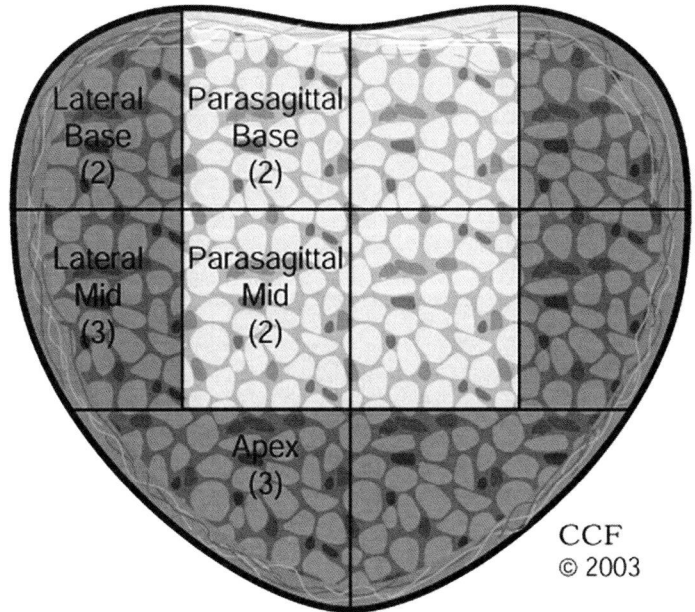

Fig. 25.2 Our current sPBx template showing reduced sampling in the medial sectors based on finding no unique cancers in those sectors, assuming that the entire apex is regarded as a lateral sector

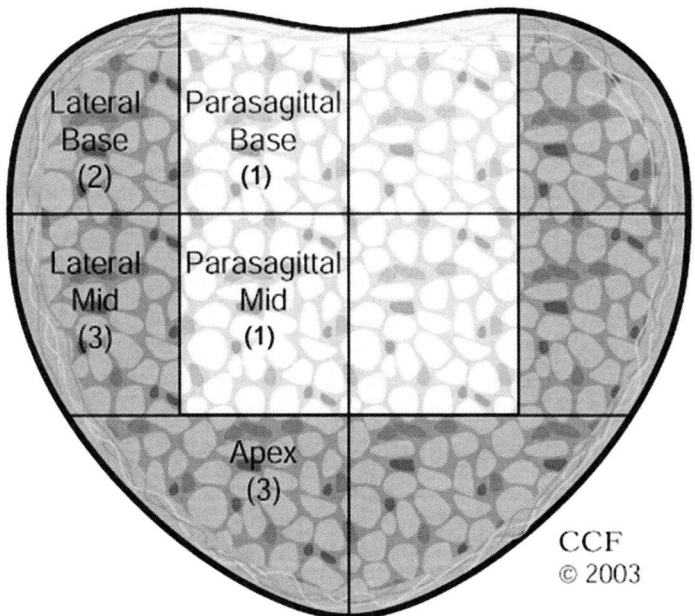

strategy [19], our own and several other series suggested that sPBx enhances cancer detection in the repeat PBx population. Recently, we compared sPBx and ePBx in 1,462 patients undergoing their first repeat PBx. The sPBx had an approximately 50% higher cancer detection rate when compared to ePBx (33% vs. 22.4%, $p < 0.0001$). Broken down by initial biopsy results, for patients with benign initial biopsy, sPBx demonstrated an almost 50% improvement (31.7% vs. 21.6% $p < 0.0002$). Moreover, for patients with HGPIN or ASAP on initial biopsy, the PCa detection rate was significantly higher in the sPBx group (38.6% vs. 25.9%, $p = 0.028$) [53].

Table 25.1 Detection rates in patients with benign, HGPIN, and ASAP findings on initial PBx

Indication	No. of pts/total no. (%)			
	Overall	Extended PBx	Saturation PBx	*p* value
Benign PBx	229/751 (30.5)	71/277 (25.6)	158/474 (33.3)	0.027
Pathological findings:				
HGPIN	50/196 (25.5)	16/74 (21.6)	34/122 (28)	0.33
ASAP/PIN 3	6/109 (33)	11/42 (26.2)	25/67 (37.3)	0.23
Totals	86/305 (28.2)	27/116 (23.3)	59/189 (31.2)	0.13

Table 25.1 displays studies that evaluated the performance of sPBx on different biopsy situations. sPBX might lead to a more accurate assessment of the extent and grade of disease in men with prostate cancer on an active surveillance protocol than traditional biopsy [54].

Risk of Detection of Insignificant Cancer; How Many Sessions Are Enough?

Several studies have shown that the chance of PCa detection drops with pursuing more repeat biopsies [55–57]. The ERSPC demonstrated PCa detection rates on biopsies 1, 2, 3, and 4 of 22%, 10%, 5% and 4%, respectively, but notably most patients underwent fewer core biopsy compared to contemporary standards.

A second biopsy is clearly a consideration for patients with persistent suspicion of PCa following one negative biopsy, but we have found that fewer than 10% of patients with two adequate prior biopsies will be found to have cancer per subsequent biopsy session, so our threshold to do so is very high, often driven by a positive PCA3. Moreover, we found that the incidence of low-grade clinically insignificant PCa was 62% in patients with two or more negative PBx, so even if cancer is present, it is unlikely to be harmful [58]. The original sPBx studies had conflicting findings with most reports suggest that sPBx does not increase the detection of clinically insignificant tumors [19, 59, 60]. In our comparison of sPBx and ePBx in 1,462 men who had one negative PBx, 38.3% patients with positive biopsy had clinically insignificant cancer. A higher percentage was detected in the sPBx group (41.2% vs.

34.6%), but this was not statistically significant (*p*=0.178) [53]. Regardless, there was a trend to increase detection of clinically insignificant cancer that we believe is real and demonstrates the potential for diagnosis for clinically insignificant disease using any biopsy protocol, especially if it is a repeat biopsy.

The big picture is that the concern of overdetection must be weighed against the risk of missing clinically significant malignancy. Regarding detection of small, potentially insignificant cancers, it is our strong belief that detection and treatment of PCa should be always considered independent processes as advocated by Carroll [61], and we actively pursue less rigorous management options such as active surveillance or focal therapy for patients with tumors that appear clinically insignificant [62].

Models for Prediction of Positive Prostate Biopsy

The challenge for all prediction models is their pertinence to the clinical question being asked. This is most clearly illustrated by considering the PCPT risk calculator. It was well designed and met rapid acceptance by many urologists, including ourselves. However, we quickly observed that it did not appear to predict the likelihood of a prostate biopsy in our own practice, so performed a validation study that confirmed our hypothesis [63]. It is critical to understand that this does not mean the PCPT risk calculator was errant. Rather, it becomes evident that it describes a different population than that seen in contemporary clinical practice. The people on whose data PCPT was built were actually not patients at all. Rather, they were human subjects in a cancer prevention trial. They presented not based on elevated PSA or abnormal DRE, but these issues actually precluded patients from being enrolled in the study, and thus in the creation of the calculator. Furthermore, the subjects were from the early PSA era before screening culled many patients from the baseline population, and the biopsies were sextant, known to miss ½–1/3 of cancers as emphasized in several parts of this book.

It is obvious in retrospect that patients presenting for clinical evaluation of elevated PSA or abnormal DRE were just not reflective of the risk calculator. When we recognized that this and most other risk calculators were based on dissimilar populations, we developed and validated a nomogram to predict the outcome of initial and repeat PBx. In the repeat biopsy nomogram, 408 men were included for creating the model and another 470 men for the validation purpose. The concordance index of the nomogram was 0.72, which was greater than any single risk factor. In the validation group, the AUC was 0.62 [64].

Furthermore, we recognized that most nomograms were designed with as much data as could be found for obvious reasons of improving prediction accuracy. Prostate volume was a key factor in most. However, we felt that this obviated most of their value if the decision for ultrasound had already been made, i.e., the threshold of invasion was already crossed too late in the process. Therefore, we developed a nomogram for initial biopsy that is based on clinical information known prior to the decision to biopsy. This had minimal negative impact on prediction accuracy and allowed the nomogram to be meaningful to real patients as they and their physicians made decisions on whether to proceed [65].

We have posted these nomograms on our website at http://www.clevelandclinic.org/lp/prostate-cancer-risk-assessment/index.html?utm_campaign=prostatecancerrisk-url&utm_medium=offline&utm_source=redirect and designed the interface so that if any information is unknown, the patient or physician can still get a prediction of prostate biopsy without meeting a "hard stop" that precludes use of other nomograms.

Key Lessons from Cleveland Clinic Prostate Cancer Diagnostics Experience

The first step in managing a negative biopsy is simply to avoid it by performing an adequate initial biopsy. For the last decade, we have used the ePBx scheme as the initial biopsy protocol on about 1,600 patients every year. Among these men, PCa is diagnosed in 49% on initial biopsy, while approximately one third of men pursuing subsequent biopsies prove to have PCa. For the past 5 years, we have added an extreme apical core to the traditional 12-core extended template based on this being the most common site of unique cancer detection, resulting in a 14-core initial biopsy strategy.

Regarding indication for biopsy, it is clear that there is no valid threshold to identify an "abnormal" PSA value to indicate either initial or repeat PBx. Thus, we usually recommend biopsy for the admittedly artificial level of 2.5 in otherwise healthy young men. If the %fPSA is less than 11–12% or PSAV more than 0.75, we are more emphatic in the recommendation. PCA3 is often used in equivocal cases where repeat biopsy is considered. Biopsy for HGPIN is individualized as described above, with delayed interval biopsy every 3 years in men with multifocal HGPIN. ASAP almost always merits at least one repeat biopsy.

Regarding patient preparation and pain management, we have demonstrated and published that the number of cores is unrelated to pain or morbidity. We recommend a single dose of fluoroquinolone and add a single dose of aminoglycoside prior to biopsy, but evolving bacterial resistance patterns necessitate reevaluating this often, and we expect this to require responsiveness on our part to changing infection rates [66, 67]. We have followed the work of Shinohara and others regarding periprostatic block and have shown that apical biopsy can be painless using either apical periprostatic block or the rectal sensation test as commented on in Dr. Shinohara's chapter. We prefer injection at the apical "Mount Everest" based on our publications showing this leads to the lowest pain scores.

The senior author recommends sPBx for all repeat biopsies, finding approximately 50% higher cancer detection rates compared to our own experience with extended repeat biopsy. The potential to detect clinically insignificant cancers is balanced by applying active surveillance to approximately ¼ of newly diagnosed prostate cancer patients, and we find this is well tolerated with patients comforted more by surveillance for low-risk disease than they are by taking an approach of avoiding biopsy because we might not want to know what is going on.

Finally, we offer risk reduction to all men following negative biopsy, but acceptance of this is relatively low in our practice.

References

1. Fleshner NE, O'Sullivan M, Fair WR. Prevalence and predictors of a positive repeat transrectal ultrasound guided needle biopsy of the prostate. J Urol. 1997;158:505–8.
2. Djavan B, Margreiter M. Biopsy standards for detection of prostate cancer. World J Urol. 2007;25(1):11–7.
3. Hong YM, Lai FC, Chon CH, et al. Impact of prior biopsy scheme on pathologic features of cancers detected on repeat biopsies. Urol Oncol. 2004;22:7–10.
4. Eskicorapci SY, Guliyev F, Islamoglu E, Ergen A, Ozen H. The effect of prior biopsy scheme on prostate cancer detection for repeat biopsy population: results of the 14-core prostate biopsy technique. Int Urol Nephrol. 2007;39(1):189–95.
5. National Comprehensive Cancer Network: National Comprehensive (2004). http://www.nccn.org/professionals/physician_gls/PDF/prostate_detection.pdf. Accessed 31 Aug 2012.
6. Scattoni V, Zlotta A, Montironi R, Schulman C, Rigatti P, Montorsi F. Extended and saturation prostatic biopsy in the diagnosis and characterisation of prostate cancer: a critical analysis of the literature. Eur Urol. 2007;52:1309–22.
7. Scattoni V, Maccagnano C, Zanni G, Angiolilli D, Raber M, Roscigno M, Rigatti P, Montorsi F. Is extended and saturation biopsy necessary? Int J Urol. 2010;17(5):447–9.
8. Presti Jr JC, O'Dowd GJ, Miller MC, et al. Extended peripheral zone biopsy schemes increase cancer detection rates and minimize variance in prostate specific antigen and age related cancer rates: results of a community multipractice study. J Urol. 2003;169: 125–9.
9. Wright JL, Ellis WJ. Improved prostate cancer detection with anterior apical prostate biopsies. Urol Oncol. 2006;24:492–5.
10. Presti Jr JC. Prostate biopsy strategies. Nat Clin Pract Urol. 2007;4:505–11.
11. Jones JS, Zippe CD. Rectal sensation test helps avoid pain of apical prostate biopsies. J Urol. 2003;170 (6 Pt 1):2316–8.
12. Moussa AS, Fergany A, Fareed K, Jones JS. Importance of additional "extreme" anterior apical needle biopsies in the initial detection of prostate cancer. Urology. 2010;75(5):1034–9.
13. Philip J, Hanchanale V, Foster CS, Javle P. Importance of peripheral biopsies in maximising the detection of early prostate cancer in repeat 12-core biopsy protocol. BJU Int. 2006;98:559–62.
14. Pelzer AE, Bektic J, Berger AP, et al. Are transition zone biopsies still necessary to improve prostate cancer detection? Results from the Tyrol screening project. Eur Urol. 2005;48:916–21.
15. Peyromaure M, Ravery V, Boccon-Gibod L. The role of the biopsy of the transitional zone and of the seminal vesicles in the diagnosis and staging of prostate cancer. Eur Urol Suppl. 2002;1:40–6.
16. Onur E, Littrup PJ, Pontes JE, Bianco Jr FJ. Contemporary impact of trans-rectal ultrasound lesions for prostate cancer detection. J Urol. 2004;172: 512–4.
17. Djavan B. Prostate biopsies and Vienna nomograms. Eur Urol Suppl. 2006;5:500–10.
18. Patel AR, Jones JS, Rabets J, et al. Parasagittal biopsies add minimal information in repeat saturation prostate biopsy. Urology. 2004;63:87–9.
19. Jones JS, Patel A, Schoenfield L, Rabets JC, Zippe CD, Magi-Galluzzi C. Saturation technique does not improve cancer detection as an initial prostate biopsy strategy. J Urol. 2006;175:485–8.
20. Lane B, Zippe C, Abouassaly R, Schoenfield L, Magi-Galluzzi C, Jones JS. Saturation technique does not decrease cancer detection during follow-up after initial prostate biopsy. J Urol. 2008;179(5):1746–50.
21. Chun FK, Epstein JI, Ficarra V, Freedland SJ, Montironi R, Montorsi F, Shariat SF, Schröder FH, Scattoni V. Optimizing performance and interpretation of prostate biopsy: a critical analysis of the literature. Eur Urol. 2010;58:851–64.
22. Scattoni V, Roscigno M, Raber M, et al. Initial extended transrectal prostate biopsy – are more prostate cancers detected with 18 cores than with 12 cores? J Urol. 2008;179:1327–31.
23. Guichard G, Larre S, Gallina A, et al. Extended 21-sample needle biopsy protocol for diagnosis of prostate cancer in 1000 consecutives patients. Eur Urol. 2007;52:430–5.
24. Catalona WJ, Smith DS, Ornstein DK. Prostate cancer detection in men with serum PSA concentrations of 2.6 ng/mL to 4.0 ng/mL and benign prostate examination. Enhancement of specificity with free PSA measurements. JAMA. 1997;277:1452–5.
25. Catalona WJ, Partin AW, Slawin KM, et al. Use of the percentage of free prostate-specific antigen to enhance differentiation of prostate cancer from benign prostatic

disease: a prospective multicenter clinical trial. JAMA. 1998;279:1542–7.

26. Chan DW, Sokoll LJ, Partin AW, et al. The use of %free PSA to predict prostate cancer probabilities: an eleven center prospective study using an automated immunoassay system in a population with nonsuspicious DRE. J Urol. 1999;161(Suppl 4):A353.

27. Letran JL, Blasé AB, Loberiza FR, et al. Repeat ultrasound guided prostate needle biopsy: use of free to total PSA ratio in predicting prostatic carcinoma. J Urol. 1998;60:426–9.

28. Morgan TO, McLeod DG, Leifer ES, et al. Prospective use of free prostate-specifi c antigen to avoid repeat prostate biopsies in men with elevated total prostate-specifi c antigen. Urology. 1996;48:76–80.

29. Lee BH, Moussa AS, Li J, Fareed K, Jones JS. Percentage of free prostate-specific antigen: implications in modern extended scheme prostate biopsy. Urology. 2011;77:899–903.

30. Lee BH, Hernandez AV, Zaytoun O, Berglund RK, Gong MC, Jones JS. Utility of percent free prostate-specific antigen in repeat prostate biopsy. Urology. 2011;78:386–91.

31. Pinsky PF, Andriole G, Crawford ED, et al. Prostate-specific antigen velocity and prostate cancer Gleason grade and stage. Cancer. 2007;109:1689–95.

32. Etzioni RD, Ankerst DP, Weiss NS, Inoue LYT, Thompson IM. Is prostate-specific antigen velocity useful in early detection of prostate cancer? A critical appraisal of the evidence. J Natl Cancer Inst. 2007;99:1510–5.

33. Keetch DW, McMurtry JM, Smith DS, et al. Prostate specific antigen density versus prostate specific antigen slope as predictors of prostate cancer in men with initially negative prostatic biopsies. J Urol. 1996;156:428–31.

34. Borboroglu PG, Comer SW, Riffenburgh RH, Amling CL. Extensive repeat transrectal ultrasound guided prostate biopsy in patients with previous benign sextant biopsies. J Urol. 2000;163:158–62.

35. Loeb S, Roehl KA, Yu X, Han M, Catalona WJ. Use of prostate-specific antigen velocity to follow up patients with isolated high-grade prostatic intraepithelial neoplasia on prostate biopsy. Urology. 2007;69(1):108–12.

36. Okada K, Okihara K, Kitamura K, Mikami K, Ukimura O, Kawauchi A, Kamoi K, Nakao M, Miki T. Community-based prostate cancer screening in Japan: predicting factors for positive repeat biopsy. Int J Urol. 2010;17(6):541–7.

37. El-Shafei A, Zaytoun O, Vargo E, Li J, Berglund R, Gong MC, Jones JS. PSA slope as a predictor of prostatic cancer & high grade cancer on repeat biopsy (in press).

38. Epstein J, Herawi M. Prostate needle biopsies containing prostatic intraepithelial neoplasia or atypical foci suspicious for carcinoma: implications for patient care. J Urol. 2006;175:820–34.

39. Joniau S, Goeman L, Pennings J, Van Poppel H. Prostatic intraepithelial neoplasia (PIN): importance and clinical management. Eur Urol. 2005;48:379–85.

40. Merrimen JL, Jones G, Walker D, et al. Multifocal high grade prostatic intraepithelial neoplasia is a significant risk factor for prostatic adenocarcinoma. J Urol. 2009;182:485.

41. Godoy G, Taneja SS. Contemporary clinical management of isolated high-grade prostatic intraepithelial neoplasia. Prostate Cancer Prostatic Dis. 2008;11(1): 20–31.

42. Schoenfield L, Jones JS, Zippe CD, et al. The incidence of high-grade prostatic intraepithelial neoplasia and atypical glands suspicious for carcinoma on first-time saturation needle biopsy and the subsequent risk of cancer. BJU Int. 2007;99:770.

43. Lee MC, Moussa AS, Yu C, Kattan MW, Magi-Galluzzi C, Jones JS. Multifocal high grade prostatic intraepithelial neoplasia is a risk factor for subsequent prostate cancer. J Urol. 2010;184(5):1958–62.

44. Thompson IM, Lucia MS, Redman MW, et al. Finasteride decreases the risk of prostatic intraepithelial neoplasia. J Urol. 2007;178:107.

45. Andriole GL, Humphrey P, Ray P, et al. Effect of the dual 5-alpha reductase inhibitor dutasteride on markers of tumor regression in prostate cancer. J Urol. 2004;172:915.

46. Price D, Stein B, Sieber P, et al. Toremifene for the prevention of prostate cancer in men with high grade prostatic intraepithelial neoplasia: results of a double-blind, placebo controlled, phase IIB clinical trial. J Urol. 2006;176:965.

47. Bostwick DG, Srigley J, Grignon D, et al. Atypical adenomatous hyperplasia of the prostate: morphologic criteria for its distinction from well-differentiated carcinoma. Hum Pathol. 1993;24:819–32.

48. Abouassaly R, Tan N, Moussa A, Jones JS. Risk of prostate cancer after diagnosis of atypical glands suspicious for carcinoma on saturation and traditional biopsies. J Urol. 2008;180:911–4.

49. Zhou M, Magi-Galluzzi C. Clinicopathological features of prostate cancers detected after an initial diagnosis of 'atypical glands suspicious for cancer'. Pathology. 2010;42(4):334–8.

50. Isariyawongse B, El–Shafei A, Jones JS. Risk of prostate cancer on third prostate biopsy following diagnosis of atypical glands suspicious for carcinoma on repeat biopsy (in press).

51. Stewart CS, Leibovich BC, Weaver AL, Lieber MM. Prostate cancer diagnosis using a saturation needle biopsy technique after previous negative sextant biopsies. J Urol. 2001;166:86–91. discussion 92.

52. Jones JS, Oder M, Zippe CD. Saturation prostate biopsy with periprostatic block can be performed in office. J Urol. 2002;168(5):2108–10.

53. Zaytoun OM, Moussa AS, Gao T, Fareed K, Jones JS. Office based transrectal saturation biopsy improves prostate cancer detection compared to extended

biopsy in the repeat biopsy population. J Urol. 2011;186:850–4. Zaytoun et al. in press.

54. Abouassaly R, Lane BR, Jones JS. Staging saturation biopsy in patients with prostate cancer on active surveillance protocol. Urology. 2008;714(4):573–7.

55. Roehl KA, Antenor JA, Catalona WJ. Serial biopsy results in prostate cancer screening study. J Urol. 2002;167:2435–9.

56. Djavan B, Ravery V, Zlotta A, et al. Prospective evaluation of prostate cancer detected on biopsies 1, 2, 3 and 4: when should we stop? J Urol. 2001;166:1679–83.

57. Lopez-Corona E, Ohori M, Scardino PT, Reuter VE, Gonen M, Kattan MW. A nomogram for predicting a positive repeat prostate biopsy in patients with a previous negative biopsy session. J Urol. 2003;170(4 Pt 1):1184–8. discussion 1188.

58. Tan N, Lane BR, Li J, Moussa AS, Soriano M, Jones JS. Prostate cancers diagnosed at repeat biopsy are smaller and less likely to be high grade. J Urol. 2008;180(4):1325–9.

59. Singh H, Canto EI, Shariat SF, et al. Improved detection of clinically significant, curable prostate cancer with systematic 12-core biopsy. J Urol. 2004;171:1089–92.

60. Meng MV, Elkin EP, DuChane J, Carroll PR. Impact of increased number of biopsies on the nature of prostate cancer identified. J Urol. 2006;176:63–9.

61. Carroll PR. Early stage prostate cancer–do we have a problem with over-detection, over treatment or both? J Urol. 2005;173(4):1061–2.

62. Jones JS. Prostate cancer: are we over-diagnosing-or under-thinking? Eur Urol. 2008;53(1):10–2. Epub 14 Sept 2007.

63. Nguyen CT, Yu C, Moussa AS, Kattan MW, Jones JS. Performance of the prostate cancer prevention trial risk calculator in a contemporary cohort of men screened for prostate cancer and diagnosed with extended prostate biopsy schemes. J Urol. 2010; 183:529–33.

64. Moussa AS, Kattan MW, Yu C, Jones SJ. Development and validation of a nomogram for predicting a positive repeat prostate biopsy in patients with a previous negative biopsy session in the era of extended prostate sampling. BJU Int. 2010;106(9):1309–14.

65. Zaytoun OM, Kattan MW, Moussa AS, Li J, Yu C, Jones JS. Development of improved nomogram for prediction of outcome of initial prostate biopsy using readily available clinical information. Urology. 2011; 78:392–8.

66. Zaytoun OM, Anil T, Moussa AS, Jianbo L, Fareed K, Jones JS. Morbidity of prostate biopsy after simplified versus complex preparation protocols: assessment of risk factors. Urology. 2011;77:910–4.

67. Zaytoun OM, Vargo EH, Rajan R, Berglund R, Gordon S, Jones JS. Emergence of fluoroquinolone-resistant *Escherichia coli* as cause of postprostate biopsy infection: implications for prophylaxis and treatment. Urology. 2011;77:1035–41.

Future Directions in Prostate Cancer Diagnosis

26

Joseph C. Klink and Eric Klein

Introduction

Since Hugh Hampton Young described his series of 111 prostate cancer patients in 1909 [1], much progress has been made in the diagnosis of prostate cancer. Many of Dr. Young's patients were diagnosed when symptoms of advanced prostate cancer developed, and many died of their disease. A century later, 80% of prostate cancers are diagnosed while still localized [2]. The prostate cancer mortality rate now stands at its lowest point in more than 70 years after falling for 14 consecutive years despite the aging of the population [2]. While many factors have contributed to these trends, earlier diagnosis has played a large role in improving outcomes.

Since 1987 when PSA was described as a potentially useful serum marker for the detection of prostate cancer [3], screening has become widespread. In fact, by 2000, 51% of men over age 65 were being screened with a serum PSA yearly [4]. This rapid adoption of widespread PSA screening caused a substantial initial

upsurge in the incidence of prostate cancer in the early 1990s, but many of these newly diagnosed cancers were low grade and low stage. Now more than two decades later, the debate continues over whether these low-grade, low-stage prostate cancers are clinically significant. Clinically significant prostate cancer is a disease which will cause symptoms, metastasis, or death if untreated.

While current practices likely "overdiagnose" low-risk prostate cancers, 12% of men present initially with locally advanced disease and 4% present with metastasis [2]. Ideally, only those men with clinically significant disease should be diagnosed, and all men with clinically significant disease should be diagnosed early while their prostate cancer is still localized and curable. The future of prostate cancer diagnosis relies on pursuing this ideal through the following goals:

1. Decrease indiscriminate screening for prostate cancer
2. Reduce the number of negative prostate biopsies performed
3. Detect all clinically significant prostate cancers

The remainder of this chapter will explore each of these goals individually and discuss discoveries and technologies on the horizon that may help us achieve these goals. Many of the advancements discussed in all of the preceding chapters of this book will play a role in shaping the future of prostate cancer diagnosis, but they will not be discussed again here.

J.C. Klink, M.D. • E. Klein, M.D. (✉)
Glickman Urological and Kidney Institute, Cleveland Clinic Lerner College of Medicine, 9500 Euclid Ave., Desk Q10-1, Cleveland, OH 44195, USA
e-mail: kleine@ccf.org

Goal 1: Decrease Indiscriminate Screening for Prostate Cancer

After the widespread adoption of PSA screening for prostate cancer, many professional organizations recommended screening nearly all men above a given age threshold, usually around 50 years old [5, 6]. For example, the American Urological Association "PSA Best Practice Policy" in 2000 stated,

> Early detection of prostate cancer should be offered to asymptomatic men 50 years of age or older with an estimated life expectancy of more than 10 years. It is reasonable to offer testing at an earlier age to men with defined risk factors, including men with a first-degree relative who has prostate cancer and African-American men. [6]

As time passed and more data became available on the benefits of screening, or lack thereof, the recommendations were updated to include fewer and fewer men [7]. In 2009, two studies were published which cast doubt on the benefits of population-wide screening for prostate cancer [8, 9]. These findings and their implications are discussed in detail in the first section of this book. Since 2009, screening recommendations have again been updated [10, 11]. The American Urological Association now recommends

> PSA screening for well informed men with an estimated ten year life expectancy who wish to pursue early diagnosis. The risks of overdetection and overtreatment should be discussed…. Early detection and risk assessment of prostate cancer should be offered to healthy, well-informed men 40 years of age or older. [11]

There has clearly been a shift toward risk stratification and only screening the higher-risk cohort. However, we cannot simply eliminate screening altogether, or we may see a rebound in prostate cancer morbidity and mortality. Bill-Axelson et al. showed that mortality was greater for watchful waiting than for radical prostatectomy in men diagnosed with early stage prostate cancer [12]. These data suggest that if we put all men on watchful waiting by default because we do not screen or diagnose them, we will miss the opportunity to cure some men of their fatal cancers. Population-level trends show decreased prostate cancer mortality starting a few years after prostate cancer screening with PSA became widespread [2]. A global reduction in screening likely would not change outcomes for a few years, but could increase mortality rates a decade from now.

Currently available tools cannot adequately differentiate between low- and high-risk men to allow highly targeted screening. In the European study of prostate cancer screening, 1,410 men would need to be screened to prevent one death [8]. In the future, this number will be reduced dramatically through several promising discoveries. First, a number of serum and urine markers of prostate cancer are under development and were discussed in Chap. 1 of this book. These markers, or new ones that have yet to be discovered, may eventually allow one test to be performed at a relatively young age that will reveal a man's lifetime risk of clinically significant prostate cancer. Men at low risk could stop screening altogether after such a test, while men at high risk could follow up much more closely. This approach has already been investigated using PSA. In a study of Swedish men, those with a PSA below 1 ng/ml at age 60 very rarely develop clinically significant prostate cancer [13]. This criteria is far from perfect, however, as many men develop prostate cancer before age 60, the criteria leave half of the population in the high-risk group, and a few men in the low-risk group will still develop metastasis and death. Improved markers with better discrimination will overcome these problems and define most men as low risk, allowing them to stop screening.

Second, genetic and epigenetic tests promise to greatly increase accuracy in predicting lifetime risk of prostate cancer, thereby reducing the need for screening. Both genetic (the order of nucleotides in DNA) and epigenetic (controlling gene expression through mechanisms not based in the DNA itself) characteristics of a man influence his cancer risk. These are areas of active research by many groups around the world. While much remains to be discovered, the following pages discuss what we do know about how genetic susceptibility and epigenetic changes may shape the future of prostate cancer diagnosis.

Genetic Susceptibility Loci and SNPs

Linkage analysis and studying familial cases of prostate cancer have had very limited success in identifying prostate cancer susceptibility genes. The genes that have been identified, such as BRCA2, dramatically increase a man's risk of developing prostate cancer, but these genes are rarely found and therefore can only explain a tiny fraction of the cases of inherited risk for prostate cancer [14].

Familial prostate cancer must rely on other mechanisms in addition to susceptibility genes. Single-nucleotide polymorphisms (SNPs) are variants in a single base in the DNA strand. More than 23 million SNPs have been identified [15]. When an SNP is associated with a disease (such as prostate cancer), the area of the DNA where the SNP is located is known as a susceptibility locus. In recent years, genome-wide association studies (GWAS) have analyzed the DNA from thousands of cancer patients and identified over 40 SNPs that significantly increase the risk of prostate cancer [16–33]. Taken together, these known SNPs likely explain 25% of familial prostate cancer cases. Some SNPs can help differentiate high-risk from low-risk prostate cancer [34, 35].

Asian-Americans have a lower incidence of prostate cancer [2]. Lui et al. studied 33 SNPs that had been identified in men of European descent and found that 11 of them were also associated with prostate cancer risk in Chinese men [36]. This shows promise for SNP-based prostate cancer risk assessments, as men at lower risk (Asian-Americans) may have fewer SNPs than their higher-risk counterparts (European-Americans or African-Americans).

In the future, studies may demonstrate that additional SNPs are relevant in prostate cancer. Once all the relevant SNPs are identified, a commercial test could be developed that rapidly and inexpensively checks each patient's DNA for these SNPs. In fact, known SNPs have already been incorporated into a model that predicts an individual's risk of developing prostate cancer in the future [37]. A patient can submit a small blood sample for SNP analysis and learn his lifetime risk of prostate cancer. As this technology advances and more SNPs are identified, the predictive ability of these tests will increase. Men at high risk of developing clinically significant prostate cancer will be identified early in life for more intensive follow-up.

Epigenetic Changes

Epigenetics is "cellular information, other than the DNA sequence itself, that is heritable during cell division." [38] Since the first epigenetic abnormality in cancer cells was described in 1983, study of this topic has greatly escalated, and we are just beginning to understand heritable phenomena that were previously unexplained by genetic mechanisms. Most known epigenetic changes can be categorized into three groups: DNA methylation, chromatin remodeling (histone code), and microRNA regulation.

DNA Methylation

DNA methyltransferases can silence genes by adding a methyl group to cytosine residues in CpG dinucleotides [39–41]. "CpG dinucleotide" refers to a cytosine nucleotide followed by a guanine nucleotide in sequence along a DNA molecule, not a cytosine-guanine base pair. Multiple CpG dinucleotides often occur together in groups called "CpG islands" [40]. About 60% of human genes have these CpG islands in their promoter regions, thereby putting many cellular processes (DNA repair, apoptosis, cell cycle, cell adherence, carcinogen metabolism) under the influence of DNA methylation [41]. Tumor suppressor genes can be inactivated by hypermethylation, and oncogenes can be activated by hypomethylation. Global and gene-specific DNA methylation alterations affect carcinogenesis [42].

DNA methylation changes have been associated with prostate cancer. Methylation of RASSF1A, RAR beta 2, GSTP1, CD44, and EDNRB has been observed in cancerous glands but not in normal tissue [43]. Given the higher incidence and worse outcomes of prostate cancer in black men [2, 44, 45], it is interesting that CD44 hypermethylation was found more frequently in black than in white men with prostate cancer [46]. Black men with prostate cancer are also more likely to have hypermethylation of GSTP1 than white or Asian men with prostate cancer, while GSTP1 hypermethylation correlates to higher stages and Gleason scores in Asian men [47]. These are just a few of the more than 50 genes that have been found to be hypermethylated in prostate cancer [39]. Several of these can be detected in serum or urine which raises the possibility of using them for screening, diagnosis, or prognosis [48–50].

Chromatin Remodeling and the Histone Code

DNA strands normally do not exist in isolation, but rather are packaged with proteins, primarily histones, into higher-order structures called chromatin. Eight histones together form a nucleosome, and 147 base pairs of DNA wrap around each nucleosome. The histone proteins, especially their N-terminus tails, are often modified in ways that affect repair, transcription, replication, or condensation of the DNA associated with the modified histones. To date, eight types of histone modifications have been identified: acetylation, methylation of lysines and arginines, phosphorylation, ubiquitylation, sumoylation, ADP ribosylation, deimination, and proline isomerization [51]. These modifications are sometimes referred to as the histone code. Acetylation of the histones by histone acetyltransferases (HAT) typically results in the DNA unraveling from the nucleosome, making it more available for transcription or modification. Acetylation is balanced with deacetylation by histone deacetylases (HDAC), which cause decreased transcription [39]. Acetylation and methylation modifications of histones have been linked to several types of cancer, including prostate cancer [42, 51].

Clinical studies of histone modifications in prostate cancer are limited. Two studies have demonstrated by immunohistochemistry of prostatectomy specimens that specific patterns of histone acetylation and methylation correlate with preoperative PSA, pT-stage, lymph node positivity, Gleason score, biochemical recurrence, and castration resistance status [52, 53]. These limited studies require confirmation and further development before becoming broadly applicable. No human studies of blood or urine markers of prostate cancer using histone modifications have been reported.

MicroRNA (miRNA) Regulation

Some noncoding segments of DNA are transcribed in the nucleus as primary microRNAs (pri-miRNA). Pri-miRNAs are cleaved in the nucleus to pre-miR and then further processed and exported to the cytoplasm to become mature miRNA. These miRNAs bind to complementary sequences on messenger RNA (mRNA) and induce a silencing complex. However, miRNAs are incompletely understood at this time. While most miRNAs reduce mRNA expression, some upregulate it or have other effects [54]. Multiple miRNAs can regulate one mRNA, and each miRNA can regulate multiple mRNAs. Greater than 30% of human genes are likely modulated by miRNA [55].

Many miRNAs have been screened by microarrays, bead-based flow cytometry, or RT-qPCR [54, 56–60], and several miRNAs have been found to be over- or underexpressed in prostate cancer. Schaefer et al. demonstrated that the overexpression of miR-183 combined with the underexpression of miR-205 discriminated between normal and cancerous prostate tissue in 85% of cases [57]. This same study showed that miR-96 overexpression was significantly correlated with biochemical recurrence. Most miRNA studies used tissue from pathology specimens or cell culture. One study, however, examined miRNA in plasma and found it remarkably stable. Mitchell et al. found miR-141 in plasma could distinguish between patients with metastatic prostate cancer patients and controls with 60% sensitivity and 100% specificity [58]. Many more miRNAs have yet to be thoroughly investigated in serum, urine, and tissue.

Development of a Clinically Useful Test

These recent discoveries of genetic and epigenetic changes in prostate cancer provide exciting prospects for changing the way we screen for and diagnose prostate cancer.

Jeronimo et al. present a flow diagram of currently known epigenetic markers showing how they could be used at each stage of prostate cancer screening, diagnosis, and prognostication [39]. Many schemes like this will be developed and refined in the coming years, with the final result likely looking very different from our current schemes.

As the fields of genetics and epigenetics mature, prospective clinical trials will be needed to confirm the predictive ability of each marker individually and of large groups of markers taken together. Ideally, *all* heritable molecular risk factors for developing prostate cancer will be characterized. Mathematical models will then be developed that weight each of the molecular markers according to their respective contributions to overall risk and produce precise numeric estimates of a man's lifetime risk of developing prostate cancer, developing metastasis, and dying from the disease.

To take advantage of these heritable factors clinically, a user-friendly clinical test will need to be developed. Cells from a man's blood or the inside of his cheek could be easily retrieved and sent to a lab. There, the DNA and epigenetic material will be extracted, amplified, and loaded on a small "chip" similar to current gene microarray chips. This one "chip" would contain thousands of microscopic dots, each with a unique probe for an SNP, DNA methylation, histone modification, or miRNA. Each probe would produce greater or lesser intensity of microscopic chemiluminescence depending on the concentration of that factor in the sample. The intensity of each microscopic dot would be read by a special machine that would calculate the relative abundance of that factor in the patient's genetic material. After the reader automatically applies a mathematical model as described above, the urologist would give his patient a customized risk assessment. "Mr. X, your lifetime risk of developing prostate cancer is 23%. Your lifetime risk of developing symptomatic metastasis is 2.1%, and your lifetime risk of dying from prostate cancer is 0.4%. Now let's talk about whether you want any prostate cancer screening in the future."

Armed with such a customized risk assessment at 30 or 40 years old, each patient, with the guidance of his urologist, could make an informed decision about screening. Decision aids based on our current limited knowledge have already been shown to be beneficial to patients [61]. When refined with exact prognostic data as described above, these decision aids will help patients make decisions about their screening with which they are comfortable. Men at low risk who have a high risk tolerance may elect to never undergo screening for the rest of their lives, while men at moderate risk who have low risk tolerance and all men at high risk may choose screening with PSA or a novel biomarker every few years.

This personalized approach to screening could bring the number needed to screen to prevent one prostate cancer death well under 100. Genetic and epigenetic testing will never predict the development of prostate cancer with complete accuracy, however, since environmental factors are also involved. Therefore, higher-risk individuals will always need to be screened.

Goal 2: Reduce the Number of Negative Prostate Biopsies Performed

This goal is closely tied to Goal 1 discussed above. Customized risk assessment based on heritable characteristics will likely allow the majority of the population to stop routine screening. As the total number of screening tests decreases, so will the *number* of false-positive tests, even if the false-positive *rate* does not change. Fewer men, therefore, would be candidates for prostate biopsy based simply on more targeted screening. As discussed in Chap. 1 of this book, new serum and urine biomarkers that have lower false-positive rates than PSA and DRE may be discovered. If 50% fewer men were screened and the screening biomarker had a 50% lower false-positive rate, three-quarters of negative prostate biopsies could be eliminated. This equates to hundreds of thousands of men avoiding the potential pain and complications of a prostate biopsy each year.

Novel imaging modalities also may decrease the number of negative biopsies performed. Prostate biopsy will always be the gold standard for diagnosis of prostate cancer, but imaging will continue to improve in its ability to predict pathology. Exciting new technologies in this field are discussed in detail in Chap. 5 of this book. New imaging modalities that are sensitive and specific for prostate tumor biology are needed. Nanotechnology holds promise in the development of these technologies.

MRI will likely become increasingly important in the coming years. Recent studies have shown that MRI may be useful in detection, grading, and staging prostate cancer [62]. As this technology becomes more accurate, prostate MRI may become the standard of care after positive screening tests and *before* biopsy. If an MRI can reliably rule out clinically significant prostate cancer, a biopsy could be avoided. Many of the characteristics of clinically significant disease—high Gleason grade, high tumor volume, and extraprostatic extension—can already be detected by MRI [63, 64]. When the sensitivity and specificity of MRI for these characteristics increase sufficiently, men with persistently elevated screening markers but negative initial evaluation (biopsy or imaging) could be followed with repeated MRIs instead of repeated biopsies.

Prostate biopsy has substantial risks and complications, including death in rare cases, as discussed in Chap. 4. The developments described above and new discoveries that we cannot predict will enable patients to avoid this morbidity in almost all cases that do not involve clinically significant prostate cancer.

Goal 3: Detect All Clinically Significant Prostate Cancers

One in six men born today in the United States will develop prostate cancer in his lifetime [65]. Given the indolent natural history of some forms of prostate cancer, many of these men will not benefit significantly from treatment [66]. A significant subset of men, however, have prostate cancers that will progress to become symptomatic, metastatic, or lethal. Identification of these men before definitive treatment currently relies primarily on biopsy Gleason grade, PSA, and clinical and pathologic characteristics. Unfortunately, these predictors frequently risk stratify men incorrectly, resulting in some patients mistakenly choosing conservative therapy when they actually have aggressive tumors. More accurate predictors will be developed in the future to allow nearly perfect discrimination between clinically significant and indolent prostate cancer.

The primary key to accurate identification of all clinically significant prostate cancers will lie in molecular analysis of biopsy specimens. Specific SNPs have been shown to correlate with aggressive prostate cancer [34, 35]. DNA methylation, histone modification, and miRNAs are implicated in the development and progression of prostate cancer [39]. While each patient caries genetic and epigenetic variants inherited from his parents in all his cells, as the prostate cells undergo malignant transformation, they will accumulate dozens or hundreds more variants which allow them to escape normal cell cycle control. A test incorporating thousands of these markers, as described above, could be validated for use on fresh biopsy tissue. This test could enumerate exactly which genetic and epigenetic changes have occurred in the cancer cells to transform them from benign to malignant. Clinical trials of this test will likely show that each cancer is not defined by one or two variants, but by an array of changes. A mathematical formula will be developed to assign the appropriate prognostic weight to each variant and thereby produce a precise prediction of the biologic behavior of that tumor. Predictions based on this panel of genetic and epigenetic tests will be much more accurate than predictions based on one or two genes in combination with clinical and pathologic variables.

Circulating tumor cells have potential for differentiating between aggressive and indolent prostate cancers. These cells are shed by the primary cancer into the bloodstream in low numbers and can be isolated using an FDA-approved assay, even when there is less than one cell per milliliter [67]. A major challenge in using circulating tumor cells as biologic markers is isolating such rare cells. Some recent technologic breakthroughs enable more efficient isolation of these cells and even allow analysis of the genetic material contained within them [68, 69]. Now that they can be isolated more easily, research into the diagnostic and prognostic value of circulating tumor cells is exploding. Much of the research is focused on breast cancer. Within prostate cancer, the research is focused on metastatic castrate-resistant disease and predicting response to chemotherapy. De Bono et al. isolated circulating tumor cells from 231 men with castrate-resistant prostate cancer before and after starting chemotherapy [67]. Those men with less than five circulating tumor cells per 7.5 ml of blood before chemotherapy had an overall survival of 21.7 months compared to 11.5 months for men with five or more cells. Patients whose number of circulating tumor cells decreased with therapy also had significantly longer overall survival than those whose cell numbers did not decrease. Response of circulating tumor cell numbers to chemotherapy was shown to be more predictive of overall survival than PSA decrement algorithms.

Circulating tumor cells were detectable in 8 of 19 patients (42%) with clinically localized disease in one study [69]. After radical prostatectomy, all but two patients had an immediate decrease in circulating tumor cells. While the follow-up was not long enough in this study to correlate circulating tumor cells with outcomes, it fuels exciting speculations. Could those patients with detectable circulating tumor cells and seemingly localized disease be those who are destined to recur after local therapy? Do those men whose circulating tumor cell numbers did not come down after prostatectomy actually have clinically undetectable micrometastatic disease? Could prostate cancer be definitively diagnosed by this blood test since the circulating cells could be considered small pieces of the tumor and therefore a tissue diagnosis? Much work remains to be done to answer these questions and determine the role circulating tumor cells will play in prostate cancer diagnosis and prognosis, but they may someday help determine which patients have clinically significant prostate cancer.

Conclusion

Predicting the future is always hard to do. The deficiencies in our current diagnostic abilities are clear, however. Future research will hopefully enable the urologic community to decrease indiscriminate screening for prostate cancer, reduce the number of negative prostate biopsies performed, and detect all clinically significant prostate cancers, among many other goals. During the next decade, disruptive technologies may dramatically change the methods we use to diagnose and treat prostate cancer in ways we cannot currently imagine. May we use each new discovery to reduce suffering and bring hope to our patients.

Editorial Commentary:

I cannot recall whom to give credit for saying something down the line of *discovery is easy, but making sense of our discoveries is hard.* However, the observation is poignant as we try to figure out how to use the diagnostic and prognostic future that is rushing at us as described in this chapter.

We are on the precipice of the era of molecular diagnostics and personalized medicine. However, the discoveries are outpacing our ability to understand their implications and to place them into the standards of care. Too often, these discoveries are thrown at us with charts, PPVs, and AUCs that look great on posters at professional meetings but become meaningless when applied to patient care. Diagnostics companies come and go without their scientific and marketing teams ever figuring out how they failed to change the field of prostate cancer diagnostics when their *p* values were <0.05. They fail by not driving their discovery through meaningful clinical questions such as "how can we identify the patient that has cancer that will harm him if unrecognized and untreated but that can be successfully managed if the patient is willing to be subject to the potential side effects incumbent to curative therapy?" Those who have answers simply seeking pertinent questions will almost surely fail, but those who figure out how to ask and answer the right questions will ultimately deliver valuable discoveries to move this challenging field forward.

–J. Stephen Jones, MD

References

1. Young HH. XV. Cancer of the prostate: a clinical, pathological and post-operative analysis of 111 cases. Ann Surg. 1909;50(6):1144–233.
2. Siegel R, Ward E, Brawley O, Jemal A. Cancer statistics, 2011: the impact of eliminating socioeconomic and racial disparities on premature cancer deaths. CA Cancer J Clin. 2011;61(4):212–36.
3. Stamey TA, Yang N, Hay AR, McNeal JE, Freiha FS, Redwine E. Prostate-specific antigen as a serum marker for adenocarcinoma of the prostate. N Engl J Med. 1987;317(15):909–16.
4. Swan J, Breen N, Coates RJ, Rimer BK, Lee NC. Progress in cancer screening practices in the United States: results from the 2000 National Health Interview Survey. Cancer. 2003;97(6):1528–40.
5. Smith RA, von Eschenbach AC, Wender R, et al. American Cancer Society guidelines for the early detection of cancer: update of early detection guidelines for prostate, colorectal, and endometrial cancers. Also: update 2001–testing for early lung cancer detection. CA Cancer J Clin. 2001;51(1):38–75. quiz 77–80.
6. American Urological Association (AUA): Prostate-specific antigen (PSA) best practice policy. Oncology (Williston Park) 14(2):267–272, 277–268, 280 passim.
7. Smith RA, Cokkinides V, Eyre HJ. American Cancer Society guidelines for the early detection of cancer, 2006. CA Cancer J Clin. 2006;56(1):11–25. quiz 49–50.
8. Schroder FH, Hugosson J, Roobol MJ, et al. Screening and prostate-cancer mortality in a randomized European study. N Engl J Med. 2009;360(13):1320–8.
9. Andriole GL, Grubb 3rd RL, Buys SS, et al. Mortality results from a randomized prostate-cancer screening trial. N Engl J Med. 2009;260(13):1310–9.
10. Wolf AM, Wender RC, Etzioni RB, et al. American Cancer Society guideline for the early detection of prostate cancer: update 2010. CA Cancer J Clin. 2010;60(2):70–98.
11. Greene KL, Albertsen PC, Babaian RJ, et al. Prostate specific antigen best practice statement: 2009 update. J Urol. 2009;182(5):2232–41.
12. Bill-Axelson A, Holmberg L, Ruutu M, et al. Radical prostatectomy versus watchful waiting in early prostate cancer. N Engl J Med. 2011;364(18):1708–17.
13. Vickers AJ, Cronin AM, Bjork T, et al. Prostate specific antigen concentration at age 60 and death or metastasis from prostate cancer: case–control study. BMJ. 2010;341:c4521.
14. Foulkes WD. Inherited susceptibility to common cancers. N Engl J Med. 2008;359(20):2143–53.
15. Pomerantz MM, Freedman ML. Genetics of prostate cancer risk. Mt Sinai J Med. 2010;77(6):643–54.
16. Kote-Jarai Z, Olama AA, Giles GG, et al. Seven prostate cancer susceptibility loci identified by a multistage genome-wide association study. Nat Genet. 2011;43(8):785–91.
17. Eeles RA, Kote-Jarai Z, Al Olama AA. Identification of seven new prostate cancer susceptibility loci through a genome-wide association study. Nat Genet. 2009;41(10):1116–21.
18. Schumacher FR, Berndt SI, Siddiq A, et al. Genome-wide association study identifies new prostate cancer susceptibility loci. Hum Mol Genet. 2011;20(19): 3867–75.
19. Eeles RA, Kote-Jarai Z, Giles GG, et al. Multiple newly identified loci associated with prostate cancer susceptibility. Nat Genet. 2008;40(3):316–21.
20. Amundadottir LT, Sulem P, Gudmundsson J, et al. A common variant associated with prostate cancer in European and African populations. Nat Genet. 2006;38(6):652–8.
21. Gudmundsson J, Sulem P, Gudbjartsson DF, et al. Genome-wide association and replication studies identify four variants associated with prostate cancer susceptibility. Nat Genet. 2009;41(10):1122–6.
22. Gudmundsson J, Sulem P, Manolescu A, et al. Genome-wide association study identifies a second prostate cancer susceptibility variant at 8q24. Nat Genet. 2007;39(5):631–7.
23. Gudmundsson J, Sulem P, Rafnar T, et al. Common sequence variants on 2p15 and Xp11.22 confer susceptibility to prostate cancer. Nat Genet. 2008;40(3): 281–3.
24. Gudmundsson J, Sulem P, Steinthorsdottir V, et al. Two variants on chromosome 17 confer prostate cancer risk, and the one in TCF2 protects against type 2 diabetes. Nat Genet. 2007;39(8):977–83.
25. Thomas G, Jacobs KB, Yeager M, et al. Multiple loci identified in a genome-wide association study of prostate cancer. Nat Genet. 2008;40(3):310–5.
26. Yeager M, Chatterjee N, Ciampa J, et al. Identification of a new prostate cancer susceptibility locus on chromosome 8q24. Nat Genet. 2009;41(10):1055–7.
27. Yeager M, Orr N, Hayes RB, et al. Genome-wide association study of prostate cancer identifies a second risk locus at 8q24. Nat Genet. 2007;39(5):645–9.
28. Zheng SL, Stevens VL, Wiklund F, et al. Two independent prostate cancer risk-associated loci at 11q13. Cancer Epidemiol Biomarkers Prev. 2009;18(6): 1815–20.
29. Sun J, Zheng SL, Wiklund F, et al. Sequence variants at 22q13 are associated with prostate cancer risk. Cancer Res. 2009;69(1):10–5.
30. Sun J, Zheng SL, Wiklund F, et al. Evidence for two independent prostate cancer risk-associated loci in the HNF1B gene at 17q12. Nat Genet. 2008;40(10): 1153–5.

31. Takata R, Akamatsu S, Kubo M, et al. Genome-wide association study identifies five new susceptibility loci for prostate cancer in the Japanese population. Nat Genet. 2010;42(9):751–4.

32. Hsu FC, Sun J, Wiklund F, et al. A novel prostate cancer susceptibility locus at 19q13. Cancer Res. 2009;69(7):2720–3.

33. Al Olama AA, Kote-Jarai Z, Giles GG, et al. Multiple loci on 8q24 associated with prostate cancer susceptibility. Nat Genet. 2009;41(10):1058–60.

34. Xu J, Zheng SL, Isaacs SD, et al. Inherited genetic variant predisposes to aggressive but not indolent prostate cancer. Proc Natl Acad Sci USA. 2010;107(5): 2136–40.

35. Duggan D, Zheng SL, Knowlton M, et al. Two genome-wide association studies of aggressive prostate cancer implicate putative prostate tumor suppressor gene DAB2IP. J Natl Cancer Inst. 2007;99(24):1836–44.

36. Liu F, Hsing AW, Wang X, et al. A systematic confirmation study of reported prostate cancer risk-associated SNPs in Chinese men. Cancer Sci. 2011;102(10):1916–20.

37. Macinnis RJ, Antoniou AC, Eeles RA, et al. A risk prediction algorithm based on family history and common genetic variants: application to prostate cancer with potential clinical impact. Genet Epidemiol. 2011;35(6):549–56.

38. Feinberg AP, Tycko B. The history of cancer epigenetics. Nat Rev Cancer. 2004;4(2):143–53.

39. Jeronimo C, Bastian PJ, Bjartell A, et al. Epigenetics in prostate cancer: biologic and clinical relevance. Eur Urol. 2011;60(4):753–66.

40. Goldberg AD, Allis CD, Bernstein E. Epigenetics: a landscape takes shape. Cell. 2007;128(4):635–8.

41. Lopez-Serra L, Esteller M. Proteins that bind methylated DNA and human cancer: reading the wrong words. Br J Cancer. 2008;98(12):1881–5.

42. Esteller M. Epigenetics in cancer. N Engl J Med. 2008;358(11):1148–59.

43. Woodson K, Gillespie J, Hanson J, et al. Heterogeneous gene methylation patterns among pre-invasive and cancerous lesions of the prostate: a histopathologic study of whole mount prostate specimens. Prostate. 2004;60(1):25–31.

44. Powell IJ, Dey J, Dudley A, et al. Disease-free survival difference between African Americans and whites after radical prostatectomy for local prostate cancer: a multivariable analysis. Urology. 2002;59(6):907–12.

45. Hamilton RJ, Aronson WJ, Presti Jr JC, et al. Race, biochemical disease recurrence, and prostate-specific antigen doubling time after radical prostatectomy: results from the SEARCH database. Cancer. 2007;110(10):2202–9.

46. Woodson K, Hayes R, Wideroff L, Villaruz L, Tangrea J. Hypermethylation of GSTP1, CD44, and E-cadherin genes in prostate cancer among US Blacks and Whites. Prostate. 2003;55(3):199–205.

47. Enokida H, Shiina H, Urakami S, et al. Ethnic group-related differences in CpG hypermethylation of the GSTP1 gene promoter among African-American, Caucasian and Asian patients with prostate cancer. Int J Cancer. 2005;116(2):174–81.

48. Ellinger J, Haan K, Heukamp LC, et al. CpG island hypermethylation in cell-free serum DNA identifies patients with localized prostate cancer. Prostate. 2008;68(1):42–9.

49. Roupret M, Hupertan V, Yates DR, et al. Molecular detection of localized prostate cancer using quantitative methylation-specific PCR on urinary cells obtained following prostate massage. Clin Cancer Res. 2007;13(6):1720–5.

50. Hoque MO, Topaloglu O, Begum S, et al. Quantitative methylation-specific polymerase chain reaction gene patterns in urine sediment distinguish prostate cancer patients from control subjects. J Clin Oncol. 2005;23(27):6569–75.

51. Kouzarides T. Chromatin modifications and their function. Cell. 2007;128(4):693–705.

52. Seligson DB, Horvath S, Shi T, et al. Global histone modification patterns predict risk of prostate cancer recurrence. Nature. 2005;435(7046):1262–6.

53. Ellinger J, Kahl P, von der Gathen J, et al. Global levels of histone modifications predict prostate cancer recurrence. Prostate. 2010;70(1):61–9.

54. Catto JW, Alcaraz A, Bjartell AS, et al. MicroRNA in prostate, bladder, and kidney cancer: a systematic review. Eur Urol. 2011;59(5):671–81.

55. Guil S, Esteller M. DNA methylomes, histone codes and miRNAs: tying it all together. Int J Biochem Cell Biol. 2009;41(1):87–95.

56. Porkka KP, Pfeiffer MJ, Waltering KK, Vessella RL, Tammela TL, Visakorpi T. MicroRNA expression profiling in prostate cancer. Cancer Res. 2007;67(13): 6130–5.

57. Schaefer A, Jung M, Mollenkopf HJ, et al. Diagnostic and prognostic implications of microRNA profiling in prostate carcinoma. Int J Cancer. 2010;126(5): 1166–76.

58. Mitchell PS, Parkin RK, Kroh EM, et al. Circulating microRNAs as stable blood-based markers for cancer detection. Proc Natl Acad Sci USA. 2008;105(30): 10513–8.

59. Carlsson J, Davidsson S, Helenius G, et al. A miRNA expression signature that separates between normal and malignant prostate tissues. Cancer Cell Int. 2011; 11(1):14.

60. Lu J, Getz G, Miska EA, et al. MicroRNA expression profiles classify human cancers. Nature. 2005; 435(7043):834–8.

61. Lin GA, Aaronson DS, Knight SJ, Carroll PR, Dudley RA. Patient decision aids for prostate cancer treatment: a systematic review of the literature. CA Cancer J Clin. 2009;59(6):379–90.

62. Villers A, Lemaitre L, Haffner J, Puech P. Current status of MRI for the diagnosis, staging and prognosis of prostate cancer: implications for focal therapy and active surveillance. Curr Opin Urol. 2009;19(3): 274–82.

63. Puech P, Potiron E, Lemaitre L, et al. Dynamic contrast-enhanced-magnetic resonance imaging evaluation of intraprostatic prostate cancer: correlation with radical prostatectomy specimens. Urology. 2009;74(5):1094–9.

64. Villers A, McNeal JE, Redwine EA, Freiha FS, Stamey TA. The role of perineural space invasion in the local spread of prostatic adenocarcinoma. J Urol. 1989;142(3):763–8.

65. Hayat MJ, Howlader N, Reichman ME, Edwards BK. Cancer statistics, trends, and multiple primary cancer analyses from the surveillance, epidemiology, and end results (SEER) program. Oncologist. 2007;12(1): 20–37.

66. Lu-Yao GL, Albertsen PC, Moore DF, et al. Outcomes of localized prostate cancer following conservative management. JAMA. 2009;302(11):1202–9.

67. de Bono JS, Scher HI, Montgomery RB, et al. Circulating tumor cells predict survival benefit from treatment in metastatic castration-resistant prostate cancer. Clin Cancer Res. 2008;14(19):6302–9.

68. Nagrath S, Sequist LV, Maheswaran S, et al. Isolation of rare circulating tumour cells in cancer patients by microchip technology. Nature. 2007;450(7173):1235–9.

69. Stott SL, Lee RJ, Nagrath S, et al. Isolation and characterization of circulating tumor cells from patients with localized and metastatic prostate cancer. Sci Transl Med. 2010;2(25):25ra23.

Index

J.S. Jones (ed.), *Prostate Cancer Diagnosis: PSA, Biopsy and Beyond*, Current Clinical Urology,
DOI 10.1007/978-1-62703-188-2, © Springer Science+Business Media New York 2013

Printed by Publishers' Graphics LLC
JCIMO140114.15.16.11